A MANUAL OF CLINICAL SURGERY

Dr. Rameshwar Naik

ALLIED HEALTH PRESS

A Manual of Clinical Surgery

Author: **Dr. Rameshwar Naik**

Allied Health Press
4164 Lakeshore Road
Burlington ON L7L 1A4
Canada
www.alliedhealthpress.com
Email: orders@arclereducation.com

ISBN: 978-1-77956-846-5

Allied Health Press publishes wide variety of books and eBooks. For more information about Allied Health Press and its products, visit our website at www.alliedhealthpress.com

ABOUT THE AUTHOR

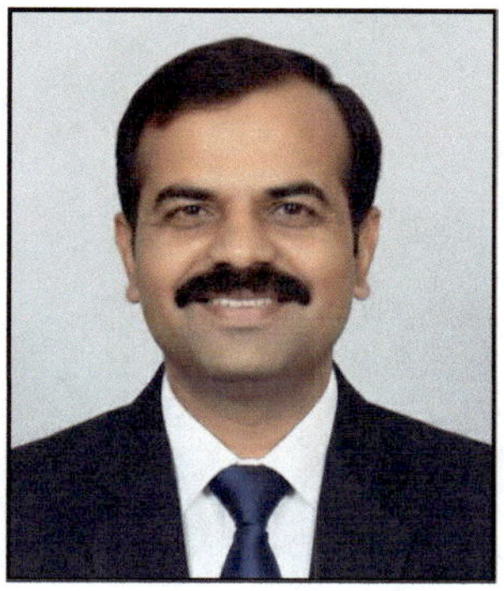

Dr. Rameshwar Naik is a medical professional involved in clinical practice, medical training, and community health activities. He is the Founder and Director of Lifeline Hospital, Parbhani, a multi-specialty healthcare center established 14 years ago that offers diagnostic, critical care, and specialized medical services. As a Consultant Physician, he manages infectious disease, cardiology, and emergency medicine cases while promoting preventive healthcare. He also serves as an Assistant Professor in the Department of Medicine at Parbhani Medical College, contributing to the training of future doctors.

He completed his MBBS from Government Medical College, Nanded, and MD (Medicine) from Sassoon Government Medical College, Pune, followed by an International Fellowship at Johns Hopkins Center for Clinical Global Health Education, USA, focusing on "Adult Management for HIV-AIDS in India." He played a key role during the Swine Flu and COVID-19 pandemics, serving as a District Task Force member and leading patient care and public health initiatives.

Dr. Naik actively conducts community health programs, notably the Arogyawari Camp at Daithana, held annually for over 15 years, offering free consultations and medicines in rural areas. He has also organized awareness drives on chronic illnesses, maternal health, sanitation, and fluoride-related diseases.

As President of the Parbhani Astronomical Society (PAS), he leads scientific outreach through the "Science on Wheel" initiative with Suhana Pravin Masalewale and is guiding the development of an International Science Park in collaboration with VNMKV, Parbhani. He has also served as Vice President of Rajmudra Patsanstha, Secretary of Jeevan Seva Sewabhavi Sanstha, and Accreditation Committee Member at VNMKV.

He has given talks on health and sanitation, including at the Newton-Bhabha Programme on Antibacterial Resistance, and contributed to local health policy discussions. His work has been acknowledged through the COVID-19 Service Award from the Government of Maharashtra, the Best Medical Practitioner Award (Sakal & ABP Group), and the Mahatma Phule Samta Parishad Puraskar (Parbhani Bhushan).

His interests include infectious disease management, preventive medicine, and public health outreach, with a focus on improving healthcare access and awareness in both urban and rural regions.

Brief Table of Contents

Getting Started with This Book

Chapter Openers

A list of Chapter Outline is presented providing a brief Introduction to what will be covered in the chapter.

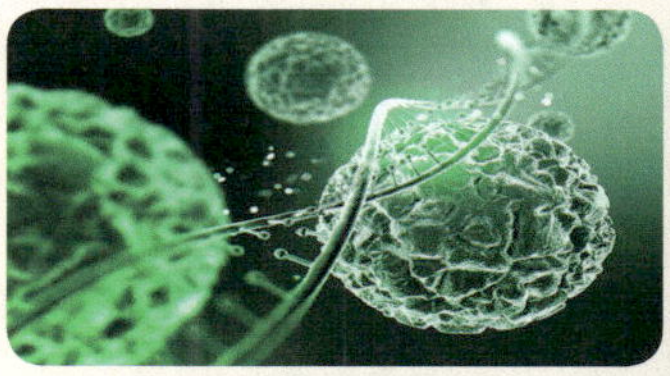

Introduction

Often referred to as the science of life, biology is a broad field of study aimed at comprehending the several kinds of life on Earth, from tiny creatures to sophisticated multicellular entities. Comprising several subfields, including molecular biology, ecology, and evolutionary biology, each of which advances our knowledge of living systems, this field clarifies the mechanisms controlling life events, including development, reproduction, and interaction with the surroundings, which is the central goal of biology. Moreover, biology fills in the void between the natural sciences and medicine by offering a necessary understanding of health, illness, and the interactions between organisms and their environments. Dealing with urgent global issues such as climate change, biodiversity loss, and new diseases depends on an awareness of these complex biological interactions, therefore highlighting the critical part biology plays in modern civilization. Fundamentally, biology explores and tests ideas about the living world using the scientific method. Through methodical observation and experimentation,

LEARNING OBJECTIVES

After studying this chapter, you will be able to:

1. Discuss the scientific method in biology;
2. Explain the cell theory;
3. Discuss the genetics and heredity;
4. Evolution and natural selection;
5. Focus on ecology and ecosystems;
6. Learn about human biology;
7. Evaluate the plant biology;
8. Explain the microbiology;
9. Focus on current trends in biology.

1.1. The Scientific Method in Biology

Learning Outcome

1. Describe the steps of the scientific method;
2. Focus on hypothesis formation;
3. Learn about experimental design.

Learning Outcomes

The beginning of each section of every chapter contains a set of Learning Outcomes that inform students of concepts they should understand. These outcomes help students understand what they should be able to do if they have mastered the material in that section.

Test Your Knowledge

Throughout each chapter, Test Your Knowledge cues you to note which topics have been covered and to self-test your understanding of the material presented.

Test Your Knowledge

1. Explain why correlation does not imply causation in scientific experiments.
2. How does the scientific method help reduce the influence of personal opinions in research?

Chapter Summary

The Summary Section appear at the end of each chapter and summarize main concepts covered throughout the chapter. These points provide key concepts in an engaging and meaningful way.

Summary

The investigation of biological principles highlights the importance of a comprehensive view of life by reflecting the intricate interactions that occur within living systems. The complexity of biology goes beyond individual species or systems, as this essay highlights; it also includes the interactions that mold ecosystems and affect biodiversity. Researchers can conduct in-depth analyses of metabolomic data using sophisticated technologies like MetaboAnalyst, which offer insights into the molecular mechanisms underlying these interactions. As demonstrated by the developments in MetaboAnalyst, for example, the integration of diverse omics data promotes a thorough understanding of metabolic pathways and helps identify important biological markers necessary for research on development and disease (Chong et al., 2018). Additionally, the phenomenon of ecological invasions is a key component of biological research and a vital field of study. The introduction of non-native species into unfamiliar habitats has significant ramifications and calls for multidisciplinary management strategies. Examining the origins and effects of these biological incursions, invasion science has become a crucial field that highlights the need to comprehend ecological dynamics and community interactions. As interest in biological invasions increases, new findings are emerging that put conventional ecological theories and practices to the test. The importance of incorporating various scientific viewpoints is shown by this developing discipline, which also highlights how invasive species shape ecosystems and advances our knowledge of ecological resilience (David et al., 2013). When taken as a whole, these discoveries from invasion science and metabolomics highlight the value of multidisciplinary biology research. Fostering cross-disciplinary collaboration and utilizing technological breakthroughs to improve our comprehension of intricate biological interactions are crucial as we look to the future of biological research. In addition to deepening our understanding of the complexities of life, this method lays the groundwork for tackling urgent environmental issues. Future studies can ensure the continued relevance of biology in a world that is constantly changing by acknowledging the interconnection of biological systems and opening the door to creative solutions that support sustainability and biodiversity conservation. We might imagine a thorough comprehension of life that serves both academia and society at large through ongoing investigation and integration of scientific knowledge.

Knowledge Assessment

The chapter includes material designed to review and reinforce each content. It includes Critical Thinking Questions to help test of your understanding of information presented in the chapter and Short answer Questions to review your understanding of the key concepts presented in the chapter.

Critical Thinking Questions

1. **Who is known as the "Father of Modern Biology"?**
   a. Aristotle
   b. Charles Darwin
   c. Gregor Mendel
   d. Louis Pasteur
2. **What is the basic unit of life?**
   a. Atom
   b. Molecule
   c. Cell
   d. Organism
3. **Which branch of biology studies the interaction of organisms with their environment?**
   a. Genetics
   b. Ecology
   c. Physiology
   d. Botany
4. **Which macromolecule is the main source of energy for living organisms?**
   a. Proteins
   b. Lipids
   c. Carbohydrates
   d. Nucleic acids
5. **DNA is primarily responsible for which function in living organisms?**
   a. Energy production
   b. Protein synthesis
   c. Storing genetic information
   d. Regulating body temperature

Short Answer Questions

1. What is biology, and why is it important to study biology?
2. What are the three main domains of life, and how are they different from one another?
3. Define homeostasis and give an example of how it works in living organisms.
4. What is the cell theory, and why is it fundamental to biology?
5. How do autotrophs and heterotrophs differ in the way they obtain energy?
6. What is the scientific method, and how is it applied in biological research?
7. Discuss how biology helps address global challenges such as climate change, disease, and food security.
8. Explain the levels of biological organization from the smallest unit to the largest. Provide examples at each level.
9. Describe the relationship between structure and function in biology, giving specific examples from cells or organs.
10. How has the discovery of genetics shaped our understanding of inheritance and variation among organisms?

Supplementary Materials

Key Terms: A list of key terms is given for quick reference

KEY TERMS FROM THIS CHAPTER

Annotation enrichment analysis	Biological structure	Cell
Cell theory	Cellular structure	Ecology
Ecosystems	Genetics	Human biology
Microbiology	Natural selection	Organism
Plant biology		

Further Resources: Recommendations for additional readings, websites, and multimedia resources.

References

1. Argelaguet, R., Velten, B., Arnol, D., Dietrich, S., Zenz, T., Marioni, J. C., Buettner, F., et al. (2018). Multi-omics factor analysis—A framework for unsupervised integration of multi-omics data sets. *Molecular Systems Biology, 14*. https://doi.org/10.15252/msb.20178124.
2. Bacher, S., Blackburn, T. M., Essl, F., & Genovesi, P. (2017). *Socio-Economic Impact Classification of Alien Taxa (SEICAT)*. https://core.ac.uk/download/286567949.pdf (accessed on 8th March 2025).
3. Barnett, R., Brace, S., Cucchi, T., & Dobney, K. (2013). *Divergent Evolutionary Processes Associated with Colonization of Offshore Islands*. https://core.ac.uk/download/20664364.pdf (accessed on 8th March 2025).

Detailed Table of Contents

CHAPTER 5

Liver, Pancreatic, and Biliary Surgery 137

CHAPTER 6

Abdominal Wall Surgery 169

CHAPTER 7

Urology Surgery 203

CHAPTER 10

Orthopedic Surgery 303

CHAPTER 11

Plastic Surgery 337

CHAPTER 12

Cardiothoracic Surgery 369

LIST OF FIGURES

PREFACE

Surgery is a hands-on field of medicine that utilizes both scientific knowledge and practical skills to treat a wide range of unique health conditions. From the beginning, surgeons have sought to make their procedures safer and more effective, and consistently pushed the limits of what can be treated. Advances in anesthesia, antisepsis, and imaging have made formerly fatal injuries a manageable issue, and the continued evolution of minimally invasive methods has reduced morbidity and accelerated convalescence. While advances were made with the aid of technology, the basic principles of surgery did not change: proper patient assessment, sound anatomical understanding, clean tissue handling, and meticulous postoperative care.

Surgical practice nowadays is the practice of sub-specialization, with the specialist working in specialized fields such as hepatobiliary or pediatric urology, but never has the sound knowledge of general principles been more crucial. Surgeons are called upon to synthesize increasingly larger amounts of evidence, make complex decisions, and manage multidisciplinary teams in an effort to achieve optimal outcomes. Along with technical skills, good surgeons acquire judgment, empathy, and adaptability—skills essential for managing intraoperative surprises, dealing with complications, and guiding patients through the emotional aspects of the operative process. Such a comprehensive volume, combining fundamentals with subspecialty data, is therefore invaluable for students and experienced practitioners.

A Manual of Clinical Surgery begins with basic surgery principles and progress through areas of anatomy and specialty procedures, concluding with chapters on quality assurance, tropical disease therapy, and recent trauma procedures. Each chapter weaves together straightforward explanations of pathophysiology with step-by-step procedural descriptions, didactic figures, and evidence-based recommendations, allowing readers to translate theory into practice. Whether you are a medical student coming face-to-face with the operating room for the first time or a consultant looking for a dependable reference, this handbook is intended to guide your clinical decision-making and technical skill acquisition.

Chapter 1 establishes the fundamental principles of surgery, such as patient assessment, preoperative preparation, aseptic technique, hemostasis, wound healing, and the management of surgical complications. Risk management, informed consent, and the use of technology in safe operating practice are emphasized.

Chapter 2 covers head and neck surgery, detailing the anatomy of the most critical structures, exposure of the thyroid and parathyroid glands, treatment of salivary gland pathology, and surgical treatment of congenital and acquired airway and cervical soft tissue lesions.

Chapter 3 covers breast and endocrine surgery, including the evaluation of breast masses, oncologic resection principles, sentinel lymph node procedures, and surgical treatment of adrenal, pancreatic, and parathyroid neoplasms. Reconstruction and aesthetic factors are also covered.

Chapter 4 covers upper gastrointestinal surgery, including esophageal resection and anastomosis, gastric ulcer repair, gastric bariatric procedures, and endoscopic technology. Preoperative optimization and postoperative nutritional protocols are highlighted.

Chapter 5 covers liver, pancreatic, and biliary surgery, detailing liver segmental anatomy, portal triad clamping, hepatic resections, steps in pancreaticoduodenectomy, and biliary reconstruction methods. The chapter addresses perioperative management of liver failure as well as pancreatic fistula prevention.

Chapter 6 details abdominal wall surgery, including descriptions of open and laparoscopic hernia repair methods, mesh choice and placement strategies, component separation methods for large defects, and the treatment of complex ventral hernias and wound dehiscences.

Chapter 7 addresses urology surgery, such as surgical treatment of renal tumors, radical prostatectomy, ureteral reconstruction, bladder surgery, and genitourinary trauma. Robotic and minimally invasive approaches are contrasted with open surgery.

Chapter 8 addresses pediatric surgery, such as congenital malformations, such as diaphragmatic hernia and intestinal atresia, neonatal surgical emergencies, and the challenges of perioperative care in infants and children. Special emphasis is placed on growth-friendly operational planning.

Chapter 9 addresses major trauma surgery and covers principles of damage control surgery, measures for control of hemorrhage, management of abdominal and thoracic trauma, and polytrauma multidisciplinary coordination. It also includes protocols for critical care and massive transfusion.

Chapter 10 addresses orthopedic surgery, describing fracture classification, fixation techniques, joint replacement basics, and procedures for limb salvage. It also covers emergency orthopedic surgeries, identification of compartment syndrome, and infection prevention in musculoskeletal trauma.

Chapter 11 covers plastic surgery principles and applications, ranging from flap design and microvascular anastomosis to the management of burns, wound reconstruction, and cosmetic surgery. The chapter combines functional and aesthetic objectives to achieve optimal patient outcomes.

Chapter 12 covers cardiothoracic surgery, with chapters on open-heart surgery, coronary artery bypass grafting, valve replacement and reconstruction, management of thoracic aneurysms, and minimally invasive lung resections. Perfusion methods and postcardiac care are addressed.

Chapter 13 covers colorectal surgery, including techniques for inflammatory bowel disease, removal of colorectal cancer, anorectal disorders, and pelvic floor dysfunction. It highlights more recovery pathways, stoma management, and measurement of functional outcome.

Chapter 14 covers peripheral vascular disease surgery, detailing bypass grafting procedures, endarterectomy, repair of aneurysms, and limb-salvage procedures. The chapter addresses the interpretation of duplex ultrasonography, anticoagulation protocols, and surveillance after surgery.

Chapter 15 reports surgery in tropical diseases, with an emphasis on operative management of endemic conditions, such as excision of hydatid cysts, filarial lymphoedema, debridement of tropical ulcers, and complications of infectious diseases. Resource-adaptive strategies are emphasized.

This book is addressed to a broad audience: students on their surgical rotation, surgical trainees seeking a dependable guide, general surgeons with wide-ranging skills, and subspecialists who desire cross-disciplinary perspectives. Anesthesiologists, surgical nurses, and allied health professionals involved in perioperative care will also find it helpful.

PRINCIPLES OF SURGERY

1

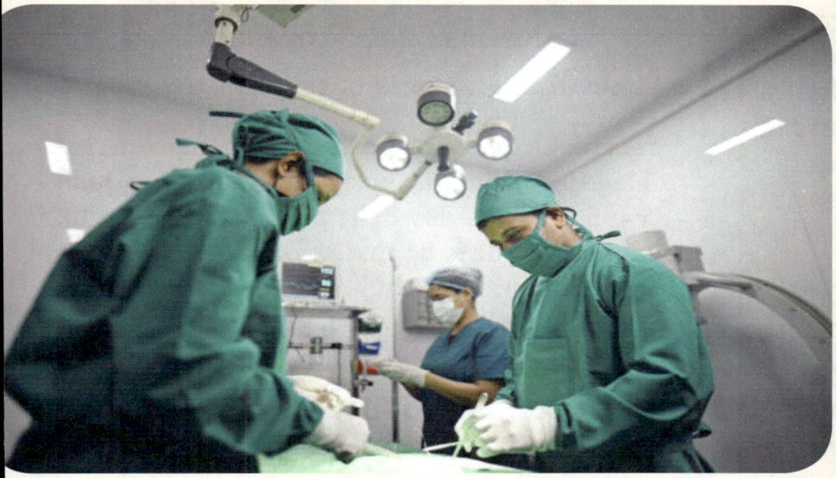

Introduction

The art of surgery encompasses a wide range of techniques and principles to ensure the safe and effective delivery of medical care. Surgery is not just about performing a technical operation, but also about understanding the biological processes underlying it, the disease process being addressed, and the therapeutic goals the procedure is designed to achieve. Surgical introduction begins with a thorough understanding of surgical anatomy, which serves as the foundation for any surgical intervention. From this, surgeons can navigate intricate pathways of anatomy with reduced trauma and improved patient outcomes. The actual surgery also involves proper comprehension of various techniques and the paradigms behind them, for instance, minimally invasive surgery, where possible. Such knowledge is essential for every surgical operator to enhance their proficiency and adapt to evolving surgical techniques, ensuring the highest possible standards of surgical efficacy and patient safety. Besides anatomical knowledge, the foundations of surgery also branch into the areas of

LEARNING OBJECTIVES

After studying this chapter, you will be able to:

1. Understand the preoperative considerations of surgery
2. Explain the surgical techniques
3. Discuss the anesthesia in surgery
4. Focus on intraoperative management of surgery
5. Learn about postoperative care of surgery
6. Evaluate the ethical considerations in surgery

patient care and preparation. Comprehensive preoperative assessment is essential since it informs surgical teams about the general health of the patients, the presence of comorbidities, and intrinsic surgical risks. Evidence-based medicine-guided evaluations enable meticulous planning and high-level risk management strategies, ultimately leading to improved patient outcomes. The preparation phase also entails acquiring informed consent, ensuring patients understand the risks, benefits, and alternatives to the planned surgical procedure. Furthermore, the inclusion of multidisciplinary team practice emphasizes the significance of effective communication among surgeons, anesthesiologists, nurses, and other healthcare professionals, ensuring seamless perioperative care and resulting in better postoperative recovery and satisfaction.

The integration of advanced technologies and procedures was revolutionary to the discipline of surgery. These advances, such as the use of laparoscopic and robotic-assisted procedures, are the trend towards minimally invasive procedures with lesser recovery periods and postoperative morbidity. Further, the development of anesthetic agents and monitoring equipment has improved the safety and efficacy of surgery. Techniques like lamellar keratoplasty, which have revolutionized corneal surgery, reveal the importance of continuous advancement in surgical methods since they yield better patient outcomes than traditional techniques (Dua et al., 2018). These kinds of advancements play around with surgical principles, especially showing the importance of being grounded in evidence-based practice and continuous learning for surgeons. Therefore, a complete introduction to surgery can no longer be simply knowledge of anatomy and technique but must include an appreciation of the dynamic manner in which surgical practice evolves to keep up with technological developments and shifting patient standards of care (Figure 1.1).

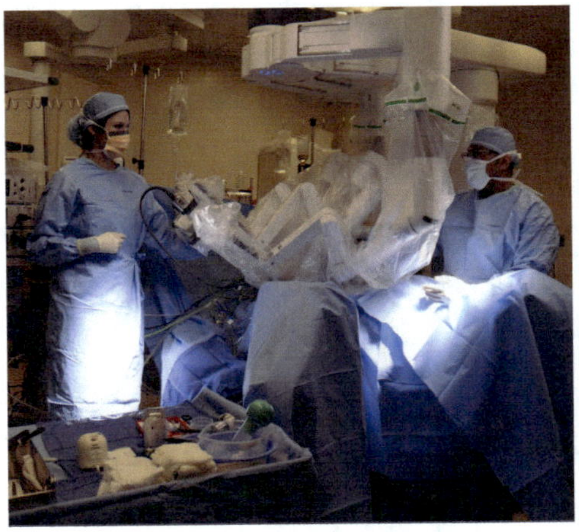

Figure 1.1. Principles of surgery.

Source: https://images.zapnito.com/cdn-cgi/image/metadata=copyright,format=auto,quality=95,fit=scale-down/https://images.zapnito.com/users/82978/posters/41a249505eb0714f45e126c0364484bb/9e866d62-8dda-4212-bf40-87a83e344e9c_large.jpg.

Definition and Scope of Surgery

The definition and scope of surgery encompass a broad range of medical interventions aimed at diagnosing, curing, and controlling various disease conditions through operative techniques. Surgery has historically been classified as either elective or emergency, but contemporary classifications have broadened these two categories into additional subsets. Elective surgery is planned and generally encompasses non-life-threatening conditions, while emergency surgery needs to be performed expeditiously to avert looming severe complications or death. Within this overall framework, various surgical specialties have evolved, each addressing specific body parts, types of diseases, or modes of surgery. The evolution of minimally invasive techniques, for instance, has significantly transformed the discipline of surgical practice, allowing for quicker recoveries, less postoperative discomfort, and shorter hospital stays. These advancements illustrate the ever-changing nature of the practice and its ongoing adaptation to meet developments in technology and patients' needs. In addition, surgery is not merely an intrusive practice; it involves a broad scope of procedures that include diagnostic surgery, therapeutic surgery, and palliative surgery. Diagnostic surgery is designed to diagnose an illness or disease more clearly, while therapeutic surgery is designed to correct or lessen health issues. Palliative surgeries, on the other hand, seek to improve the quality of life of dying patients through relief of symptoms and not for curative intent. The evolution of surgical procedures, such as Transanal endoscopic surgery, shows how expert techniques are developed to manage special clinical situations. As the recent trend has demonstrated, a professional agreement has been established to ensure consistent practice in this area, allowing surgeons to possess the necessary guidelines and information to perform these procedures effectively (N/A, 2023). This moving definition and scope of surgery demonstrate the delicate relationship between innovation and patient-focused practice in contemporary medical practice. Apart from the technical aspects, the extent and meaning of surgery also encompass ethical considerations and multidisciplinary practice. The role of various health professionals, such as nurses, anesthetists, and specialists in rehabilitation medicine, underscores the importance of a collaborative team effort to achieve optimal patient outcomes (Christopher et al., 2023). Consensus-driven standards in pediatric trauma care, for example, emphasize the treatment of patients holistically by engaging a variety of viewpoints from a cross-section of disciplines. This interdependent model helps create best practice guidelines for surgical interventions and ensures that all facets of a patient's health are addressed throughout the surgical process. With the advancement of surgical methods, the need to integrate ethical practice, evidence-based practice, and collaborative practice grows, further solidifying surgery's central role in the delivery of integrated healthcare.

Historical Evolution of Surgical Practices

The evolution of surgical procedures in history is marked by profound advances that have transformed medical interventions. Surgical techniques, which were simple and, in most instances, dangerous in the past, have undergone vast improvements through the application of scientific inquiry and technological progress. Ancient civilizations, in the early days of surgery, typically involved simple wound healing and amputations, and had high mortality as a result of infections without anesthesia. But the Renaissance introduced a new age by a greater understanding of human anatomy through dissections and greater precision in surgery. New innovator Andreas Vesalius broke through the dominant misconceptions, and with them, contemporary surgical education and practice were established. The gradual acceptance of antiseptic techniques in the 19th century revolutionized surgery by significantly reducing postoperative infections and deaths, further propelling the field into a new era of safety and efficacy. The last few decades have witnessed a revolution in surgical procedures, driven by the adoption of technology and innovation. The universal acceptance of minimally invasive surgeries has made patients recover faster with less trauma, a complete change from the old methods of open surgery. Innovations such as laparoscopy and robotic surgery represent the pinnacle of this trend, enabling surgeons to perform complex procedures with greater accuracy and less pain for the patients. Moreover, the field has been advanced by imaging advancements, such as MRI and CT scans, which facilitate more precise preoperative planning and intraoperative guidance. This era of technological advances in surgery has not only improved surgical success rates but also revolutionized patient care models, emphasizing the importance of precision, efficiency, and personalized treatment paradigms. The historical trajectory is that of a steadfast commitment to the promotion of surgical practice through research and the discovery of new techniques. Another essential evolution of surgical practice is evident in trauma care innovations, particularly in the creation and application of damage control surgery (DCS). This technique was formulated as a creative response to the unique issues posed by traumatic trauma, under which early intervention is required in a bid to prevent complications and save lives. Initially developed from techniques used during World War II, the principles of damage control have evolved over the years, transitioning from traditional techniques to more sophisticated ones that focus on early stabilization of patients. The adoption of DC into advanced surgical scenarios is a testament to today's medicine's can-do spirit, wherein more and more surgeons utilize this method to correct various types of injuries beyond abdominal injuries. The knowledge of trauma patient physiology and progressive resuscitation has set the need for adjusting surgical approaches towards optimal patient outcomes, reflecting a continuous process of learning and innovation in surgical practice (Ball et al., 2017) (Figure 1.2).

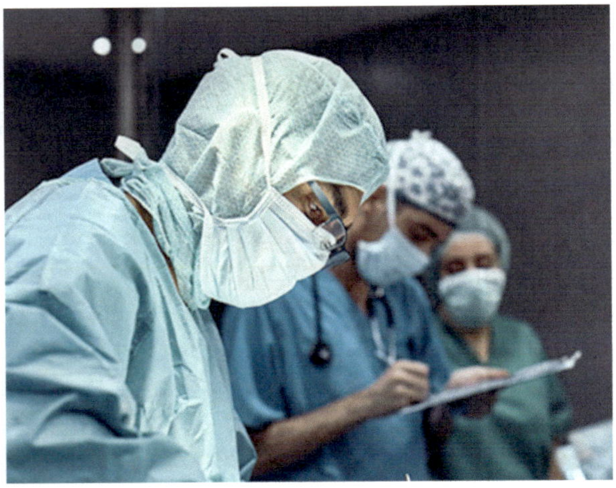

Figure 1.2. Surgical practices.

Source: https://www.hopkinsmedicine.org/-/media/images/health/2_-treatment/surgical-care/methods-of-surgery-teaser.jpg.

Importance of Surgery in Modern Medicine

The contribution of surgery to modern medicine cannot be overstated, for it is an essential intervention for most conditions that conservative therapies alone cannot adequately treat. Surgical practices have evolved over the years, with technological advancements enabling minimally invasive procedures that dramatically minimize recovery time and improve success rates in surgery. Such technologies not only enhance the precision and effectiveness of surgical interventions but also significantly reduce morbidity and mortality rates compared to standard open surgery. For instance, operations such as laparoscopic surgery enable smaller incisions, resulting in less pain and quicker discharge from the hospital, thereby emphasizing the importance of ongoing surgical innovation in enhancing patient care and outcomes in modern healthcare (Modarai et al., 2022). Furthermore, surgery brings value-altering implications to the treatment of life-threatening diseases, particularly in trauma and emergency medicine. Acute appendicitis, hemorrhagic shock, and traumatic injury are some of the life-threatening conditions that often necessitate immediate surgical intervention to prevent death. By the swift application of surgical practices, patients can be stabilized, and complications significantly reduced. The ability to react effectively through surgical means not only saves lives but also underscores the extreme need for surgical competence within healthcare systems. Training for surgeons-in-the-making is therefore still crucial, equipping medical professionals with competency to function in complex surgical environments and respond to the challenges of contemporary medicine (Buchbinder et al., 2020). Aside from its life-saving capability, surgery also plays a tremendous role in enhancing the quality of life of millions of individuals. Surgical interventions such as joint replacement, weight loss surgery, and pain management interventions have the ability to greatly alleviate pain and enhance the functionality of patients in general. Such interventions alter lives by restoring mobility, enhancing physical function, and enabling patients to be more actively involved in their daily activities. The role of surgery is vital in the era of an aging population, where degenerative disease and chronic illness are prevalent. As surgical procedures improve and become more widespread, the public health contribution of surgery also expands, reaffirming its central position in promoting well-being and longevity in today's society (Modarai et al., 2022).

1.1. Preoperative Considerations

Learning Outcome

1. Describe the patient assessment and evaluation
2. Focus on the informed consent process
3. Learn about preoperative preparation and optimization

Preoperative planning is an integral part of the success of surgical procedures, providing a basis that can significantly impact the outcome of surgery. The first principal component of this process involves patient assessment, which includes evaluating the patient's past medical history, active comorbidities, and psychosocial issues. Thorough patient assessments enable the surgical staff to identify possible risk factors that may complicate or complicate surgery, as well as recovery. Furthermore, patient selection best practices for minimally invasive surgery determine today's standards for achieving an optimal result. For example, whether the patient is anatomically suited for the procedure and whether there are significant comorbidities must be carefully evaluated to reduce the risk of intra- or postoperative complications (Agnihotri et al., 2016). Hence, meticulous preoperative assessment guarantees a more potent surgical plan that enhances patient safety and the success of the procedure. The importance of personalized preoperative planning is further established when considering special populations, that is, the elderly. With the aging population growing, there is a pressing need to implement complete geriatric assessment in an effort to provide proper surgical care. This multidimensional tool takes into account relevant issues such as frailty, nutrition, and social support structures, which are of major importance in determining surgical risk and outcome in older adults. Despite the recognized benefits, implementation of these assessments is abysmally low among oncogeriatric patients. Implementation obstacles are likely to relate to the time-consuming nature of such evaluations, which form the foundation of resistance from clinicians to implement them as standard preoperative practice (Lampugnane et al., 2017).

Education, overcoming these obstacles, could promote more extensive use of geriatric assessment, eventually enhancing surgical outcomes in a high-risk patient group. Moreover, proper preoperative communication between patient and surgical team is an imperative that contributes to the overall surgery experience. Adequate communication of expectations during, before, and after surgery minimizes patient anxiety and enables patient-centered decision-making. This conversation must cover not only the technical details but also the risks, benefits, and potential courses of recovery specific to the individual patient. The operating room staff must engage patients in communication about their values and preferences to ensure patient-centered care, especially when treating intricate cases with comorbid conditions or unique personal circumstances. Prioritizing these interactions will enable the operating room staff to establish patient trust and optimize compliance with preoperative preparation, thus optimizing outcomes. Lastly, a comprehensive preoperative strategy that comprises evaluation, special population assessment on an individual basis, and communication is integral to the art of surgery (Figure 1.3).

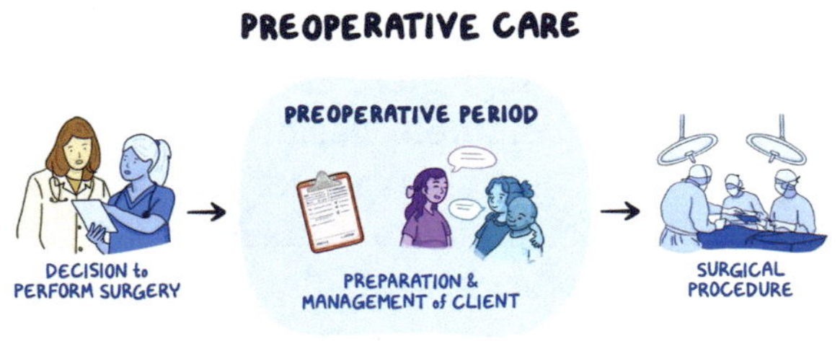

Figure 1.3. Preoperative care.

Source: https://d16qt3wv6xm098.cloudfront.net/cMQjO-Y9Qjy_j6OtmiPkudniTWqqz_z2/_.jpg.

1.1.1. Patient Assessment and Evaluation

In surgical practice, comprehensive patient evaluation and assessment are pivotal in ensuring the realization of desired outcomes. This is achieved through a comprehensive history and physical examination, which enables the surgeon to gain an understanding of the patient's medical history, conditions, and personal needs. Appropriate assessment enables the identification of potential risk factors that could complicate surgery, thereby providing a safer platform for the procedure under specific circumstances. Furthermore, evaluating the patient's psychological and emotional readiness for surgery is necessary as such determinants play significant roles in recovery and satisfaction. Through this exhaustive evaluation, clinicians can develop a therapeutic relationship with patients, fostering trust and enhancing overall communication during the surgery.

Apart from initial assessment, continued evaluation is paramount in preoperative preparations. This period typically involves interdisciplinary collaboration, in which surgeons work together with anesthesiologists, nurses, and other health care providers to coordinate care. Patient evaluation should involve risk stratification and identification of potential complications that may arise following surgery. Utilization of evidence-based practice in this evaluation process decreases the chances of adverse events, which is of the highest priority to assure patient safety. Part of an overarching strategy, in that feedback from the patients regarding their symptoms and expectations ensures that the operative process is aligned with their goals and, as a result, enhances the overall value of the care provided.

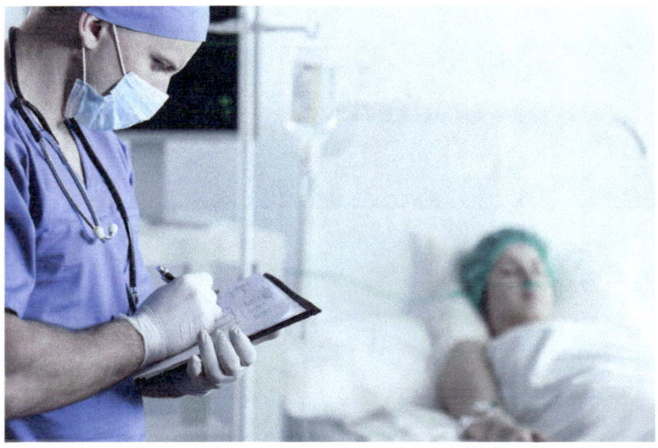

Figure 1.4. Pre and post-surgical evaluations.

Source: https://coremedplus.com/wp-content/uploads/2023/05/iStock_72742951_XXLARGE-5764b8093df78ca6e42d0b8e.jpg.

Postoperative assessment is also essential in that it provides early diagnosis of complications and informs proper adjustments in the recovery program of the patients. Observation of vital signs, the integrity of the surgical wound, and pain may provide essential information on the patient's healing process. Involving patients in the postoperative assessment also promotes responsibility and allows them to voice concerns that may arise following surgery. Advanced operations, like three-dimensional gluteoplasty for aesthetic procedures, require accurate evaluation of the anatomical structures around it so that optimal results are obtained while meeting patient expectations. This continuous cycle of assessment not only reinforces the principles of patient-centered care but also demonstrates the surgical team's commitment to medical excellence and patient comfort (Figure 1.4).

1.1.2. Informed Consent Process

Informed consent is a fundamental aspect of ethical surgical practice, the core of which is the relationship between patient autonomy and physician responsibility. A prerequisite of the process is the adequate provision of information to patients regarding their planned surgical interventions, including the risks, benefits, and alternatives to the proposed surgical intervention. Transparency is essential not only for establishing trust with patients but also for enabling patients to make knowledgeable healthcare decisions. In the surgical context, specifically within the Enhanced Recovery After Surgery (ERAS) program, informed consent is even more significant, as patients are actively engaged in shared decision-making. Clinical evidence supports increasing informed consent by ensuring that patients receive proper education, which has been proven to enhance recovery and satisfaction with care for patients undergoing surgery. Thus, the informed consent process extends beyond legal obligation and becomes an integral part of patient-centered surgical care (Michael et al., 2024). In addition to patient education, the informed consent process must incorporate a clear communication plan that addresses patients' values and preferences. Surgeons not only have to deliver medical facts but also probe the psychosocial and emotional sides of surgery. This is a holistic approach to doing things that creates a better patient care environment, enabling patients to speak up about their concerns and questions. Good communication is under the umbrella of trust maintenance in the physician-patient relationship, as espoused by the General Medical Council's guidelines (N/A, 2021). Surgeons should demonstrate empathy and interest when consulting with patients, making a conscious effort to ensure that patients understand what is being said. The inclusion of electronic devices, such as patient portals and preoperative education apps, can even streamline this process, thereby enhancing engagement and improving care pathway compliance. By developing these communication tools, the informed consent process not only meets ethics but also best practice standards in surgical care. Ultimately, the process of informed consent is an evolving component that is subject to ongoing assessment and adjustment based on emerging practices and patient needs. As surgical methods change and new treatment modalities are developed, the consent process must reflect updates in risks and benefits derived from current evidence-based standards. Participation in quality improvement initiatives, such as those encouraged through auditing against ERAS guidelines, can help define areas for improvement in the informed consent process, ensuring it remains timely and effective. This ongoing review of informed consent is situated within clinical governance structures, which prioritize quality assurance in surgical care (N/A, 2021). By enabling a culture of ongoing improvement and accountability, informed consent is more than merely a safeguard of patient autonomy but also a cornerstone of sound and safe surgical care that respects the diverse needs of patients who are being taken through operative procedures.

1.1.3. Preoperative Preparation and Optimization

The preoperative optimization and preparation phase is crucial for enhancing the surgical outcome. This phase is essential and involves extensive evaluations based on the individual patient's needs, which can include a comprehensive medical assessment and preoperative optimization of current states of health. An Enhanced Recovery After Surgery (ERAS) protocol is crucial for optimizing the process. As also indicated by studies evaluating AI-generated clinical advice according to expert consensus for ERAS, formal preoperative planning can result in improved patient outcomes (e.g., ChatGPT's alignment in 82.9% of questions tested shows promise in guiding preoperative planning) (Wang et al., 2025). Emphasis on patient education, risk stratification, and preoperative optimization enables patients to be in optimal health status during surgery, leading to an improved response to surgery and reduced postoperative complications. Optimal preoperative optimization also requires thoughtful planning of anesthesia and pain control management. Preoperative planning is necessary to address potential issues with anesthesia, such as underlying conditions or complications. A systematic review comparing ERAS protocols demonstrated that preoperative pain control is crucial in minimizing postoperative pain and accelerating recovery (Wang et al., 2025). Furthermore, equilibrating anesthetic practice with comorbid patient conditions is needed; maximizing these techniques leads to fewer complications. Various recommendations have been set in literature, but none of them have applied to specific patient circumstances to maximize anesthesia safety and effectiveness intraoperatively, and thereby the overall success of surgery. Second, emphasis should lie on the special requirements of surgical procedures, particularly in oral and maxillofacial surgery. For instance, in odontogenic cysts, preoperative optimization can decrease infection and delayed complications. Preparing conditions for surgery is of utmost significance, as the conditions themselves can actually direct the process of healing and, indirectly, influence patients' well-being. Effective control of such conditions requires a combination of surgical expertise and preoperative optimization aimed at enhancing local tissue perfusion, which is crucial for the healing process following intervention. Encouraging a comprehensive understanding of preoperative principles thus provides a safe basis for surgical interventions, enabling patients to benefit from the most favorable outcomes (Figure 1.5).

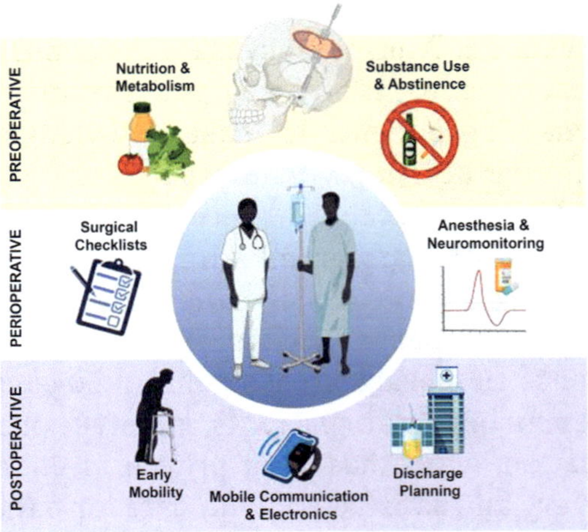

Figure 1.5. Enhanced recovery after surgery (ERAS).

Source: https://ars.els-cdn.com/content/image/1-s2.0-S1878875022004090-gr1.jpg.

Test Your Knowledge

1. What are the patient's comorbid conditions, and how might they affect surgical risk and anesthesia planning?
2. Has the patient provided informed consent after understanding the risks, benefits, and alternatives of the surgery?

1.2. Surgical Techniques

Learning Outcome

1. Explain the open surgery vs. minimally invasive surgery
2. Define the standard surgical instruments and their uses
3. Discuss the role of technology in surgical procedures

Surgical practice includes a broad range of practice necessary for the effective conduct of surgical operations. From minimally invasive approaches, such as laparoscopy, to traditional open surgery, the choice of surgical technique reflects a balance between the surgeon's skill and the patient's particular condition. Aesthetic sensibility also applies, particularly in fields such as plastic surgery, where ideals of beauty influence the choice of surgery to be conducted. This intersection of aesthetic practice and medical need raises important questions regarding the motivations behind surgical procedures: are they solely for the restoration of health, or do they serve to express society's values of beauty? Appreciation of this duality is essential for surgeons to reconcile their scientific and aesthetic procedures, not only meeting the medical needs but also considering the long-term repercussions of their surgical techniques (Edmonds et al., 2008). Moreover, the ethical implications of surgical techniques cannot be overlooked. The rapid rate of progress in surgical technology has introduced with it novel modalities that challenge traditional ethical paradigms. As highlighted in current debates, as in the Islamic law code of qiṣāṣ, there are ethical issues when surgical procedures can be used for purposes other than healing, such as punishment. When, for instance, there are instances of grievous injury, where the onus is on medical professionals to act with retributive justice, the erosion of trust within the doctor-patient relationship becomes an issue. Surgeons, therefore, have to deal with not only technical competence but also navigate complex ethical landscapes, ensuring that their practices align with the Hippocratic Oath and overall medical ethics. The responsibility to prioritize patient interests, even in culturally diverse environments, is paramount in developing the primary principles that direct surgical practice (Dabbagh et al., 2016). Lastly, progress in surgery involves an ongoing investment in education and adaptation by the medical community. Continued training fosters a culture of excellence and creativity that is safely, essential for safely integrating new technologies and methods into practice. Surgical residencies and continuous professional development are primary considerations in ensuring surgeons have access to the latest information and methods. These education systems should give equal weight to ethical considerations as technical education, equipping surgeons to make effective decisions that harmonize medical standards and social values. Equilibrium in surgical education ultimately enhances the quality of care and supports the complex decisions surgeons must make. By combining surgical dexterity with a solid ethical foundation, the practice of medicine can foster not only surgical proficiency but also a deeper understanding of the complex nature of surgery as both a science and a human endeavor (Edmonds et al., 2008; Dabbagh et al., 2016) (Figure 1.6).

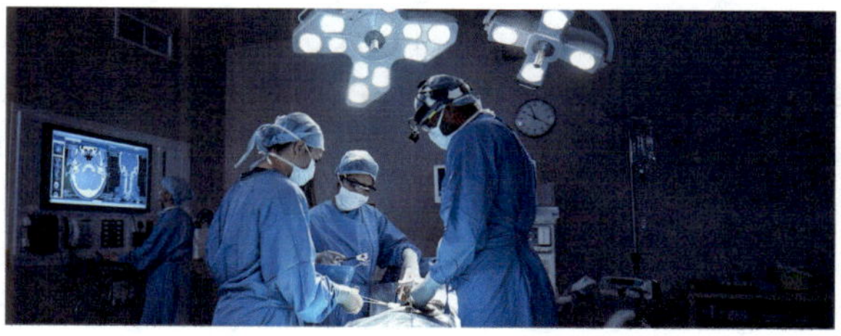

Figure 1.6. Common surgical procedures.

Source: https://www.hopkinsmedicine.org/-/media/images/health/2_-treatment/surgical-care/common-surgical-hero.jpg?h=500&iar=0&mh=500&mw=1300&w=1297&hash=FD277EB2AEE62E1B53537767AEE778CE.

1.2.1. Open Surgery Versus Minimally Invasive Surgery

Among surgical operations, the case in support of open surgery and against minimal invasive surgery (MIS) is increasingly gaining ground, given continued advances in surgical techniques. Open surgery has traditionally been defined by larger incisions that allow direct access to the surgical site, enabling extensive manipulation of tissues and organs. Although this approach often yields longer recovery times, increased postoperative pain, and greater complication rates in the form of scarring or infection, minimally invasive procedures employ smaller incisions and refined instruments so that surgeons may perform operations with less trauma to the tissues. This shift in philosophy toward less invasive interventions aligns with the principles of patient-centered care, prioritizing optimal outcomes and shorter recovery times.

The advantages of minimally invasive surgery are eminently illustrated in interventions such as mitral valve repair and replacement. As described in the literature, techniques for these cardiac interventions are evolving at an accelerating rate with a focus on successful outcomes at lesser morbidity (Agnihotri et al., 2016). Minimally invasive methods not only provide quick postoperative recovery but also achieve maximum patient satisfaction by limiting visible scarring and lowering trauma to surrounding tissues. Moreover, the potential for standardizing patient evaluation and procedure techniques has the potential to foster the widespread application of these practice methods, thereby reinforcing optimal practice among the surgical community (Agnihotri et al., 2016). Such concurrence is significant as it enhances the safety and efficacy of the procedures, ultimately leading to better patient outcomes. Despite the apparent benefits of minimal invasive techniques, open surgery remains an essential option in some complex situations, where full exposure is an absolute condition for successful intervention. Surgeons must carefully evaluate each patient's individual case, including the degree of complexity of the operation, anatomical problems, and overall condition. In some cases, the benefits of open surgery, that is, direct vision and haptic feedback, dominate those of minimally invasive interventions. As surgical method evolves, technique choice needs to be grounded in an environment of empirical recommendations and tailored patient care in a manner to offer all possibilities in the quest for optimal surgical outcomes. Balancing these techniques remains a cornerstone of contemporary surgery, as the specialty evolves towards more advanced therapies.

1.2.2. Common Surgical Instruments and Their Uses

Surgery relies heavily on a variety of specialized equipment, each of which is designed to perform specific functions with the highest level of precision and efficiency. These general surgical instruments include scalpels, scissors, forceps, and clamps, each of which serves a distinct role in surgical procedures. For instance, scalpels are primarily used for making incisions, while scissors assist in cutting tissue, sutures, and other materials. Forceps are a gripping instrument that enables the surgeon to hold and manipulate tissues during procedures. Knowledge of each individual's use guarantees surgical precision and patient safety. Inappropriate application of these generic instruments not only enhances surgeons' maximum dexterity but also significantly contributes to the successful outcome of the surgical procedure, highlighting the delicate interaction between their choice and surgical outcomes. Among the many devices employed in surgery, hemostatic devices stand out due to their central role in controlling bleeding during surgery. Clamps, such as hemostatic forceps, are fundamental in closing vessels and controlling hemorrhage, allowing for an unrestricted surgical field. Electrocautery units have also become indispensable equipment that employ heat energy to coagulate tissue and cut through tissue while simultaneously minimizing blood loss. Successful hemostasis significantly affects technical complexity and surgical duration since it reduces the risk of postoperative morbidity in the condition of preventing hematomas and bleeding.

Thus, proficiency in hemostatic control with these instruments has become a fundamental principle in modern surgical practice, demonstrating the significance of skill with surgical instruments in delivering optimal patient outcomes. Additionally, advances in surgical technology have introduced new tools that enhance the performance of previous surgical methods. Laparoscopic technology, for example, offers minimally invasive procedures that reduce patient recovery time and hospital length of stay. Combining high-definition cameras, graspers, and energy sources within a single system enables surgeons to perform delicate procedures through small incisions with reduced trauma to the surrounding tissues. These innovations require constant training and education of operating teams to maintain efficient use. As learned from recent guidelines, the creation and application of new operating instruments should be followed by rigorous tests of their effectiveness, safety, and usability in diverse clinical situations (Matthew et al., 2021). Moreover, the consideration of such advancements is crucial in fields like head and neck surgery due to the existence of separate anatomical concerns (David et al., 2020). The continuous evolution of surgical equipment is thus an essential aspect of the fundamentals of surgery that optimizes patient care and outcomes (Figure 1.7).

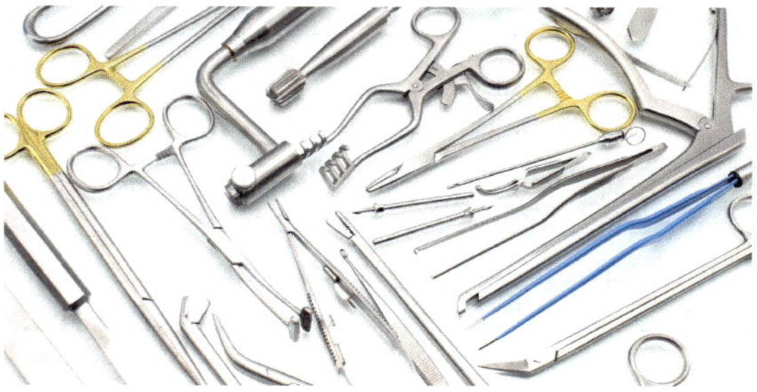

Figure 1.7. Standard surgical instruments with their uses.

Source: https://rigorinstruments.com/wp-content/uploads/2023/07/post-image-1.jpg.

1.2.3. Role of Technology in Surgical Procedures

The application of technology to surgeries has revolutionized the face of modern surgery, where precision has been enhanced and patient outcomes have been improved. Surgical equipment has undergone dramatic advancements with the emergence of robots, imaging devices, and minimally invasive procedures. Robotic surgery, for instance, enables surgeons to perform complex surgeries with greater dexterity and enhanced visualization. These systems provide high-definition 3D images of the area to be operated on, thereby reducing the margin of error that is likely to exist in open surgery. Evidence suggests that these types of technologies not only improve surgery safety but also lead to reduced recovery periods and hospitalization for patients, aligning with the objectives of Enhanced Recovery After Surgery (ERAS) protocols, which emphasize timely efficiency and patient-focused care (Michael et al., 2024). Technology even extends its influence outside the operating room, influencing preoperative assessment and postoperative monitoring. Computer networks, including electronic medical records and telemedicine systems, facilitate end-to-end care coordination for meticulous and patient-specific preoperative evaluations. Technology in the form of wearable devices has emerged as a novel tool for monitoring patients vital signs and parameters of recovery remotely so that clinicians can address potential complications before they arise. These technologies enable greater patient engagement by allowing for real-time monitoring of recovery progress, a fundamental component in the application of ERAS protocols. Patient participation in their own surgery results in better outcomes due to enhanced decision-making and tailored perioperative strategies (Skjold et al., 2020).

Ultimately, technology is revolutionizing the educational processes for surgical trainees. Traditional surgical training models, which utilize the "see one, do one, teach one" approach, are being revised due to the widespread adoption of simulation technologies and virtual reality. These new instructional tools enable surgical residents to practice techniques and procedures in a simulated environment, optimizing their skills before entering the operating room. In addition, feedback and observation systems are supported by digital platforms, enabling more formalized assessments of surgical skills acquisition. Competency-based education facilitates this shift in ensuring that effective training engages residents in deliberate practice, thereby enabling them to perform a range of surgical procedures safely and independently throughout their training (Skjold et al., 2020).

Test Your Knowledge

1. What anatomical landmarks must be identified to ensure proper surgical access and minimize complications?
2. Which surgical approach (open, laparoscopic, robotic) is most appropriate for this procedure, and why?

1.3. Anesthesia in Surgery

Learning Outcome

1. Explain the types of anesthesia: general, regional, and local
2. Define the anesthesia administration and monitoring
3. Describe the risks and complications associated with anesthesia

The application of anesthesia in surgery is a cornerstone of modern surgical practice, enabling safe and compassionate patient care. Anesthesia is employed to abolish pain and suffering, allowing for various types of surgery, ranging from minor procedures to complex surgeries. Evolutions of anesthesia in the past have been remarkable, beginning with rudimentary techniques and progressing to general, regional, and local anesthesia, all adapted to specific surgical needs. Under appropriate anesthesia, surgeons can carry out surgical procedures with accuracy, making intraoperative pain and anxiety management more efficient and thereby enhancing patient outcomes and satisfaction. The development of anesthetic drugs and technology has also reduced the risks associated with surgery, making previously complicated procedures more achievable and safer than before. Acharya Sushrutas contribution to surgical concepts like anesthesia is considerable in the context of emergency surgery. His seminal work, the Sushruta Samhita, laid the foundation for understanding various ailments that are amenable to surgery and their corresponding modes of treatment. In the book, Sushruta specified the need for anesthesia, highlighting its utility in life-or-death surgeries conducted by surgeons. His holistic approach encompassed not just the physical act of surgery but also the necessity of preparing patients mentally and physically in advance, emphasizing the interconnectedness of pain relief and the success of surgery. Key practices instituted by Sushruta, such as the use of herbal remedies for pain relief, represent early attempts to understand and minimize patient pain. His established principles remain applicable, resonating with present practice that emphasizes patient care in surgical disciplines.

In current surgical practice, new uses of anesthesia continue to evolve, leveraging advancements in technology and techniques to enhance patient safety and comfort. For instance, improvements in monitoring systems used during anesthesia have improved the ability to tailor anesthetic treatment to individual patient needs. This individualized titration of care minimizes surgery-related risks and complications, ensuring compliance with principles for successful pain management. In addition, the multidisciplinary profession of anesthesia encompasses not only the delivery of anesthetic drugs but also preoperative assessment and postoperative care, both of which are essential in providing a comprehensive view of the patient's surgical experience. The historical context provided by writers like Sushruta underscores the ongoing significance of anesthesia in surgery, tracing how underlying principles continue to guide and evolve modern practices, and in the process, transform surgery into a more accessible and streamlined branch of medicine (Figure 1.8).

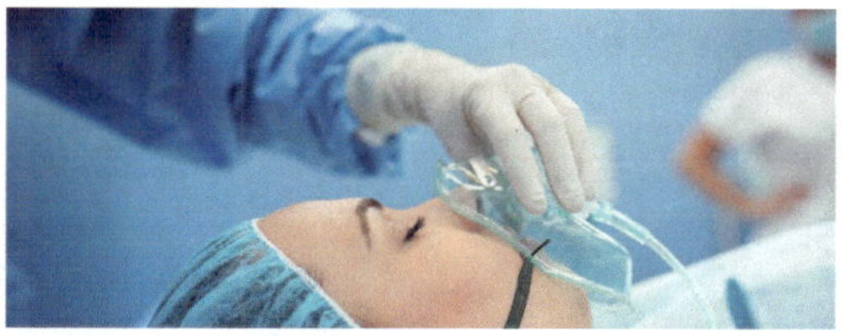

Figure 1.8. Anesthesia in surgery.

Source: https://www.hopkinsmedicine.org/-/media/images/health/_-images-to-be-filed/surgeonadjustsmaskonpatienthero.jpg?h=500&iar=0&mh=500&mw=1300&w=1297&hash=C3E081A71D824668F99FBDF94DCA588B.

1.3.1. Types of Anesthesia: General, Regional, and Local

Administering anesthesia during surgery is crucial for preserving the patient's safety and comfort. Anesthesia can be broadly categorized into general, regional, and local anesthesia. General anesthesia results in the rendering of the patient completely unconscious and insensitive, and therefore, it is applied in extensive surgery. It is usually administered through inhalation or intravenous methods and should be taken with care due to associated risks such as reactions to anesthetic substances and long recovery times. An illustration is provided for the operations performed on the distal radius; evidence shows that general anesthetics play a significant role in operating time and complications, thus the choice should be carefully considered depending on the patient's condition (Halvachizadeh et al., 2025). It is essential that surgical teams understand the nuances of general anesthesia, as understanding them can lead to better patient outcomes and a more robust safety profile during the execution of complex procedures. Regional anesthesia, by contrast, involves blocking sensation in a specific section of the body, allowing patients to remain awake and active during their treatment. Such a technique is increasingly becoming popular in certain forms of surgery, such as orthopedics, where localized procedures are dominant. The circumstantial advantages of regional anesthesia include fewer systemic effects compared to general anesthesia and reduced postoperative complication rates, such as nausea and vomiting (Valente et al., 2025). A good example is in breast surgery, where interventions such as interpectoral and serratus plane blocks can effectively manage pain while mitigating cardiac complications, particularly in patients with comorbidities such as heart failure. Regional anesthesia is thus not only safer for specific populations but also allows faster recovery, further underlining its growing role in modern surgical practice. Local anesthesia, the third type, anesthetizes explicitly a small area of the body, and it is employed for minor surgery such as dental treatment or skin biopsies. This method involves direct injection of anesthetic medications into the area of treatment with minimal or no effect on the rest of the body when the patient is awake. Local anesthesia shortens the recovery period and causes minimal systemic effects, thereby enhancing patient satisfaction and reducing overall healthcare costs. It is limited in its use to minimally invasive procedures due to its localized action. The choice between local, regional, and general anesthesia ultimately depends on several variables, including the nature and complexity of the procedure, patient condition, and anticipated recovery course, which underscores the need for an individualized anesthesia plan in surgical planning.

1.3.2. Anesthesia Administration and Monitoring

Anesthesia administration is a critical element of surgery that significantly impacts patient safety and surgical outcomes. The selection of anesthetic agents varies according to several factors, including the type of surgery, patient history, and anticipated postoperative care. Tailoring the anesthesia strategy can significantly enhance patient comfort and decrease the risk of adverse outcomes. For instance, in transplant surgery, as characterised in experimental models, a diligent anesthesia regimen involving repeated drug dosing has been shown to enhance hemodynamic stability and operative efficiency (Banner et al., 1989). Not only does such anaesthesia attention facilitate the surgery, but it also affects the recipient's recovery course and outcome. Monitoring is also equally important in anesthesia administration as it ensures the patient's stability throughout the surgical process. Continuous monitoring of vital signs, including blood pressure, heart rate, and oxygen saturation, is necessary to detect any hemodynamic instability or adverse effects of anesthesia. In complex operating rooms, where rapid procedures may be required, this careful monitoring enables the anesthesiologist to make rapid adjustments to anesthetic levels and other aspects, thereby providing optimal physiological status. Further, technological progress in monitoring has improved the ability to assess the patient's status in real-time, which leads to evidence-based clinical decisions during surgery (Pozek et al., 2018). Therefore, successful monitoring is crucial to surgical efficacy and safety. Ideas about multimodal analgesia are increasingly focal to modern anesthesia practice, especially in the effort to minimize opioid consumption in the postoperative phase. Rationale for utilizing multiple modalities of analgesia—for example, regional anesthesia and adjuvant medications—will help to restrict opioid addiction, thereby reducing the danger of chronic postoperative pain and opioid dependence. According to the evolving perioperative care model, anesthesiologists are now being urged to collaborate with surgical teams in developing customized pain management plans. Not only does this enhance the initial postoperative experience, but it also addresses the issue of generalized opioid exposure in surgical patients (Pozek et al., 2018). Thus, the underlying principles of anesthesia management and monitoring are a key component of establishing surgical outcomes and optimizing patient care in an advanced surgical environment (Figure 1.9).

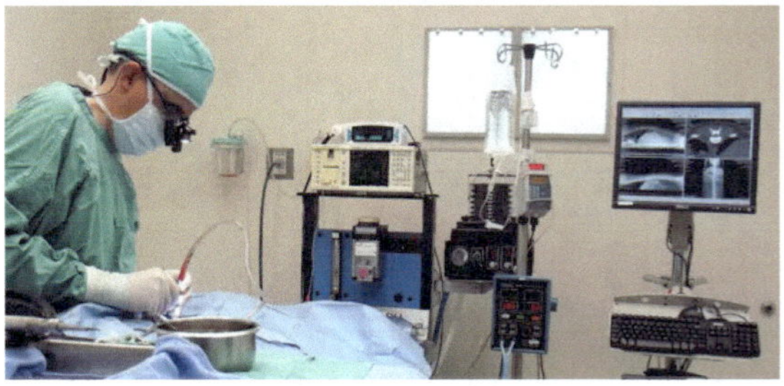

Figure 1.9. Anesthesia monitoring.

Source: https://vetneuro.com/wp-content/uploads/2016/06/IMG_5684edited.jpg.

1.3.3. Risks and Complications Associated with Anesthesia

Administration of anesthesia is a critical element of every surgical procedure, but one with innate risks and complications that must be adequately managed appropriately. One of the primary concerns is the risk of respiratory complications, which can occur in both general anesthesia and regional anesthesia. For instance, airway obstruction in the form of action on the respiratory musculature by the anesthetic or patient, or the patient's operative position during surgery, presents a risk. Risk of respiratory complications is particularly high in the presence of underlying lung disease, and so perioperative care becomes more complex. Intraoperative hypoxia may, in turn, lead to severe neurological dysfunction or death if not recognized and treated. As highlighted in the literature, recovery programs with an early mobilization and patient activation focus have been promising in restricting such complications, and thus the importance of including best practices in anesthesia management to improve surgical outcomes (Michael et al., 2024).

Another critical risk about anesthesia includes cardiovascular complications that can present as myocardial infarction, arrhythmia, or hemodynamic instability during or after surgery. These are most frequent in patients with pre-existing cardiovascular disease and need to be thoroughly preoperatively evaluated to risk-stratify. Some variables, including age, comorbid conditions, and anesthetic type, can be involved in the increase of these cardiovascular risks. Anesthesiologists need to employ perioperative hemodynamic monitoring and management strategies to optimize patient stability during surgery. Also, the inclusion of evidence-based practice, as highlighted in guideline documents, to counteract these cardiovascular risks, and it is able to ensure that patients undergo optimal parameters throughout the surgical process (Lori et al., 2021).

Finally, post-anesthesia complications, such as postoperative nausea and vomiting (PONV), are possible complications that can extend recovery and raise healthcare costs. PONV is annoying to patients and theoretically can lead to complications such as dehydration, electrolyte imbalance, and even wound dehiscence secondary to vomiting-induced increased intra-abdominal pressure. There are several risk factors for PONV, including the type of surgery and whether or not the patient has a history of motion sickness. Therefore, prophylactic measures, including multimodal antiemetic therapy and adherence to Enhanced Recovery After Surgery (ERAS) protocols, are crucial in preventing these unwanted outcomes. The effective execution of these strategies further highlights the importance of continuous innovation in anesthetic practice, ultimately enhancing patient care and postoperative recovery following surgical interventions (Michael et al., 2024).

Test Your Knowledge

1. What type of anesthesia is most suitable for this surgical procedure?
2. How is the patient monitored intraoperatively to ensure anesthetic safety?

1.4. Intraoperative Management

Learning Outcome

1. Identify the surgical team roles and responsibilities
2. Define the sterile techniques and infection control
3. Describe the handling complications during surgery

Intraoperative care is a crucial aspect of surgical principles, as it has a direct impact on patient outcomes and the overall success of the surgical procedure. The intraoperative care involves a series of practices and protocols that are followed to achieve maximum patient safety and surgical effectiveness. Surgeons are responsible for ensuring sterility, anesthesia, and appropriate instrumentation. Adherence during this stage can diminish the intraoperative risk of complications and enhance recovery time. Additionally, constant intraoperative monitoring of vital signs is essential to record any fluctuations that may indicate distress or complications, allowing for instant action to correct them. Intraoperative management, as it should be, is a cornerstone, reinforcing the belief that whole surgical care goes beyond performing technically to include constant monitoring of patient health while doing so. Use of advanced technologies and methods in intraoperative management has revolutionized surgery. Endoscopic interventions, for instance, have greatly enhanced exposure of critical anatomical sites without inflicting trauma to tissues. This type of approach is well illustrated in pituitary surgery, where the differentiation between endoscopic and microscopic techniques is significant in ensuring maximum tumor resection with minimal trauma to surrounding healthy tissue. Awareness of each technique's nuances enhances intraoperative decision-making, directly affecting patient outcomes. Additionally, intraoperative imaging modalities, such as fluoroscopy and intraoperative ultrasound, are increasingly utilized in the operating room. These technologies provide real-time feedback, allowing the surgical team to make informed decisions regarding tumor margins and resection strategies, ultimately enhancing the safety and efficacy of the procedure (Evans et al., 2018). Secondly, intraoperative care is not just the technical execution of surgery; it demands effective communication and coordination of the entire operating team. Effective teamwork and clear roles are essential, as each member contributes to the success of the procedure. Anesthesiology, surgical support, and the nursing staff must work in harmony to achieve a smooth process, manage complications, and respond to any unforeseen issues that may arise throughout the procedure. Preoperative briefings conducted on a regular basis can establish shared expectations and clarify tasks, resulting in improved intraoperative dynamics. Additionally, intraoperative decision-making protocols and emergency procedures are crucial for maintaining patient safety. As is the case in the study of heterogeneous tumors, including gastrointestinal stromal tumors, the ability to manage such complexities well highlights the importance of systematic intraoperative management protocols (Alecu et al., 2019) (Figure 1.10).

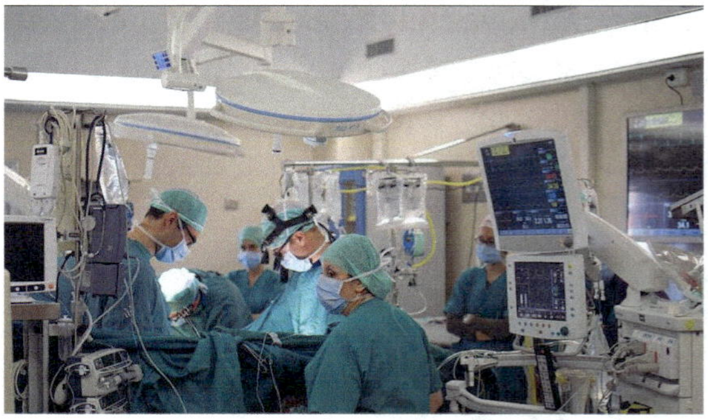

Figure 1.10. Intraoperative nursing care.

Source: https://wtcs.pressbooks.pub/app/uploads/sites/47/2023/12/Cardiac_surgery_operating_room.jpg.

1.4.1. Surgical Team Roles and Responsibilities

The operating staff operates as a cohesive entity, with every member fulfilling a specialist role to ensure patient safety, in addition to achieving overall success in surgical procedures. This staff has traditionally included the surgeon, surgical assistant, the anesthesiologist, and the nursing staff, all of whom contribute as a group to the surgical procedure. The surgical team is typically led by the surgeon, who takes charge of conceptualizing and conducting the operation. The surgical assistant provides valuable assistance, helping with suturing and tissue handling. The anesthesiologist, on the other hand, plays a special role in managing the patient's pain and life functions throughout the procedure. This allocation of duty reflects the harmony that is required to achieve optimal patient outcomes and realizes the necessity for effective communication and regard for each position in the surgical hierarchy, in the end improving procedural efficiency and effectiveness. Over the last several years, the incorporation of advanced providers, such as physician assistants (PAs) and nurse practitioners (NPs), onto surgical teams has become increasingly prevalent. These trained professionals, commonly referred to as "advanced providers," are crucial to operations by augmenting the capabilities of surgeons and enhancing the quality of care in surgical units. By their active participation in preoperative, intraoperative, and postoperative care, PAs and NPs enable surgeons to focus on complex surgical procedures. At the same time, patients get complete and attentive care during their operation. Thus, studies aimed at such integration have suggested increased efficiency and patient outcomes, supporting the usefulness of diverse skill sets in the operating room. Such improvements in surgical team operations verify growing awareness of the imperative to incorporate advanced providers into comprehensive care.

Organized models for functional improvement must successfully integrate advanced providers as members of surgical teams and foster improved coordination among these practitioners and surgical residents. As suggested by recent publications, attempts at constructing collaborative partnerships among surgical team members can have the potential to significantly impact the educational environment for surgical residents and patient care in general. By establishing systematized professional development activities and designating explicit leadership roles to surgical advanced providers, hospitals can establish a culture of continuous improvement in practice and education of surgeons. This not only broadens the practice scope of PAs and NPs but also enhances surgical residents' education, better preparing them to practice in more multidisciplinary healthcare environments. The evolving roles and responsibilities of surgical team members thus emphasize the importance of flexibility and lifelong learning in the practice of surgery (Bonica et al., 2017; Dunnington et al., 2018).

1.4.2. Sterile Techniques and Infection Control

Practice of sterile techniques is central to the surgical setting as it has direct implications on patient safety and overall surgery efficiency. Sterile techniques form the basis of infection prevention, which isolates pathogens from sterile environments. The principles of maintaining sterile fields, using aseptic equipment, and proper hand care are all pivotal in eliminating the risk of SSIs. It is estimated that SSIs impact a large number of surgical patients, increasing the duration of hospitalization and additional healthcare costs. Therefore, initiating strict sterilization protocols not only serves the interest of patient outcomes but also decreases the strain on the healthcare system. Furthermore, adherence to sterile procedures results in patient confidence, as it fosters trust in the safety measures adopted during surgical operations, thereby ensuring adherence to medical practice ethics in surgery. Infection control procedures extend beyond the operating room to preoperative, intraoperative, and postoperative phases. Preoperative awareness of skin preparation and prophylactic antibiotics is a fundamental components that assist in reducing the risk of infection. Furthermore, during the surgical procedure, careful adherence to protocols such as limiting traffic flow into the operating theater and using sterile drapes is crucial in creating a zone free from microbes. The team's work is vital, as each member must be familiar with conducting such procedures and be thorough in their execution. With continued education and training in the practice of infection control, surgical teams will be well-positioned to ensure high standards of quality at all phases of surgical care. This is crucial in preventing infection and achieving optimal surgical outcomes.

The management of postoperative infection is a vital infection control intervention that necessitates commitment and effort from healthcare professionals. Identifying the early symptoms of infection, such as redness, swelling, and discharge from surgical wounds, is crucial for early intervention. Simple postoperative advice, including instructions on wound care, recognizing infection symptoms, and follow-up, is also crucial for healing. The integration of digital health technology, such as telemedicine, also offers an opportunity for closer monitoring and early detection of complications following surgery. It is particularly necessary in the wake of the increasing reliance on evidence-based medicine and open reporting measures, as highlighted by the revised ARRIVE guidelines (Percie et al., 2020). Adopting active infection control measures is imperative for enhancing the standards of surgical care in terms of long-term patient safety and satisfaction within the health system (Figure 1.11).

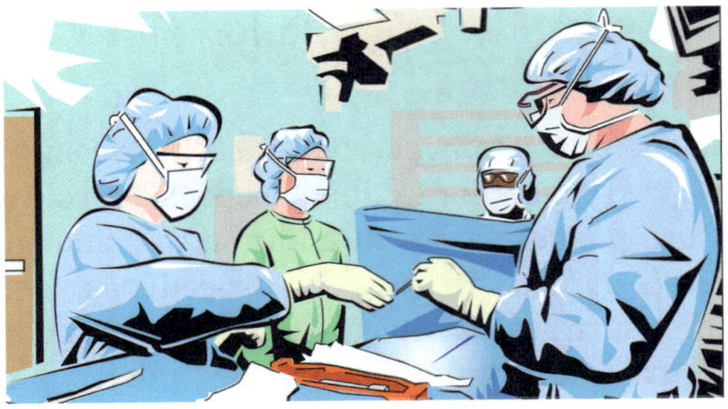

Figure 1.11. Sterile technique.

Source: https://aornjournal.onlinelibrary.wiley.com/cms/asset/7e7cfab6-73d5-4612-8505-3d98c0d5ad76/aorn13849-fig-0004-m.jpg.

1.4.3. Handling Complications During Surgery

Surgical complication management is an indispensable aspect of patient safety provision and optimization of surgical performance. Surgeons must remain vigilant for the potential of intraoperative complications that can arise unpredictably due to various factors, including patient anatomy, surgical technique, and instrument handling. For instance, minimally invasive surgery (MIS) has transformed procedures for surgery by lowering trauma and making recovery times shorter; however, it is also accompanied by problems, like unanticipated bleeding or anatomical issues that will complicate procedures (Qadrie et al., 2025). Surgeons who are skilled in knowing these complications and possess the capacity to mitigate them in real time significantly reduce risks for patients. An active strategy, accompanied by extensive preoperative assessment and realistic contingencies, including the potential for conversion to open surgery, is essential for safeguarding patient outcomes. Another integral component of surgical complication management is the surgeons' skill and ongoing education regarding complex surgical techniques. The training curve of various procedures, specifically in methods like manual minor incision cataract surgery (MSICS), emphasizes that surgeons strive towards refining their skills and employing severe preventive measures to ward off risks. Training in recognizing potential complications, such as rupture of the posterior capsule or corneal burns, is imperative (Shetty et al., 2023). Surgeons should also work with multidisciplinary teams for efficient preoperative planning, considering patient background, anatomical complexity, and the selection of appropriate instruments. This collaboration is held accountable for enhanced decision-making during surgery with enhanced speed, and it has the potential to improve patient safety greatly.

Finally, technology application and the use of new surgical instruments are also crucial in avoiding surgical complications. Advances in imaging and robotic-assisted surgical equipment enhance visualization and precision, allowing surgeons to navigate difficult anatomical landscapes with increased confidence. Regular maintenance and calibration of surgical instruments are essential for preventing equipment breakdown, which can lead to procedural complications (Qadrie et al., 2025). Additionally, ensuring smooth communication among surgical teams ensures that all teams are synchronized in response mechanisms for potential intraoperative complications. By implementing these strategies, the surgery practice can continue to evolve, with an emphasis on addressing challenges in the complication area and striving for greater safety and efficacy in patient care.

Test Your Knowledge

1. How is blood loss estimated and managed during surgery?
2. What measures are taken to maintain aseptic technique throughout surgery?

1.5. Postoperative Care

Learning Outcome

1. Describe the recovery room protocols
2. Define the pain management strategies
3. Discuss the monitoring for complications of surgical care

Better patient outcomes and lower postoperative complications are reliant on successful postoperative care. In this context, surgical wound care plays a primary role. In the 90-day economic model, improved wound closure techniques, such as the Skin Closure System, were found to significantly reduce direct costs and the utilization of post-acute care services. The study proposed potential savings of $56.70 to $79.62 per patient, and when scaled up to a few surgeries, can result in substantial hospital budgetary savings. These findings underscore the importance of evaluating different surgical protocols not just in terms of their immediate efficacy but also in terms of their long-term impact on recovery and healthcare spending, thus solidifying the principle that postoperative care must balance both clinical and financial dimensions to enhance patient care as a whole (Ferko et al., 2018). Along with managing wounds, the use of holistic assessments in individually crafted postoperative care is even more critical, especially for an elderly population. Since many surgeries are done on older patients, the inclusion of pre-surgical geriatric evaluation can allow for the detection of certain risk factors that could make recovery difficult. Although there could be several advantages to these kinds of assessments, they are not used as frequently, mainly because they are time-consuming. Research has shown that targeted education interventions for healthcare professionals on key aspects of these evaluations can enhance postoperative outcomes. This paradigm shift emphasizes not only expert surgical procedures but also a strategic focus on tailored patient evaluation to optimize postoperative treatment outcomes and efficiency (Lampugnane et al., 2017). Furthermore, postoperative care plans can be enhanced by a multidisciplinary approach, in which collaborative working among various healthcare professionals becomes the priority. Physicians' assistants, nurses, and physical therapists can collaborate to provide care for the complex requirements of surgically recuperating patients. Personalized discharge plans, tailored to the patients' living setup and support system, are crucial in preventing readmissions. Evidence-based attempts to standardize postoperative care pathways also provide a guarantee against non-compliance with best practices so that each patient receives follow-up treatment as required. Emphasizing continuity of care following surgery not only increases patient satisfaction but also reinforces the leading principle that successful surgical outcomes rely on having an even, proactive postoperative strategy oriented towards patient safety and welfare (Lampugnale et al., 2017; Ferko et al., 2018) (Figure 1.12).

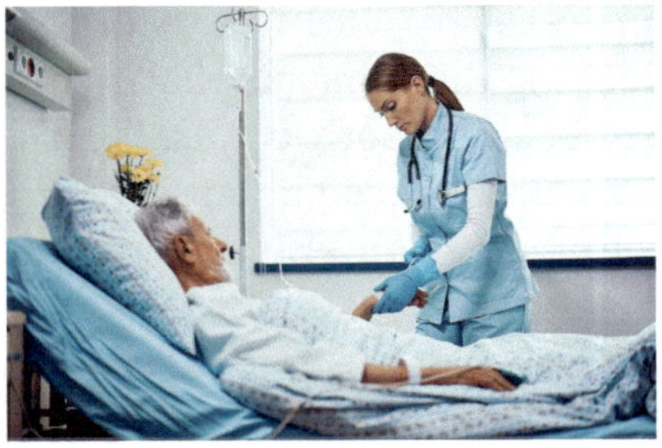

Figure 1.12. Importance of post-operative care.

Source: https://sukinohealthcare.com/wp-content/uploads/2023/06/Post-operative-cares.jpg.

1.5.1. Recovery Room Protocols

The recovery room is a critical juncture in the surgical process, where patients transition from the phases of anesthesia to a state of stability as the discharge decision is made. Adherence to strict recovery room protocols is essential to ensure patient safety and optimize results. These protocols often include continuous observation of vital signs, assessment of pain levels, and evaluation of the anesthesia's effect. It is also crucial that recovery room personnel are adequately trained to recognize complications and respond promptly. By managing any resultant immediate postoperative complications—respiratory compromise or bleeding, for instance—healthcare providers can dramatically reduce the recovery times of patients, reduce complications, and enhance overall satisfaction. The development of these protocols based on evidence and best practice enables an environment controlled by patient health requirements first and foremost, and with a reduction in the risks of recovery from anesthesia. The integration of standardized recovery room procedures also enhances the efficacy of surgical services. For instance, the use of Enhanced Recovery After Surgery (ERAS) principles is a step towards multidisciplinary practices that cover preoperative awareness, optimized surgical practice, and postoperative care. ERAS protocol utilizes a combination of strategies, such as early mobilization and standardized pain management protocols, in an attempt to facilitate quicker recovery and discharge. With the adoption of these evidence-based practices for care, medical professionals are able to achieve shorter recovery times and reduced hospital stays, ensuring a smoother workflow of patients. The proper application of ERAS principles has been widely documented, positively impacting patient outcomes and highlighting the importance of organized methods in surgical recovery processes (Aktimur, 2021). Better communication between surgical teams also improves the validity of the protocol in recovery settings. The need for particular vigilance towards recovery room complications cannot be overemphasized. Such a case includes the infrequent but severe phenomenon of bilateral simultaneous postoperative endophthalmitis (BSPOE), which underscores the utmost need for adherence to prescribed surgical procedures. While uncommon, this condition usually results from violations of recommended procedures, especially in cases such as immediately sequential bilateral cataract surgery (Chen et al., 2021). Understanding of the pathogenesis and outcome of such complications directs enhanced recovery processes and highlights the importance of strict postoperative monitoring. Through a robust protocol system, healthcare teams are well-positioned to significantly limit the risks of postoperative infection and improve patient visual outcomes. In the end, adherence to strict recovery room protocols not only guards against recognized complications but also facilitates an environment of continuous enhancement in surgical care delivery.

1.5.2. Pain Management Strategies

Effective pain management in the operating room is crucial, as it significantly influences patient outcomes and recovery experiences. There are various methods to minimize pain, beginning with multimodal analgesia that employs multiple medications and modalities to attack numerous pain pathways. Employing non-opioid analgesics, regional anesthetics, and adjuvant therapy, clinicians can effectively reduce the consumption of opioids while maximizing the relief of pain. Such a method not only diminishes the dangers of opioid use but also directly tackles pain at its site of origin, permitting faster recovery times for patients. Involving patients in their pain management plans also encourages compliance and enables them to describe their symptoms more clearly. This inter-disciplinary approach is highly congruent with best up-to-date evidence-based practice within surgery, supporting individualization of approaches to each patient's requirements for optimum pain control. Hypnosis is introduced as a possible adjunct treatment for pain reduction, particularly in small-scale procedures. Evidence has found that hypnosis can decrease pain considerably more than traditional management, and thus it has a valuable tool to offer clinicians when wishing to optimize patients' comfort. A meta-analysis of 29 randomized controlled trials demonstrated that hypnosis not only alleviates pain but also equals other psychological and behavioral treatments. The patients who received numerous sessions of hypnosis before surgery had the most significant levels of pain relief, justifying early intervention in pain management plans.

This finding highlights the importance of more research to explore the effects of hypnosis in more types of surgical procedures. As the clinical community increasingly understands pain control, the introduction of new methods, such as hypnosis, can complement standard practice and enhance surgical performance (Elkins et al., 2014). Chronic postsurgical pain management is another aspect that needs to be considered in surgical practice. Few patients experience residual pain following surgery related to prolonged opioid use, with profound implications. These also consist of preoperative opioid use, anxiety, and drug abuse, which all refer to an interdisciplinary approach by the surgeons and anesthesiologists to mitigate the long-term opioid exposure. Individualized analgesic plans and the utilization of regional anesthesia can significantly decrease opioid use and prevent the progression to chronic pain management. An enhanced recovery pathway, which streamlines the care process, is a crucial factor in optimizing surgical outcomes. By incorporating detailed pain management practices on an individual patient basis, health professionals can significantly improve postoperative outcomes and minimize the risk of chronic pain (Pozek et al., 2018) (Figure 1.13).

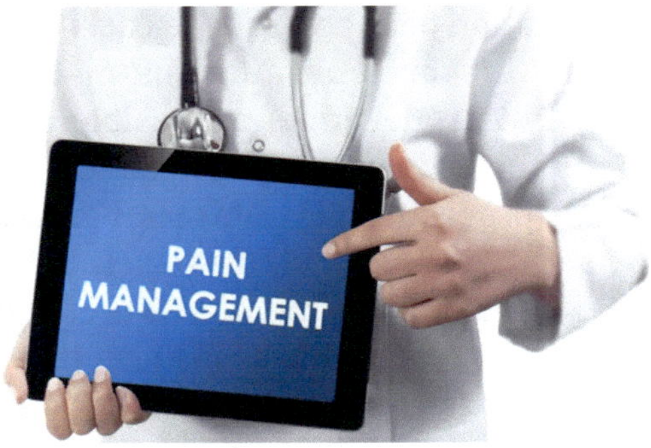

Figure 1.13. Managing pain after surgery.

Source: https://www.healthywomen.org/media-library/pain-management.jpg?id=27865001&width=1200&height=800&quality=85&coordinates=0%2C24%2C0%2C24.

1.5.3. Monitoring for Complications

Complication monitoring is an essential component of operative care, requiring an organized approach to maximize patient outcomes and minimize the possibility of harm. Effective postoperative monitoring involves vigilant attention to vital signs, wound appearance, and patient-reported symptoms to identify untoward events in their early stages. Vigilance is of utmost importance because infection, hemorrhage, and thromboembolic complications can significantly influence recovery pathways. By implementing monitoring protocols for routine check-ups, surgical teams can detect complications early, thereby reducing avoidable morbidity and mortality rates. Moreover, systematic monitoring enables the collection of data that can inform improvements in subsequent surgical procedures and patient care protocols, underscoring the importance of comprehensive postoperative care in the art of surgery (Vahanian et al., 2021). The utilization of advanced technologies in monitoring complications represents a paradigm shift in surgical management. For instance, real-time monitoring systems with AI are capable of processing huge amounts of information from surgical parameters and patient vital signs. These systems enhance the precision of clinical assessments by identifying deviations from normal recovery patterns, thereby leading to anticipatory compensation for imminent complications. Development initiatives, such as the Smart Tissue Autonomous Robot (STAR), illustrate the union of robotics with monitoring capabilities to create safer surgery environments, wherein autonomous systems can aid in evaluating operative areas (Sandip et al., 2019). The adoption of such technology marks the beginning of a paradigm shift in which monitoring procedures become increasingly sophisticated through algorithm-driven information that detects complications before they worsen. Moreover, interdisciplinarity plays a crucial role in monitoring postoperative complications. Surgeons, nurses, and other medical staff must communicate on an ongoing basis to provide a united effort towards patient care. This includes scheduling regular team meetings to check on patient status and address any emerging issues that may arise, thereby fostering a culture of shared responsibility in monitoring results. Education and training regarding the identification of specific complication indicators allow the entire healthcare team to possess the necessary skills in responding appropriately and effectively. Furthermore, the identification and implementation of standard practices across healthcare facilities can even render monitoring practices more efficient, establishing a system that facilitates uniform and high-quality surgical care (Vahanian et al., 2021).

Test Your Knowledge

1. What are the key signs to monitor for early detection of postoperative complications?
2. How is pain managed in the immediate postoperative period?

1.6. Ethical Considerations in Surgery

Learning Outcome

1. Describe the ethical dilemmas in surgical decision-making
2. Define the patient autonomy and surgical interventions
3. Identify the role of ethics committees in surgical practices

Ethical surgery is a multi-sided business of moral premises that guide practitioners as they make decisions that serve patients' welfare. At the heart of these is the Hippocratic Oath, which binds practitioners to the commitment not to harm and to what is best for the patient. Surgeons must grapple with multiple challenges, particularly when operations are performed for both medical and cosmetic purposes. For instance, dermatologists often face the dilemma of reconciling curative care with the allure of cosmetic treatments, as these treatments pose a threat to the ethical principles that govern their practice. Such dualism is gravely ethically challenged, particularly inasmuch as it concerns the potential manipulation of patients' perception of beauty and health, introducing issues of autonomy and informed consent into the surgical process (Lowe et al., 2017). Moreover, the commodification of surgery, particularly in areas such as dermatology, complicates the ethical issue. As aesthetic demands grow, physicians are likely to be inclined towards profit motives at the expense of care, leading to ethical breaches that deteriorate respect for the medical community. The practice tends to promote a culture that conflates beauty with perfection, thereby exerting undue pressure on patients to conform to societal standards. By profiting from these procedures, surgeons risk compromising their professional ethics to a market-driven philosophy that will prioritize appearance over the health and well-being of patients. These challenges necessitate robust ethical principles, as their absence would result in significant harm not only to patients but also to society at large, rendering a revision of current practice within the surgical team unavoidable (Lowe et al., 2017). Also, the field of psychosurgery provides a new layer of ethical complications, namely when it comes to the historical intervention into mental health problems through surgical means. According to Dr. Kanoti, the surgeon's history is problematic from an ethical standpoint, as it involves questions regarding consent, the possibility of coercion, and the long-term impact of such intervention on a patient's autonomy. Ethics must take into account the psychological implications of procedures, whether the patients are making autonomous choices without external coercion. With continued progress in the field, there must also be continued ethical consideration and vigilance to ensure new methods, particularly those that blur the lines with mental health, are grounded in respect for patient autonomy and dignity. This critical appraisal will outline the future of surgery, ensuring that its practitioners remain committed to ethical procedures that prioritize not only the success of the operation but also the overall health of the patient (Figure 1.14).

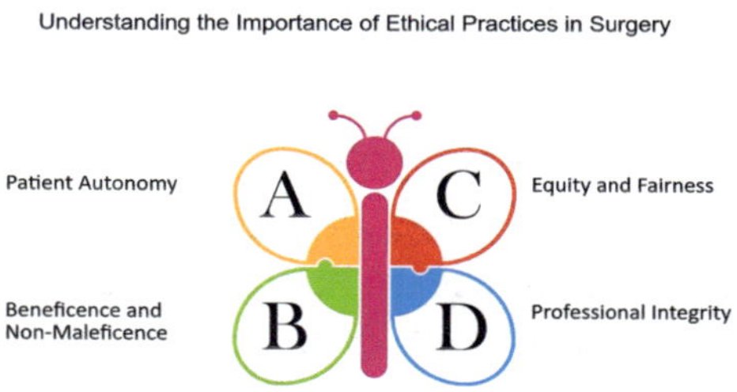

Figure 1.14. Ethical considerations in surgery.

Source: https://fastercapital.co/i/Surgical-Ethics--Ethical-Practices-in-Surgery--The-FRCS-Commitment--Understanding-the-Importance-of-Ethical-Practices-in-Surgery.webp.

1.6.1. Ethical Dilemmas in Surgical Decision-Making

The moral issues in surgical decision-making are typically due to the competing principles of patient autonomy, beneficence, and non-maleficence. Surgeons must navigate the delicate balance between respecting a patient's preferences and providing the best care in surgical practice. Jehovah's Witness patients are a special ethical concern since they do not receive blood transfusions. Surgeons must ensure the doctrine of informed consent and ensure patient safety in procedures with the risk of massive hemorrhage. As stated, respect for a patient's autonomy is the prevailing ethical guideline, which demands complete disclosure of surgery risks and the patient's decision so that an informed decision can be made (Lobo et al., 2016). Such conversations can empower patients while ensuring that operating teams are still accountable and vigilant when operating on such complex ethical grounds. The intersection of technological advances and patient treatment also muddies ethical decision-making in the operating room. The development of new healthcare technologies—particularly in fields such as fetal medicine—has been accompanied by a plethora of ethical dilemmas, whereby judgments must be made under circumstances of questionable prognostic predictions and complex risk assessments. Doctors have to deal with the dilemmas of direct interventions on fetuses, including ethical reflection on the maternal-fetal relationship and implications of newly available procedures. This shifting environment brings to the fore the necessity for solid ethical principles that will be capable of guiding surgeons in achieving the balance between surgical interventions' potential benefits and the risk and uncertainty linked to them. These principles are crucial in promoting ethical practice focused on patients' well-being while being capable of coping with developments in medical technology (Williams et al., 2006).

Lastly, the role of multidisciplinary teams in resolving ethical dilemmas cannot be overlooked. Collaboration among various specialties enables surgeons to consider diverse ideas and perspectives when handling complex cases. For instance, when a surgical team is working on a patient who cannot agree on suggested interventions due to personal beliefs, they must engage with ethicists, psychologists, and spiritual care workers. This interprofessional practice not only improves decision-making but also allows for a better understanding of the patient's values and requirements. By integrating various viewpoints, the operating room team is in a better position to address the psychosocial needs of care, reestablishing the relationship of trust and respect necessary to solve ethical dilemmas effectively. Finally, these interprofessional conversation sessions allow for a more integrated ethical model of surgical practice, ensuring that patient-centered care remains at the forefront in surgical decision-making (Figure 1.15).

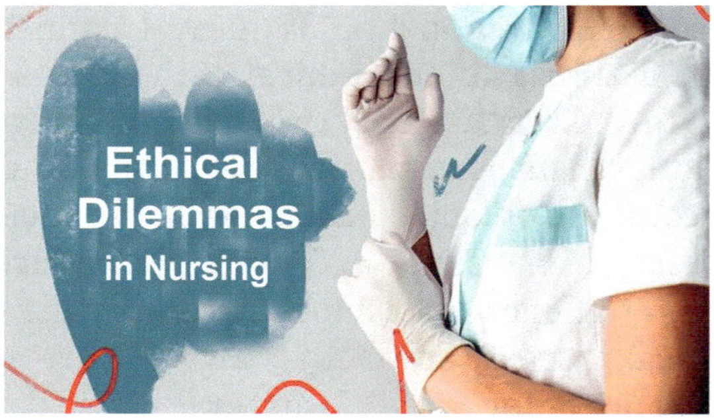

Figure 1.15. Ethical dilemmas in nursing.

Source: https://cdn.prod.website-files.com/5e5d43546b94f97f39c228fa/6690efedfb9e1cb7abcf1c3c_banner%20%20Ethical%20Dilemmas%20in%20Nursing-(Compressify.io).webp.

1.6.2. Patient Autonomy and Surgical Interventions

The principle of patient autonomy is central in surgical practices, particularly as it relates to informed consent and decision-making. Unlike the traditional physician-centered era, when surgeons' authority was largely in command, the modern practice of surgery emphasizes respect for patient decisions and wishes. The new format recognizes that patients have the right to be informed about their condition, treatment alternatives, and even surgery outcomes. By engaging patients in decision-making, healthcare practitioners establish trust and reinforce the patient's journey. Surgical operations are usually complex and carry inherent risks; therefore, it is imperative that patients fully understand the implications of their choices. Empirical evidence confirms that when patients are actively engaged, they tend to adhere more closely to treatment suggestions and express greater satisfaction with their treatment. Hence, adhering to surgical procedures according to the standards of patient autonomy is the foundation of modern medicine. Automation and technological advancements in surgery have also created additional issues related to patient autonomy, particularly in robotic surgery and autonomous devices. The application of robotic technology offers several advantages, including precision and efficiency in surgical procedures. These systems, as cited in the literature, can operate with sub-millimeter precision, employ real-time bio signals, and offer computer-guided treatment using a range of imaging modalities (Das et al., 2017). However, the increased use of automated systems raises ethical concerns regarding patient autonomy. Patients must be taught not just about the procedure that they will undergo but also the extent to which automation will be taking care of them. The issue is how to keep patients in command of health decisions, particularly when faced with complex robotic surgeries that may cause them to feel disconnected from the operating procedure. Moreover, contemplation of unique patient groups, like the oncogeriatric population, highlights the complexity of upholding autonomy in surgical interventions. Since the population of older persons in the United States continues to grow, cancer diagnosis among elderly patients is more common, thereby creating a pressing need for personalized surgical care (Lampugnane et al., 2017). While detailed pre-surgery assessments to determine the most suitable interventions are critical, the majority of oncogeriatric patients are not assessed due to insufficient time during clinical practice. This deficiency presents a challenge to geriatricians and surgeons in striking a balance between the intricacies of patient autonomy and the essence of surgical decision-making. Through educational interventions that emphasize the value of geriatric assessment, future clinicians can work towards equipping themselves with the competence required to respect patient autonomy while navigating the complexities of surgical involvement. This approach can ultimately lead to improved outcomes for this patient population, who are at risk, by making patient preferences the center of the surgical planning process.

1.6.3. The Role of Ethics Committees in Surgical Practices

Inclusion of ethics committees in surgical practice is a primary vehicle for upholding patient welfare and guiding clinical decision-making. The function of these committees is to manage extremely complex ethical dilemmas that may arise during the conduct of surgical operations, particularly in cases involving end-of-life care, informed consent, and patient autonomy. Having an ethics committee allows surgical teams the chance to debate challenging instances that might otherwise create ethical dilemmas, encouraging an interdisciplinary forum in which diverse perspectives are weighed. Not only does this enhance quality in surgical care, but it also ensures practice is guided by formalized ethical guidelines and patient-centered values inherent within surgical specialties. Furthermore, ethics committees play a crucial role in the consideration and implementation of new surgical technologies and strategies. By adhering to guidelines like those from France's National

Authority for Health, best care standards must be adopted for evaluating the efficacy and ethical implications of new surgical techniques. By utilizing comparative effectiveness studies, ethics committees can inform surgeons and health care organizations whether it is ethical to implement new technology in practice. This function is crucial not only for the individual outcomes of patients but also for maintaining the integrity of the surgical profession and adhering to evidence-based practices that advance safety and efficacy (Xerri et al., 2009). Additionally, the bioethics mediation process in such committees helps resolve conflicts that arise between healthcare professionals, patients, and their families. By establishing a system of principled resolution, ethics committees create formal channels for resolving disputes that can impede surgical operations or patient decisions. This is important where disagreements of opinion may arise regarding a patient's potential treatments or operations. The principles developed in bioethics provide a platform for gaining consensus, thereby creating a communicative and respectful environment for all parties involved in surgical care. Such a process not only resolves short-term ethical issues but also creates an ethos of ethical behavior that sustains trust in surgery (Dubler et al., 2011).

Test Your Knowledge

1. How is informed consent ethically obtained before a surgical procedure?
2. What ethical principles guide decisions in life-threatening surgical emergencies without patient consent?

SUMMARY

The debate about surgical principles is worthy of emphasizing the overall significance of surgical accuracy and patient safety. As surgical techniques and technology evolve, the well-being of the patient remains paramount. The introduction of minimal invasive methods, for example, proves to be a shift towards practices emphasizing reduced morbidity and faster recovery. Such enhancements not only demonstrate the technical skill of the surgeons but also evidence a dedication to ethical practice. Sticking to the principles of surgery ensures that patient outcomes are optimized, as evidenced by many successful approaches. Additionally, a superior grasp of the principles of surgery is most crucial for effectively managing complex cases that present much complexity. GISTs management is an example where the significance of complete surgical resection with clear margins is highlighted. In this, the surgeon needs to take on a delicate balance between tumor integrity and the integrity of adjacent tissue in an effort to yield long-term results for patients. Oncological surgery principles come into play at this critical juncture, as strict adherence to techniques ensures optimal patient outcomes. This careful navigation of surgical dilemmas is a classic illustration of the necessity for underlying principles to guide all surgical decision-making in the operating room, highlighting the requirement for ongoing re-education and training. Furthermore, surgical techniques must also consider the patient's psychological and aesthetic concerns, particularly those procedures that impact body image. Techniques such as three-dimensional gluteoplasty (3-DGP) exemplify the fusion of surgical skill and artistic expertise, delivering patients with more personalized results tailored to their desires for body enhancement. Empathy with the patient's perspective enhances the practice of surgery, reinforcing the idea that surgery isn't just an expert procedure but a whole practice directed at improving quality of life. As the profession continues to evolve, embracing both the science and art of surgery will be essential in addressing the diverse needs of patients, ultimately encapsulating the practice of surgery: to heal and empower.

In surgery, knowledge of the essential principles that guide practice is paramount in ensuring patient safety and optimal outcomes. A key principle is learning from errors using a systems approach. This approach requires practitioners to own up to mistakes without blaming individual workers ex post facto. Instead, building a Just Culture opens a platform for open discussion of mistakes, allowing for continuous learning and improvement. When such surgical errors occur, the issue at hand should be discussed not just in terms of pointing to a human error, but rather in exploring the intricacies that led to such consequences. Such a system-focused approach not only helps combat the fear of reporting errors but also fosters a safety- and quality-improvement-friendly environment (Bowie et al., 2016). Another critical aspect of surgical principles is the emphasis on detail in ensuring effective communication during transitions of care, particularly during handoff activities. Ineffective handoffs may lead to significant harm, such as retained foreign bodies, which can irreparably harm patients. The use of standardized communication methods, such as handoff safety checklists, has been shown to lead to astounding leaps in the quality of nurse-to-nurse communication in the operating room. Research has shown that the application of these checklists can enhance nurse satisfaction and ensure the accurate transfer of key information from shift to shift (Rowe et al., 2015). Not only does this enhance the effectiveness of operations, but it is also a patient safety mechanism, highlighting the significance of standard practice in the operating environment.

Lastly, unevenness in the conduct of surgery among staff must be understood and addressed accordingly. Surgeons often face innovative challenges and stressful conditions that require adaptability in decision-making and execution. Such fluctuations in performance, while sometimes interpreted in a negative light, may be necessary to accommodate patient-specific needs and effectively address unforeseen complications. Simulation training and courses can be practical in exposing surgical teams to dealing with such dynamic environments without forgoing established protocols and best practices. In the long term, rigorous training, coupled with continuous feedback and a positive culture, fosters flexibility without compromising patient care quality, allowing surgical principles to thrive in complex healthcare systems (Bowie et al., 2016).

KEY TERMS FROM THIS CHAPTER

- Anesthesia principles
- Electrosurgery
- Hemostasis
- Infection control
- Patient safety
- Preoperative care
- Sterilization
- Asepsis
- Fluid and electrolyte balance
- Incision planning
- Minimally invasive surgery
- Postoperative care
- Shock management
- Surgical anatomy

CRITICAL THINKING QUESTIONS

1. **Which of the following is the most effective method to achieve surgical asepsis?**
   a. Wearing gloves only
   b. Using sterile drapes
   c. Proper hand scrubbing and sterile technique
   d. Application of an antiseptic to the surgical site
2. **Which phase of wound healing is characterized by fibroblast proliferation and collagen deposition?**
   a. Inflammatory phase
   b. Maturation phase
   c. Proliferative phase
   d. Hemostasis phase
3. **What is the primary goal of preoperative evaluation?**
   a. To decide the cost of surgery
   b. To select the surgeon
   c. To identify and optimize risk factors
   d. To schedule the operation
4. **Which of the following is NOT a part of the WHO Surgical Safety Checklist?**
   a. Time-out before incision
   b. Confirmation of patient identity
   c. Pre-anesthesia fasting instructions
   d. Counting instruments and sponges
5. **Which surgical wound class is associated with the highest risk of infection?**
   a. Clean
   b. Clean-contaminated
   c. Contaminated
   d. Dirty

Short Answer Questions

1. Define the term "asepsis" and explain its significance in surgical practice.
2. What are the key differences between clean, clean-contaminated, contaminated, and dirty surgical wounds?
3. Describe the physiological response to surgical trauma. What are the implications for perioperative care?
4. List and explain the principles of hemostasis in surgery. Why is meticulous hemostasis essential?
5. Outline the key steps in preoperative assessment and their purpose in surgical planning.
6. Discuss the concept of the "surgical safety checklist." How does it reduce perioperative complications?
7. Explain the principles of wound healing. What factors may impair wound healing in surgical patients?

Answers to Critical Thinking Questions

1. (c); 2. (c); 3. (c); 4. (c); 5. (d)

REFERENCES

1. Wolfe, J. A., Malaisrie, S. C., Farivar, R. S., Khan, J. H., Hargrove, W. C., Moront, M. G., Ryan, W. H., Ailawadi, G., Agnihotri, A. K., Hummel, B. W., Fayers, T. M., Grossi, E. A., Guy, T. S., Lehr, E. J., Mehall, J. R., Murphy, D. A., Rodriguez, E., Salemi, A., Segurola, R. J., . . . Goldman, S. M. (2016b). Minimally Invasive Mitral Valve Surgery II surgical technique and postoperative management. *Innovations Technology and Techniques in Cardiothoracic and Vascular Surgery, 11*(4), 251–259. https://doi.org/10.1097/imi.0000000000000300Aktimur, R. (2021). Enhanced recovery after surgery in bariatric and metabolic surgery. *Annals of Laparoscopic and Endoscopic Surgery, 6*, 48–48. https://doi.org/10.21037/ales-19-254.
2. Alecu, L., Nitipir, C., Slavu, I., Stanculeanu, S., et al. (2019). *Laparoscopic resection of gastric GISTs. Where do we stand now? A single-centered experience.* https://core.ac.uk/download/232440347.pdf (accessed on 12th July 2025).
3. Ball, C. G., Fabian, T. C., Feliciano, D. V., Ivatury, R., et al. (2017). *History of the innovation of damage control for management of trauma patients: 1902–2016.* https://core.ac.uk/download/84402892.pdf (accessed on 12th July 2025).
4. Banner, B., Enrichens, F., Ferla, G., Kahn, A., et al. (1989). *A modified technique of orthotopic transplant of the kidney in rabbits.* https://core.ac.uk/download/12204382.pdf (accessed on 12th July 2025).
5. Bergenholtz, G., Hørsted-Bindslev, P., & Reit, C. (2018). *Textbook of endodontology.* Wiley eBooks. https://doi.org/10.1002/9781394323081.
6. Blugerman, G., D'Angelo, J. A., Habbema, L., Lisborg, M., et al. (2011). *Application of the liposuction techniques and principles in specific body areas and pathologies.* https://core.ac.uk/download/17179833.pdf (accessed on 12th July 2025).
7. Bonica, M., & Students of Health Management 721.01. (2017). *Healthcare management primer.* University of New Hampshire. https://core.ac.uk/download/215509297.pdf (accessed on 12th July 2025).
8. Bowie, P., McNab, D., Morrison, J., Ross, A., et al. (2016). *Understanding and responding when things go wrong: Key principles for primary care educators.* https://core.ac.uk/download/46165173.pdf (accessed on 12th July 2025).
9. Buchbinder, R., Underwood, M., Hartvigsen, J., & Maher, C. G. (2020). The *Lancet* Series call to action to reduce low value care for low back pain: An update. *Pain, 161*, S57–S64. https://doi.org/10.1097/j.pain.0000000000001869.
10. Burton, M. J., Ramke, J., Marques, A. P., Bourne, R., Congdon, N., Jones, I., Ah Tong, B. A. M., et al. (2021). The Lancet Global Health Commission on global eye health: Vision beyond 2020. *The Lancet Global Health, 9*, e489–e551. https://doi.org/10.1016/s2214-109x(20)30488-5.
11. Chen, M. Y., Qi, S. R., & Arshinoff, S. A. (2021). Bilateral simultaneous postoperative endophthalmitis: Review of cases reported over the past 50 years. *Journal of Cataract & Refractive Surgery, 48*, 850–854. https://doi.org/10.1097/j.jcrs.0000000000000875.
12. Dabbagh, H., Koenig, H. G., & Tabriz, A. A. (2016). *Medical ethics in Qiṣāṣ (eye-for-an-eye) punishment: An Islamic view; an examination of acid throwing.* https://core.ac.uk/download/186331225.pdf (accessed on 12th July 2025).

13. Darzi, A., Hettiaratchy, S., Hughes-Hallett, A., Kwasnicki, M., et al. (2016). *Fifty years of innovation in plastic surgery*. https://core.ac.uk/download/77010125.pdf (accessed on 12th July 2025).
14. Das, N., & Yip, M. (2017). *Robot autonomy for surgery*. http://arxiv.org/abs/1707.03080 (accessed on 12th July 2025).
15. Dua, H. S., Singh, N. P., & Said, D. G. (2018). Lamellar keratoplasty techniques. *Indian Journal of Ophthalmology, 66*, 1239–1239. https://doi.org/10.4103/ijo.ijo_95_18.
16. Dubler, N. N. (2011). *A "principled resolution": The fulcrum for bioethics mediation*. https://core.ac.uk/download/62552950.pdf (accessed on 12th July 2025).
17. Dunnington, G., Hockaday, M., Smith, C., Torbeck, L., et al. (2018). *Optimizing the integration of advanced practitioners in a department of surgery: An operational improvement model*. https://core.ac.uk/download/161229732.pdf (accessed on 12th July 2025).
18. Edmonds, A. (2008). *Beauty and health: Anthropological perspectives*. https://core.ac.uk/download/29049646.pdf (accessed on 12th July 2025).
19. Elkins, G., Fisher, W., Johnson, A., Kekecs, Z., et al. (2014). *Hypnosis for acute procedural pain: A critical review*. https://core.ac.uk/download/77011633.pdf (accessed on 12th July 2025).
20. Evans, J. J., Farag, A., Farrell, A., et al. (2018). *Principles of pituitary surgery*. https://core.ac.uk/download/155271643.pdf (accessed on 12th July 2025).
21. Ferko, N., Flener, J., Gargiulo, J., Hogan, K., et al. (2018). *A US hospital budget impact analysis of a skin closure system compared with standard of care in hip and knee arthroplasty*. https://core.ac.uk/download/213444689.pdf (accessed on 12th July 2025).
22. Grant, M. C., Crisafi, C., Alvarez, A., Arora, R. C., Brindle, M. E., Chatterjee, S., Ender, J., et al. (2024). Perioperative care in cardiac surgery: A joint consensus statement by the Enhanced Recovery After Surgery (ERAS) Cardiac Society, ERAS International Society, and The Society of Thoracic Surgeons (STS). *The Annals of Thoracic Surgery, 117*, 669–689. https://doi.org/10.1016/j.athoracsur.2023.12.006.
23. Halvachizadeh, S., Dreifuss, M., Rauer, T., Kaiser, A., Ubmann, D., Pape, H.-C., & Allemann, F. (2025). Does the AO/OTA fracture classification dictate the anesthesia modality for the surgical management of unstable distal radius fractures? A retrospective cohort study in 127 patients managed by general vs. regional anesthesia. *Patient Safety in Surgery, 19*. https://www.semanticscholar.org/paper/46782955c682b9ba7102e37fe9a79a6ee48f208e (accessed on 12th July 2025).
24. Kanoti, G. A. (1974). *Surgical control of behavior*. https://core.ac.uk/download/67761662.pdf (accessed on 12th July 2025).
25. Khafizova, F. A., Sabitova, A. I., Sagetdinov, I. G., & Gabdrafikov, D. R. (2024). Optimization of endodontic dental treatment using modern diagnostic methods in preoperative preparation. *NAUKA MOLODYKH (Eruditio Juvenium)*. https://www.semanticscholar.org/paper/881e81923d98ef67dcab55742d61ea08c8b8ef7f (accessed on 12th July 2025).
26. Kitsiou, A., Caforio, A. L. P., Porta-Sanchez, A., Vahanian, A., Iung, B., Carrera, C., Szymanski, C., et al. (2013). *ESC core curriculum for the general cardiologist (2013)*. https://core.ac.uk/download/55756305.pdf (accessed on 12th July 2025).
27. Kumar, P. H., & Sharma, R. (2020). *A review on contribution of Acharya Sushruta in emergency surgical conditions*. https://core.ac.uk/download/333820259.pdf (accessed on 12th July 2025).

28. Lampugnale, C. A. (2017). *Surgical assessment of the geriatric oncology patient.* https://open.bu.edu/bitstream/2144/26707/5/Lampugnale_bu_0017N_13146.pdf (accessed on 12th July 2025).

29. Lerner, L. B., McVary, K. T., Barry, M. J., Bixler, B. R., Dahm, P., Das, A. K., Gandhi, M. C., et al. (2021). Management of lower urinary tract symptoms attributed to benign prostatic hyperplasia: AUA guideline part II—Surgical evaluation and treatment. *The Journal of Urology, 206*, 818–826. https://doi.org/10.1097/ju.0000000000002184.

30. Lobo, D. N., Han, S., Horstmann, W., Rollins, K. E., Inumerable, R., Trzciński, R., Contractor, U., et al. (2016). *Major abdominal surgery in Jehovah's Witnesses.* https://core.ac.uk/download/156744288.pdf (accessed on 12th July 2025).

31. Lowe, B. (2017). *Slathered, zapped, nipped, and tucked: An ethical analysis of cosmetic dermatology.* https://core.ac.uk/download/129153456.pdf (accessed on 12th July 2025).

32. Modarai, B., Haulon, S., Ainsbury, E., Böckler, D., Vañó-Carruana, E., Dawson, J., Farber, M. A., et al. (2022). Editor's choice – European Society for Vascular Surgery (ESVS) 2023 clinical practice guidelines on radiation safety. *European Journal of Vascular and Endovascular Surgery, 65*, 171–222. https://doi.org/10.1016/j.ejvs.2022.09.005.

33. Panesar, S. S., Cagle, Y., Chander, D., Morey, J., Fernandez-Miranda, J. C., & Kliot, M. (2019). Artificial intelligence and the future of surgical robotics. *Annals of Surgery, 270*, 223–226. https://doi.org/10.1097/sla.0000000000003262.

34. Percie du Sert, N., Ahluwalia, A., Alam, S., Avey, M. T., Baker, M., Browne, W. J., Clark, A., et al. (2020). Reporting animal research: Explanation and elaboration for the ARRIVE guidelines 2.0. *PLoS Biology, 18*, e3000411–e3000411. https://doi.org/10.1371/journal.pbio.3000411.

35. Pfister, D. G., Spencer, S., Adelstein, D. J., Adkins, D. R., Anzai, Y., Brizel, D. M., Bruce, J. Y., et al. (2020). Head and neck cancers, version 2.2020, NCCN clinical practice guidelines in oncology. *Journal of the National Comprehensive Cancer Network, 18*, 873–898. https://doi.org/10.6004/jnccn.2020.0031.

36. Pozek, J.-P. J., Schwenk, E. S., & Viscusi, E. R. (2018). *Managing prolonged pain after surgery: Examining the role of opioids.* https://core.ac.uk/download/213444274.pdf (accessed on 12th July 2025).

37. Qadrie, Z., Maqbool, M., Dar, M., & Qadir, A. (2025). Navigating challenges and maximizing potential: Handling complications and constraints in minimally invasive surgery. *Open Health, 6*. https://www.semanticscholar.org/paper/1a0e933a2131922fa770e51f4ca9d163222e1772 (accessed on 12th July 2025).

38. Rowe, S. T. (2015). *Improve intra-operative nurse-to-nurse communication using a safety checklist.* https://core.ac.uk/download/70419776.pdf (accessed on 12th July 2025).

39. Shetty, P., Bhalerao, S., Vuyyuru, S., Thigale, U., & Tara, D. (2023). Maximizing surgical safety: Approaches to prevent intraoperative complications in manual small incision cataract surgery (MSICS). *Indian Journal of Ophthalmology, 72*, 151–151. https://www.semanticscholar.org/paper/21c8cc5e73ea5f609b97965482d9e102d3c4d559 (accessed on 12th July 2025).

40. Skjold-Ødegaard, B., & Søreide, K. (2020). Competency-based surgical training and entrusted professional activities – Perfect match or a Procrustean bed? *Annals of Surgery, 273*, e173–e175. https://doi.org/10.1097/sla.0000000000004521.

41. Snyder, C. W., Kristiansen, K. O., Jensen, A. R., Sribnick, E. A., Anders, J. F., C. X., E. B., et al. (2023). Defining pediatric trauma center resource utilization: Multidisciplinary consensus-based criteria from the Pediatric Trauma Society. *Journal of Trauma and Acute Care Surgery, 96*, 799–804. https://www.semanticscholar.org/paper/68c6e1f7c7f519e624b5cdc7c760f68cc3a05d2b (accessed on 12th July 2025).

42. Vahanian, A., Beyersdorf, F., Praz, F., Milojevic, M., Baldus, S., Bauersachs, J., Capodanno, D., et al. (2021). 2021 ESC/EACTS guidelines for the management of valvular heart disease. *European Heart Journal, 43*, 561–632. https://doi.org/10.1093/eurheartj/ehab395.

43. Valente, L., Caciolo, F., Antonellis, M., Fiorini, M., Quinzii, M., Regolo, R., Zazzaro, A., et al. (2025). Breast cancer surgery in heart failure patients: Role of loco-regional anesthesia. *European Heart Journal Supplements*. https://www.semanticscholar.org/paper/17ee647ff3879ad0f2cfa69ba741db75644c1c5b (accessed on 12th July 2025).

44. Wang, R., Situ, X., Sun, X., Zhan, J., & Liu, X. (2025). Assessing AI in various elements of enhanced recovery after surgery (ERAS)-guided ankle fracture treatment: A comparative analysis with expert agreement. *Journal of Multidisciplinary Healthcare, 18*, 1629–1638. https://www.semanticscholar.org/paper/3c3a61ea672c3d430c3a48711b8498ef12b1b620 (accessed on 12th July 2025).

45. Williams, C. (2006). *Dilemmas in fetal medicine: Premature application of technology or responding to women's choice?* https://core.ac.uk/download/338116.pdf (accessed on 12th July 2025).

46. Xerri, B., & Rochaix, L. (2009). *National Authority for Health: France*. https://core.ac.uk/download/71353349.pdf (accessed on 12th July 2025).

HEAD AND NECK SURGERY

2

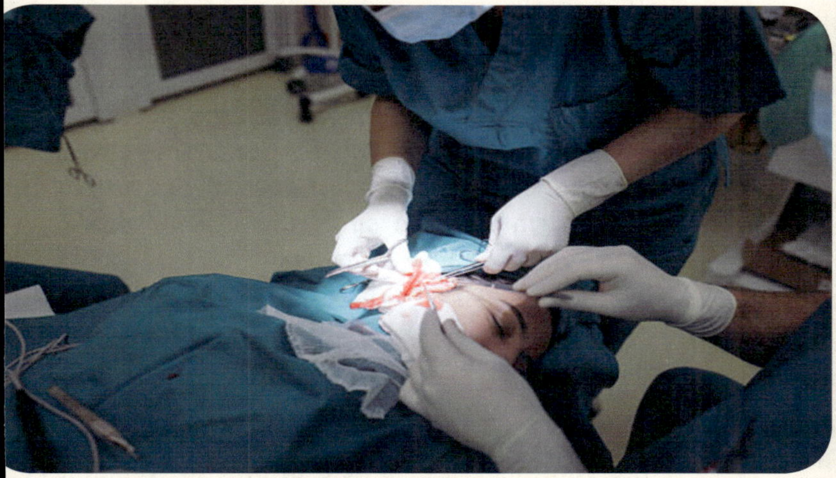

LEARNING OBJECTIVES

After studying this chapter, you will be able to:

1. Understand the anatomy of the head and neck
2. Explain the types of head and neck surgeries
3. Discuss the indications for surgery
4. Focus on surgical techniques for the head and neck
5. Learn about preoperative considerations of head and neck surgeries
6. Evaluate the postoperative care of head and neck surgeries

Introduction

The specialty of head and neck surgery represents a subspecialty within the broad practice of surgery, focusing on the treatment of a diverse group of conditions affecting this anatomically complex area. As the gateway to vital physiological functions such as breathing, swallowing, and speech, surgical attention in this area cannot be overstressed. This subspecialty encompasses the treatment of both benign and malignant diseases, often requiring multidisciplinary approaches that integrate surgical techniques with oncologic principles. The intricate anatomical relationships and functional significance of the head and neck render it essential that surgeons have complete knowledge of both normal anatomy and disease. These abilities are not only necessary for ensuring successful patient outcomes but also for maintaining quality of life that is consistently endangered by disease in this area. In the subspecialty area of head and neck surgery, the integration of new methods and technological advances has radically altered treatment paradigms. For instance, the use of brachytherapy in the management of recurrent head and neck carcinoma (RHNC) has been a landmark development. Thirty studies show that brachytherapy, when used as an adjunct to resection, augments local regional control as well as survival compared to standard re-irradiation methods, indicating its potential for success in curing complex cases (Bar-Ad et al., 2018). Thus, advancements in surgical oncology not only improve therapeutic outcomes but also contribute significantly to the long-term care of once troublesome or intractable conditions. The psychological and cosmetic implications of head and neck conditions, augmented by the ramifications of surgical treatment, are also compounded by the effects of scarring, particularly in the forehead region. Scarring in this region presents special challenges that require specific management protocols.

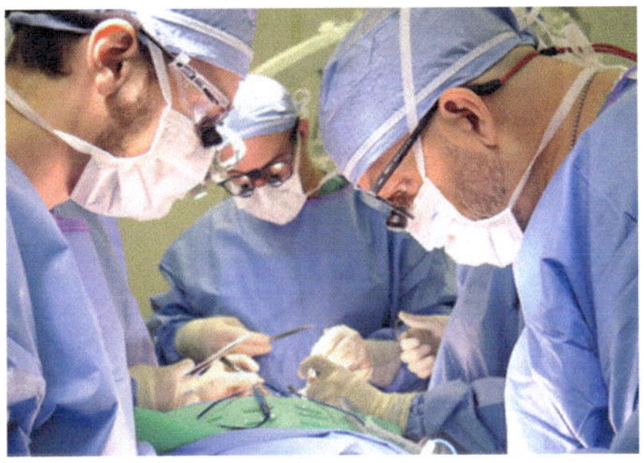

Figure 2.1. Head and neck surgery.

Source: https://static.wixstatic.com/media/690369_2e53ff439a3c4be1a91e318591cfb604~mv2.png/v1/fill/w_616,h_434,al_c,lg_1,q_85,enc_avif,quality_auto/WhatsApp%20Image%202023-10-31%20at%201_44_21%20PM.png.

Resolving such issues is of prime importance not only in surgical terms but also for the preservation of the patient's mental health. Creation of protocols, as the subsite-based treatment algorithm for scalp injuries, demonstrates the value of individualized treatment in ensuring better aesthetic results and practical treatment approaches for scar management (Bryant et al., 2017). Thus, head and neck surgery not only addresses the medical aspect of disease, but it also acknowledges the central role of psychological support and aesthetic concerns in the overall treatment and healing processes (Figure 2.1).

Definition of Head and Neck Surgery

Head and neck surgery is a surgical specialty that encompasses a wide range of surgical procedures for the treatment of conditions affecting the complex anatomical regions of the head and neck. The field of the specialty not only treats diseases such as tumors, infections, and congenital anomalies but also performs reconstructive surgery to restore shape and function. Surgeons in this specialty are taught to perform a broad spectrum of operations, from removing malignancies of the oral cavity and pharynx to reconstructive surgery following resection. With current imaging and surgical methods, head and neck surgeons emphasize patient-centered care by considering both the physiological and aesthetic impact of their interventions. As this field of practice remains dynamic, the use of technology in surgery continues to be fundamental in providing accuracy and improving patient outcomes.

One such evolution of head and neck surgery is the use of preoperative virtual surgical planning, namely, in mandibular defect reconstruction with free bone flaps. By using 3D-printed patient-specific models and cutting guides, surgeons can maximize operating times and reduce surgery-related complications caused by ischemia. Not only does this technique improve complex reconstructions, but it also maximizes surgeons' potential to create more precise anatomical positioning, which is crucial for achieving optimal functional and aesthetic results. The facts supporting 3D-aided surgery all indicate a tendency towards higher-level procedures, while ensuring the utmost standards of patient safety and surgical effectiveness.

These advances reflect the innovative spirit of head and neck surgery coupled with its capacity to adopt state-of-the-art techniques in the quest for optimal patient care (Lasse et al., 2024).

Aside from surgery, preserving the parathyroid glands during thyroid surgery is a crucial concern in head and neck surgery. Accidental injury or devascularization of parathyroid glands leading to hypoparathyroidism results in significant morbidity. Emerging technologies, such as near-infrared autofluorescence (NIRAF), offer promising tools for identifying and protecting the parathyroid gland during operation. By enhancing the visibility of these structures, surgeons can effectively minimize the risk of postoperative complications. With the incorporation of novel technologies into daily practice continuing, increased demand for standardized protocols for testing their efficacy is imminent. The long-term consequences of these technologies on surgical training and patient outcomes need to be investigated in future studies (Karcioglu et al., 2023).

Importance in the Medical Field

The significance of head and neck surgery in the medical field cannot be overstated, particularly since it encompasses a complete spectrum of illnesses relating to important anatomical and functional structures. The complexity of the head and neck region, where vital organs such as the airway, esophagus, and speech and swallowing mechanisms lie, necessitates sophisticated surgical interventions. These surgeries address benign and malignant neoplasms, congenital abnormalities, and trauma, and are aimed at reestablishing function and quality of life in patients. Multidisciplinary treatment needs, which are commonly inherent to these conditions, such as the coordination of otolaryngologists, oncologists, and plastic surgeons, reflect the fine balance of expertise necessary to achieve optimal patient outcomes. Furthermore, technologies employed to enhance surgical techniques, such as minimally invasive surgery and robotic-assisted surgery, have revolutionized the practice of head and neck surgery. Not only do they reduce postoperative morbidity and improve recovery, but they also offer enhanced cosmetic outcomes, a consideration that is particularly important when the fields are socially prominent and highly visible.

The blending of high-tech imaging modalities the potential for accuracy in diagnosis as well as surgical planning, and thus to be able to spare those subtle structures while achieving complete resection of the tumor. This refinement in surgical technique reflects the evolving nature of medical skills, moving towards patient-centered care and improved functional reconstruction in the treated. In addition, conditions like eosinophilic granulomatosis with polyangiitis highlight the role of head and neck surgeons in diagnosing complex diseases that may present with symptoms of a multifaceted nature.

A systematic review of recent literature on the disease indicates that a high proportion of patients present with head and neck manifestations, suggesting the potential for early treatment and diagnosis by otolaryngologists. Thus, consultation with rheumatologists and specialists becomes essential as a majority of these patients are responsive to steroid treatment, while others may require surgery for managing complications effectively (Basnyat et al., 2016). The necessity of an interdisciplinary solution to handle such cases underscores the importance of head and neck surgery within the broader context of medical science, as it not only addresses the problem but also averts the long-term consequences of various health-related issues (N/A, 2001) (Figure 2.2).

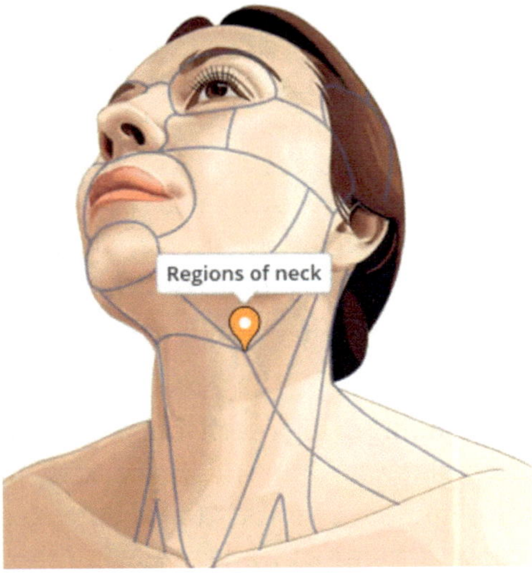

Figure 2.2. Neck region.

Source: https://cdn1.imaios.com/i/imaios-images/web/images/eanatomy/modules/mouth-oral-cavity- illustrations/images/v2/cfbdba9f8ef735323d007db29da37906e083ebbfc9c2bbcc904b79720b9a7860?ar=640:670&bg= FFFFFF&fit=crop&p64= NTcwLDgzMg&t=UmVnaW9ucyBvZiBuZWNr&tx=570&ty=832&w=350&wk=1&s=917226c45e88870760cbd87054361f1e.

Overview of Surgical Procedures

The field of head and neck surgery encompasses a vast array of surgical procedures specifically designed to address both aesthetic and reconstructive issues in this complex anatomical region. Surgical techniques are remarkably varied, ranging from relatively straightforward procedures like excisional biopsies to more advanced operations, such as microvascular reconstruction. The principal surgeries are rhinoplasty, which restores the nose's form to facilitate cosmetic or functional correction, and facelifts, intended to rejuvenate the facial structure by tightening loose tissues. Additionally, provisions are also made for significant reconstructive efforts following resections for skin cancers, where advanced techniques are used to restore function and form. The integration of new technology, such as minimally invasive techniques and advanced imaging capabilities, continues to revolutionize these operations, providing improved patient outcomes and recovery rates as clinicians remain at the forefront of surgical innovation and technique improvement (Barnes et al., 2016). Apart from cosmetic surgery, the operation of RHNC has begun to recognize the importance of multimodality therapy, including the use of brachytherapy. This localized radiation delivery through implanted radioisotopes has shown promise in enhancing oncologic outcomes in combination with surgery. Literature synthesis suggests that brachytherapy, when combined with surgical resection, can result in improved local and regional control, as well as survival outcomes, compared to standard reirradiation modalities such as external beam radiotherapy. The addition of brachytherapy to surgery provides medical professionals with the opportunity to give patients an adjunctive therapy that minimizes complications without sacrificing effectiveness (Bar-Ad et al., 2018). Thus, head and neck surgical procedures are becoming increasingly advanced to incorporate newer approaches that enhance therapeutic results, with a priority on patient safety. Finally, the ongoing evolution of head and neck surgical techniques underscores the dynamic nature of the field, as it is characterized by progressive enhancements in techniques and technology. As an example, the advances in minimally invasive surgical procedures, such as endoscopic surgery, have revolutionized the management of most head and neck illnesses. Not only do these techniques minimize patient trauma, but they also increase recovery rates and shorten hospitalization periods. Moreover, intraoperative navigation technology has enhanced the precision of surgery, allowing more accurate resections and better preservation of essential structures. As the practice evolves, the inclusion of multidisciplinary information across various specialties, such as otolaryngology, plastics, and oncology, further diversifies surgical practices, ultimately resulting in improved patient satisfaction and outcomes through personalized care techniques (Barnes et al., 2016).

2.1. Anatomy of the Head and Neck

Learning Outcome

1. Describe the primary structures of head and neck surgery
2. Focus on the functional significance of head and neck surgery
3. Learn about common pathologies of head and neck surgery

Head and neck anatomy is a complex interplay of structures required for various surgical processes. Minimal awareness of these anatomical components is vital to head and neck surgeons who need to work through this intricate landscape during surgery. Key structures include the skeletal support provided by the skull and cervical vertebrae, which offer protection and support to the brain, as well as essential vascular and neural pathways. Soft tissues, including nerves, blood vessels, and muscles, closely interact with bones to facilitate various functions, such as movement, sensation, and blood supply. Understanding the spatial interaction between these structures minimizes operative complications and optimizes patient outcomes.

With the evolution of surgical techniques comes the requirement for precision in identifying and preserving critical anatomic landmarks, thus emphasizing the importance of detailed anatomical knowledge in head and neck surgery. In addition to standard surgical anatomy, new techniques for training and educating head and neck surgeons have been developed using animal models to complement knowledge gaps. Research has established the porcine model as an outstanding method for replicating human anatomy in surgical training, offering unique insights into the nuances of head and neck anatomy. Through conducting regulated dissections, characteristics such as sternum-chin length, chin-chin length, and prelaryngeal muscle length were measured, resulting in a comprehensive resident manual. The structural similarity between swine and human subjects highlights the effectiveness of the model, enabling residents to gain valuable hands-on experience in acquiring surgical skills. This approach not only enhances the understanding of anatomical relationships but also helps build confidence among residents as they proceed to real-world surgical issues (Alcalá Rueda et al., 2023).

The importance of being aware of the anatomy of the neck and head is also present in the field of dental rehabilitation, particularly in patients that are recovering from head and neck cancer. The way in which radiation therapy interacts with the oral tissues, including damaged anatomy and susceptibility to complications, makes treatment planning for rehabilitation with dental implants more complicated. Literature has shown that implant-supported dentures can also significantly improve the quality of life in such individuals, offering both functional and esthetic benefits. However, there are significant challenges, including the risk of osteoradionecrosis, among others, which necessitate a careful assessment of existing anatomical conditions and the multidimensional risk of implant placement. Therefore, medical practitioners must integrate a conceptual understanding of head and neck anatomy into their practice to customize optimal treatment schedules for rehabilitation without compromising the risks associated with treating irradiated tissues (Chan et al., 2013) (Figure 2.3).

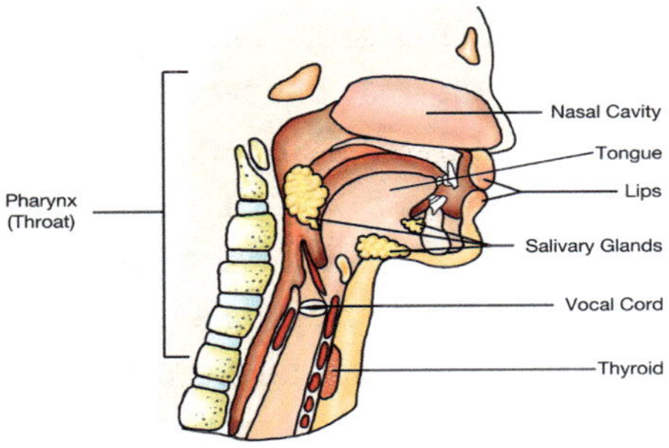

Figure 2.3. Anatomy of the head and neck.

Source: https://www.oncolink.org/var/site/storage/images/media/images/overview-head-and-neck/370947-1-eng-US/overview-head-and-neck.jpg.

2.1.1. Major Structures Involved

In neck and head surgery, knowledge about the major anatomical structures is necessary to deliver successful surgical outcomes. The procedure typically involves a complex interrelationship of multiple tissues, including skin, muscle, vascular systems, and nerves. The complexity of the head and neck region is essentially a result of its compact bundle of significant structures, such as the oral cavity, pharynx, larynx, and their respective vessels and nerves. Knowledge of these structures is essential to enable surgeons to drive through the surgical field effectively without unduly damaging surrounding tissues. Surgeons also utilize advanced imaging modalities to assess these structures preoperatively, ensuring accurate planning and increasing the chances of successful patient outcomes. Such accuracy is not only critical for standard procedures but also for complex oncologic procedures that can involve extensive resections and reconstructions. Involvement of major vascular structures, such as the carotid arteries and prominent veins, is a significant factor in head and neck surgery. Not only are these vessels most critical to oxygenation and nutrition delivery, but they also have a high probability of bleeding on surgical dissection. Anticipation for vascular complication control must be prepared for so that unexpected bleeding results in significant morbidity. Surgeons must also recognize the vascular anatomy, including any possible variation among patients. In recent studies, newer methods, such as intraoperative ultrasound, have been advocated to better identify vessels and aid in surgical navigation. In addition, the novel application of technology, including convolutional neural networks, has potential in predicting surgical outcomes from preoperative factors, thus optimizing planning by verifying clinically sound cohorts from extensive dataset analysis (Culié et al., 2022).

Nerve preservation is another central area of research in head and neck surgery, due to the presence of numerous nerves responsible for critical functions, such as motor control and sensation. Key structures such as the facial nerve and hypoglossal nerve must be identified and preserved during surgery to prevent postoperative complications such as paralysis or dysphagia. Surgeons employ anatomical landmarks and intraoperative nerve monitoring to minimize the risk of nerve injury. Evidence suggests that the use of standardized protocols for nerve identification has led to lower postoperative complication rates, underscoring the importance of education and training in this area (Archer et al., 2021). Continued focus on these critical structures engaged allows for more targeted surgical techniques that aim to maximize patient outcome while minimizing the inevitable risks associated with intricate surgery in this delicate region.

2.1.2. Functional Significance

Head and neck surgery consists of a series of operations that serve basic functional functions, most notably in locations that are essential to communication, eating, and respiration. The functional significance of these operations is best understood by considering the quality of life of the patient. For instance, treatment of head and neck cancers with surgical intervention not only aims to remove cancerous tissues but also tries to preserve significant structures such as the oral cavity and larynx, which are integral to speech and swallowing. Preservation of these functions is essential since derangement may lead to long-term issues, seriously affecting a patient's social as well as emotional life. Thus, a comprehensive surgical approach that focuses on restoring function following surgery remains at the center of head and neck surgical procedures. Once again emphasizing the functional significance, elective revision procedures often address complications of the initial therapy, such as those found in the setting of head and neck cancer. Revision of previous surgeries may offer better oncologic outcomes in addition to restoring the functional capabilities of the areas of interest. For example, studies have found that patients undergoing revision surgery can experience improved overall survival if certain critical variables, including tumor stage and site, are well controlled (Monteiro et al., 2023). Such interventions therefore have the potential to alleviate quality-of-life issues due to persisting symptoms or complications following past surgery. Analyzing the functional outcome following revision surgery is a crucial component in determining patient satisfaction and success in head and neck surgery. Additionally, an understanding of functional significance in head and neck surgery extends beyond strictly anatomical issues; it involves a systemic analysis that considers the psychological and social recovery of the patient. Such surgeons not only need to consider surgical correction but also the impact of these surgeries on daily routines, such as eating, speaking, and social interaction. After all, the successful restoration of functions is closely associated with increased self-esteem and social integration of the patients. Therefore, a multidisciplinary management incorporating speech and swallowing therapy becomes essential in the postoperative period. Generally, an emphasis on functional significance in head and neck surgery highlights the need for ongoing research to delineate a framework that optimizes both oncologic and functional outcomes, since the pervasive impact of such surgical interventions continues (Belluzzi et al., 2019) (Figure 2.4).

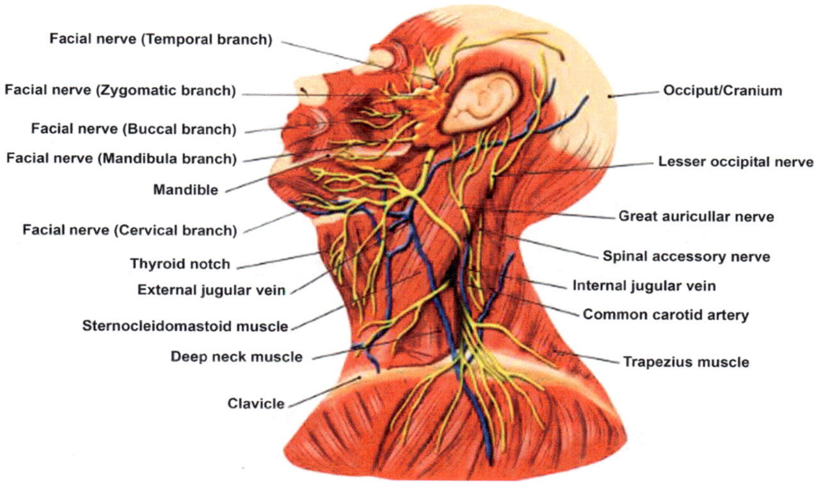

Figure 2.4. Functional significance for head and neck.

Source: https://encrypted-tbn0.gstatic.com/images?q=tbn:ANd9GcTNGbITFsu6TDREuCxk3byrgZvntzDMUf-_-TD1eQQe4-p5LUeX.

2.1.3. Common Pathologies

In head and neck surgery, common pathologies are a broad array of conditions that need precise diagnosis and management. Tinnitus is now one of the most frequent presenting symptoms in patients and is often found in association with other underlying conditions such as auditory nerve damage or ototoxicity. Tinnitus patients are usually severely distressed, with psychiatric comorbidities adding to the complexity of their management. Disturbing as it is, some of these individuals can develop sudden attacks, which take them to emergency rooms for emergency medical attention. The literature indicates that appropriate medical or surgical management is vital for maintaining auditory functions and addressing associated psychological problems. The nature of tinnitus thus requires a systematic diagnostic and therapeutic regimen to minimize the morbidity and mortality of affected individuals (Altissimi et al., 2016). Another frequent pathology in this field is obstructive sleep apnea syndrome (OSAS), which is secondary to various respiratory sleep disorders. OSAS in children is of special significance, with a prevalence of about 2%, most notably among children aged between 2 and 8 years. The disease's pathophysiology has a clear relation with adenoid tissue size in children, along with prevalent pediatric risk factors for upper airway obstruction during sleep. The following complications are significant, impacting not only the quality of sleep but also abnormal growth and development in children. As OSAS is better understood, particularly in the pediatric environment, it becomes increasingly more critical that clinicians adopt a considered approach to the diagnosis and treatment of this condition, which is often quite distinct from adult presentations (Bellini et al., 2019). The overlap of these common pathologies, tinnitus and OSAS, illustrates the intricacies of head and neck surgery. Each illustrates how structural, functional, and psychological forces converging affect patient morbidity and quality of life. Management of tinnitus must be multimodal, addressing both auditory symptoms and associated psychological morbidity, while management of OSAS frequently includes surgery to correct anatomical defects that lead to airway obstruction. Surgeons and clinicians in this field should therefore be vigilant and informed about the evolving diagnostic methods and treatment options available. In this way, they can provide quality care, even amidst the challenges posed by these common yet complicated head and neck diseases (Figure 2.5).

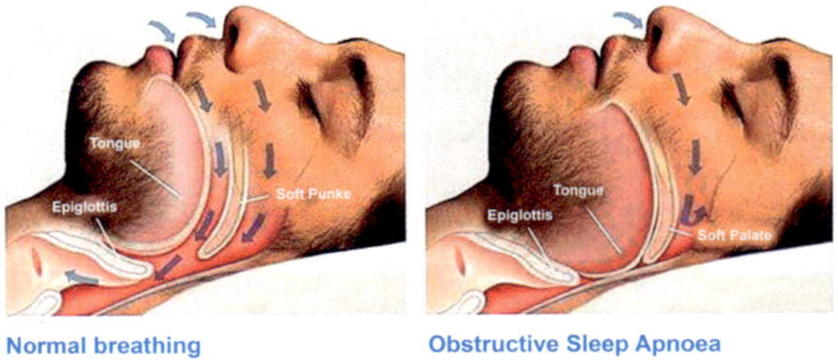

Figure 2.5. Obstructive sleep apnea syndrome (OSAS).

Source: https://www.shalby.org/wp-content/uploads/2017/10/OSAS2-.jpg.

Test Your Knowledge

1. What are the major branches of the external carotid artery?
2. Which cranial nerve is responsible for facial muscle movement?

2.2. Types of Head and Neck Surgeries

Learning Outcome

1. Explain the oncological Surgery
2. Define the reconstructive surgery
3. Discuss the cosmetic surgery

Head and neck surgeries include a wide variety of procedures aimed at treating various conditions, ranging from benign tumefactions to neoplastic tumors. Some of the most common ones are oncological surgeries, whose primary purpose is to excise malignant tumors found in areas such as the oral cavity, pharynx, or larynx. These procedures are highly reliant on precise diagnostic imaging and staging to determine the extent of the malignancy as well as the potential for resection. A case in mind is the management of advanced-stage head and neck cancers that are often considered unresectable due to their aggressive nature. Research has established that even for stage IVb patients, reasonable survival rates can be achieved through surgical treatment, with significantly better mean survival rates than palliative treatment alone, thus necessitating informed decision-making in oncological surgery (Kidwai et al., 2016).

In addition to oncological surgeries, reconstructive surgeries also constitute a significant component of the spectrum of head and neck surgeries. Following tumor resection, patients sometimes require reconstructive techniques to restore anatomical form and function. Flap reconstruction, where tissue is taken from one part of the body to fill defects, thus restoring both functional compromise and psychological well-being, can be encompassed. Emotional distress is vast among head and neck cancer patients following surgery through evidence, and the necessity for incorporating psychological care within treatment regimens. Furthermore, consultations suggest that the response of healthcare providers to emotional cues from patients plays a crucial role in determining their healing process, underscoring the central importance of emotional health in surgical care (Friderichs et al., 2014).

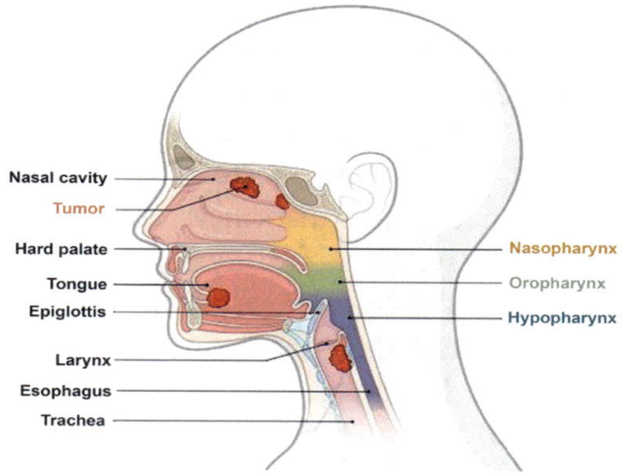

Figure 2.6. Types of head and neck.

Source: https://cdn.prod.website-files.com/621e95f9ac30687a56e4297e/64a8d0e7994b58201f15124d_V2_1611169468660_87faee49-e9c1-4904-885a-28af8205c88e.png.

A second critical area of head and neck surgery is functional treatment of conditions caused by diseases such as sleep apnea and thyroid disease. Procedures like uvulopalatopharyngoplasty (UPPP) are done to decrease obstructive sleep apnea by removing excess tissue in the throat. Likewise, thyroidectomy is done to address thyroid nodules or cancers, with the conservation of hormone levels and voice function often being accomplished upon its laparoscopic execution. Because these procedures are formulated to correct one functional disruption at a time specifically, their success is determined by both the surgical technique employed and the aggregate pre-operative assessment of the patient's health. Thus, meeting aesthetic as well as functional demands renders head and neck surgery a multidimensional field requiring an interdisciplinary approach involving surgeons, oncologists, and psychological support systems (Figure 2.6).

2.2.1. Oncological Surgery

Oncologic surgery within head and neck surgery is at the core of head and neck cancer treatment of this complex area of anatomy. Not only is surgery in this region aimed at excising cancers, but also at preserving critical structures to maintain functional continuity, including the airway, swallowing functions, and cosmesis. Advances in surgical intervention technology have significantly improved survival rates for patients with head and neck cancer (HNC), according to a population-based study using data from the Swedish Head and Neck Cancer Register (SweHNCR). A notable reduction in six-month mortality rates was observed over time. This decline, from 4.7% to 2.5% during the period 2008–2020, highlights the impact of prior interventions and improved therapy protocols, underscoring the crucial role of effective and timely oncological surgery in enhancing patient survival (Talani et al., 2024). The details of oncologic surgery also involve the need for precise preoperative planning and intraoperative precision, particularly in recognizing vital structures that may be damaged during tumor extirpation. Surgeons must have a fine sense of the anatomy of the head and neck to avoid complications such as hypoparathyroidism caused by inadvertent loss of parathyroid glands during thyroid surgery. New imaging technologies, such as near-infrared autofluorescence (NIRAF), appear to aid in the detection and salvage of such glands, thereby decreasing postoperative morbidity. With the use of such technologies during surgical procedures, surgeons of head and neck oncology can maximize salvage protocols, ultimately leading to improved postoperative quality of life for patients (Karcioglu et al., 2023). Furthermore, multidisciplinary treatment of head and neck cancer also imposes the integration of oncologic surgery with other therapies, including radiation and chemotherapy. This is a coordinated approach in managing the multifocal nature of head and neck cancers, where surgical resection alone might be inadequate for maximum disease control. For instance, those who are at higher risk of premature mortality due to extensive disease, as quantified by their WHO performance status, require an intensive treatment regimen that may also consist of neoadjuvant therapies before surgery. A strategy of this kind not only extends survival rates but also imposes the discipline of optimizing surgical care in response to the needs and presentation of individual patients, thus enhancing the efficacy of oncological surgery in this complicated arena (Talani et al., 2024) (Figure 2.7).

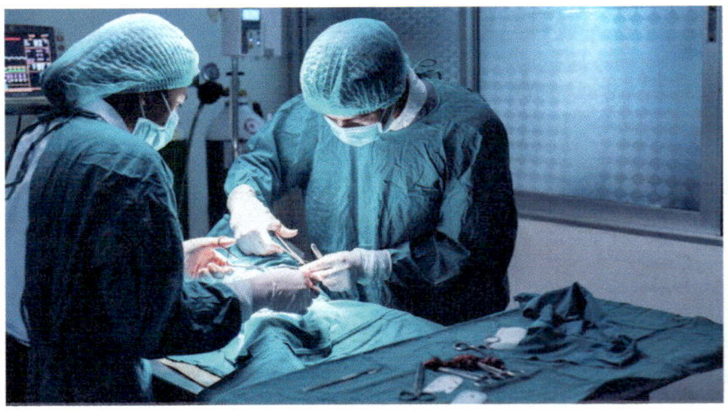

Figure 2.7. Surgical oncology.

Source: https://www.krupamayihospitals.in/wp-content/uploads/2023/06/Onco-Surgery.jpg.

2.2.2. Reconstructive Surgery

Reconstructive surgery in the field of head and neck surgery is an essential leap in patient management, particularly for patients with severe trauma or malignancies. This field focuses significantly on the reestablishment of form and function through novel techniques and materials. Medical rapid prototyping (MRP) models have evolved into a revolutionary method for mandibular reconstruction in cancer patients. Recent studies prove that the preoperative fabrication of reconstruction plates made by computer-aided design and additive manufacturing has displayed superior operative results. Surprisingly, patients treated with such sophisticated MRP-model-based prebent plates exhibit superior mandibular symmetry when compared to those undergoing traditional treatment, ultimately resulting in an enhanced quality of life and self-esteem in the postoperative phase (Koji et al., 2014). Despite the advanced technology and surgical techniques, successful scarring management remains problematic, particularly in the forehead region. The forehead region is a challenging area for reconstruction due to its visibility and functional role in facial expression. It demands a methodical approach to scar management to achieve optimal aesthetic results and reduce patient distress. Recent publications suggest that a stepwise treatment protocol explicitly tailored for forehead injuries can be a factor towards improved patient outcomes. Not only does this make use of best practices in surgical technique, but it also demands patient-specific care, thereby addressing the distinctive requirements of every patient (Bryant et al., 2017). Using these measures in reconstructive strategies maximizes the success of surgical interventions in head and neck surgery. The use of advanced technology in reconstructive surgery reduces the therapeutic process, enabling surgeons to provide precise and personalized treatment. Technologies like CAD/CAM not only enhance surgical planning but also reduce the operation time taken for complex reconstructive operations. Furthermore, the application of these technologies suggests a general trend in modern medicine towards patient-centered care, in which the recovery of function is complemented by a serious attention to aesthetics. With head and neck surgery increasingly being coupled with new materials and techniques, surgical precision and patient needs are the blend that matters. Hence, the future of developing reconstructive surgery promises much to significantly enhance both functional rehabilitation and emotional well-being of patients subjected to the trauma of head and neck pathology (Figure 2.8).

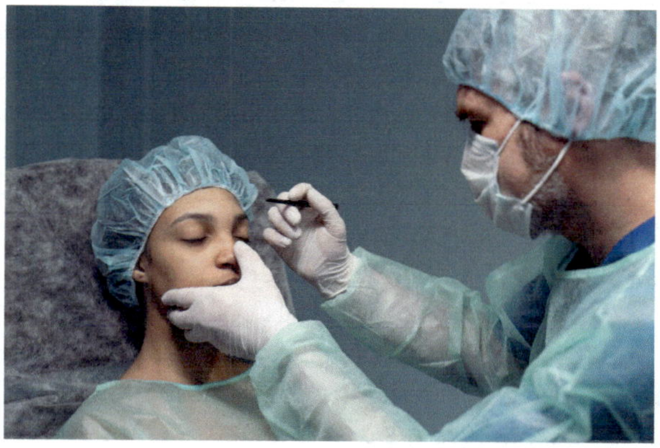

Figure 2.8. Reconstructive surgery within the realm of head and neck surgery.

Source: https://parashospitals-web.s3.ap-south-1.amazonaws.com/blogs/March2024/1711106487Plastic%20Surgery.jpg.

2.2.3. Cosmetic Surgery

The arena for cosmetic surgery within head and neck surgery encompasses a variety of procedures aimed at enhancing aesthetic appearance and optimizing quality of life in patients. Surgical procedures of this nature are often motivated by aesthetic desires rather than medical indications, providing the patient with a vehicle for self-expression and enhancing self-esteem. Rhinoplasty, facelifts, and eyelid surgery are among the most popular procedures, used to redefine or revitalize facial contours. With growing demand for cosmetic surgery, updates on novel surgery methods and developments become worth their weight in gold to professionals operating in this field. The integration of new technology and methodologies significantly enhances the precision and overall outcome of such procedures, ensuring that patient satisfaction takes precedence in the ever-evolving landscape of cosmetic treatment, as outlined in the current volume of literature (N/A, 2021). In recent decades, interest has shifted to the multi-specialty nature of facial plastic surgery, which encompasses the blending of material from various specialties, including otolaryngology and oral maxillofacial surgery. This collaboration not only enhances the qualifications of surgeons but also addresses a broader range of patient issues, as it offers comprehensive treatment plans that incorporate both reconstructive and cosmetic objectives. The advancements in cosmetic techniques, such as minimally invasive surgery and the use of injectable materials like BOTOX Cosmetic, reflect a shift toward less invasive procedures and more natural, subtle results. As discussed in Barnes et al. (2016), the field's dynamism is demonstrated through ongoing research and development, further molding the future of cosmetic and reconstructive surgery in the head and neck area. The role of cosmetic surgery in the context of head and neck surgery transcends physical appearance; it is a transformation of existence, as it affects how individuals perceive themselves and their place within society. In addition to the physical transformation, psychological benefits are also realized through these procedures, including enhanced self-esteem and improved social relationships. Surgeons need to be not only technically proficient but also well-grounded in understanding patient motivations and expectations. This psychological component is generally addressed through extensive consultations before surgery, leaving patients with realistic expectations and enabling them to make well-informed decisions about their aesthetic procedure. With improvements in the specialty, the requirement to balance aesthetic needs with ethical expectations remains of the highest concern, necessitating cautious practices and reiterating the need for an integrated ethos in patient treatment in cosmetic surgery, as discussed further in N/A (2021).

Test Your Knowledge

1. What is the primary indication for a radical neck dissection?
2. Which type of surgery is commonly performed for obstructive sleep apnea in the oropharynx?

2.3. Indications for Surgery

Learning Outcome

1. Explain the tumor removal
2. Define the trauma repair
3. Describe the congenital anomalies

The role of surgery in head and neck surgery is complex, considering several clinical presentations and etiologies. One of the most common indications for surgery is the occurrence of neoplastic processes, most importantly cancers of the oropharynx, larynx, and thyroid. Surgical procedures like transoral robotic surgery (TORS) have been highlighted for their effectiveness in treating tumors of these areas. For instance, TORS for cT1-T2 oropharyngeal cancers is an operation commonly performed by head and neck surgeons, offering improved exposure intraoperatively and potentially better postoperative outcomes compared to conventional operations. These advancements underscore the importance of evaluating the role of surgical intervention as a crucial component in the treatment of malignancies in the head and neck region, thereby providing patients with the opportunity for an improved quality of life after treatment (Allison et al., 2024).

Aside from oncologic purposes, surgery also addresses functional dysfunction from other conditions. In otolaryngology, chronic rhinosinusitis with polyposis has emerged as a disease where surgery significantly improves a patient's quality of life. Endoscopic sinus surgery is then usually the preferred treatment when medical treatment is unsuccessful and nasal polyps play a role in continued symptoms. Clinical evidence suggests that perioperative systemic corticosteroids may be beneficial in this scenario to reduce postoperative edema and accelerate healing. This highlights the role of surgery in alleviating chronic symptoms, which can have a profound impact on daily life and overall well-being. Therefore, surgery may prove to be a viable option worth considering in chronic otolaryngologic disorders (Allison et al., 2024).

For pediatric patients, in addition to oncological and functional diseases, surgical intervention is also required for the management of obstructive sleep apnea (OSA). Aforementioned situations, such as adenoid hypertrophy and tonsillar enlargement, lead to significant airway obstruction, which necessitates surgical procedures like adenotonsillectomy. Prevalence of sleep-related breathing disorders necessitates early surgical treatment to prevent long-term morbidity from health issues, which involve cardiovascular anomalies and developmental delay. Moreover, the increasing realization of surgical procedures, such as TORS for the management of sleep apnea through base of tongue resection, indicates the dynamic character of surgical indications in head and neck surgery. This is a shift from the traditional application of surgery as an ultima ratio to the application of surgery as an active agent in the treatment of intricate health issues in diverse patient populations (Lechien et al., 2024) (Figure 2.9).

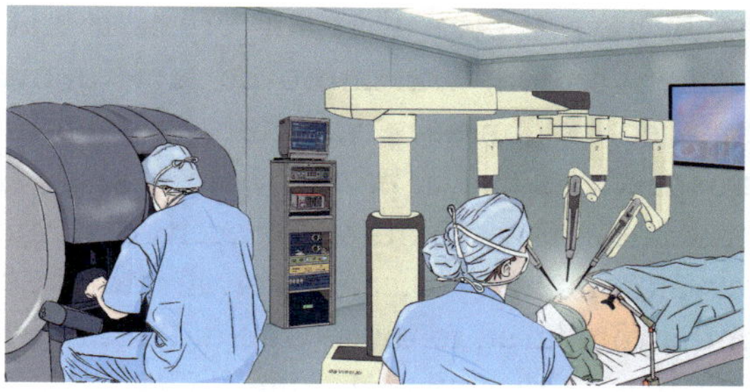

Figure 2.9. Transoral robotic surgery.

Source: https://www.entuk.org/_userfiles/pages/images/conditions/transoral_robotic_surgery_torsupdated.jpg.

2.3.1. Tumor Removal

Surgical resection of head and neck neoplasms is an essential component of treatment regimens for malignant lesion control. Tumor resection typically involves meticulous surgical debridement of the involved tissues to achieve clear margins and minimize the risk of recurrence. In high-stage lesions, where tumors extensively invade locally, the ease of complete resection is significantly heightened. Furthermore, the subtle topographic anatomy of the neck and head necessitates oncologic effectiveness balanced against functional preservation, prompting the need for innovative approaches, such as organ-preserving techniques. For instance, studies have shown that certain adjunct therapies, such as hyperthermia combined with brachytherapy, may favorably enhance outcomes in well-chosen patients following tumor excision. These multimodal strategies emphasize the evolving extent of head and neck surgery as practitioners strive to optimize survival and quality-of-life metrics after treatment (Bar-Ad et al., 2016).

Added to the degree of complexity in the treatment of head and neck cancer is the tumor staging, particularly those staged as IVb, commonly labeled as unresectable due to their virulent presentation. Such tumors are of particular challenge not only in surgical outcomes but also in overall patient prognosis.

Studies have proven that surgery is a viable treatment option, with improved survival rates compared to non-surgical interventions. In a retrospective survival pattern among stage IVb tumor patients, patients who received surgical interventions had a mean survival rate of 29.5 months compared to those who did not receive surgical intervention, with a mere 20.83 months (Kidwai et al., 2016). This evidence indicates the potential for surgery as part of multimodal treatment plans regardless of the impression of unresectability for advanced-stage head and neck cancers.

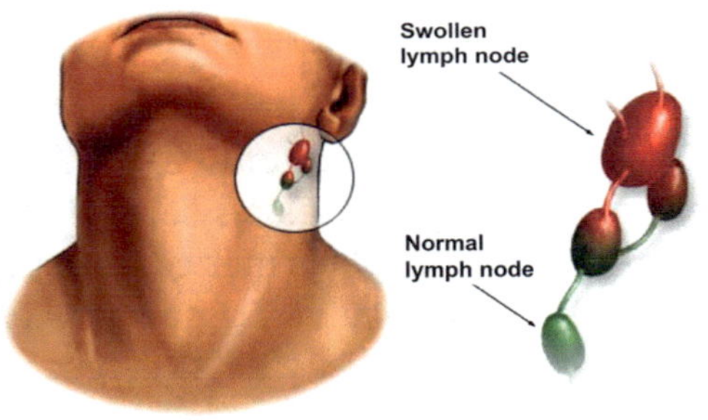

Figure 2.10. Tumor removal.

Source: https://www.cvsurgicalgroup.com/wp-content/uploads/2016/01/lymph-node.jpg.

New surgical techniques and supportive treatments are on the horizon, which serve to improve methods for tumor removal. For instance, the integration of high-dose-rate (HDR) brachytherapy and brachytherapy implants can optimize targeting of radiation with minimal collateral damage to surrounding normal tissues. This technique not only permits precise dosing but also provides a promising approach to augment local disease control, as well as to enhance surgical resection. Furthermore, exploration of hyperthermia technologies in combination with surgical techniques has gained momentum, providing a promising new front in head and neck oncology. By applying thermal enhancement in the operating bed, adjuvant treatments would be much improved in effectiveness, with accompanying improvements in long-term results and survival rates among patients undergoing complex tumor excisions (Bar-Ad et al., 2016). Collectively, these technologies represent a paradigm shift in head and neck tumor management, where the intersection of surgical skill and new therapies leads to improved patient care (Figure 2.10).

2.3.2. Trauma Repair

Trauma reconstruction in head and neck surgery presents unique challenges that are specific to certain techniques and methods. The facial tissues' intricate anatomy and function require close attention to detail during reconstruction. Management of scars is a critical consideration following traumatic injuries, particularly those of the forehead and surrounding regions. Effective trauma repair involves the application of a methodical approach, as outlined in the literature, emphasizing the need for individualized treatment algorithms based on the singular characteristics of the injury. The integration of current best practices, as demonstrated in Bryant et al. (2017), enables surgeons to navigate the complexities associated with traumatic injuries in this delicate area, ultimately leading to increased patient satisfaction and improved outcomes following surgery. The second significant feature of trauma repair is the use of appropriate reconstructive modalities that take into account both soft tissue and aesthetic considerations. For head and neck surgery, traumatic wounds create extensive defects that predispose to severe functional impairments as well as psychosocial morbidity in patients. Exposure of deeper structures, for instance, necessitates complex coverage solutions, which also indicates the need for reconstructive modalities, such as free flap procedures. The challenge is further amplified when dealing with extensive wounds that require reconstructive measures, such as in the case of Achilles tendon injuries, where reconstructive modalities, such as the anterolateral thigh (ALT) flap, are involved. This method is not only intended to safeguard the integrity of the area but also to sustain mobility, as discussed in Chou et al. (2013), which highlights the importance of using the correct method based on the characteristics of the injury and patient needs. The psychological impact of facial trauma also needs consideration while rehabilitating. Head and neck injury patients can develop severe emotional trauma as a result of an alteration in function and appearance. Trauma repair is thus not only the physical reconstruction, but an overall strategy of patient care, including psychological intervention alongside surgical management. Involvement of multidisciplinary teams comprising psychologists and social workers can significantly enhance recovery. By creating a supportive environment, caregivers can buffer the psychological effects typically associated with trauma, so that functional and aesthetic needs are more integrated into the treatment plan. Ultimately, effective restoration of trauma in head and neck surgery depends on an embracing understanding of these complementary components, so that patients can recover at their best through the healing of traumatic experiences.

2.3.3. Congenital Anomalies

Congenital head and neck malformations consist of a wide range of developmental defects that are encountered at birth or arise subsequently in life. Such defects most often result from disruptions during the initial stage of embryonic development, with a particular fondness for those structures derived from branchial arches. The most frequent pediatric head and neck tumors among these malformations are branchial cleft cysts. Their diagnosis is primarily based on a proper understanding of the embryological processes and a careful evaluation of clinical presentations. Such cystic masses can be mistaken for other conditions and require the cautious use of imaging modalities, such as computed tomography and magnetic resonance imaging, to make the correct diagnosis. Lastly, proper diagnosis and treatment are critical, since operative removal remains the cornerstone treatment for effectively addressing these congenital defects (N/A, 2018). Going beyond their physical manifestations, congenital anomalies have broader consequences, influencing surgical results and management plans for patients in head and neck surgery. Interestingly, patients with craniofacial deformities have considerable complications, with significantly higher rates of postoperative complications, most notably infections. A study on the Nationwide Inpatient Sample confirmed that these patients also had a rate of infectious complications at 7.4%, a stark contrast to 0.6% in the absence of these abnormalities. Further, the economic burdens of surgical interventions for individuals with craniofacial abnormalities are significant, with their average hospital costs totaling $139,317 compared to $56,189 for their peers. Thus, the surgical complexity of congenital anomalies necessitates a multidisciplinary approach for optimal surgical management and minimizing associated risks (Allareddy et al., 2018).

Moreover, long-term consequences of congenital anomalies in the head and neck region highlight the urgent necessity of early intervention and later management. Early diagnosis and operative correction can significantly improve functional and cosmetic outcomes, thereby optimizing the quality of life for individuals involved. Close follow-up is essential, as patients may experience recurring problems or develop other diseases, necessitating further surgical and therapeutic interventions. Due to the severity of these anomalies, interdisciplinary treatment involving otolaryngologists, surgeons, and orthodontists is necessary. It enables a unified treatment plan tailored to the specific needs of each patient, ultimately leading to improved health outcomes and enhanced social integration. The nuanced intersection of clinical skill and patient-centered care underscores the challenges and achievements of treating congenital anomalies in head and neck surgery (Figure 2.11).

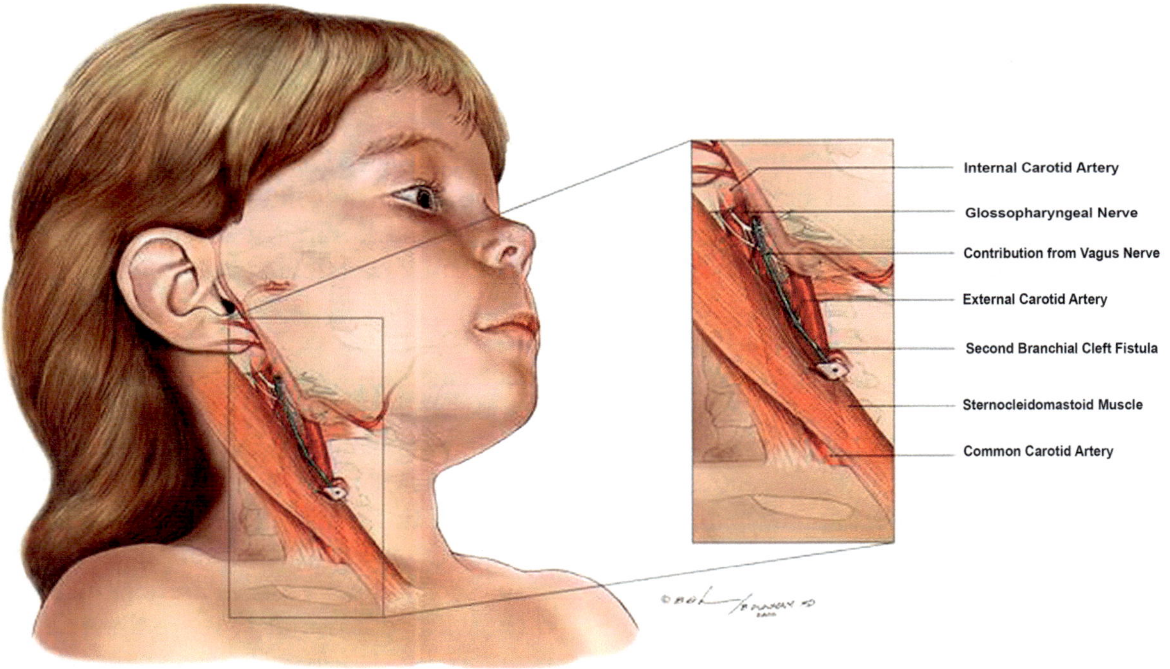

Figure 2.11. Congenital malformations of the neck.

Source: https://entokey.com/wp-content/uploads/2017/03/A190217_1_En_8_Fig5_HTML.gif.

Test Your Knowledge

1. What clinical signs indicate the need for emergency abdominal surgery?
2. When is surgical intervention preferred over conservative management in gallstone disease?

2.4. Surgical Techniques

Learning Outcome

1. Describe the open surgery in the head and neck
2. Define the endoscopic surgery in the head and neck
3. Discuss the robotic-assisted surgery in the head and neck

In head and neck surgery, the choice of surgical approach is paramount to achieving the best patient outcomes. Advances in minimally invasive surgery, such as robotic-assisted surgery, have significantly enhanced recovery time and postoperative complication rates. The techniques provide precision within sensitive structures, avoiding trauma to surrounding tissues and preserving function to the fullest extent. For instance, these approaches can be particularly valuable in OSCC patients, when standard methods would require aggressive resections that severely compromise function and aesthetics. Furthermore, the shift toward more effective recovery strategies following surgery emphasizes the importance of implementing these new techniques, underscoring the need for regular training and surgical team adjustments to deliver the highest quality care for head and neck surgery patients. Complete assessment and planning play a crucial role in the efficient utilization of surgical strategies in head and neck surgery. A multidisciplinary group of oncologists, radiologists, and reconstructive surgeons is invaluable in offering personalized surgical planning, considering the complexity of head and neck anatomy. Accurate tumor localization and assessment of vital structures are facilitated by the application of advanced imaging modalities such as CT and MRI scans, which inform the surgical plan. Particularly, one must be cautious when planning intervention, considering the impact of radiotherapy on tissue healing and integrity. This is particularly true in the patient with a history of head and neck carcinoma who is susceptible to osteoradionecrosis. These are fine points that, if understood, guarantee that surgical plans are tailored to the patient's own physiological and pathological parameters, with resultant improvement in outcomes and reduction of morbidity. Apart from technical choice and meticulous preoperative planning, postoperative management is also an essential part of the overall success of surgical treatments of head and neck surgery. The postoperative course of recovery after surgery typically presents formidable challenges like pain management, nutritional rehabilitation, and monitoring for potential complications. The impact of such interventions on function and quality of life calls for an aggressive rehabilitative plan. For instance, OSCC resection patients can exhibit significantly altered swallowing habits and taste abilities, which greatly impact the quality of their lives. In line with a more recent focus, new approaches, such as saliva liquid biopsy, demonstrate novel paradigms for managing oral cancer patients. These procedures not only facilitate early diagnosis and prognostic evaluation but are also less invasive, representing a potential opportunity for monitoring postoperative disease progression (Campisi et al., 2019). Hence, integrating these sophisticated components into the operation is vital to enhance recovery and promote overall patient care in head and neck surgery.

2.4.1. Open Surgery

Open surgery remains a fundamental technique employed in head and neck surgery, particularly for conditions that necessitate broad exposure and dissection of anatomical structures. The operation is typically requested in the presence of complex pathologies, such as thyroid malignant neoplasms or ectatic lesions requiring extensive resections. While less minimally invasive than some other techniques, open surgery provides surgeons with unimpaired vision and tactile sensations, which perhaps better fit fine performances in sensitive procedures. The broad exposure gained with open techniques is significant when addressing issues with critical structures like nerves and blood vessels. In addition, surgeons can utilize newer adjuncts, such as intraoperative imaging and neuromonitoring, which can potentially radically improve patient outcomes. In spite of advances in minimally invasive alternatives, the safety and efficacy of open techniques ensure they are an irreplaceable part of the head and neck surgical armamentarium. Likewise, in open head and neck surgery, the choice of anesthetic management is also crucial. The inherent issues of the surgical field, including anatomic distortion and risk of airway compromise, necessitate a tailored anesthetic approach. Appropriate airway management is at the core of patient safety, particularly concerning intraoperative airway obstruction, bleeding, and operative contamination. Techniques such as cuffed tracheal tubes, supplemented by other modalities like jet ventilation or laryngeal masks, are employed to ensure stable airway management during these procedures. Airway plans between the anesthetic and surgical team should be clearly communicated preoperatively. This collaborative approach not only optimizes patient outcomes but also prepares the group for unforeseen complications that may arise in the intricate and often complicated settings of head and neck surgery (Abdul-Rahman et al., 2020).

Even though open surgery has benefits, more discussion is ongoing about its competition with robotic-assisted techniques in thyroid surgery. While robotic procedures have demonstrated several advantages, including enhanced visualization and precision, they typically accompany increased operative time. Open surgery remains, nonetheless, unreplaceable due to its established safety and its ability to cope with diverse surgical challenges, especially in complex cancer. Moreover, the cosmetic and functional outcomes associated with open methods, particularly regarding recovery times and postoperative quality of life, should not be underestimated. As both surgical modalities continue to develop, it is increasingly vital that the practitioner can discern the proper indications for application of each technique. Ultimately, the integration of robotic technology into the surgical field may complement traditional open approaches with a more individualized approach to patient care for much head and neck pathology (정웅윤, 2013) (Figure 2.12).

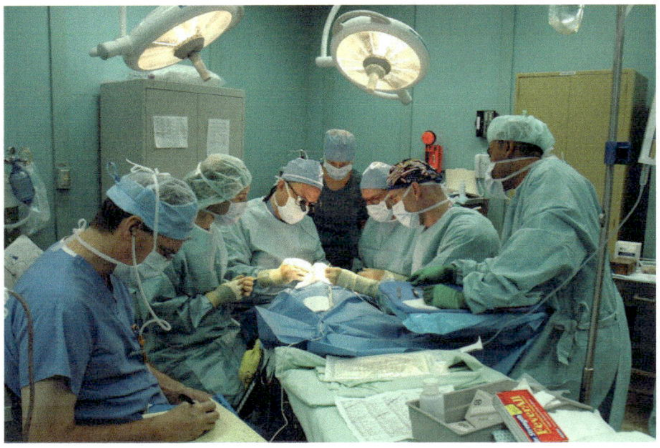

Figure 2.12. Open surgery in head and neck surgery.

Source: https://www.acmehospital.com/asset/img/PageHeader_img/head-neck.jpg.

2.4.2. Endoscopic Surgery

Endoscopic surgery has revolutionized the management of head and neck operations by offering a choice of minimal invasiveness, unlike traditional open surgical procedures. With the help of high-resolution imaging modalities, such as endosonography, it becomes feasible for surgeons to visualize the fine anatomy of the upper airway —namely, the oral cavity, pharynx, and larynx —in excellent detail. Technological advances in probe technology over the past few years have provided greater imaging resolution, which raises the potential for diagnosing several conditions affecting the salivary glands and other head and neck anatomy. This evolution is essential as it becomes possible to detect conditions earlier and with better surgical therapy and significant improvement in patient outcomes. The integration of all these technologies not only makes surgical operations easier but also reduces recovery times, allowing patients to resume their normal lives more quickly and efficiently. Furthermore, endoscopic procedures used in oncology, particularly in head and neck cancers, have shown considerable promise. For instance, endoscopic endolaryngeal ultrasound is crucial in diagnosing small tumors of the larynx and ascertaining the extent of cancer invasion, a significant aspect in planning proper management. Another example is carcinoma of the oral tongue, where surgical planning includes thorough tests on tumor invasiveness; endosonography has been very helpful. It provides an accurate assessment, which allows surgical excisions to be more precise, hence reducing recurrence. In addition, the method has demonstrated outstanding effectiveness in identifying small tumors in challenging cases, such as HPV-positive oropharyngeal carcinomas, thereby further solidifying the role of endoscopic surgery in maximizing oncologic management within the head and neck practice (Brandt et al., 2024).

The beneficial outcomes associated with endoscopic techniques underscore their effectiveness in treating head and neck carcinomas. Research has established that early diagnosis using minimally invasive techniques, such as narrow-band imaging and magnifying endoscopy, is associated with improved treatment outcomes and survival rates. In one such study on superficial head and neck carcinoma (SHNC), patient outcomes following endoscopic resection were very encouraging, with the five-year disease-specific survival rate being 100% (Okabe et al., 2022). Predictor variables such as tumor thickness, lymphatic invasion, and vessel classification by narrow-band imaging were significant predictors of risk for cervical lymph node metastasis and therefore had an impact on surgical planning. With the ongoing advancement of endoscopic surgery, its translation into clinical practice has the potential to enhance diagnostic yield and therapeutic effect in head and neck surgery (Figure 2.13).

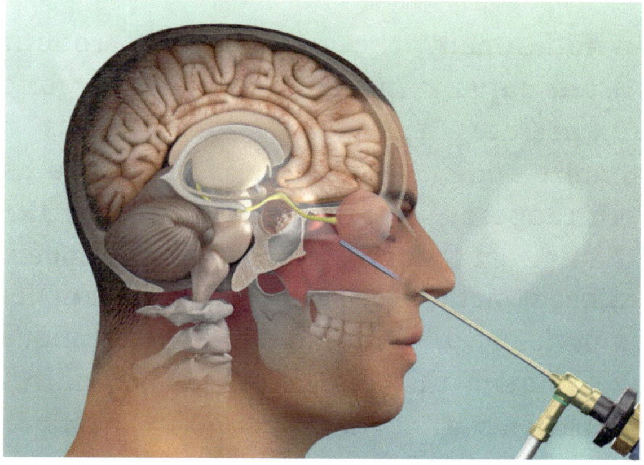

Figure 2.13. Endoscopic endonasal surgery.

Source: https://www.pacificneuroscienceinstitute.org/pituitary-disorders/wp-content/uploads/sites/3/2020/02/14-190_SAINT-JOHNS-KEYHOLE-SURGERY_ENDONASAL-Adenoma1.jpg.

2.4.3. Robotic-Assisted Surgery

Robotic-assisted surgery has revolutionized head and neck surgery, enabling surgeons to achieve greater precision and control over complex procedures. The advanced technique utilizes a robotic system that provides a three-dimensional visualization of the field, enabling precise dissection and enhanced visualization of critical anatomy. Thus, surgeons may perform intricate maneuvers with greater delicacy than is possible with traditional methods, particularly in limited spaces prevalent in head and neck surgery. The emergence of robotic technology is increasingly founded on clinical data that attest to the fact that such advancements yield better patient outcomes, for example, reduced blood loss, less postoperative pain, and shorter recovery times. Interestingly, otolaryngology robotics represents a watershed moment in the direction of increasingly minimally invasive surgical interventions, instilling a culture that prioritizes patient safety and comfort at all costs, thereby revolutionizing treatment regimes in the most complex cases (Ferraz et al., 2012).

Additionally, the application of robotic-assisted surgery in head and neck surgeries demonstrates the ability of robotics to minimize complications. For instance, the use of intraoperative nerve stimulation (IONS) technology in robotic thyroidectomy has been a significant method for preserving vocal function. Comparisons of nerve stimulation techniques have shown the effectiveness of indirect stimulation via the vagus nerve, with reduced recurrent laryngeal nerve (RLN) damage for patients following surgery (Lang et al., 2011). Through real-time monitoring of nerve integrity, surgeons can proactively act during dissection and thereby avoid worse postoperative vocal cord function. This not only impacts postoperative quality of life but also provides evidence of an increasing need to incorporate advanced technological solutions into surgical work for patient protection. Briefly, robotic surgery represents a paradigm shift in head and neck surgical procedures characterized by its ability to boost operating precision, improve patient outcomes, and reduce complications. Ongoing research and the application of technology, such as IONS, further indicate the potential of these methods, necessitating further research into their cross-sectional integration into various fields of surgery. As the profession evolves, professionals must stay current with new technology through ongoing exposure to emerging technologies and by adopting advanced patient treatment techniques. Combining robotics with traditional surgical techniques enables improved therapeutic means through creating a future-driven course of head and neck surgery consistent with advancements in medical technology and patient-centered models of healthcare (Ferraz et al., 2012).

Test Your Knowledge

1. What are the key steps in performing a tracheostomy?
2. How is the facial nerve preserved during parotid gland surgery?

2.5. Preoperative Considerations

Learning Outcome

1. Describe the patient evaluation of head and neck surgery
2. Define the imaging and diagnostics of the head and neck
3. Discuss the risk assessment of head and neck surgery

Preoperative factors in the pre-surgery preparation for head and neck surgery are very crucial to ensure maximum results in surgery. Their evaluation begins with a thorough history and physical examination. They enable the detection of risk factors, such as other accompanying medical conditions that may complicate surgery or anesthesia. For example, patients with severe comorbidities such as cardiovascular or respiratory disorders need careful observation and intervention, if necessary, before surgery. The surgical team must develop individualized plans based on each patient's profile, considering the unique patient's particular needs and health condition. Preoperative imaging examinations and laboratory tests also guide the type of surgery and operation, allowing for the recognition of any anatomical variations that may impact the procedure. This thoughtful process of assessment is standard practice in developing a comprehensive treatment plan to optimize patient safety and perioperative outcomes. Another critical consideration during the preoperative phase is modifiable risk factor management. For patients undergoing surgery for head and neck cancer, optimal nutrition is of the highest priority because it directly influences recovery and healing of wounds. Early nutritional intervention can help mitigate risks related to malnutrition, which may lead to postoperative complications. Additionally, the cessation of tobacco and alcohol consumption before surgery has been shown to decrease complications significantly, shorten healing time, and improve surgery outcomes in general. The Society for Head and Neck Anesthesia emphasizes the importance of these lifestyle modifications in its consensus statements, which strongly encourage clinicians to take collective responsibility for educating patients on adopting health-protective behaviors before surgery (Le et al., 2024). The presence of well-educated and supported patients on such modifications further encourages a multidisciplinary style of care in the preoperative setting. Furthermore, the specific surgical procedure in question also has its own preoperative planning issues, namely anesthesia and airway management. For the head and neck procedures with high tumor burden, careful preplanning of airway access is essential because patients may present anatomical challenges to routine intubation techniques. Techniques such as awake fiberoptic intubation or tracheostomy may be indicated in complex cases to ensure patient safety during anesthesia induction. Additionally, the integration of point-of-care ultrasound has transformed preoperative practice for head and neck surgeons by allowing direct real-time assessment of tumor characteristics and planning of incisions (Harleen et al., 2024). This new imaging technique not only enhances the accuracy of surgical procedures but also enables the creation of individualized treatment plans tailored to the unique anatomical situation of each patient. In this manner, careful attention to these variables in the preoperative stage is essential in reducing complications and maximizing successful outcomes in head and neck surgery.

2.5.1. Patient Evaluation

A comprehensive assessment of the patient is at the heart of head and neck surgery practice, as it informs treatment and optimizes postoperative recovery. Evaluation typically begins with a thorough assessment of the physical and psychosocial factors that influence the patient. Head and neck cancers are multifaceted and necessitate an ideal appreciation of the demands of every individual patient, for instance, how the disease impacts speech and swallowing functions. Studies of recent literature reveal that a lack of systematic rehabilitation programs, combined with inadequate multidisciplinary organization, can lower the success rate of surgical procedures. By recognizing the value of comprehensive examinations and addressing systemic issues, healthcare providers can develop more personalized treatment programs with better functional outcomes and a higher quality of life for patients after glossectomy and other head and neck surgeries (McMillan et al., 2025).

One potential area for optimizing patient evaluation in this discipline is the incorporation of advancements in machine learning. The models utilize varying data modalities to predict post-treatment complications such as dysphagia and dysphonia and offer clinicians valuable information that aids treatment planning. According to studies, machine learning algorithms can provide standardized measures of swallowing function and voice, which are significant in determining head and neck cancer patients. As such, technological innovations keep increasing; they can not only facilitate improved patient examinations but also help in early screening for diseases such as laryngeal cancer. The challenge remains in providing valid and generalizable machine learning findings; thus, the suggestion of large data sets and clinical trials for their effective implementation (Srinivasan et al., 2023). In addition to technological advancements, the integration of interprofessional personnel in patient evaluation significantly enhances the management of conditions resulting from head and neck surgery. Interdisciplinary practice among surgeons, restorative dentists, and speech pathologists is crucial in designing and developing effective intraoral prostheses that facilitate speech and swallowing rehabilitation. The Prosthetic Rehabilitation for Speech and Swallowing (PReSS) model demonstrates how a systematic approach can methodically meet patient needs through assessment, prosthetic development, and the functional incorporation of these devices into the natural course of daily life. By tapping into interdisciplinary knowledge, healthcare professionals can better maximize recovery pathways, thereby ensuring increased patient involvement and satisfaction during the rehabilitation process. This collaborative platform promotes a comprehensive approach to patient care, ensuring that personal obstacles are not only identified but also addressed effectively (McMillan et al., 2025) (Figure 2.14).

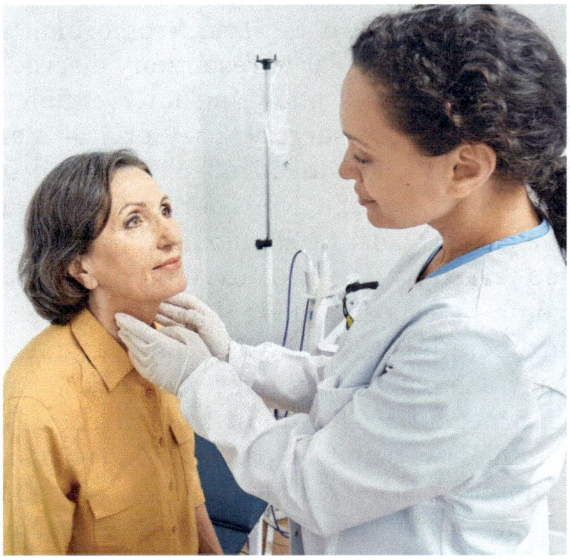

Figure 2.14. Patient evaluation in head and neck surgery.

Source: https://www.datocms-assets.com/113066/1641411686-head-and-neck-cancer-evaluation-and-surgery.jpg?auto=format,compress&w=1340.

2.5.2. Imaging and Diagnostics

In head and neck surgery, imaging and diagnostics play a pivotal role in the treatment and care of disorders of this anatomically delicate region. New imaging devices, such as optical coherence tomography (OCT), offer non-surgical modalities that enhance the visualization of tissue microanatomy. Based on near-infrared light, OCT creates high-resolution cross-sectional images that enable clinicians and surgeons to differentiate between abnormal changes and standard tissue architecture. The capability to measure multiple layers of tissue, such as the keratin cell layer and epithelial structures, enables the early detection and prompt intervention of oral pathology, which is crucial for improving patient outcomes. Current studies highlight the effectiveness of OCT in differentiating between non-malignant and malignant lesions, which validates its use as a valuable diagnostic adjunct for head and neck surgical procedures (Al-Delayme et al., 2012). In addition, the value of advanced imaging modalities extends beyond OCT with the development of new diagnostic technologies that are cost-effective and efficient. Such innovations, typically founded on tissue biochemical and physical changes, aim to detect malignancy before clinical onset. Optical methods complement each other to provide real-time tissue assessment and instantaneous feedback to clinicians regarding tissue health. The evolving world of imaging and diagnostics is underscored by recent collaborations in interdisciplinary platforms, as indicated by flagship conferences such as the Third Scientific Meeting of the Head and Neck Optical Diagnostics Society. Such partnerships promote a comprehensive understanding of optical diagnostics and their multiple applications, which bodes well for a promising future of *in situ* and real-time diagnostic potential in head and neck surgery (Amelink et al., 2011). With the latest imaging technologies, the translation of such systems to the practice of medicine becomes a viable prospect. The broad applicability of techniques like OCT not only enhances diagnostic data but also influences surgical planning and postoperative care. Moreover, the evolution of diagnostic algorithms derived from imaging findings continues to improve the identification of pathological processes of oral tissues. The challenge is to enhance the resolution of such technologies to provide accurate cellular and subcellular information, which is crucial for grading dysplastic lesions with precision. Clinical trials and ongoing research are necessary to determine the efficacy of these imaging modalities, ensuring they meet the stringent standards in surgical oncology and enabling enhanced patient management strategies in head and neck surgery (Al-Delayme et al., 2012) (Figure 2.15).

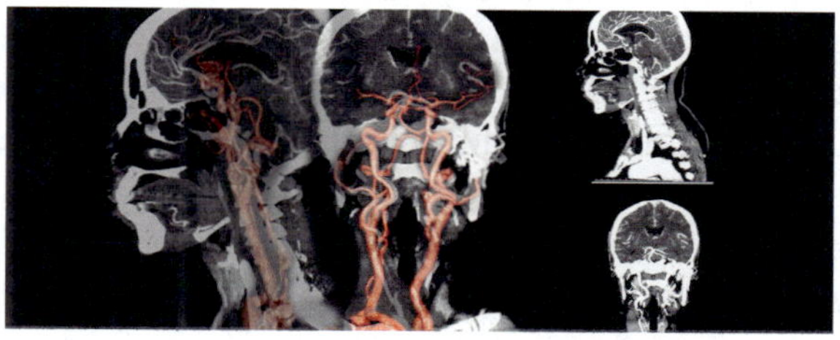

Figure 2.15. Imaging and Diagnostics in head and neck surgery.

Source: https://www.ucsfhealth.org/-/media/project/ucsf/ucsf-health/medical-tests/hero/ct-angiography-head-and-neck-2x.jpg?rev=ed81b8d16414455aa0286673bfa185c8.

2.5.3. Risk Assessment

Effective risk assessment is crucial in head and neck surgery, particularly due to the anatomical complexities of the region. The complexity of operations within the region necessitates knowledge of both physical and biological factors that have the potential to impact patient outcomes. A thorough preoperative evaluation, including assessment of frailty and comorbid conditions, is crucial for predicting complications. Frailty has been recognized through current studies as a valuable predictor of adverse postoperative outcomes and thus should be included in the risk assessment process. The integration of frailty assessment into clinical assessment can provide useful information to surgical teams to improve decision-making and refine patient management algorithms in head and neck oncology (Carvalho et al., 2021). A comprehensive identification of risk factors not only maximizes preoperative planning but also assists in tailoring postoperative care protocols for improved overall patient safety and outcomes. Furthermore, the association of specific surgical methods with patient comorbidities complicates risk evaluation in head and neck surgery. Individualized surgical techniques require consideration of specific health profiles that include existing conditions or potential impacts on healing and recovery, such as vascular disease or endocrine disorders. Evaluation of such factors is significant in predicting postoperative complications, including infection and prolonged recovery periods. Recent literature shows that patients with increased frailty scores experience complications and mortality after head and neck surgery at a greater rate. These findings underscore the importance of employing a multifaceted risk assessment methodology that integrates objective clinical data and subjective clinical judgment to inform surgical treatment and postoperative care (Belluzzi et al., 2019). By resolving these intricacies in an organized manner, health care providers can enhance the validity of their risk estimates and, consequently, the results of surgery. In addition to frailty and comorbidities, the socioeconomic situation of patients undergoing head and neck surgery must also be considered during risk assessments. Patient access to healthcare resources, patient support systems, and patient education can have a significant impact on both preoperative and postoperative cases. Being aware of the socioeconomic status allows surgical teams to avoid potential obstructions to recovery, such as transportation issues or breakdowns in follow-up care. It has been shown that a global approach with the incorporation of social determinants in the risk assessment process increases patient participation and compliance. Thus, incorporating variables such as social support and socioeconomic status strengthens the rationale for an expansive risk assessment. This approach not only prepares surgical teams for the upcoming challenges in the operating room but also aids long-term success of treatment outcomes, ultimately improving the quality of care provided to patients in head and neck surgery (Carvalho et al., 2021).

Test Your Knowledge

1. What imaging studies are essential before planning head and neck tumor surgery?
2. How does airway assessment influence the anesthetic plan in head and neck procedures?

2.6. Postoperative Care

Learning Outcome

1. Describe the recovery process for head and neck surgery
2. Define the complications and management for head and neck surgery
3. Identify the follow-up protocols for head and neck

Postoperative care is a critical component of the recovery process following head and neck surgery. Not only does it cover pain management and complications, but it also promotes good communication among patients and healthcare workers. Ineffective communication can lead to confusion regarding postoperative expectations, potential complications, and aftercare measures. Research has shown that inadequate patient education and consent processes are responsible for significant shares of malpractice suits in operating rooms, particularly for conditions like vestibular schwannomas. Actually, 44% of malpractice claims against doctors are a result of complications after surgery, which highlights the need for improved communication and documentation procedures by healthcare teams (Abouzari et al., 2019). Through attention to these factors, medical professionals can control risks, ensuring that patients are thoroughly educated and in a position to participate in their recovery process actively. Another critical aspect of head and neck surgery postoperative management relates to nutritional care. These patients typically experience transient or chronic dysphagia and oral intake impairment secondary to swelling, pain, or functional impairment. The utilization of tailored nutritional strategies is key in promoting recovery and preventing malnutrition during this vulnerable period. For instance, the utilization of enteral feeding methods may prove critical for patients with limited ability to restore oral intake. In addition, evidence-based evaluation following surgery can identify patients at risk for complications, for example, implant loss, particularly among those undergoing ablative therapy for oral cancer (Agresti et al., 2015). These evaluations are to be followed by frequent observations of dietary intake to ensure that all patients' nutritional needs are being met and that they are recovering. Emotional and psychological counseling also make up an essential aspect of postoperative care for head and neck surgical patients.

The extent of surgical involvement in this region does tend to affect patients' self-esteem and induce a lot of psychological trauma. Healthcare providers should be sensitive to these emotional challenges and offer mental health support resources. The provision of counseling services and peer support groups can do much to address the psychosocial dynamics of recovery. Greater physician sensitivity to these areas can result in a more holistic treatment approach, leading to improved overall outcomes. In addition, recognizing and addressing the emotional consequences of a patient's condition are likely to ensure better compliance with postoperative care instructions, thereby facilitating an easier recovery process (Figure 2.16).

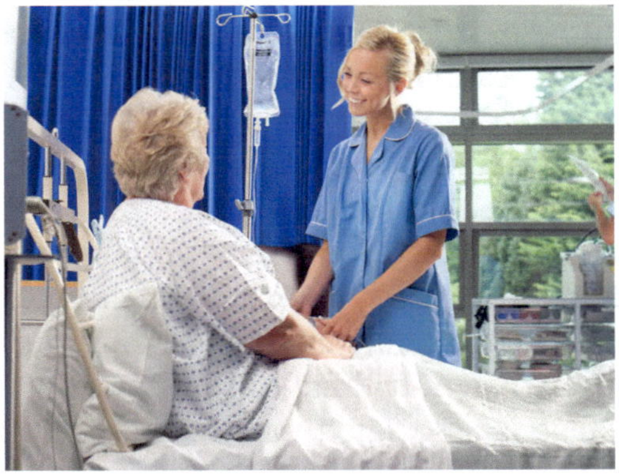

Figure 2.16. Postoperative care.

Source: https://media.post.rvohealth.io/wp-content/uploads/2020/08/postoperative-care_thumb.jpg.

2.6.1. Recovery Process

The recovery process of head and neck surgery is a complex process of physical, psychological, and nutritional rehabilitation. Patients experience significant discomfort and swelling at the surgical site during the early phases. This necessitates optimal pain management measures and monitoring for potential complications such as infection and hematoma. In conjunction with physical recovery, patients may experience difficulty with changes in their speech or swallowing capabilities, making involvement in speech and language therapy a crucial component of their healing process. These therapies aim to restore functionality and improve the quality of life, fostering a sense of satisfaction and alleviating concerns about communication difficulties. As these areas become entwined, medical professionals typically prioritize a patient-directed framework, allowing for customized interventions that target unique needs throughout this pivotal time of recovery. Nutritional support is a crucial component during the healing process in head and neck surgery. Given that surgical interventions may involve swallowing obstruction or taste disturbances, dietary adjustments are necessary. Soft and high-calorie diets are usually recommended by the nutritionist to trigger recovery and ensure adequate caloric intake. Therapeutic fluid inclusion is also likely to simplify swallowing while maintaining hydration status, which has a role in healing. With patient progression, gradual food reintroduction occurs in most cases, often at the request of speech therapists in order to assess safety upon ingestion. Evidence suggests that nutritional optimization during this stage is associated with increased healing and a shorter hospital stay, further supporting the case for a targeted approach to nutrition in recovery from head and neck surgery (Copeland et al., 2018). Psychosocial problems are a significant part of the recovery process following head and neck surgery because patients are likely to face not only physical but also psychological and emotional adjustments. Anxiety about the possible modifications that may occur to their appearance following surgery is expected to induce shyness and isolation, impacting the mental well-being of the patient. Multidisciplinary support systems, including those of social workers, psychologists, and peer support groups, become integral parts of the recovery process to overcome such problems. Opening lines of communication and providing facilities for mental health care encourage patients to voice their anxieties and fears. These interventions ultimately develop resilience and create a therapeutic setting, demonstrating that holistic recovery extends far beyond physical rehabilitation (N/A, 1989). The interplay of these conflicting factors underscores the necessity for an integrated rehabilitation strategy in head and neck surgery to treat all facets of a patient's condition.

2.6.2. Complications and Management

Management of complications after head and neck surgery is a multifaceted problem with a strong influence on patient outcomes. A significant concern is the risk of flap hypoperfusion during microvascular reconstructive surgery, particularly with free flaps. Anesthetic management in such surgeries should be optimal, as recent evidence suggests that inadequate control of hemodynamic variables can lead to severe adverse events related to flap viability. The systematic review conducted within the past seven years highlights the need for a multidisciplinary approach to enhance recovery pathways, thereby reducing the likelihood of complications. In addition, the use of standardized intraoperative anesthetic management would decrease the occurrence of critical events, such as flap failure, underscoring the need for ongoing discussion among surgical teams regarding best practices in hemodynamic monitoring during such complex operations (GM et al., 2018). Dysphagia is another frequent complication developing in patients treated for head and neck cancers. It is an illness generally resulting from a surgical operation like laryngectomy or pharyngectomy and subsequent radiation therapy, and can severely handicap a patient's lifestyle. Treatment is typically in the form of esophageal dilation to overcome hypopharyngeal stenosis, but this too is not entirely risk-free. There can be complications of esophageal perforation and mediastinitis, which shows the fine line on which these patients are being treated. Surprisingly, in some cases, these patients could have cervical spine osteomyelitis as a late complication of the dilation of the esophagus. These events contribute significantly to the clinical presentation, and follow-up with caution and a thorough understanding of the patient's surgical history is necessary to establish effective management and rule out the likelihood of severe complications (Cognetti et al., 2014).

As head and neck surgery advances, so should the techniques for managing complications. Identification of the complexities of various operations emphasizes the necessity of taking particular precautions to minimize risks. Improved recovery pathways, which integrate preoperative, intraoperative, and postoperative care, have been recognized as vital tools for optimizing overall outcomes. Optimization of hydration and nutrition before operation may enable enhanced healing patterns. In contrast, new monitoring techniques during operation, such as utilization of the Hypotension Probability Indicator, may enhance intraoperative stability. Lastly, an engaged style of complication management, firmly grounded in interaction among experts, education, and adherence to evidence-based standards, is crucial in facilitating patient recovery and the long-term success of head and neck surgeries (GM et al., 2018) (Figure 2.17).

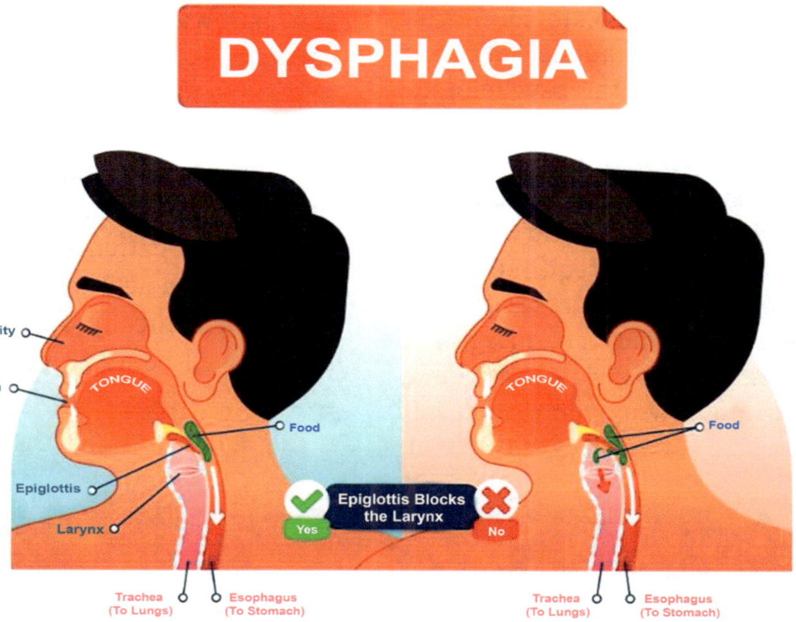

Figure 2.17. Cervical disc disease and difficulty swallowing cervicogenic dysphagia.

Source: https://www.caringmedical.com/wp-content/uploads/2022/12/cervicogenic-dysphagia-1024x774.jpg.

2.6.3. Follow-Up Protocols

In head and neck surgical practice, there is a need to establish robust follow-up systems that ensure optimal patient outcomes. After surgical interventions, patients are likely to have a range of complications that make close observation necessary. Follow-up visits provide an opportunity to assess healing, identify early signs of recurrence, and evaluate postoperative complications. Furthermore, such protocols have undergone significant transformations in response to challenges such as the COVID-19 pandemic, necessitating modifications to follow-up practices to promote patient and healthcare worker safety. These changes can include reduced face-to-face contact and increased telemedicine consultations, with improved continuity of care at a lower risk of exposure. As noted, enforcing such protocols is essential not only in the observation of patients during unprecedented circumstances, but also in solidifying the vitality of healthcare systems in handling follow-ups in a surgical context (Cascone et al., 2020). In addition to monitoring the surgical site and complications, follow-up protocols must also address the psychological aspects of patients undergoing head and neck surgery. Most patients possess a unique set of emotional and psychological issues following surgery, particularly when aesthetic outcomes are involved. The commitment required during the follow-up visit involves addressing these psychological aspects, as they are integral to the recovery process. Psychosocial support may play a crucial role in follow-up compliance and patient satisfaction. Thus, it is essential for healthcare providers to incorporate discussions on emotional well-being, lifestyle modifications, and care services into the follow-up visit process. The combined approach provides a caring atmosphere of trust, hence facilitating improved recovery outcomes among patients undergoing the intricacies of head and neck procedures (Chinn et al., 2020).

Finally, the effective implementation of follow-up protocols also relies on effective communication among multi-disciplinary teams. Effective interaction among surgeons, nurses, nutritionists, and mental health professionals enhances the quality of perioperative care, allowing for the consideration of all elements of a patient's overall health. Ongoing team meetings to discuss progress and evolving patient needs can enable timely interventions and tailored follow-up protocols. Furthermore, the inclusion of patient feedback in these meetings can lead to more patient-centered care pathways that address particular patient concerns. As health systems continue to develop protocols in response to shifting challenges, such as those faced during the COVID-19 pandemic, maintaining a patient-centered focus will be paramount. Maintaining this focus on cooperative, patient-centered care will ensure that head and neck surgery follow-up protocols are both clinically appropriate and improve overall well-being and healing (Cascone et al., 2020).

Test Your Knowledge

1. What are the signs of hematoma formation after neck surgery?
2. How is airway patency monitored in the immediate postoperative period?

SUMMARY

The specialty of head and neck surgery encompasses a range of complex challenges with significant implications for patient outcome and quality of life. The intricacies of the treatments themselves, and those of anatomical structure reconstruction in particular, require an in-depth knowledge of many risk factors. As noted in the literature, various risk factors contribute to unfavorable outcomes, such as surgical site infections and flap loss, highlighting the need for surgeons to remain vigilant in detecting and managing risks efficiently (Tsai et al., 2025). With advancements in surgical techniques and postoperative treatment protocols, patient management and outcomes can be optimized, with a special focus on continually improving surgical interventions. Moreover, integration of palliative care as part of head and neck surgery highlights the patient-centered focus during treatment planning. Implementation of palliative treatments, even in cases where curative treatment would be restricted, has been shown to increase survival and overall quality of life for the patients (Townsley et al., 2024). Such an approach requires the actions of multi-disciplinary teams composed of surgeons, oncologists, and palliative care specialists, who, in conjunction, ensure that therapeutic decisions are made based on the preferences and requirements of the patients. Such collaboration not only encourages holistic patient care but also forms an environment where subtle planning can be undertaken to address the multifaceted aspects of head and neck diseases. Regarding the dynamism of head and neck surgery, ongoing research and innovation are of utmost significance. Combining evidence from institutional reports and meta-analyses allows strengthening the knowledge regarding the effectiveness of operations and their resulting complications (Tsai et al., 2025). Although definitive conclusions may be elusive, the cumulative evidence serves as a basis for establishing future protocols. Progress in the field is centered on the implementation of adaptive practices that have a focus on patient safety and satisfaction. Ultimately, continued discovery in both the surgical and palliative realms will continue to reiterate the critical truth that head and neck surgery should be not only a technically focused discipline but a caring field as well, one that strives to optimize patient outcomes and experiences.

Within head and neck surgery, understanding the relationship between procedural risk and outcome is paramount. A systematic study has begun to quantify the adverse effects of surgery, in this case, among sensitive patient populations such as pregnant women. A recent survey of non-obstetric surgery during pregnancy highlighted that such surgery, while sometimes unavoidable, is not without risks. Specifically, the findings indicated that non-obstetric surgery had an association with adverse birth outcomes, although the absolute risk remained low. This advanced consciousness enables clinicians to navigate the complexities of surgical selection by weighing the advantages and disadvantages of potential complications, thereby facilitating enhanced patient counseling and informed consent processes (Aylin et al., 2016).

One key step towards maximizing patient care for head and neck surgery is to consider novel models of care. There was evidence from a systematic review about nurse-managed cancer survivorship programs, which showed their capacity to improve patient-reported outcomes for cancer survivors, including head and neck cancer survivors. Among various studies, the participants who received nurse-managed care had improved cognitive and social functioning. These findings point to a pathway for enhancing post-treatment quality of life, which is crucial given the protracted recovery issues that are typically associated with head and neck surgery patients. Implementation of such support care models has the potential to mitigate some of the side effects traditionally associated with surgical interventions (Berg et al., 2019). Moreover, the evolving era of head and neck surgery demands the ongoing evaluation of technological integration with patient management modalities. With the advancement of surgical techniques, the need for post-operative care is further established. The risks that have been identified in studies, like increased risks of preterm delivery in association with surgical procedures in pregnancy, highlight the greatest need for proper follow-up care uniquely created for the distinct needs of these patients. Furthermore, the advantages of the survivorship programs by nurses can impact a broad variety of post-operative recovery in several surgical procedures. As research continues to advance, patient-centered outcomes will be a key factor in the direction of future practice in head and neck surgery to ensure a proportionate approach that emphasizes both the effectiveness of surgery as well as quality of life (Aylin et al., 2016; Berg et al., 2019).

KEY TERMS FROM THIS CHAPTER

- Airway management
- Cranial nerve injury
- Facial nerve preservation
- Laryngectomy
- Neck dissection
- Parotidectomy
- Reconstructive flap surgery
- Cervical lymph nodes
- Endoscopic sinus surgery
- Head and neck cancers
- Microlaryngoscopy
- Oropharyngeal carcinoma
- Pharyngectomy
- Salivary gland tumors

CRITICAL THINKING QUESTIONS

1. **Which nerve is most commonly injured during thyroidectomy?**
   a. Vagus nerve
   b. Hypoglossal nerve
   c. Recurrent laryngeal nerve
   d. Glossopharyngeal nerve
2. **Which of the following is the most reliable initial diagnostic tool for a solitary thyroid nodule?**
   a. CT scan
   b. Thyroid scintigraphy
   c. MRI
   d. Fine needle aspiration cytology (FNAC)
3. **The most common histological type of salivary gland tumor is:**
   a. Warthin's tumor
   b. Mucoepidermoid carcinoma
   c. Adenoid cystic carcinoma
   d. Pleomorphic adenoma
4. **Which of the following symptoms is most suggestive of a malignant laryngeal tumor?**
   a. Recurrent sore throat
   b. Hoarseness lasting more than 3 weeks
   c. Postnasal drip
   d. Episodic ear pain
5. **A 55-year-old male with a painless, slowly growing mass in the parotid region likely has:**
   a. Parotid cyst
   b. Acute sialadenitis
   c. Pleomorphic adenoma
   d. Lymph node metastasis

Short Answer Questions

1. What are the typical clinical signs of a malignant thyroid nodule?
2. Describe the classification and staging system used for head and neck squamous cell carcinoma.
3. Explain the indications and potential complications of neck dissection.
4. What are the anatomical boundaries of the anterior and posterior triangles of the neck?
5. Discuss the evaluation and management of a patient presenting with hoarseness lasting more than two weeks.
6. What is the role of fine needle aspiration cytology (FNAC) in the diagnosis of head and neck masses?
7. Compare and contrast the surgical approaches for parotid gland tumors.
8. What are the possible causes and surgical treatments of obstructive sleep apnea in the context of head and neck surgery?
9. Explain the significance of perineural invasion in head and neck cancers.
10. Describe the basic principles of airway management in patients with upper airway obstruction due to head and neck pathology.

Answers to Critical Thinking Questions

1. (c); 2. (d); 3. (d); 4. (b); 5. (c)

REFERENCES

1. Khan, M. J., Tageldin, T., Farooqi, M. W., Khamash, O. Q., Shahid, U., Abdul-Rahman, M. E., Elarref, M., & Hassan, J. (2020). Principles of anesthesia and airway management in head and neck surgery. In *IntechOpen eBooks*. https://doi.org/10.5772/intechopen.95029Abouzari, M., Birkenbeuel, J., Cheung, D., Djalilian, H., et al. (2019). *Medical malpractice of vestibular schwannoma: A 40-year review of the United States legal databases*. https://core.ac.uk/download/305124340.pdf (accessed on 12th July 2025).

2. Agresti, A., Garg, A., Korfage, A., Barber, A. J., Polimeni, A., Misch, C. E., Misch, C. E., et al. (2015). *Survival of dental implants in patients with oral cancer treated by surgery and radiotherapy: A retrospective study*. https://core.ac.uk/download/54520092.pdf (accessed on 12th July 2025).

3. Alcalá Rueda, I., Bogoya Castaño, A., Cenjor Español, C., Sánchez Barrueco, A., et al. (2023). *Everything but the squeal: A guide for head and neck surgery training on the live porcine model*. https://core.ac.uk/download/648147647.pdf (accessed on 12th July 2025).

4. Al-Delayme, R., Hamdoon, Z., Hopper, C., Jay, A., et al. (2012). *Structural validation of oral mucosal tissue using optical coherence tomography*. https://core.ac.uk/download/16220461.pdf (accessed on 12th July 2025).

5. Allareddy, V., Fletcher, S., Metalwala, Z., Okunseri, C., et al. (2018). *Orthognathic surgical outcomes in patients with and without craniofacial anomalies*. https://core.ac.uk/download/213086834.pdf (accessed on 12th July 2025).

6. Altissimi, G., Cianfrone, G., Ciofalo, A., Greco, A., et al. (2016). *When alarm bells ring: Emergency tinnitus*. https://core.ac.uk/download/54538689.pdf (accessed on 12th July 2025).

7. Amelink, A., Amelink, A., Brunsting, A., Gillenwater, A., Sharwani, A., Sharwani, A., El-Naggar, A. K., et al. (2011). *The future of medical diagnostics: Review paper*. https://core.ac.uk/download/1899260.pdf (accessed on 12th July 2025).

8. Archer, N., Zebic, L., Turton, N., Higginson, J., Idle, M., Praveen, P., Martin, T., et al. (2021). An evaluation of the clinical utility of C-reactive protein and antibiotic use in patients undergoing major head and neck reconstructive surgery with outcome assessment. *Oral and Maxillofacial Surgery, 26*, 455–461. https://www.semanticscholar.org/paper/99d6b754d9f3c7610840ae37a2ae373abcb39852 (accessed on 12th July 2025).

9. Aylin, P., Balinskaite, V., Bennett, P., Bottle, A., et al. (2016). *Estimating the risk of adverse birth outcomes in pregnant women undergoing non-obstetric surgery using routinely collected NHS data: An observational study*. https://core.ac.uk/download/77021205.pdf (accessed on 12th July 2025).

10. Bar-Ad, V., Cognetti, D., Curry, J., Doyle, L., et al. (2018). *A systematic review of treating recurrent head and neck cancer: A reintroduction of brachytherapy with or without surgery*. https://core.ac.uk/download/213444412.pdf (accessed on 12th July 2025).

11. Barnes, C., Chuang, J., & Wong, B. (2016). *Overview of facial plastic surgery and current developments*. https://core.ac.uk/download/617032104.pdf (accessed on 12th July 2025)..

12. Basnyat, S., Goldfarb, J. M., Nyquist, G. G., Rabinowitz, M., et al. (2016). *Head and neck manifestations of eosinophilic granulomatosis with polyangiitis: A systematic review*. https://core.ac.uk/download/83049399.pdf (accessed on 12th July 2025).

13. Bellini, C., Cammaroto, G., Colizza, A., de Vincentiis, M., et al. (2019). *Risk factors for obstructive sleep apnea syndrome in children: State of the art.* https://core.ac.uk/download/231747914.pdf (accessed on 12th July 2025).

14. Belluzzi, E., Biz, C., De Cicco, M., Fantoni, M., et al. (2019). *Long-term radiographic and clinical-functional outcomes of isolated, displaced, closed talar neck and body fractures treated by ORIF: The timing of surgical management.* https://core.ac.uk/download/224995443.pdf (accessed on 12th July 2025).

15. Berg, M., Bulsara, M., Monterosso, L., Platt, V., et al. (2019). *Systematic review and meta-analysis of patient-reported outcomes for nurse-led models of survivorship care for adult cancer patients.* https://core.ac.uk/download/213607897.pdf (accessed on 12th July 2025).

16. Brandt, M., Garset-Zamani, M., Bozzato, A., Weimer, J., Arens, C., Dietrich, C. F., Todsen, T., et al. (2024). Endosonography in head and neck imaging and surgery. *Ultraschall in der Medizin – European Journal of Ultrasound, 46*, 224–244. https://www.semanticscholar.org/paper/913f044ce1ade205057247ff5689726c4c373da0 (accessed on 12th July 2025).

17. Bryant, L. M., Heffelfinger, R. N., & Sanan, A. (2017). *Management of forehead scars.* https://core.ac.uk/download/83049612.pdf (accessed on 12th July 2025).

18. Campisi, G., Cristaldi, M., Di Fede, O., Giuliana, G., et al. (2019). *Salivary biomarkers for oral squamous cell carcinoma diagnosis and follow-up: Current status and perspectives.* https://core.ac.uk/download/286528275.pdf (accessed on 12th July 2025).

19. Carvalho, A. C. A., Mahl, C., Martins Filho, P. R., Mendes, R., et al. (2021). *Frailty and risk of complications in head and neck oncologic surgery: Systematic review and dose-response meta-analysis.* https://core.ac.uk/download/570980458.pdf (accessed on 12th July 2025).

20. Cascone, P., Fontanari, M., Maffia, F., Mercuri, L., et al. (2020). *Impact of COVID-19 on maxillofacial surgery practice: A worldwide survey.* https://core.ac.uk/download/323192162.pdf (accessed on 12th July 2025).

21. Chan, H.-L., MacEachern, M., Oh, T.-J., Tanaka, T., et al. (2013). *Updated clinical considerations for dental implant therapy in irradiated head and neck cancer patients.* https://deepblue.lib.umich.edu/bitstream/2027.42/99596/1/jopr12028.pdf (accessed on 12th July 2025).

22. Chinn, S. B., Clayburgh, D., Davies, L., Givi, B., et al. (2020). *Safety recommendations for evaluation and surgery of the head and neck during the COVID-19 pandemic.* https://core.ac.uk/download/322846968.pdf (accessed on 12th July 2025).

23. Chou, S., Osman, S., Rosing, J., Sahar, D., et al. (2013). *Total posterior leg open wound management with free anterolateral thigh flap: Case and literature review.* https://core.ac.uk/download/323068446.pdf (accessed on 12th July 2025).

24. Cognetti, D. M., Curry, J. M., D'Souza, D., et al. (2014). *Cervical spine osteomyelitis after esophageal dilation in patients with a history of laryngectomy or pharyngectomy and pharyngeal irradiation.* https://core.ac.uk/download/46973320.pdf (accessed on 12th July 2025).

25. Copeland, J., Duinkerken, K., & Kelsey, L. (2018). *Jefferson Digital Commons quarterly report: April–June 2019.* https://core.ac.uk/download/220159103.pdf (accessed on 12th July 2025).

26. Culié, D., Schiappa, R., Contu, S., Scheller, B., Villarmé, A., Dassonville, O., Poissonnet, G., et al. (2022). Validation and improvement of a convolutional neural network to predict the involved pathology in a head and neck surgery cohort. *International Journal of Environmental*

Research and Public Health, 19. https://www.semanticscholar.org/paper/29d97ee542f76ba1494480befdbeb4f8f542d57d (accessed on 12th July 2025).

27. Ferraz, A. R., Nguyen, H. T., Oliveira, C. M., Rahbar, R., et al. (2012). *Robotic surgery in otolaryngology and head and neck surgery: A review*. https://core.ac.uk/download/28940482.pdf (accessed on 12th July 2025).

28. Friderichs, S., Ghazali, N., Grosset, D., Humphris, G., et al. (2014). *How head and neck consultants manage patients' emotional distress during cancer follow-up consultations: A multilevel study*. https://core.ac.uk/download/30320273.pdf (accessed on 12th July 2025).

29. Ikeda, A. K., Gray, R., Lee, V., Johns, J. D., Briggs, S. E., Raol, N., Megwalu, U., et al. (2024). Perioperative use of systemic steroids within otolaryngology–head and neck surgery: Evidence-based guidance for clinicians. *Otolaryngology–Head and Neck Surgery*. https://www.semanticscholar.org/paper/0531e9aa73424c73ff34b0a88aedc30711e226fd (accessed on 12th July 2025).

30. Karcioglu, A. S., Triponez, F., Solórzano, C., Iwata, A. J., Ahmed, A. A. A., Almquist, M., Angelos, P., et al. (2023). Emerging imaging technologies for parathyroid gland identification and vascular assessment in thyroid surgery: A review from the American Head and Neck Society Endocrine Surgery Section. *JAMA Otolaryngology–Head & Neck Surgery*. https://www.semanticscholar.org/paper/992f68d79f1e88af9e84b8f1ba34f7211cd60960 (accessed on 12th July 2025).

31. Kidwai, N. (2016). *Stage T4B head and neck cancer survival outcome comparisons based on treatment modality: Is surgery a viable treatment option?* https://open.bu.edu/bitstream/2144/16169/1/Kidwai_bu_0017N_11136.pdf (accessed on 12th July 2025).

32. Koji, A., Masaki, A., Hiroki, B., Shogo, H., Takaaki, I., Kaoru, S., Mitsuru, S., et al. (2014). *Mandibular reconstruction using plates prebent to fit rapid prototyping 3-dimensional printing models ameliorates contour deformity*. https://core.ac.uk/download/56657307.pdf (accessed on 12th July 2025).

33. Lang, B. H. H., & Wong, K. P. (2011). *Feasibility on the use of intraoperative vagal nerve stimulation in gasless, transaxillary endoscopic, and robotic-assisted thyroidectomy*. https://core.ac.uk/download/38036151.pdf (accessed on 12th July 2025).

34. Le, J., Ponto, J., Ying, Y., & Morlandt, A. (2024). Perioperative management for microvascular free tissue transfer for head and neck reconstruction – Commentary. *Journal of Diagnostics and Treatment of Oral and Maxillofacial Pathology*. https://www.semanticscholar.org/paper/30cec1260bbb6a549999adb7353f018559905094 (accessed on 12th July 2025).

35. Lechien, J., Hamdan, A.-L., Fakhry, N., Vaira, L., Iannella, G., Gengler, I. M., Michel, J., et al. (2024). Perception of young European otolaryngologists toward transoral robotic surgery in head and neck oncology and surgery. *Journal of Clinical Medicine, 13*. https://www.semanticscholar.org/paper/59c91fcced25a4fbc5a105c0393489b34d6e5b09 (accessed on 12th July 2025).

36. McMillan, H., Montgomery, P., & Cardoso, R. (2025). Prosthetic Rehabilitation for Speech and Swallowing (PReSS): A novel, interdisciplinary approach to head and neck cancer survivorship. *Current Opinion in Otolaryngology & Head and Neck Surgery, 33*, 142–148. https://www.semanticscholar.org/paper/e990be2065789ebf3ae7db39beba3154a203c03d (accessed on 12th July 2025).

37. Monteiro, E., & Sousa-Machado, A. (2023). *Elective revision surgery in head and neck cancer patients: A retrospective analysis at an oncology center in Porto, Portugal*. https://core.ac.uk/

download/614511087.pdf (accessed on 12th July 2025).

38. Okabe, R., Ueki, Y., Ohashi, R., Takeuchi, M., Hashimoto, S., Takahashi, T., Shodo, R., et al. (2022). Predicting cervical lymph node metastasis following endoscopic surgery in superficial head and neck carcinoma. *Frontiers in Surgery, 8*. https://www.semanticscholar.org/paper/0bebef6cd964f08bc131b2a174d84d57f24c6279 (accessed on 12th July 2025).

39. Petersen, L. Ø., Kiil, B., Gade, S. D., Jakobsen, A., & Krag, A. (2024). 3D-assisted surgery for reconstruction in the head and neck area. *Ugeskrift for Laeger, 186*(36). https://www.semanticscholar.org/paper/20ff838cf12276ab3ebae654ac7cb7d04eef94e4 (accessed on 12th July 2025).

40. Prucher, G. M., Caporali, L., Lauretta, M. P., et al. (2018). *Anesthetic challenges in microsurgical flap reconstruction: A systematic review*. https://core.ac.uk/download/188826841.pdf (accessed on 12th July 2025).

41. Sethi, H. K., & Fundakowski, C. E. (2024). Preoperative approach and technical considerations in parotid surgery. *Gland Surgery, 13*, 2414–2419. https://www.semanticscholar.org/paper/d427e28fd189694d40f502c8b30ab99c68b88000 (accessed on 12th July 2025).

42. Srinivasan, Y., Liu, A., & Rameau, A. (2023). Machine learning in the evaluation of voice and swallowing in the head and neck cancer patient. *Current Opinion in Otolaryngology & Head and Neck Surgery, 32*, 105–112. https://www.semanticscholar.org/paper/8be42b13d12c2243be6ce8ad27ffbc127990091a (accessed on 12th July 2025).

43. Talani, C., Högmo, A., Laurell, G., Mäkitie, A., & Farnebo, L. (2024). Six-month mortality has decreased for patients with curative treatment intent for head and neck cancer in Sweden. *PLOS ONE, 19*. https://www.semanticscholar.org/paper/57cc3ac69415ad7a9f2d7edd0f086d32224a3741 (accessed on 12th July 2025).

44. Townsley, R., Tan, J., Edy, E., Lim, A. E., & McMahon, J. D. (2024). A case series of interventions and outcomes in patients with laryngeal squamous cell cancer. *The Journal of Laryngology & Otology, 138*, 961–964. https://www.semanticscholar.org/paper/afd154eac912f6eb8ed2bf7b9e608e50f85a9241 (accessed on 12th July 2025).

45. Tsai, C.-H., Yang, C., Liu, Y.-C., Chen, C.-L., & Kao, H. (2025). Risk factors of free flap outcomes after head and neck cancer surgery: A multivariable analysis from a single center experience. *Microsurgery, 45*. https://www.semanticscholar.org/paper/b39a4fc00eec66faf06724b59c09516ec8737c01 (accessed on 12th July 2025).

BREAST AND ENDOCRINE SURGERY

3

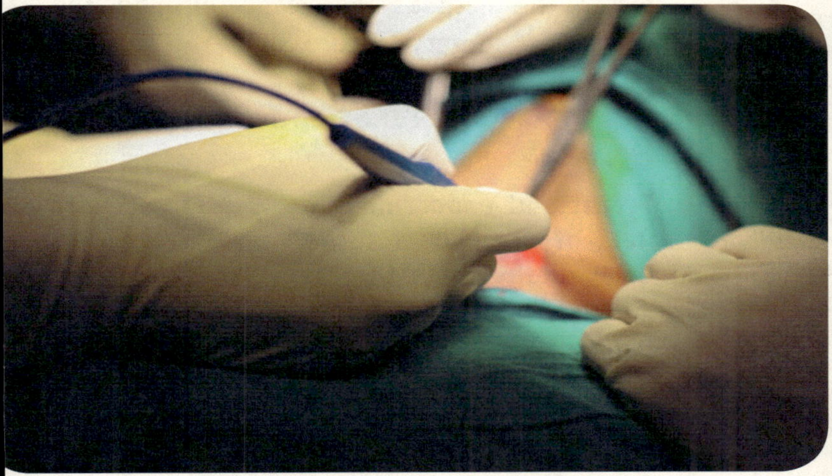

LEARNING OBJECTIVES

After studying this chapter, you will be able to:

1. Understand the anatomy of the breast
2. Explain the common breast conditions
3. Discuss the techniques in breast surgery
4. Focus on endocrine system overview
5. Learn about surgical interventions in endocrine disorders
6. Evaluate the postoperative care and complications

Introduction

Breast and endocrine surgery is a subspecialty of surgical practice that addresses various pathologies of the breast and endocrine system. The last decades have brought significant advances in surgical techniques and technology, which have improved patient outcomes by decreasing complications and shortening recovery periods. The specialty addresses a wide range of conditions from benign neoplasms and hormonal disorders to cancerous conditions such as breast cancer and thyroid cancers. Understanding the complexity of such procedures is essential, considering that they often require an interdisciplinary team that may include oncologists, endocrinologists, and surgeons to deliver comprehensive patient care. Minimally invasive procedures have revolutionized traditional surgical approaches by enabling finer procedures that prioritize patient safety and healing. A key aspect of breast and endocrine surgery is the identification and management of varied risk factors and genetic predispositions that influence patient outcomes. Genetic markers and screening devices have assumed increasing significance in assessing the risk of contracting particular cancers, such as breast cancer due to BRCA mutations, or assessing thyroid nodules to determine malignancy risk. By integrating genetic counseling and surgical planning, clinicians can deliver tailored interventions that match individual patient profiles, maximizing the success of treatment. Biomarkers in related oncologic diagnoses, such as head and neck squamous cell carcinoma, are the subject of a critical examination, highlighting the importance of understanding how specific biomarkers can indicate disease outcome and, consequently, affect surgical procedures and follow-up care (Mathew et al., 2017). Furthermore, multidisciplinary communication cannot be overstressed in regard to enhancing the quality of care in breast and endocrine surgery. Communication among a multi-specialty team of health practitioners—surgeons, medical oncologists, pathologists, and radiologists—facilitates comprehensive assessment that is essential for the formulation of well-informed treatment plans.

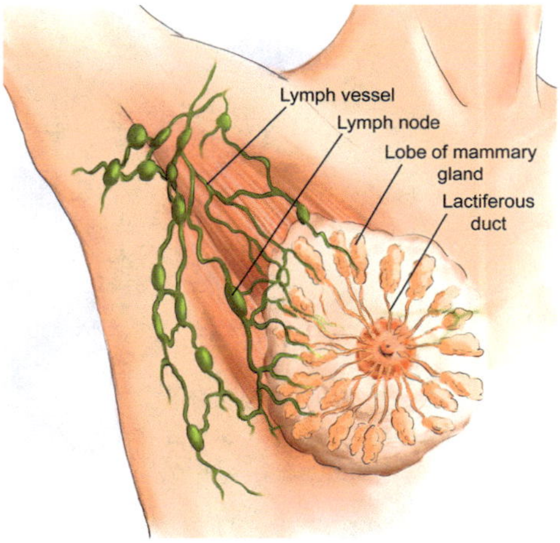

Figure 3.1. Breast cancer surgery.

Source: https://drandrewkiu.com.au/wp-content/uploads/2016/10/breast-cancer-surgery-1.jpg.

Each specialty contributes feedback that guides the surgical plan from preoperative evaluation to postoperative management. For instance, plans for surgery can be optimized based on imaging protocols or pathological examination that shows a risk of recurrence or metastasis. Through the emphasis placed on this multidisciplinary management, not only is the efficacy of interventions promoted, but so are contemporary medical practices that accommodate patient-centered care as well. As the subspecialty progresses, it is crucial to have an obligation of education and research that fosters the methods and science of endocrine and breast surgery (Figure 3.1).

Definition of Breast and Endocrine Surgery

Breast and endocrine surgery is a specialty field of practice in surgery that deals with the pathologies of the breast and endocrine system. This field of surgery deals particularly with diseases such as breast cancer, thyroid diseases, and other tumors of the endocrine glands. Surgeons who work in this specialty are educated to perform a range of procedures, from minimally invasive surgeries such as biopsies and lumpectomies to more advanced surgeries such as mastectomies or total thyroidectomies. The purpose of such operations is not only to cure malignant and benign diseases but also to enhance the quality of life of the patient by offering reconstructive options and supportive therapy that can minimize the psychological impact of such diseases. The use of advanced techniques and technologies consistently redefines surgical practice, improving outcomes and reducing recovery times for patients. In breast surgery, the focus is again aimed at the comprehensive treatment of breast disease, particularly cancer. Breast cancer has become one of the most prevalent types of cancer, and thus early detection and intervention strategies are adopted. Surgeons use multimodal approaches, in which surgical resection is complemented by adjuvant therapy, such as chemotherapy and radiotherapy, that are effective in improving prognosis and survival rates. The specialty has also embraced breast conservation methods with dramatic improvements to allow patients to stay away from more invasive surgical procedures whenever it is feasible. The research and application of genomic treatments and genetic testing continue to evolve, providing data that guides surgical decisions and personalized treatment protocols, ultimately resulting in enhanced patient outcomes in this life-enhancing area of medicine. Endocrine surgery encompasses operations for the treatment of glands that secrete hormones, including the thyroid, parathyroid, adrenal glands, and pancreas. The pathophysiology of endocrine disorders necessitates a comprehensive understanding of the hormonal pathways and their underlying mechanisms. Endocrine surgeons must not only confront the surgical aspect but also the potential endocrine dysfunctions following surgery. For instance, thyroid tissue resection causes hypothyroidism, requiring lifetime hormone replacement therapy, and parathyroid surgery can cause postoperative disturbances of calcium metabolism. As highlighted by recent works, the medical community appreciates the importance of a multidisciplinary strategy that entails blending surgical expertise with endocrinology to optimize patient care and health outcomes. Furthermore, ongoing studies related to the natural history of endocrine tumors and their hereditary syndromes are essential in the development of effective diagnostic and therapeutic strategies, such that surgical intervention is timely and adequate.

Importance of Surgical Intervention in Endocrine Disorders

Surgery plays a significant role in the treatment of endocrine diseases, particularly when the treatment with drugs is not effective or feels insufficient. Conditions such as hyperparathyroidism and thyroid nodules often necessitate surgery to cure the underlying pathology effectively. For instance, parathyroidectomy will ameliorate hypercalcemia and associated morbidity, significantly improving the quality of life of a patient and preventing long-term complications like osteoporosis and kidney stones. Likewise, thyroidectomy may play a role in those cases when thyroid nodules turn out to be malignant or may have potential malignancy. Not only does the procedure alleviate symptoms, but it also improves the prognosis of the patient when he or she is diagnosed with cancer of the thyroid gland. Through regular endocrine restoration by surgery, medical professionals can offer a better overall outcome for patients suffering from these complex conditions. Within the field of gender-affirming treatment, surgery belongs to hormonal management among transgender patients, paralleling endocrine treatment objectives. The Endocrine Society highlights the importance of multidisciplinary work, focusing on the fact that surgeries must be tailored to satisfy the unique physiological requirements of transgender individuals. Procedures such as breast augmentation or chest masculinization have a profound effect on the psychological and sociocultural aspects of an individual's transition, thereby enhancing mental health outcomes. As recorded in existing literature, the psychosocial benefits of such treatments can lead to a remarkable reduction in anxiety and depression levels among patients and thus signify that surgical interventions are not elective but instead necessary components of holistic care for patients with endocrine conditions calling for gender affirmation (Arcelus et al., 2018). Besides, technological advances in endocrine surgery not only enhance survival but also reduce the psychosocial effects of oncologic treatments. Breast cancer care is the best example, as modern surgical techniques have significantly altered to enhance aesthetic and functional outcomes for survivors. The continued emphasis on integrating patient-reported outcomes (PROs) into practice reminds surgeons of the long-term effects that surgical choices can have on quality of life following treatment. Problems with extended iatrogenic side effects of cancer treatments require surgical intervention as a measure for remedies against complications of past therapies. By carefully monitoring such consequences and implementing surgical measures when needed, practitioners can improve more holistic care, ultimately enhancing both physical and emotional well-being for patients facing the aftermath of endocrine disease and its treatments (Ahles et al., 2014) (Figure 3.2).

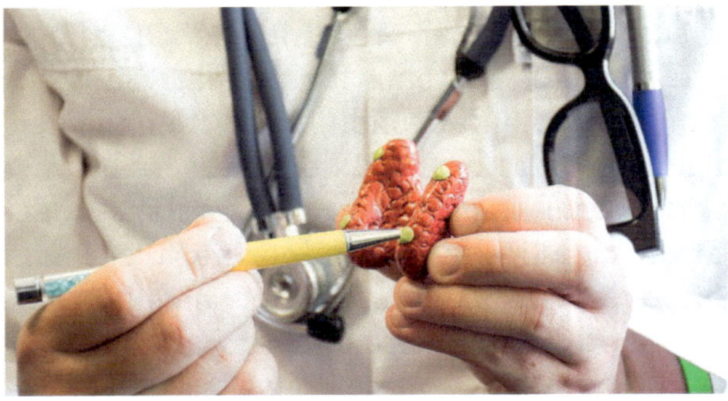

Figure 3.2. Exploring endocrine surgery.

Source: https://www.fortishealthcare.com/drupal-data/2024-07/Endocrine-Surgery.jpg.

3.1. Anatomy of the Breast

Learning Outcome

1. Describe the structure and function of breast tissue
2. Focus on blood supply and lymphatic drainage
3. Learn the common anatomical variations

The composition of the breast is complex, comprising several tissues that work together to facilitate its primary functions, primarily associated with lactation. The breast is made up of glandular tissue, composed of lobules and ducts, and adipose tissue, which provides structural support and shape to the breast. The milk-producing glands are located in the lobules, while the ducts transport milk to the nipple during breastfeeding. In addition, ligaments and connective tissues like Cooper's ligaments hold the breasts in place and provide the breasts' integrity. For surgical operations within breast surgery, it is essential to understand this complex anatomical composition, as it enables surgeons to maneuver the different components and preserve the integrity of surrounding tissues as much as possible during operations such as mastectomies or lumpectomies. Careful consideration of anatomical structures ensures effective surgical outcomes and preserves as much breast tissue as possible during the procedure. In addition to the structural components, the vascular and lymphatic systems play significant roles in the anatomy of the breast. The internal thoracic artery and lateral thoracic artery mainly supply the breast tissue with blood through their branches. Lymphatic drainage is also essential as it facilitates the drainage of interstitial fluid and protects against infection by filtering lymph through the lymph nodes. Drainage usually occurs under a pattern that communicates with axillary, supraclavicular, and internal mammary lymph nodes. Therefore, in breast surgical interventions, caution should be exercised not to traverse these lymphatic and vascular channels to prevent such complications as lymphedema or unnecessary bleeding. A good understanding of these anatomical facts is essential to the accurate performance of procedures such as sentinel node biopsies and axillary lymphadenectomies, which are cornerstone procedures in breast cancer patient treatment. Progress in breast surgery procedures has necessitated an ongoing dialogue among the medical profession regarding best practices and patient-centered care. There are various methods to support different clinical scenarios, with an emphasis on the importance of tailored treatment planning based on the anatomy of each patient. For instance, breast-conserving surgeries such as lumpectomy are more frequent in the setting of early breast cancer, while modified radical mastectomies are more appropriate for locally advanced disease. The resection margin problem remains a topic of controversy, and studies continue to be conducted in an effort to establish the ideal criteria for surgical excision. In addition, advances in sentinel lymph node biopsy highlight the need to minimize the impact of surgery on lymphatic function. In parallel with advancing surgery techniques is the establishment of standards of care to ensure that they remain consistent with current evidence-based practice guidelines. Such adaptability illustrates the discreet interaction between breast anatomy and strategic decision in endocrine and breast surgery (Domschke et al., 2012) (Figure 3.3).

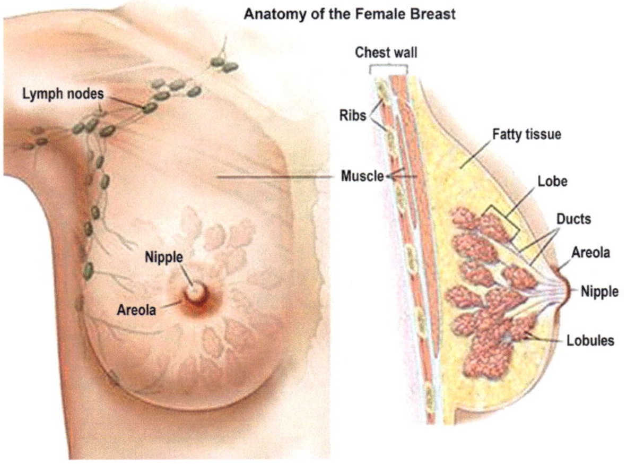

Figure 3.3. Anatomy of the breast.

Source: https://training.seer.cancer.gov/images/breast/female-breast-anatomy.jpg.

3.1.1. Structure and Function of Breast Tissue

The structural organization of the breast tissue is essential to its multifunctionality, particularly lactation and overall hormonal regulation. Composed of glandular tissue, adipose tissue, and connective tissue, the breast not only offers a site for milk formation but is also an endocrine organ. The glandular tissue, in the form of lobules, secretes and synthesizes milk during lactation, whereas fatty tissue provides the breasts with physical support and an energy reserve. Stromal cells, including fibroblasts and immune cells, play important roles in maintaining tissue integrity and responding to hormonal changes. The interaction between these varied components imparts sufficient development and operation at different stages of life, such as puberty, pregnancy, and menopause, which depicts the dynamic nature of breast tissue and its invaluable contribution to women's health. In addition to its structural complexity, breast tissue is endowed with remarkable functional capacities, which are primarily regulated under hormonal control. Estrogen and progesterone, which are released from the ovaries, also play significant roles in the growth of breasts and onset of lactation in mammary glands. Throughout the menstrual cycle, hormone levels fluctuate, resulting in cyclical breast phenomena such as swelling and tenderness. During pregnancy, the elevated level of estrogen and progesterone stimulates the further growth of alveolar cells, preparing the breasts to produce milk. Additionally, the interaction of these hormones with local growth factors is responsible for determining the features of breast tissue, specifically ductal expansion and lobulogenesis. This understanding of hormonal interaction is crucial in the management of breast health disorders like breast cancer, which may result from alterations in hormonal homeostasis and tissue regulation. The discovery of breast tissue's structural and functional properties also affects breast cancer research and treatment strategies. Recent research has revealed some of the key knowledge gaps in our comprehension of how cellular and genetic properties start and cause breast cancer that must be explored in-depth. For instance, advances in understanding the molecular mechanisms of ductal elongation and branching could reveal future therapeutic targets for early breast cancer treatment. Knowledge about the psychosocial aspects of breast health, including the influence of obesity on hormonal homeostasis as well as the role of breast tissue, is increasingly relevant. As obesity has been classified as a global epidemic, it becomes imperative to determine the impact of excess adiposity on breast tissue histological characteristics and risk for cancer (Kyrou et al., 2010). Closing these research gaps would potentially lead to better patient management, risk stratification, and customized treatment options in endocrine and breast surgery (Cox et al., 2008) (Figure 3.4).

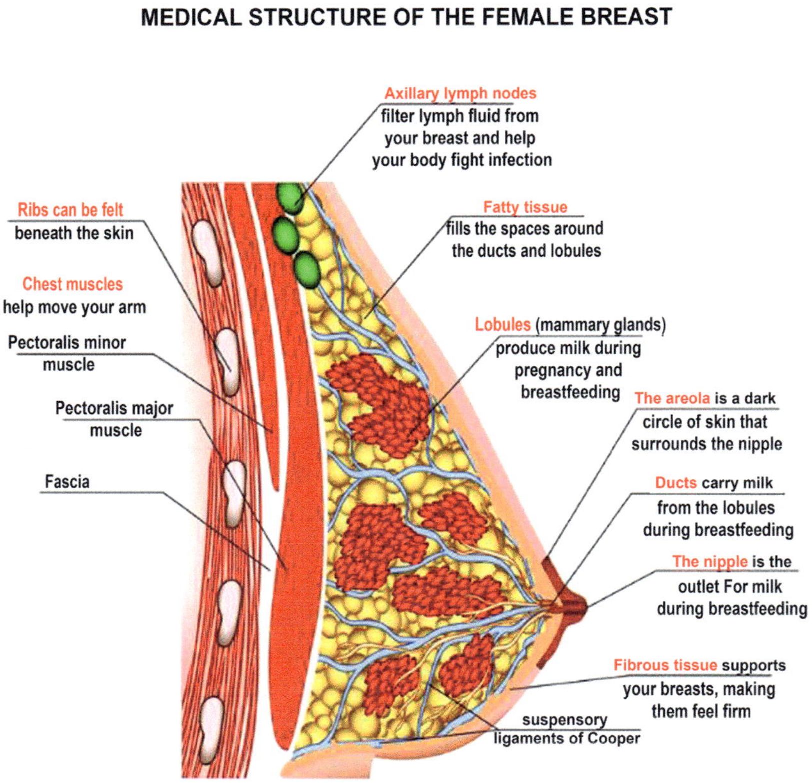

Figure 3.4. Breast tissue anatomy & physiology.

Source: https://www.jackiebellnaturalhealth.com/uploads/3/8/3/1/38313077/5403342_orig.jpg.

3.1.2. Blood Supply and Lymphatic Drainage

Understanding the blood supply and lymphatic drainage of the breast is crucial in breast and endocrine surgery practice, as it is relevant to operation outcomes, potential complications, and management. The internal mammary artery, the lateral thoracic artery, and the thoracoacromial artery give the major vascular supply to the breast through their branches. These vessels supply adequate perfusion for normal physiological breast tissue function and pathology. Insufficient blood supply can lead to necrotic tissue, which is a barrier to post-operative recovery and leads to morbidity. Such precise understanding of these vascular networks is essential in assisting surgeons to prevent complications such as flap failure after reconstructive surgeries and promising interventions in oncologic surgery. In addition to the blood supply, the lymphatic drainage system is also vital in breast surgery. Most of the lymph drainage of the breast is done by the axillary lymph nodes. In surgeries such as axillary lymph node dissection (ALND) or sentinel lymph node biopsy, care must be taken to ensure that the integrity of the lymphatic system is not compromised to prevent postoperative complications, such as lymphedema. Studies indicate that identification rates of lymphatics via procedures such as indocyanine green (ICG) fluorescence imaging are highly effective, which consequently translates to improved patient outcomes owing to less damage to the surrounding lymphatic structures. The procedure also finds it feasible to spare the lateral group of lymph nodes, which serves to maintain lymphatic function while also mitigating the risk of metastasis for patients with early-stage breast cancer (Jyothsna et al., 2016). Surgical complications after the operation, like the formation of seromas, can particularly affect recovery and hospital stay following breast surgery. Seromas are often formed due to impaired blood and lymphatic supply during surgery, as reported in studies demonstrating the efficacy of methylprednisolone injections in the wound bed to reduce the incidence of seroma formation (Maran et al., 2017). These interventions have a straightforward impact on the patient's recovery by resolving complications that prolong hospital stays and induce further morbidity. Understanding the interactions between blood supply, lymphatic drainage, and post-operative complications maximizes surgical planning and eventually provides improved patient outcomes for breast and endocrine surgery. Through the integration of various techniques and pharmacologic measures, surgeons can better neutralize the risks of these physiological systems.

3.1.3. Common Anatomical Variations

Anatomical differences have significant implications in endocrine and breast surgery, both in terms of surgical technique and patient prognosis. Genetic factors, developmental abnormalities, or environmental conditions may bring about anatomical differences. For example, the presence of accessory breast tissue, or polymastia, may complicate operations. Surgeons must be adept at identifying these kinds of anatomical differences so that they can adjust their methods accordingly. In cases where breast tissue prolapses beyond the normal limits, extensive preoperative imaging may be necessary to delineate the extent of tissue involvement. Additionally, recognition of such variations may prevent procedural complications, such as mastectomies or lumpectomies. Thus, awareness of these common anatomical variants is essential for optimizing surgical practice and delivering comprehensive patient care under the auspices of breast and endocrine surgery. In addition to accessory breast tissue, variations in the underlying vascular and lymphatic drainage must be considered when operating. Anatomical discrepancies in vascular anatomy have the potential to alter the planned surgical procedure and impact both the aesthetic and functional success of surgery. Surgeons must bear these variations in mind to escape the risk of ischemia or compromised lymphatic drainage leading to long-term complications of lymphedema. The ability to recognize and accommodate blood supply variation not only enhances surgical precision but also increases patient satisfaction with the surgical outcome. As surgical procedure evolves, integrating knowledge of such anatomical particulars remains essential. Ultimately, careful preoperative study using high-quality imaging and surgical mapping can predict such variation and modify surgical treatment to account for it. Finally, the subspecialty of breast and endocrine surgery must also deal with congenital anatomical disorders, specifically those affecting sex characteristic development. Disorders such as disorders of sex development (DSDs) present special challenges that require multidisciplinary treatment. Knowledge about how anatomical abnormalities might affect hormonal control and breast development is essential in the successful planning of management. It requires an interdisciplinary approach for collaboration among surgeons, endocrinologists, and other physicians. As there has been a shift in attitude towards gender diversity within society, an increasing demand to design individualized treatment plans that include both medical and psychosocial aspects of treatment, particularly in infants with non-typical genitalia (Ahmed et al., 2017). Assuming that clinicians possess the ability to manage such variations confidently, a cooperative environment is created for families, which ultimately leads to better-informed decision-making on surgical options in complex cases (Figure 3.5).

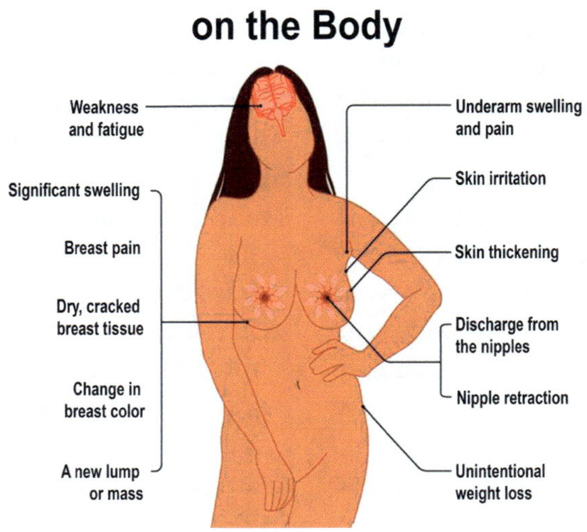

Figure 3.5. Breast cancer affects the body.

Source: https://media.post.rvohealth.io/wp-content/uploads/2024/02/effects-of-breast-cancer-on-the-body-social-1080x1080-2-1-732x549.jpg.

Test Your Knowledge

1. What is the primary blood supply to the breast?
2. Which lymph nodes are primarily involved in breast drainage?

3.2. Common Breast Conditions

Learning Outcome

1. Explain the benign breast diseases
2. Define the breast cancer statistics and types
3. Discuss the risk factors associated with breast conditions

Breast care is a significant field of concern in endocrine surgery, as many common breast conditions have devastating impacts on women's quality of life and must be addressed with care. The most frequent among them are benign processes such as mastitis, fibrocystic changes, and fibroadenomas, which can present from pain and inflammation to masses on exam. Mastitis, for instance, is excellently associated with lactation and can lead to infections that need clinical intervention as well as occasional surgery. Surgical practitioners need to be aware of such benign processes to differentiate them from malignant breast pathology, which is treated more aggressively. Appropriate screening procedures and educational outreach are thus important in enabling early detection and effective management of common breast diseases in the population. With progress in medical science, the management of breast cancer, along with benign conditions, has evolved to include newer modalities. In hormone receptor-positive breast cancers, particularly in the age of COVID-19, there has been a notable trend toward the use of neoadjuvant endocrine therapy, which allows for deferral of surgeries and safely manages malignancy. Such a strategy not only decreases the frequency of hospital encounters but also provides an effective way to manage luminal-like tumors without compromising patient safety during challenging times. This evolving treatment scenario underscores the necessity of continuous medical education and adaptability on the part of healthcare workers to remain responsive to their patients' needs while delivering evidence-based treatment against a backdrop of evolving situations, as specified in studies of breast cancer care amidst emergencies such as pandemics (Martí et al., 2020). Follow-up care among breast cancer survivors cannot be overemphasized. Studies have shown that women who have undergone treatment for initial breast cancer have an increased risk of developing a second independent breast cancer for a duration of at least 20 years after initial diagnosis. Follow-up by surveillance mammography and self-examination has been proven to improve outcomes since earlier detection has a better survival rate. Additionally, alternative follow-up methods outside clinics have been well-received by patients and offer an active approach to long-term care. Randomized controlled trials remain underpowered to deliver finalizing evidence concerning the survival benefits of these alternative follow-up methods (David et al., 2012). Therefore, optimizing follow-up care through patient education and customizing monitoring techniques is of the greatest priority for improving survival and quality of life in this population (Figure 3.6).

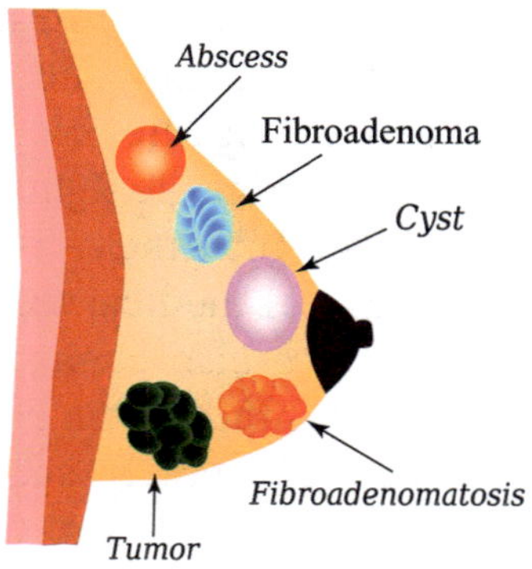

Figure 3.6. Breast conditions.

Source: https://www.breastdoctorpune.com/wp-content/uploads/2024/08/Benign-breast-disease.jpg.

3.2.1. Benign Breast Diseases

Benign breast disease is a heterogeneous group of disorders that, while not cancerous, has a significant impact on the physical and psychological well-being of affected persons. They include conditions like fibrocystic changes, benign neoplasms like fibroadenomas, and mastitis, among others. They all exhibit distinct clinical features and have specific treatment implications. For instance, while fibrocystic changes typically present with cyclical breast pain and tenderness, fibroadenomas may be incidentally diagnosed during routine clinical or imaging examinations. The prevalence of these conditions necessitates effective diagnosis and management methods to alleviate symptoms and possibly avert complications. Psychological distress associated with benign breast disorders, often based on fear of malignancy, further highlights the need for open communication and patient support by clinicians who manage such problems. Technological advances in imaging have revolutionized the diagnostic process in benign breast disease to the extent that differentiation from malignant disease can be made accurately. Mammography and ultrasound are thus the critical technologies in this context, allowing clinicians to assess the nature of breast lesions and guide management strategies. In cases where the outcome is uncertain, additional interventions such as needle biopsies will be employed to determine benign pathology and reassure patients. Integrative treatments, which involve the use of medical treatment in addition to surgery, are also commonly used, particularly where symptomatic relief is of primary importance. Conversely, some benign diseases are merely monitored over time without immediate intervention, illustrating the extent to which management depends on patient-specific circumstances and desires. It indicates the importance of understanding benign breast diseases within the context of breast and endocrine surgery in general.

Research into benign breast diseases is still advanced, with continuing attempts to define risk factors and design specific therapies. While conditions in themselves are rarely life-threatening, their interaction with hormonal factors, including estrogen and progesterone, is currently under research. For example, the role of endogenous hormonal changes in conditions such as mastitis and fibroadenomas may yield new treatment options, thereby enhancing patient outcomes. Furthermore, possible complications from certain benign conditions demand ongoing education and awareness for practitioners and patients. In this regard, integrating findings from related fields, such as studies on finasteride in hormonal modulation and its effects as described in Banu et al. (2016), and emerging interventions such as percutaneous radiofrequency thermal ablation for the therapy of nodules as described in Assanti et al. (2012), may lay the foundation for improved management of benign breast diseases. Overall, continued discovery and adaptation in paradigms of treatment and diagnosis are required to battle the complexity associated with benign breast diseases.

3.2.2. Breast Cancer Statistics and Types

Breast cancer is still one of the leading cancers among women worldwide. Recent statistics still show that about 1 in 8 women in the United States will have breast cancer at some time during their lifetime. The rate of incidence, however, still varies significantly among different populations based on age, race, and socioeconomic status. Notably, socioeconomic inequalities have been demonstrated in the survival rates of cancer, most clearly in the case of breast cancer, in which survival rates have shown a clear pattern of improvement over the decades. According to a study tracking patterns in socioeconomic survival disparities from 1973 to 2004, disparities in survival from breast cancer decreased from −10% to −6%, indicating that improvements in treatment have benefited a broader cross-section of socioeconomic groups. These variations underscore the importance of equitable access to healthcare facilities that facilitate timely diagnosis and therapeutic opportunities (Barbiere et al., 2011). Histologies of breast cancer also exhibit high variation, with hormone receptor status playing a pivotal role in the administration of treatment. Approximately 80% of breast cancers are estrogen receptor-positive (ER+), which means that endocrine therapy (ET) forms an integral component in treating them. Treatment of ET can include a number of approaches, such as selective estrogen receptor modulators (SERMs), aromatase inhibitors (AIs), and ovarian function suppression. The value of these treatments is realized once it is understood how efficiently they suppress recurrence rates; an example of this is that tamoxifen users have a significantly reduced likelihood of developing invasive and in situ breast cancers when treatment duration is extended to 10 years. Such treatment modalities also emphasize the individualized techniques adopted in both surgical and nonsurgical treatments, detailing the importance of hormone receptor status in determining the patient's outcome (Basso et al., 2015). The history of the development of breast cancer treatment has also called for reflection on innovative therapies, especially in instances of endocrine-resistant cancers. Even though old treatments have had success in most, approximately one-third of breast cancer cases progress to a resistant phase for standard endocrine therapies. Novel agents, such as cyclin-dependent kinase 4/6 and mammalian target of rapamycin (mTOR) inhibitors, are being discovered in addition to existing therapies. These advances aim to enhance therapeutic outcomes in women with advanced breast cancer, amounting to a revolution in treatment philosophy that not only emphasizes surgical therapy but also total medical management. In the face of improving survival rates and new treatment modalities, understanding how breast cancer subtypes and treatment algorithms co-exist becomes ever more critical in the environment of breast and endocrine surgery (Basso et al., 2015) (Figure 3.7).

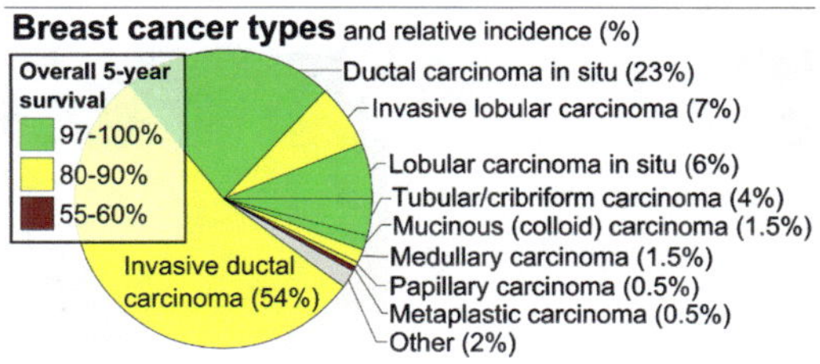

Figure 3.7. Breast cancer statistics and types.

Source: https://upload.wikimedia.org/wikipedia/commons/b/bd/Pie_chart_of_incidence_and_prognosis_of_histopathologic_breast_cancer_types.png.

3.2.3. Risk Factors Associated With Breast Conditions

An exploration of risk factors for breast disorders touches upon many biological, environmental, and lifestyle variables and is therefore an umbrella area of study. Of special interest, indeed, have been risk factors such as age, genetic predisposition, and history, each of which has been found to exert a significant influence upon breast issues. Females carrying mutations in genes such as BRCA1 and BRCA2, for instance, are at a great risk of developing breast cancer; thus, genetic testing and personalized health interventions are vital. Moreover, age remains a prime factor, with risk for breast concerns increasing immensely after 40 years, alongside menopause and hormonal changes. This intersection of age and genetics points to the need for targeted screening programs in high-risk groups to allow for the early diagnosis and intervention against probable breast diseases. Lifestyle variables such as diet, exercise, and exposure to environmental toxins also contribute to the risk profile for breast disorders. Evidence shows that a diet rich in saturated fat and poor in fruit and vegetable consumption is linked to breast cancer risk. Physical activity, on the other hand, exhibits a protective influence, with studies showing lower rates among individuals who exercise. Along with this, exposure to pollutants in the environment, such as those present in certain industrial chemicals, has likewise been linked to hormonal imbalances that could exacerbate breast health issues. Overall, the intersection of lifestyle and environmental exposures is a primary field of research for differentiating and addressing risk factors attributable to breast disorders. Public health strategies that involve thorough planning must be implemented to inform women about these modifiable risks and encourage healthier behaviors to reduce their overall risk. More clinically, chemotherapy and radiation, while effective for the control of breast cancer, have associated risks that can impact long-term health and cellular senescence. Evidence shows that breast cancer survivors who have received such treatments have evidence of DNA damage and altered telomerase activity, indicating potential long-term effects on their health after treatment. The interaction of the treatments and markers of inflammation, such as Interleukin-6 and C-reactive protein, adds another layer of complexity as to how previous therapies may influence the overall breadth of breast health. This calls for sophisticated evaluation of long-term health risks to survivors, particularly the risk of secondary cancers and management of chronic disease. An interdisciplinary effort, bringing together skills in oncology, endocrinology, and nutrition, is needed to develop post-treatment care recommendations that can effectively address these complex health issues while promoting the health of survivors.

Test Your Knowledge

1. What are the typical features of a fibroadenoma on clinical examination?
2. How is mastitis commonly managed in lactating women?

3.3. Techniques in Breast Surgery

Learning Outcome

1. Explain the lumpectomy and mastectomy
2. Define the sentinel lymph node biopsy
3. Describe the reconstruction options post-surgery

Surgical techniques for breast surgery have been significantly advanced in recent years to not only provide improved survival rates but also the general health and well-being of the patient. From mastectomy to lumpectomy, the surgical process differs based on the individual's specific needs, based on tumor size, cancer stage, and preference. New developments in onco-plastic surgery enable the synthesis of oncologic and plastic surgical concepts, allowing for the preservation of both breast function and aesthetic appeal. Multidisciplinary consultation among oncologists, radiologists, and plastic surgeons is an integral part of the decision-making process for surgery, ensuring optimal care. By considering patients' and, especially, older women's preferences and expectations, who as individual patients present special challenges in treatment, clinicians can better customize surgical approaches to each patient and maximize outcomes (Audisio et al., 2009).

In addition to traditional surgery, modern-day breast surgery has also benefited from emerging technology such as intraoperative imaging and minimally invasive surgery. Procedures like wire localization for the removal of tumors and sentinel lymph node biopsy refine surgical accuracy, minimizing recovery time and postoperative complications. These procedures are of most significant benefit in treating patients with early-stage breast cancer, where maintaining breast tissue is optimal. Additionally, the use of robotic-assisted surgery provides another measure of accuracy, resulting in minimal scarring and facilitating a quicker recovery. This development in methods underscores the need to harmonize oncological justification with aesthetic results, thereby catering to the psychological well-being of patients as they undergo treatment (Ahles et al., 2014).

Postoperative rehabilitation and care have also emerged as key elements in the continuum of the treatment of breast cancer. Enhanced Recovery After Surgery (ERAS) protocols center on maximizing postoperative outcomes through multimodal pain control and early mobilization regimens. This approach not only facilitates quicker recovery but also minimizes complications of prolonged immobilization. Further, the inclusion of psychosocial support in the model of surgery acknowledges the profound emotional impact of breast cancer diagnoses and therapies. The follow-up survivorship programs after surgery help to deal with long-term issues such as the effect of treatments on quality of life, which can vary from physical, psychological, to sexual functioning. Therefore, it is needed to continue studying such integrative strategies in breast surgery to maximize patient care and increase overall survival rates (Ahles et al., 2014) (Figure 3.8).

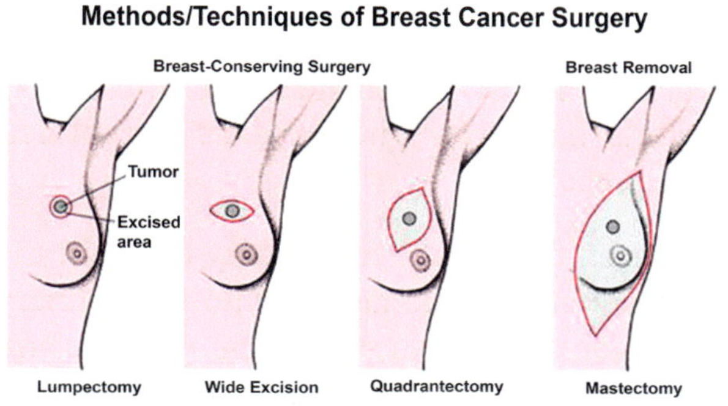

Figure 3.8. Methods techniques of breast cancer surgery.

Source: https://www.medifee.com/images/surgery/methods-techniques-of-breast-cancer-surgery.png.

3.3.1. Lumpectomy and Mastectomy

The choice between mastectomy and lumpectomy is a key decision in the operation to treat breast cancer that impacts clinical results as well as the quality of life of a patient. Lumpectomy, or breast-conserving surgery, is designed to remove the cancerous lesion while sparing as much normal breast tissue as possible. This method has gained popularity due to its association with reasonable survival rates and a minimally invasive approach, thus becoming the preferred treatment for a majority of early-stage breast cancer patients. Studies indicate that when used in combination with radiation therapy, lumpectomy offers equal efficacy to mastectomy in disease-free survival, thus proving the merit of individualization in terms of treatments based on patient choice as well as tumor-related factors. However, conditions such as margin clearance and potential need for re-excision remain crucial in deciding on surgical options, particularly when presenting tumors are complex (Domschke et al., 2012).

Conversely, sources suggest that mastectomy is the complete or partial removal of both or one breast and may be recommended due to some reasons including size and extent of the cancer, personal choice, and inherited factors. Modified radical mastectomy is commonly performed in locally advanced breast cancer, providing a primary resection of the tumor with the additional control of regional spread in the form of axillary node removal. Evolution during the past two decades about surgical and reconstructive procedures has improved aesthetic outcomes and patient satisfaction, excluding the prevailing myth that mastectomy leads to poorer psychosocial outcomes than breast-conserving surgery. The decision to follow a mastectomy is typically made in patients with increased risk factors, like BRCA mutations or contralateral breast cancer, and involves an individualized, evidence-based sequence of breast surgery based on modern clinical guidelines (Domschke et al., 2012).

Research has discussed the effectiveness of preoperative therapies, such as targeted agents, which can influence surgical outcomes. For instance, patients with breast cancer and HER2-positive tumors who receive neoadjuvant therapy have improved outcomes with the addition of early surgical intervention. Research indicates that such patients have low rates of local-regional recurrence (LRR) when treated with targeted therapy like trastuzumab combined with lumpectomy, which suggests that systemic treatment tailored to the patient can enhance the result of breast-conserving surgery. An in-depth understanding of the interface between surgical methods and new treatment protocols is essential to enable clinicians to provide optimal care and achieve patient-centered outcomes. As new therapeutic options continue to evolve, surgeons must be adaptable in their practices to modify surgical options in correlation with individual patient characteristics and ongoing research updates.

3.3.2. Sentinel Lymph Node Biopsy

In endocrine and breast surgery, sentinel lymph node biopsy (SLNB) is a vital technique to assess lymphatic spread in patients with breast cancer. Axillary lymph node dissection was the traditional method used before its advent, which was associated with substantial morbidity. SLNB offers a more discriminatory method, with the potential to detect and excise the first node(s) draining the tumor bed and avoid unnecessary surgery. The procedure not only reduces potential risks such as lymphedema but also provides critical staging information to guide adjuvant therapy. With improved surgical technique, the importance of maintaining strict stepwise guidelines for the performance of SLNB cannot be overstated, especially in the elderly, where comorbidities may complicate decision-making for invasive procedures. Contemporary literature appeals for tailored surgical strategies, particularly for elderly women with breast cancer who may have varying tumor biology and overall health profiles. Evidence indicates that older women tend not to receive the usual treatment common among younger populations, emphasizing the need for personalized treatment routes that take into consideration patient preference and comorbidities (Audisio et al., 2009). Sentinel lymph node biopsy can play an influential role within personalized treatment, allowing surgeons to balance successful treatment of cancer with avoidance of overtreatment among susceptible patients.

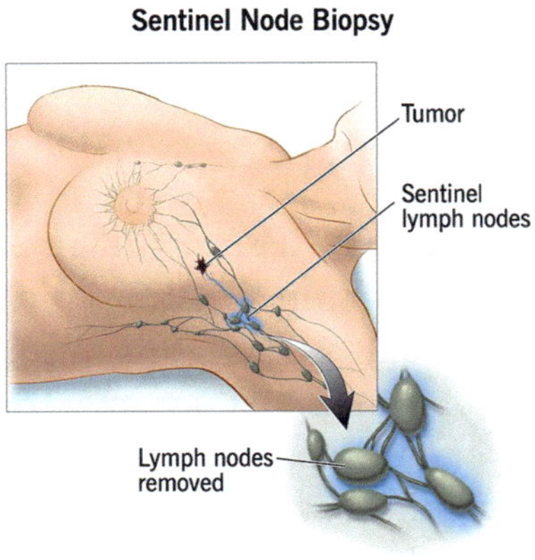

Figure 3.9. Sentinel node biopsy (SLNB).

Source: https://my.clevelandclinic.org/-/scassets/images/org/health/articles/sentinel-node-biopsy.

Given that treatment efficacy relies on the interplay of multiple factors, multidisciplinary discussions among surgical teams, geriatricians, and oncologists should be encouraged to achieve optimal outcomes and synchronize therapeutic options with the patient's values. Despite improved surgical techniques like SLNB, there remains an immense lacuna of dedicated research on surgery-oriented treatment for breast cancer. The integration of surgical expertise into the broader dialogue on the management of breast cancer is paramount to maximizing care for patients. Surgeons are primarily the first point of contact for breast cancer patients and therefore have a pivotal role to play in educating and guiding clinical studies focusing on surgery. Prioritization of studies that estimate the effectiveness and implications of sentinel lymph node biopsy will enable surgeons to contribute to the development of a more nuanced model of breast cancer treatment regimens. Continued research on the outcomes associated with SLNB, together with advancements in surgical technology, will be critical in addressing the gaps in existing research and improving the quality of care for all breast cancer patients (Figure 3.9).

3.3.3. Reconstruction Options Post-Surgery

Reconstructive postoperative choices are a part of the overall treatment plan of patients who undergo breast surgery, particularly after mastectomy due to cancer. Not only do the choices offer a solution to the physical transformation following the surgery, but they also play a crucial role in psychological recuperation and social life for the patient. Implant-based and autologous tissue reconstruction are the two primary types of reconstruction. Implant-based reconstruction involves the use of silicone or saline implants to restore breast shape and volume and is usually done in one or two surgeries. Autologous reconstruction involves using tissue from the patient's abdomen, thighs, or back. Both procedures have their unique benefits and drawbacks, where patient education is crucial, and an individualized approach must be used to decide on the most appropriate action based on certain conditions and preferences. The decision-making process following surgery is often influenced by several variables, including patient age, overall health, and personal preferences regarding cosmetic appearance and recovery. In elderly female breast cancer patients, changes associated with aging, as well as comorbidities that restrict possibilities for surgery, generate complicating variables. Research indicates that the majority of older patients are not automatically provided with the standard care typically received by younger patients, yet again highlighting the importance of individually tailored treatment schemes for this patient cohort. Multidisciplinary teams comprising geriatricians, surgeons, and oncologists are all-critical in formulating these personalized treatment and reconstruction plans, ensuring that older patients are knowledgeable and actively involved in their treatment options, addressing gaps in shared decision-making in this age group (Audisio et al., 2009).

Finally, the psychological impact of breast surgery and subsequent reconstruction cannot be underestimated. Studies have suggested that such successful reconstruction has the power to significantly enhance a patient's body image, self-esteem, and general quality of life. This is particularly relevant in a society where physical looks can have the potential to influence perceptions about femininity and identity significantly. In assisting women with post-surgical recovery, awareness of reconstruction options is essential in enabling women to make suitably informed choices that correlate with personal goals and emotional requirements. Regular reinforcement with counseling and patient education programs is crucial for making patients confident regarding their reconstruction choices. Thus, marrying surgical skills with an understanding of the psychological ramifications solidifies the foundation of better care in breast and endocrine surgery (Ndongo et al., 2010).

Test Your Knowledge

1. What are the key steps in performing a modified radical mastectomy?
2. How is sentinel lymph node biopsy performed and interpreted?

3.4. Endocrine System Overview

Learning Outcome

1. Identify the major glands of the endocrine system
2. Define the hormonal regulation and its significance
3. Describe the common endocrine disorders

The endocrine system, through its complex network of organs and glands, plays a crucial role in regulating a wide range of physiological processes by releasing hormones. Hormones are molecular messengers released into the blood to convey messages to target organs, facilitating growth, metabolism, and reproduction activities. All glands within the endocrine system, including the pituitary, thyroid, adrenal, and pancreas, secrete specific hormones that are required to orchestrate various body functions. For instance, the endocrine system causes the thyroid gland to release thyroxine, which regulates metabolism, and the adrenal glands release cortisol, a hormone that helps the body respond to stress. The intricate interplay of these hormonal messages is what maintains homeostasis and overall health, and therefore the endocrine system plays a vital role in many body functions and is a critical factor in surgical procedures, particularly in breast and endocrine surgery. Understanding the role of endocrine processes is crucial, especially in the context of breast surgery. Imbalances of endocrine activity can have a substantial effect on the growth and health of breast tissue. Estrogen, a steroid hormone produced primarily by the ovaries, has been shown to influence breast development as well as the tumorigenesis of breast cancer. Alteration of estrogen levels can increase tumorigenesis, which is why surgical interventions that take into consideration hormonal pathways become necessary. Moreover, therapy for such conditions as estrogen receptor-positive breast cancer requires a multidisciplinary approach, balancing surgical techniques with endocrine therapy regimens. The understanding of endocrine dynamics thus not only directs surgical choice but also highlights the importance of individualized treatment protocols in breast cancer that increasingly rely on hormonal assessment to enhance further patient outcomes. Recent research has emphasized the importance of personalized hormone therapy, particularly for populations such as transgender women and others who receive hormonal therapy for gender-affirmation. Evidence has illustrated how feminizing gender-affirmation hormone therapy can significantly improve quality of life, mental status, and breast development in transgender patients and therefore requires surgeons to consider these factors during endocrine treatment (Defreyne et al., 2019).

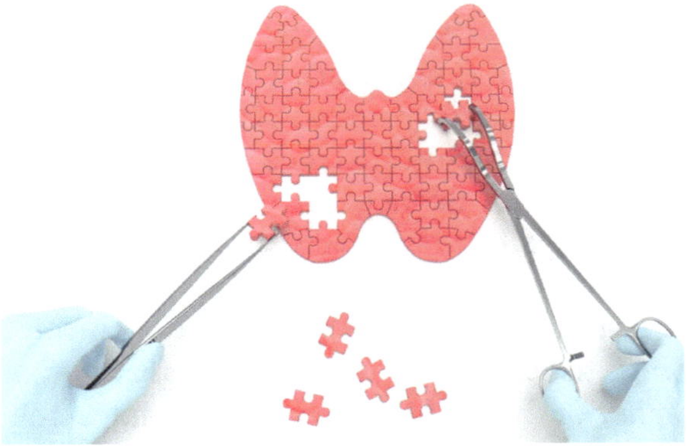

Figure 3.10. Endocrine and breast surgery.

Source: https://www.specialty-hospital.com/uploads/images/services/1/184_28.jpg.

In addition, controversy regarding the impact of hormone therapy on conditions such as breast cancer reveals the complex relationship between hormones and overall health. The incorporation of hormonal consciousness into surgery promotes a more comprehensive approach to patient care, with consideration given to outcomes that extend beyond the surgery itself (Gidron et al., 2011). As such, a good understanding of the endocrine system is increasingly essential for surgeons who practice breast and endocrine surgery (Figure 3.10).

3.4.1. Major Glands of the Endocrine System

The endocrine system comprises numerous major glands that regulate various physiological functions of the body. They include the pituitary, thyroid, adrenal, pancreas, and gonads, all of which participate in the intricate hormonal balancing act required for homeostasis. The pituitary gland, often referred to as the master gland, regulates the other endocrine glands and plays a crucial role in growth, metabolism, and reproduction. When applied to breast and endocrine surgery, knowledge of these glands' role can place hormonal effects in perspective about the development of conditions like endocrine disease or breast cancer. For example, the interaction between the pituitary, thyroid, and ovarian hormones can have a significant impact on breast tissue physiology, potentially guiding surgical intervention and treatment. Appreciation of these glands' functions, therefore, becomes clear in the realization of better patient care within the context of surgical settings. The thyroid gland also maintains metabolism and energy by producing hormones. It's thyroxine (T4) and triiodothyronine (T3) hormones that play a central role in keeping body functions like growth, temperature control, and all bodily functions running. Thyroid dysfunction can lead to significant complications that include breast health and endocrine function as a whole. Hypothyroidism or hyperthyroidism diseases may alter estrogen metabolism, thereby affecting the physiology of breast tissue and causing an enhancement of breast pathology risk. In both breast and endocrine surgery, clinicians must assess thyroid function in advance to ensure optimal patient outcomes. Treatment of endocrine diseases can significantly influence postoperative care and surgical indications, underscoring the need for a multidimensional approach in endocrine surgery that encompasses the evaluation of interrelated gland functions (Quindlen et al., 2019).

The adrenal glands, located on top of the kidneys, are responsible for secreting hormones that control stress responses and metabolic function. Cortisol, a critical hormone released by the adrenal cortex, regulates metabolism, immune response, and blood pressure, while adrenaline, produced by the adrenal medulla, plays a crucial role in the fight-or-flight response. The consequences of adrenal pathology can be pretty high, particularly on breast and endocrine function. For example, excess cortisol production influences estrogen levels, thereby influencing breast tissue with potential for increased cancer risk. Therefore, surgeons who perform breast and endocrine operations must consider adrenal function during diagnosis and treatment plans. Understanding the role of these glands not only enhances surgical decision-making but also highlights the interconnectedness of the endocrine system in maintaining health and disease management (N/A, 2001).

3.4.2. Hormonal Regulation and Its Significance

Hormonal regulation is crucial in the maintenance of the homeostasis of numerous physiological processes, with a significant effect on endocrine and breast function. These hormones, such as estrogen, progesterone, and testosterone, are critical to the growth and differentiation of the breast tissue and influence normal physiology and pathological conditions such as breast cancer. Estrogen, for instance, stimulates cell proliferation, a two-edged sword with respect to breast health: required for normal breast growth, excessively exuberant estrogen signaling can propel malignant transformation of cells. The identification of hormone mechanisms can facilitate the identification of selective therapy and prevention strategies in the management of breast cancer, emphasizing the importance of hormonal balance for health and disease. By understanding such interactions, clinicians can adjust treatment protocols in such a way as to substantially enhance outcomes among patients. The interaction between hormone regulation and cancer is illustrated through the study of vitamin D receptor (VDR) in adrenocortical carcinoma. Downregulation of VDR represents a potential mechanism by which hormonal dysregulation can contribute to malignancy. Loss of VDR expression due to epigenetic modifications, such as methylation, suggests that hormonal signal transduction pathways may be disrupted in certain cancers, including breast cancer.

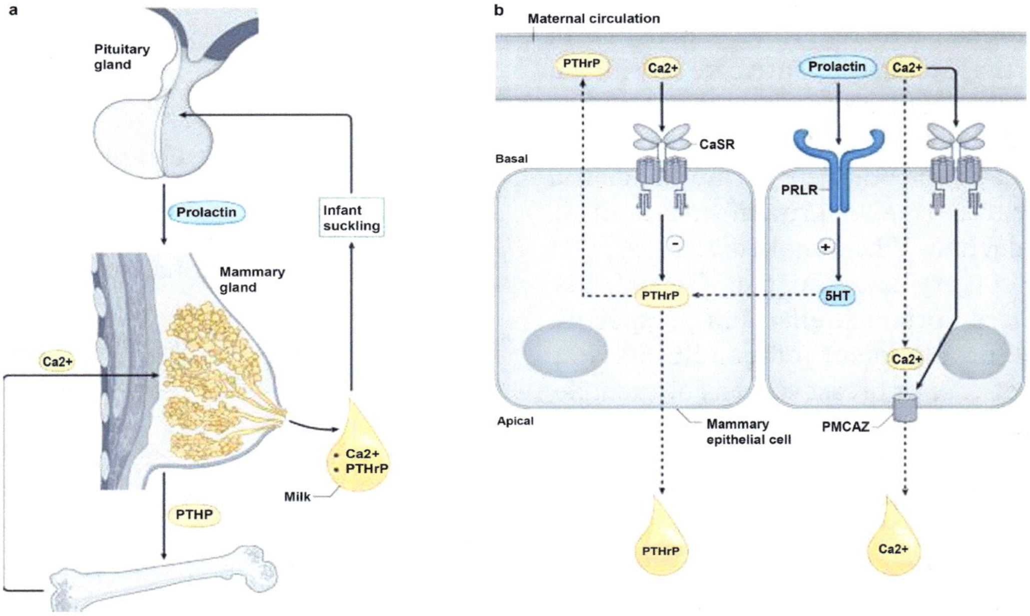

Figure 3.11. Hormonal regulation of mammary gland development and lactation.

Source: https://media.springernature.com/lw685/springer-static/image/art%3A10.1038%2Fs41574-022-00742-y/MediaObjects/41574_2022_742_Fig4_HTML.png.

This underlines the need further to investigate the role of the hormonal microenvironments in oncogenesis. Furthermore, targeting these pathways could potentially offer new therapeutic strategies for the management of both breast and endocrine-related cancers. It is essential to understand the subtleties of hormonal regulation towards the development of effective treatments and diagnostic tools since it may help identify patients at higher risk by virtue of hormonal imbalance. The expression level of specific proteins, such as SMUG1 in breast cancer, also shows how hormonal control intersects with cancer prognosis and treatment response. Decreased levels of SMUG1 have been associated with aggressive tumor behavior and a decrease in patient survival, which emphasizes the relevance of hormonal regulation in tumor biology. Importantly, this study also suggests that levels of SMUG1 can predict the efficacy of adjuvant therapies, including endocrine and chemotherapy treatments. As such, hormonal control is not only implicated in cancer progression but also in therapy outcomes, emphasizing the significance of optimizing our existing understanding of such relationships. By recognizing the importance of hormonal regulation to breast disease and health, healthcare providers are better able to organize treatment modalities, thus improving patient prognosis and quality of care in endocrine and breast surgery practice (Abdel-Fatah et al., 2013; Cappellesso et al., 2015) (Figure 3.11).

3.4.3. Common Endocrine Disorders

Endocrine disorders are fraught with a broad array of complications, particularly those involving breast health and operative outcomes. One significant concern is the disruption of hormone balance, which can lead to a multitude of abnormalities, such as breast enlargement in men or inappropriate mammary gland function in women. Hyperprolactinemia can cause galactorrhea or spontaneous breast enlargement and, therefore, necessitates careful endocrine evaluation. In addition, thyroid illness, such as hypothyroidism or hyperthyroidism, can also greatly influence breast tissue, both metabolically and hormonally. These endocrine ailments not only complicate physical well-being but also introduce complexities to mental status, as hormonal imbalance can exacerbate anxiety and affect quality of life, necessitating a multidisciplinary treatment in the case of breast and endocrine surgical treatments. The relationship between endocrine disease and reproductive health is clearly seen in conditions such as polycystic ovary syndrome (PCOS) where there is a disruption in the balance of hormones that may lead to ovulatory dysfunction and infertility. Women with PCOS are prone to abnormal breast development and changes in mammary tissue due to elevated levels of androgens. Moreover, the psychological consequences associated with these endocrine diseases may lead to immense stress and depression, further exacerbating health issues. Effective management measures, possibly including drug therapy and lifestyle adjustments, are essential. For example, insulin-sensitizing agents, such as those used in cases of insulin resistance, can enhance ovarian function. Care of these issues in the context of breast and endocrine surgery is crucial because appropriate preoperative assessment and individually adapted treatment plans enhance results and optimize patient care, particularly for patients planning surgery who are affected by such hormonal illnesses. Moreover, treatment of endocrine disorders due to gender identity has emerged into the limelight in recent years, a paradigm shift in the way transgender and nonbinary individuals have been treated. Gender-affirming treatment with hormonal interventions, as outlined in the most recent guidelines, is pivotal to the treatment of transgender women, playing an essential role in physical alteration connected with gender identity. Estrogen therapy in combination with androgen blockers leads to breast development in transgender women, profoundly altering their physical features and enhancing psychological well-being. Conversely, transgender men typically undergo testosterone treatment that prompts effects in harmony with their gender identity. However, the side effects of such therapies, such as the risk of venous thromboembolism, along with a host of psychological effects ranging from depression, require vigilant monitoring. Such knowledge educates practitioners on how to provide holistic care and obtain informed consent before initiating treatment, ultimately safeguarding patients' health during transition (Banu et al., 2016; Arcelus et al., 2018).

Test Your Knowledge

1. Which gland regulates metabolism through the secretion of thyroxine (T4)?
2. What hormone does the pancreas release to lower blood glucose levels?

3.5. Surgical Interventions in Endocrine Disorders

Learning Outcome

1. Describe the thyroid surgery: indications and techniques
2. Define the adrenal gland surgery: procedures and outcomes
3. Discuss the parathyroid surgery: diagnosis and treatment

Operations are the key to treating endocrine diseases, specifically conditions such as thyroid nodules, adrenal adenomas, and pituitary adenomas. Thyroidectomy through lobectomy and total thyroidectomy is performed regularly for both malignant and benign nodules to eliminate presenting signs and avert malignancy. In hyperthyroidism, surgery can provide curative treatment in the long run, particularly when patients have been intolerant to drugs or radioactive iodine treatment. Moreover, the particular nature of the endocrine disorder often dictates the most appropriate operation, further emphasizing the need for careful preoperative work-up that might be complemented with imaging studies and endocrine function tests. Last but not least, surgical interventions aim not only to remove diseased tissue but also to regulate hormonal levels, thus highlighting the interplay between surgery and endocrine treatment in the correction of such disorders. Endocrine surgery effects extend beyond tumor removals; it is also an essential aspect of gender-affirming gender transition surgery for transgender persons. The evidence indicates that surgeons and endocrinologists collectively facilitate the transitional process by carrying out gender-affirming surgeries that align physical characteristics with gender identification. Breast enhancement in transgender women and mastectomy in transgender men are such surgeries, paired with hormonal therapy to produce results. The guidelines of The Endocrine Society favor the need to reveal potential risks like venous thromboembolism as well as other complications of cross-sex hormones (Arcelus et al., 2018). Not only does this coordination enhance the physical transition process, but it also significantly benefits better mental health outcomes due to lower depression and anxiety levels post-surgery. In addition, the evolving landscape of survivorship care for surgical patients with endocrine disorders reflects a growing appreciation of the multidimensional impact of therapy.

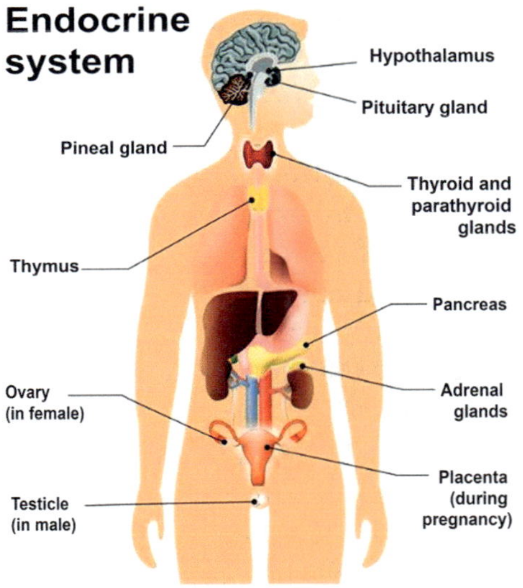

Figure 3.12. Surgical interventions in endocrine disorders.

Source: https://www.news-medical.net/image-handler/picture/Endocrine%20organs%20-%20%20Designua_thumb.jpg.

For surgery of breast cancer, for example, one must keep in mind not just the physical outcomes but also the psychosocial impacts faced by survivors. Although improvements have considerably improved survival in surgery techniques and adjuvant therapy, there are limitations in sexual, functional, and emotional health after treatment. There is an urgent need for robust quality-of-life monitoring using patient-reported outcomes (PROs), as traditional clinical measures often fail to account for these burdens (Ahles et al., 2014). Through the integration of comprehensive survivorship care plans, including emotional and psychological care, the health system can ensure better long-term care for the patients following endocrine surgery, thereby enhancing their overall quality of life (Figure 3.12).

3.5.1. Thyroid Surgery: Indications and Techniques

Thyroid surgery encompasses a range of operations primarily performed to manage various thyroid disorders of the thyroid gland, including nodular goiter, thyroid malignancy, and hyperthyroidism, among others. Among the most significant indications for surgery are thyroid nodules with suspicious features as shown on imaging or cytology, warranting further evaluation. In addition, those patients who have big goiters may form compressive symptoms, such as dysphagia or respiratory compromise, that need surgery to re-establish the pathway. In a few cases, the refractory quality of hyperthyroidism to medical therapy may also necessitate the application of surgery. It needs to be understood that such indications in the quest to have a uniform practice in the care of patients, where surgery must be only as needed, and in the interest of patients' general well-being and health. The techniques employed in thyroid surgery have undergone significant changes, particularly driven by advances in technology and surgical practice. The recent past has witnessed the evolution of less invasive techniques such as the minimally invasive video-assisted thyroidectomy (MIVAT) and others based on endoscopic techniques. They are directed towards reducing postoperative pain, scarring, and facilitating a quicker recovery to normal activity compared to open surgery. A case in point would be the MIVAT technique that allows for more diminutive sites of incision, which can lead to improved cosmetic outcomes and quicker recovery to regular activity. Furthermore, the choice of operative technique is generally determined by the type of disease to be treated, the surgeon's operative expertise, and patient preferences, illustrating the importance of individualized treatment protocols in thyroid surgery. Through determination of the patient's individual factors, healthcare workers can enhance both the effectiveness and safety of the surgical procedures. Notably, the choice of operative techniques also involves a thorough evaluation of potential complications and patients' long-term outcomes. Evidence indicates that while minimally invasive methods have several advantages, they also come with a couple of disadvantages, such as prolonged operation times and postoperative pain in some cases, particularly with more complex procedures, like the transaxillary method (Lang et al., 2013). Complications, such as recurrent laryngeal nerve (RLN) injury, may also occur regardless of the surgical technique used, underscoring the importance of experience in the surgical procedure. Follow-up and observation of the patient repeatedly after surgery are essential to assess the efficacy of the method used and the quality of life after surgery. Proper planning and execution of thyroid surgeries are thus vital to ensure patient safety along with optimal therapeutic outcomes (Figure 3.13).

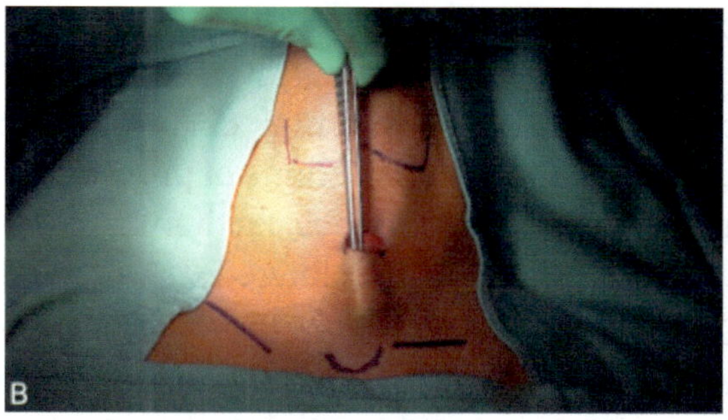

Figure 3.13. Minimally-invasive video-assisted thyroidectomy (MIVAT).

Source: https://ars.els-cdn.com/content/image/3-s2.0-B978032366127000034X-f34-06b-9780323661270.jpg.

3.5.2. Adrenal Gland Surgery: Procedures and Outcomes

In surgical endocrinology, surgery of the adrenal glands has become a leading branch with the increasing incidence of adrenal tumors like pheochromocytomas and other functioning masses. Laparoscopic adrenalectomy is currently considered the gold standard in the treatment of benign adrenal masses with a size less than 6 cm. The technique is minimally invasive with reduced rates of morbidity, less blood loss, and quicker recovery compared to open surgery. As alluded to in recent reviews, effective preoperative assessment is essential and involves clinical examination, laboratory work, and imaging studies for diagnosis and surgical care. This preoperative planning is crucial to operative success and highlights the role of multidisciplinary teams in managing such complex cases (Avenia et al., 2018).

The technical ability of laparoscopic adrenalectomy has significantly advanced in recent years, enhancing procedural outcomes. With skilled hands, the operative time for this operation has been significantly reduced, as evidenced by studies that reflect a considerable improvement after the surgeons' learning curves. The initial series of operations, for instance, tends to have longer operative times and more blood loss; however, with the improvement of surgical techniques, safety and efficiency increase. This type of learning curve highlights the need for a minimum volume of procedures to achieve maximum outcomes, further supporting the importance of specialized training and expertise in high-volume operating centers. Such facilities are increasingly recognized as a necessary component for the treatment of adrenal pathologies, where postoperative complications are minimized through close collaboration between endocrine surgeons, anesthesiologists, and endocrinologists (Avenia et al., 2018). Postoperative outcomes following adrenal gland surgery are generally favorable, particularly in terms of the return of endocrine function to normal. Literature has a high success rate in restoring patients with functioning tumors to normal hormone levels following laparoscopic adrenalectomy with low complications in a minimal number of cases. The safety record of the procedure is evidenced by the rarity of significant complications, making it increasingly appealing as a treatment option for adrenal disease. Furthermore, pre-operative medication and individualized care plans have been shown to optimize results in specific conditions, including Conn's syndrome and Cushing's disease. Not only do these developments improve the intra-operative period of recovery, but they also contribute to longer-term management regimens for the surgical patient of the adrenal gland, affirming the relevance of procedural development in endocrine surgery.

3.5.3. Parathyroid Surgery: Diagnosis and Treatment

Parathyroid disorders are primarily diagnosed by measuring calcium and parathyroid hormone (PTH) levels in the blood. Hyperparathyroidism, where there is elevated calcium and increased levels of PTH, typically calls for surgical intervention, especially where patients have symptoms or complications such as kidney stones or osteoporosis. A thorough clinical evaluation, comprehensive patient history, and physical examination are essential to establish the underlying etiology of the disorder accurately. Imaging techniques, including ultrasound and sestamibi scan, play an essential role in localizing preoperative sites of abnormal parathyroid glands. These diagnostic modalities not only enhance the surgical plan but also ensure safe and effective treatment outcomes, as knowledge of parathyroid anatomy can decrease intraoperative complications. Accordingly, complete diagnostic evaluations are integral to maximal surgical care in such individuals with presumptive parathyroid disease. Surgery for parathyroid disease is most commonly parathyroidectomy, which aims to remove the hyperfunctioning gland(s) to correct calcium homeostasis. The method of surgery—whether traditional open or minimally invasive—is dependent on a variety of factors, including patient health, multigland disease, and the surgeons' expertise. Minimally invasive parathyroidectomy is more commonly associated with smaller incisions and decreased recovery times, emphasizing advances in surgical technology and techniques. Furthermore, intrasurgical monitoring of PTH provides immediate feedback regarding the success of the procedure, allowing surgeons to confirm successful resection of hypersecreting glands. As described in existing literature, such innovations allied with traditional surgical techniques have the potential to enhance postoperative outcomes and patient safety, emphasizing the dynamic evolution of parathyroid surgery in clinical practice. In addition to surgery, postoperative care and observation are also crucial for managing potential complications and achieving long-term success. Transient hypocalcemia may develop in postoperative patients, which must be carefully monitored with serum calcium levels and supplemented as required. The use of autofluorescence (AF) imaging techniques intra-operatively has been encouraging in facilitating the distinction between parathyroid glands and thyroid tissue, as well as in preserving gland function without increasing complication rates. AF technology, although still in its infancy in the field of endocrinology, represents a significant new advance in surgical techniques and underscores the multidisciplinary nature of parathyroid surgery. As patient management and the technique of surgery both improve and diversify with our understanding, the prospects for patients who have parathyroid surgery become brighter by the day, paving the way for improved diagnosis, treatment, and recovery in the field of breast and endocrine surgery (Figure 3.14).

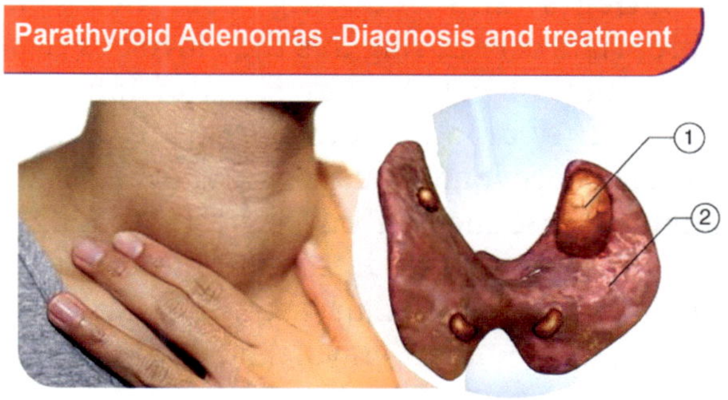

Figure 3.14. Parathyroid adenomas diagnosis and treatment.

Source: https://www.drvpareek.com/wp-content/uploads/2021/04/Parathyroid-Adenomas-Diagnosis-And-Treatment.jpg.

Test Your Knowledge

1. What are the indications for thyroidectomy in patients with thyroid nodules?
2. Which complications are most commonly associated with parathyroid surgery?

3.6. Postoperative Care and Complications

Learning Outcome

1. Describe the recovery process after breast and endocrine surgery
2. Define the potential complications and their management in breast and endocrine surgery
3. Identify the importance of follow-up care of breast and endocrine surgery

Postoperative care of endocrine and breast surgery is crucial to sustaining recovery in patients and reducing complications. Appropriate care during this time involves close observation of patients for signs of infection, hemorrhage, or other undesirable reactions, which may occur after surgery. In the meantime, patients are educated on self-care practices, such as proper wound dressing and recognizing unusual symptoms that require immediate consultation with a physician. Additionally, establishing a multidisciplinary team comprising surgeons, nurses, and pharmacists is crucial for ensuring comprehensive postoperative care. Collaboration has the potential to identify and prevent early risk factors, thereby enhancing patient outcomes and the quality of care. The patient's comorbidities and age significantly impact the likelihood of postoperative complications following breast cancer surgery. From studies, elderly patients, especially those aged over 85 years, have a statistically significant risk increase for developing complications (Accurso et al., 2013). Preconditions such as polypharmacy and the presence of multiple chronic conditions only contribute to these dangers, with those patients who have three or more comorbidities having an increased risk of postoperative complications (Accurso et al., 2013). Preoperative examinations thus need to closely evaluate these dangers to implement suitable intervention measures, which may include altered surgical procedures or enhanced postoperative monitoring. Identification and prevention of these complications are critical in the management of patient treatment and for optimizing surgical outcomes. Postoperative complications not only endanger the recovery of the patient but also can harm long-term survival as well. Complications are strongly associated with compromised global survival for patients who have had breast surgery (Accurso et al., 2013). This worse prognosis is not simply because of the complications per se but also because of intrinsic geriatric parameters, such as functional status and comorbidity, that in turn can influence recovery trajectories. Thus, early intervention in these problems during the recovery process is required to improve not only the short-term postoperative course but also the long-term health outcomes for patients. Lastly, operating teams must be well aware of the complexities involved in postoperative care if complications are to be minimized and best recovery pathways encouraged for women undergoing breast and endocrine surgery (Figure 3.15).

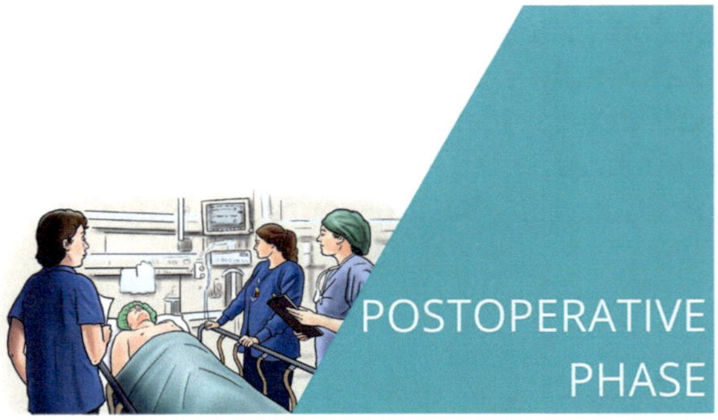

Figure 3.15. Postoperative phase of breast.

Source: https://i.ytimg.com/vi/C4-nwpkEEq0/maxresdefault.jpg.

3.6.1. Recovery Process After Breast and Endocrine Surgery

The recovery process after breast and endocrine surgery is a multifaceted process incorporating physical, emotional, and psychological aspects. The patient tends to experience a range of postoperative symptoms, including pain, swelling, and lethargy, which are natural responses to surgical trauma. The control of pain is crucial, as it not only boosts comfort but also enables one to participate in rehabilitation procedures necessary for restoring strength and mobility. Postoperative expectations need to be presented to the patient clearly so that anxiety is minimized and follow-through with recovery orders can be encouraged. Additionally, incorporating physical therapy into the recovery model can significantly enhance mobility and accelerate recovery, allowing patients to transition directly from the hospital to home care. In addition to physical rehabilitation of the patient, psychological considerations also play a powerful role in the healing process overall. For instance, women who receive breast cancer diagnoses commonly face emotional problems such as depression and anxiety. Researchers have found that childhood experiences of maltreatment can affect psychological resilience and coping in adult life, perhaps further affecting the course of recovery from breast surgery. Specifically, one study demonstrated that lower optimism and mindfulness mediate the relationship between childhood maltreatment and higher depressive symptoms in women with breast cancer (Asher et al., 2017). Therefore, provision of psychological support through counseling or support groups is important because it increases emotional well-being and can lead to improved treatment adherence and overall health outcomes. Also, the need for follow-up cannot be overstated after endocrine and breast surgery during postoperative recovery. Follow-up clinical checkups are a must in order to monitor for potential complications or disease recurrence, most importantly in the case of breast cancer, in which the detection of potential problems at an early stage can significantly improve prognosis. A good follow-up schedule ensures that healthcare providers can promptly intervene on issues arising post-surgery, such as wound healing or lymphedema complications. The patients should also be instructed in self-monitoring skills to detect abnormal symptoms early on (Ndongo et al., 2010). Lastly, a collaborative effort among healthcare professionals, patients, and their families can create a recovery-conducive environment, enabling patients to regain their health and quality of life.

3.6.2. Possible Complications and Their Management

In endocrine and breast surgery, surgical procedure-related complications must be evaluated carefully and managed effectively. Of these complications, postoperative wound infections are frequent and can cause significant morbidity. Patient age, comorbid illnesses, and the type of surgical intervention are risk factors for infection. The operating team must maintain strict aseptic technique intra-operatively and instruct patients in wound care after surgery. Furthermore, the use of prophylactic antibiotics minimizes infection rates, particularly in high-risk patients. Utilization of a multidisciplinary approach with infection control practitioners can enhance infection control when an infection occurs, thereby improving patient outcomes. Prevention of risk of surgical site infection through rigorous preoperative preparation and stringent postoperative watchfulness is imperative in the practice of endocrine and breast surgery. Hematoma formation is a severe complication of breast and endocrine operations and results from either suboptimal hemostasis or postoperative bleeding. Hematoma leads to protracted pain, delay in wound healing, and potential requirement for reoperation, complicating recovery. Effective management begins with meticulous surgical technique to avoid complications of bleeding, and post-operative monitoring is essential to be able to detect evidence of hematoma early. In those patients in whom hematomas are recognized, early intervention is necessary. This can be observed with supportive care or, in more severe cases, operative evacuation to decompress and restore normal anatomy. Patients should be taught about postoperative signs and symptoms of hematoma to allow them to report complications early if they arise. As a whole, anticipatory practice and patient education are key components in reducing the risk of hematoma formation in this specialty area of surgery. The synergy of age and postoperative complication management is a unique challenge in the management of breast cancer, particularly in older women, who typically respond differently to surgery. As explained, the majority of women over the age of 70 might not get standard treatment due to interrelated factors such as co-morbid conditions and patient preferences, which eventually make outcome prediction challenging. It is paramount that care teams use this comprehensive assessment that considers both the physiological impact of aging and patient autonomy in treatment. A multidisciplinary team, integrating geriatricians, can enhance decision-making with individualized and sensitive treatment plans that are cognizant of the complexity of older patients. With more aged populations, research on the preferences and results for such populations is still essential, with the focus still being on evidence-based practice in the care of potential complications of surgical procedures (Audisio et al., 2009).

Hence, understanding such dynamics also guides improved patient care as well as tailored interventions that nullify risks based on age.

3.6.3. Importance of Follow-Up Care

Follow-up care is an essential component of the therapeutic continuum for patients undergoing breast and endocrine procedures. It serves a twofold function: not only does it help keep track of recovery from surgery, but it also plays a significant role in the provision of long-term treatment plans. For instance, patients on aromatase inhibitors (AIs) may have varied problems leading to non-adherence, like misunderstanding the significance of their therapy. The study reveals that persistent and non-persistent women on AIs share the same information needs regarding expected side effects and symptom control. This suggests that successful follow-up care, characterized by effective communication, can significantly impact adherence to invasive therapy and, consequently, patient outcomes (Green et al., 2019). By making patients available for individualized follow-up consultations, health professionals can guide women through the complexities of medication taking and facilitate better decision-making regarding their well-being. A further critical element of follow-up after breast and endocrine surgery is attention to surveillance for complications or recurrence. Regular follow-up visits provide clinicians with the opportunity to conduct thorough examinations, which allow for the recognition of any resulting surgical complications or new illnesses in a timely manner. For the patient's part, this not only reassures them regarding their recuperative process but also stimulates active cooperation with their health. In particular, transgender women undergoing feminizing gender-affirming hormone therapy (GAHT) have particular health issues, such as cardiovascular disorders as well as breast cancer-associated complications (Defreyne et al., 2019). Such particular risks can be addressed through follow-up treatment that includes tailored interventions to mitigate the long-term health implications. Consequently, an effective follow-up plan emerges as a crucial requirement to ensure the patient's survival following surgery. Moreover, post-operative follow-up care is also key to enhancing patients' quality of life. It is a platform where psychosocial care can be provided by health workers, not just focusing on physical healthcare but also on the emotional and psychological needs of the patients. The holistic care is of top priority, particularly for those struggling with complex identities or social understandings of their health. In breast and endocrine surgery, patients experience a spectrum of emotions related to body image, femininity, and social acceptance that deeply impact their psychological health. An official follow-up program can offer counseling facilities and create milieux that validate patients' experiences. These types of extensive care measures to empower patients throughout their process, reminding them to come back for follow-up as well as enhancing overall satisfaction with their surgical outcome (Green et al., 2019). Follow-up may then transform the post-operative experience into a more fully supportive one by addressing physical and psychological aspects of care for the patients (Figure 3.16).

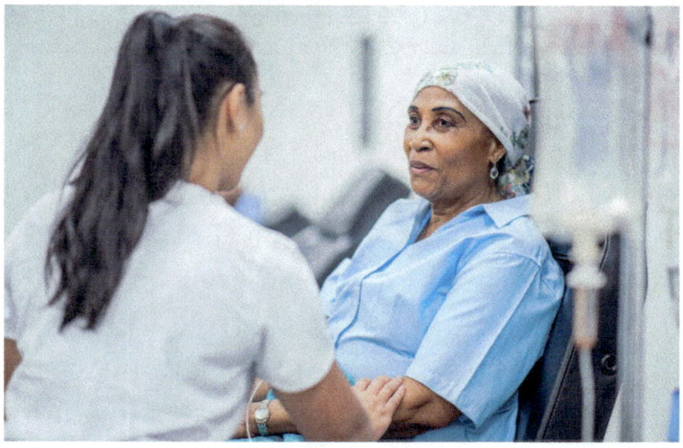

Figure 3.16. Follow-up care of the continuum of treatment for patients.

Source: https://www.novanthealth.org/globalassets/image-field/1-full-width-size-image/images-size-2800x1800/care-images/woman-patient-nurse-cancer-support-2800-1800px.webp.

Test Your Knowledge

1. What are the early signs of hypocalcemia following parathyroid surgery?
2. How is thyroid hormone replacement managed after total thyroidectomy?

SUMMARY

The area of breast and endocrine surgery has advanced, indicating the necessity of patient-specific treatment plans. The use of endocrine therapy, particularly in patients with estrogen receptor-positive (ER-positive) breast cancer, reflects the significant contribution made by customized care. Research indicates that therapies such as primary letrozole therapy are beneficial for old patients who are not satisfactory candidates for surgery. Primarily, a pilot study demonstrated that patients who received letrozole had a clinical response in 60% of cases, which justified its implementation as a first-line treatment among this group of people. Therefore, the above examples suggest that progress in surgical and endocrine treatment can meet various needs of patients, finally improving outcomes and quality of life among breast cancer patients (Agarwal et al., 2014). Furthermore, the long-term consequences of therapies such as radiation and chemotherapy need careful consideration during breast cancer survivorship. There is emerging evidence that suggests these treatments can have permanent effects on cellular aging biomarkers, which possess the potential to influence patient health years after their initial treatment. Studies have revealed that patients who are being treated with chemotherapy and/or radiation have higher levels of DNA damage and lower telomerase activity compared to those being treated with surgery alone. This indicates that there is a requirement for ongoing care and follow-up for survivors of breast cancer, placing healthcare providers in the position of remembering not only short-term outcomes but also long-term treatment effects (Bower et al., 2017). Lastly, the research findings of the studies mentioned earlier affirm the multi-faceted approach required in breast and endocrine surgery. As intra-operative techniques develop, the interaction between hormonal therapy is vital in managing complex cases, especially in high-risk patients. Interestingly, personalized medicine is increasingly becoming an issue as there are diverse reactions among patients to endocrine treatment, as well as their individual experiences with post-treatment illness. As research evolves, it will be essential to measure clinical efficacy and quality of life indicators, ensuring that the benefits of breast and endocrine surgery echo throughout the patient's lifetime. At the intersection of surgical expertise and endocrine therapy, future trends in the area will be shaped, underscoring the importance of global care strategies in enhancing patient outcomes.

In mapping the multifaceted landscape of breast and endocrine surgery, specific dominant themes emerge that reflect both the advances in medical research and the strategic imperative for investment. The primary contribution of medical research charities, particularly within the UK, is the proof of the case for continued investment to identify the causes of disease and develop new treatments. This is a significant investment as medical research charities give more than £1 billion annually, with Cancer Research, UK giving more than £350 million alone to support cancer research. The Office of Health Economics states that funding from various sources increases cooperation and innovation, noting that a decline in government funding would slow overall advances in cancer treatment and outcomes. Therefore, maintaining multiple lines of funding is essential for formulating inclusive research programs that can improve diagnosis and treatment for breast and endocrine surgery (Crane et al., 2014). Endocrinologists' practice in the multidisciplinary management of healthcare requires hormonal therapy as an essential component, particularly in transgender and gender nonbinary individuals. Proof affirms that gender-affirming hormone therapy results in substantial physical and psychological health gains. Endocrine Society guidelines advocate for the utilization of specific treatment regimens among transgender women and men, specifically estrogens and testosterone, both utilized to create desired changes in the body such as breast development, deepening of voice, and redistribution of fat. Not only are these treatments meant to bring bodily aesthetic enhancements, but also to mitigate mental health issues that commonly co-occur with gender dysphoria. Discussion about potential side effects, such as the risk of venous thromboembolism in trans women, is crucial to ensure patient safety and informed consent in the context of breast and endocrine surgery (Arcelus et al., 2018).

As breast and endocrine surgery evolves in the future, there is a need for future research to establish long-term outcomes and enhance treatment protocols. The discussion regarding gender-affirming therapies indicates that there is an urgent need for more comprehensive research comparing the physical and psychosocial impacts of hormone therapy in different populations, including those of nonbinary individuals. Similarly, charity-funded research studies have identified measurable impacts on treatment outcomes that ultimately benefit a larger population of patients. In the coming years, there will be a need to integrate data from both endocrinology and cancer studies to further advance personalized treatment practices. Through closing gaps in evidence and fostering collaboration among various stakeholders, the paradigm of breast and endocrine surgery can be significantly changed, ultimately leading to improved patient outcomes and universal healthcare equity (Crane et al., 2014; Arcelus et al., 2018).

KEY TERMS FROM THIS CHAPTER

- Adrenalectomy
- BRCA mutation
- Breast reconstruction
- Goiter
- Hormonal evaluation
- Insulinoma
- Mastectomy
- Axillary dissection
- Breast carcinoma
- Fibroadenoma
- Graves' disease
- Hyperparathyroidism
- Lumpectomy
- Medullary thyroid cancer

CRITICAL THINKING QUESTIONS

1. **Which of the following is included in the "Triple Assessment" of a breast lump?**
   a. MRI, FNAC, and clinical exam
   b. Ultrasound, mammogram, and MRI
   c. Clinical exam, imaging, and FNAC/core biopsy
   d. CT scan, biopsy, and serum CA-125
2. **Which breast cancer subtype is most likely to be estrogen receptor (ER) positive?**
   a. Triple-negative carcinoma
   b. HER2-positive carcinoma
   c. Inflammatory breast carcinoma
   d. Luminal A subtype
3. **Which electrolyte abnormality is commonly associated with primary hyperparathyroidism?**
   a. Hypocalcemia
   b. Hyperkalemia
   c. Hypercalcemia
   d. Hyponatremia
4. **The most common cause of thyrotoxicosis in young women is:**
   a. Toxic adenoma
   b. Thyroid carcinoma
   c. Graves' disease
   d. Subacute thyroiditis
5. **A 40-year-old woman undergoes total thyroidectomy and develops hoarseness of voice postoperatively. The most likely nerve injured is:**
   a. Superior laryngeal nerve
   b. Phrenic nerve
   c. Recurrent laryngeal nerve
   d. Hypoglossal nerve

Short Answer Questions

1. What are the key differences between fibroadenoma and breast carcinoma in terms of clinical presentation and investigation?
2. Describe the Triple Assessment approach in the evaluation of a breast lump.
3. What are the indications for breast-conserving surgery versus mastectomy in breast cancer?
4. Explain the role of sentinel lymph node biopsy in breast cancer management.
5. Describe the clinical features and biochemical diagnosis of primary hyperparathyroidism.
6. What are the complications of total thyroidectomy, and how are they prevented intraoperatively?
7. Discuss the differences between Graves' disease and toxic multinodular goiter in terms of clinical features and management.
8. Outline the surgical management options for a patient with medullary thyroid carcinoma.

Answers to Critical Thinking Questions

1. (c); 2. (d); 3. (c); 4. (c); 5. (c)

REFERENCES

1. Abdel-Fatah, T. M. A., Albarakati, N., Bowell, L., Agarwal, D., Moseley, P., Hawkes, C., Ball, G., Chan, S., Ellis, I. O., & Madhusudan, S. (2013). Single-strand selective monofunctional uracil-DNA glycosylase (SMUG1) deficiency is linked to aggressive breast cancer and predicts response to adjuvant therapy. *Breast Cancer Research and Treatment, 142*(3), 515–527. https://doi.org/10.1007/s10549-013-2769-6Accurso, A., Amato, B., Compagna, R., Rispoli, C., Pagano, G., Rengo, G., et al. (2013). *Breast cancer surgery in elderly patients: Postoperative complications and survival.* https://core.ac.uk/download/55113861.pdf (accessed on 12th July 2025).
2. Agarwal, V., Cawkwell, L., Drew, P. J., Fox, J., et al. (2014). *Clinical response to primary letrozole therapy in elderly patients with early breast cancer: Possible role for p53 as a biomarker.* https://core.ac.uk/download/151156899.pdf (accessed on 12th July 2025).
3. Ahles, T., Fellowes, J., Fleissig, A., Hermelink, K., Janelsins, M., Jenkins, V., Mann, E., et al. (2014). *Psychosocial/survivorship issues in breast cancer: Are we doing better?* https://core.ac.uk/download/30609789.pdf (accessed on 12th July 2025).
4. Ahmed, S. F., & Markosyan, R. (2017). *Sex assignment in conditions affecting sex development.* https://core.ac.uk/download/150597685.pdf (accessed on 12th July 2025).
5. Aigner, F., Pratschke, J., Schumann, T., Stockmann, M., et al. (2020). *Recent advances and the potential for clinical use of autofluorescence detection of extra-ophthalmic tissues.* https://core.ac.uk/download/323257980.pdf (accessed on 12th July 2025).
6. Albain, K. S., Barry, W. T., Bellon, J. R., Burstein, H. J., et al. (2019). *Local-regional recurrence in women with small node-negative, HER2-positive breast cancer: Results from a prospective multi-institutional study (the APT trial).* https://core.ac.uk/download/224407472.pdf (accessed on 12th July 2025).
7. Arcelus, J., Gooren, L., Klink, D., T'Sjoen, G., et al. (2018). *Endocrinology of transgender medicine.* https://core.ac.uk/download/162667742.pdf (accessed on 12th July 2025).
8. Asher, A., Bower, J. E., Boyle, C. C., Crespi, C. M., et al. (2017). *Childhood maltreatment, psychological resources, and depressive symptoms in women with breast cancer.* https://core.ac.uk/download/286729277.pdf (accessed on 12th July 2025).
9. Assanti, A. P., Colao, A., Del Prete, M., Faggiano, A., et al. (2012). *Thyroid nodules treated with percutaneous radiofrequency thermal ablation: A comparative study.* https://core.ac.uk/download/159268412.pdf (accessed on 12th July 2025).
10. Association of Breast Surgery Surgical Gap Analysis Working Group, Benson, J. R., Carmichael, A. R., Cutress, R. I., et al. (2018). *Opportunities and priorities for breast surgical research.* https://core.ac.uk/download/159767346.pdf (accessed on 12th July 2025).
11. Audisio, R. A., Reed, M. W. R., & Wyld, L. (2009). *The role of surgery in the treatment of older women with breast cancer.*
12. Avenia, N., Bellastella, G., Candela, G., Clarizia, G., et al. (2018). *Single center experience with laparoscopic adrenalectomy on a large clinical series.* https://core.ac.uk/download/pdf/154859595.pdf (accessed on 12th July 2025).
13. Baccari, P., Cappabianca, S., D'Andrea, A., Falcone, M., et al. (2016). *Pancreatic tumors imaging: An update.* https://core.ac.uk/download/98333045.pdf (accessed on 12th July 2025).

14. Banu, P., Bălălău, C., Constantin, V. D., Motofei, I., et al. (2016). *The postfinasteride syndrome: An overview*. https://core.ac.uk/download/144552981.pdf (accessed on 12th July 2025).

15. Barbiere, J. M., Baum, M., Coleman, M. P., Lyratzopoulos, G., et al. (2011). *Changes over time in socioeconomic inequalities in breast and rectal cancer survival in England and Wales during a 32-year period (1973–2004): The potential role of health care*. https://core.ac.uk/download/13093422.pdf (accessed on 12th July 2025).

16. Basso, S. M. M., Lumachi, F., & Santeufemia, D. A. (2015). *Current medical treatment of estrogen receptor-positive breast cancer*. https://core.ac.uk/download/53525256.pdf (accessed on 12th July 2025).

17. Bower, J. E., Breen, E. C., Carroll, J. E., Chapman, J. M., et al. (2017). *Biomarkers of aging associated with past treatments in breast cancer survivors*. https://core.ac.uk/download/323078736.pdf (accessed on 12th July 2025).

18. Cappellesso, R., Fallo, F., Fassina, A., Guzzardo, V., et al. (2015). *Methylation status of vitamin D receptor gene promoter in benign and malignant adrenal tumors*. https://core.ac.uk/download/80156880.pdf (accessed on 12th July 2025).

19. Cox, A., Howell, A., Kamb, A., Maurice, A., Moyer, A., Renwick, A., Rodger, A., et al. (2008). *Evaluation of the current knowledge limitations in breast cancer research: A gap analysis*. https://core.ac.uk/download/51353.pdf (accessed on 12th July 2025).

20. Crane, P., Farrell, C., Garau, M., Grassano, N., et al. (2014). *Exploring the interdependencies of research funders in the UK*. https://core.ac.uk/download/30608686.pdf (accessed on 12th July 2025).

21. David, A., Moadel, A. B., Winzelberg, A. J., Sandgren, A. K., Association of Breast Surgery at BASO, Pestalozzi, B., Andersen, B. L., et al. (2012). *Options for early breast cancer follow-up in primary and secondary care: A systematic review*. https://core.ac.uk/download/9562640.pdf (accessed on 12th July 2025).

22. Defreyne, J., Iwamoto, S. J., Motmans, J., Rothman, M., et al. (2019). *Health considerations for transgender women and remaining unknowns: A narrative review*. https://core.ac.uk/download/237010802.pdf (accessed on 12th July 2025).

23. Domschke, C., Fuchs, V., Golatta, M., Heil, J., et al. (2012). *Extent of primary breast cancer surgery: Standards and individualized concepts*. https://core.ac.uk/download/32585121.pdf (accessed on 12th July 2025).

24. Gidron, Y., Kishore, U., Nowicky, A. V., Parton, A., et al. (2011). *Hemispheric lateralization and immune function: A systematic review of human research*. https://core.ac.uk/download/20496329.pdf (accessed on 12th July 2025).

25. Green, E., Khakshooy, S., Pieters, H. C., Sleven, M., et al. (2019). *A qualitative comparison of how older breast cancer survivors process treatment information regarding endocrine therapy*. https://core.ac.uk/download/323079874.pdf (accessed on 12th July 2025).

26. Jyothsna, M. (2016). *Feasibility and oncological safety of axillary reverse mapping in early breast cancer, using premixed serum and indocyanine green dye fluorescence technique and an in-house near-infrared fluorescence imaging system and methylene blue dye: ARM study*. https://core.ac.uk/download/235659072.pdf (accessed on 12th July 2025).

27. Kyrou, I., & Weickert, M. O. (2010). *Clinical problems caused by obesity*. https://core.ac.uk/download/46324.pdf (accessed on 12th July 2025).

28. Lang, B. H. H., & Wong, K. P. (2013). *Endoscopic thyroidectomy: A literature review and update.* https://core.ac.uk/download/38015984.pdf (accessed on 12th July 2025).

29. Maran, N. R. (2017). *Prospective study to evaluate the prophylactic effects of Inj. Methyl prednisolone against seroma formation in post modified radical mastectomy patients.* https://core.ac.uk/download/288215926.pdf (accessed on 12th July 2025).

30. Martí, C., & Sánchez-Méndez, J. I. (2020). *Neoadjuvant endocrine therapy for luminal breast cancer treatment: A first-choice alternative in times of crisis such as the COVID-19 pandemic.* https://repositorio.uam.es/bitstream/10486/691074/1/neoadjuvant_marti_ECM_2020.pdf (accessed on 12th July 2025).

31. Mathew, R. T. (2017). *The prognostic role of VEGF in head and neck squamous cell carcinoma.* https://open.bu.edu/bitstream/2144/23808/5/Mathew_bu_0017N_12667.pdf (accessed on 12th July 2025).

32. Ndongo, B. C., Mballa, G. A. E., Hyder, A. A., Juillard, C., et al. (2010). *Patterns of injury and violence in Yaoundé, Cameroon: An analysis of hospital data.* https://core.ac.uk/download/323075033.pdf (accessed on 12th July 2025).

33. Quindlen, K. A. (2019). *Reflexology.* https://cupola.gettysburg.edu/cgi/viewcontent.cgi?article=1840&context=student_scholarship (accessed on 12th July 2025).

UPPER GASTROINTESTINAL SURGERY

4

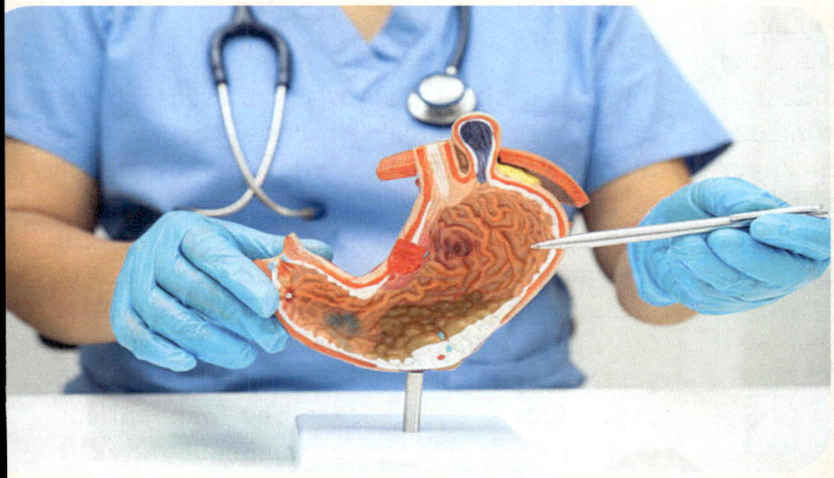

LEARNING OBJECTIVES

After studying this chapter, you will be able to:

1. Understand the anatomy of the upper gastrointestinal tract
2. Explain the indications for upper gastrointestinal surgery
3. Discuss the types of upper gastrointestinal surgical procedures
4. Focus on preoperative assessment and preparation
5. Learn about surgical techniques and approaches
6. Evaluate the postoperative care and complications

Introduction

Upper gastrointestinal (UGI) surgery is a collection of operations on the upper part of the gastrointestinal tract, including the esophagus, stomach, and the first segment of the small intestine or the duodenum. The subspecialty is crucial in the management of an extensive range of disorders such as malignancies, peptic ulcer disease, and severe gastroesophageal reflux disease. The evolution of UGI surgery as a distinct specialty has its roots in advances in surgery techniques and technologies, specifically in minimally invasive surgery, that have created more opportunities for patient care. With further advancements in the specialty, more emphasis is given to the synchronization of surgical methods with evidence-based practice to enhance patient outcomes and reduce complications. The complexity of these procedures requires a thorough understanding of both anatomy and the physiological effects of surgical intervention. The increasing prevalence of disease of the upper gastrointestinal tract, together with advances in technology, has resulted in greater involvement being given to the use of imaging and diagnostic methods in the planning of surgical treatment. For instance, GIUS is strongly promoted for application in clinical practice, and professional working groups such as the European Federation of Societies for Ultrasound in Medicine and Biology are mobilizing its use in UGI investigation. As previously reported, the GIUS working group aims to develop guidelines for clinical use that enhance the interpretation of ultrasound findings, ultimately providing timely and effective surgical treatment (Calabrese et al., 2016). These developments constitute a significant milestone toward the application of sophisticated imaging modalities in preoperative evaluation, thereby maximizing surgical planning and patient care in upper GI surgery. Furthermore, integration of quality improvement programs into surgical practice and training has emerged as essential in UGI surgery.

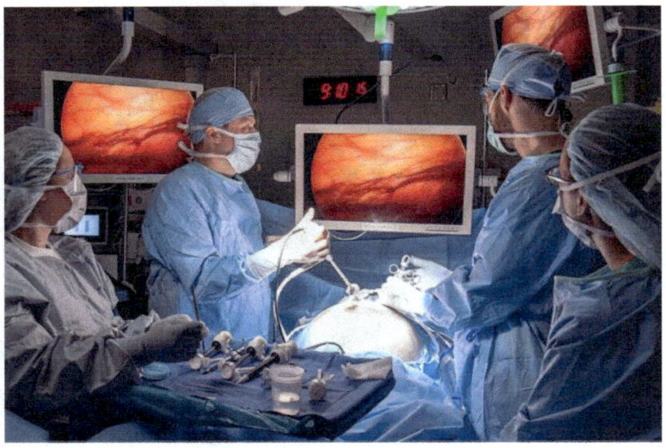

Figure 4.1. Upper-GI-surgery.

Source: https://www.hillsgastrocare.com/wp-content/uploads/2022/08/Upper-GI-Surgery-672x448.jpg.

Educational schemes that encourage medical students to become involved in quality improvement programs and learn from a series of cases not only enhance learning but also improve overall surgical practice. As the deliberations on the involvement of medical students in comparable schemes suggest, fostering a culture of responsibility and continuous learning enables surgeons to respond more effectively to the complexities of UGI surgical procedures and patient care (N/A, 2018). By focusing on these areas, the specialty not only enhances surgical technique but also educates future surgeons to meet the challenges presented by upper gastrointestinal disease, and ultimately leads to healthier results (Figure 4.1).

Definition of Upper Gastrointestinal Surgery

Upper gastrointestinal surgery is a subspecialty branch of surgical practice focused on the care of conditions affecting the upper gastrointestinal tract, including the esophagus, stomach, and duodenum. It is a surgical specialty with numerous procedures aimed at managing benign and malignant diseases of the upper gastrointestinal organs, including gastroesophageal reflux disease (GERD), peptic ulcers, and cancers. The interventions performed can range from minimally invasive techniques, such as laparoscopy, to more significant open surgery with a longer recovery time. The increased prevalence of upper gastrointestinal disease generates a need for continuous innovation in surgical procedures, making the importance of proficiency in both newer and older technologies crucial to obtaining the best patient outcomes in this high-priority area of healthcare. Additionally, the conditions of diseases frequently encountered in upper gastrointestinal surgery often require multidisciplinary care. Surgeons typically collaborate with gastroenterologists, oncologists, radiologists, and nutritionists to provide comprehensive patient care tailored to individual needs. For instance, pancreatic neuroendocrine neoplasms do not only require surgery but also specialized diagnostic and therapeutic strategies, exemplifying the intricate nature of such cases (Almar et al., 2019). The coordination of various health professionals guarantees that each patient is provided with whole well-being, not only the surgical issues, but also the general implications of their disease, including dietary plan and mental attention. This multidisciplinary approach is particularly crucial in treating patients whose conditions have complex aspects that require more than simple surgeries. In addition to the technical expertise required, upper GI surgery necessitates a thorough understanding of potential complications and risks associated with surgical intervention. Surveillance of healthcare-associated infections (HAIs) has been further highlighted in surgical settings, underscoring the need for rigorous infection control measures to minimize surgical risks (Allardice et al., 2008). Surgeons must be able to recognize postoperative complications, such as leakage, infection, or anastomotic failure, that can have a direct impact on patient recovery. Defining upper gastrointestinal surgery, thus, extends beyond the procedure; it means adopting a systems approach to patient safety, postoperative care, and compliance with protocols to enhance outcomes. This comprehensive approach not only improves the surgeons' position but also elevates the standard of care that is provided within the profession.

Significance in Medical Practice

The specialty of upper gastrointestinal surgery has much to do with the practice of medical axioms where the worth of collaborative approaches is evident. The blending of theoretical theories into the surgical practice is a clear indication of this association. The theoretical concept of surgery, for instance, as envisioned at universities such as the University of Marburg, emphasizes interdisciplinary collaboration among clinical surgeons and basic scientists. Through data analysis, decision trees, and algorithms, operating teams can optimize diagnostic and therapeutic strategies. This formalized communication facilitates ongoing research and stimulates innovation of surgical methods, which in turn leads to improved patient outcomes. With the continuous evolution of upper gastrointestinal surgery, this collaboration continues at the forefront, ensuring that scientific advancements are paired with practicality in the clinical setting (Lorenz et al., 1989). Endoscopic interventions have had a profound impact on upper gastrointestinal surgery and reflect the significance of medical technology in the practice of medicine. As endoscopy advances, surgeons can utilize advanced diagnostic and therapeutic devices designed to significantly improve patient care. For example, chromoendoscopy and magnification endoscopy allow better visualization of lesions, facilitating early diagnosis with more precision. Alongside, therapeutic techniques such as EMR and dissection have also moved beyond the traditional surgery by successfully treating diseases that would otherwise involve invasive surgery. This has long-term implications on the recovery time of patients and the overall efficacy of the intervention, illustrating how emerging endoscopic modalities are redefining surgical patterns and projecting their integral place in the larger scheme of medical treatment (Arebi et al., 2005). Additionally, upper gastrointestinal surgery is highlighted as crucial due to its significant impact on patient safety and quality of care. Within the practice of surgery, strict training and adherence to codified guidelines play a crucial role in reducing complications and improving surgical outcomes. O'Brien and Anderson highlight the practice's ongoing improvement by demonstrating the development of organized training programs, as colonoscopy, as an expression of a commitment to excellence. These courses emphasize the development of technical competence and diagnostic ability, ensuring that the surgeons become more equipped to handle the complications of gastrointestinal illness. Patient-centered care, achieved through continuous education and integration with technology, emphasizes the importance of upper gastrointestinal surgery in delivering better medical practice. As operation techniques develop and progress, the focus is always firmly centered on improving health outcomes and surgical practice (Lorenz et al., 1989; Arebi et al., 2005) (Figure 4.2).

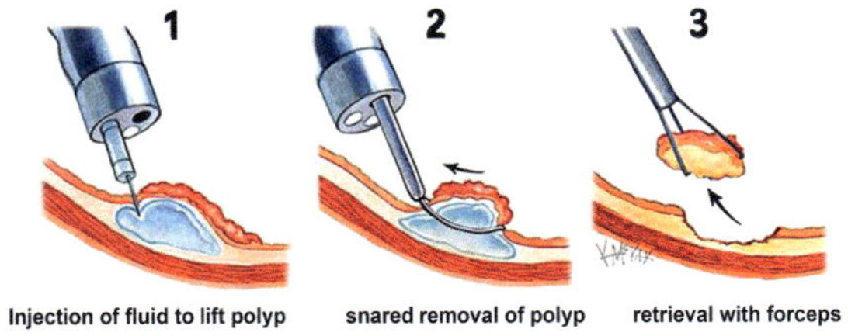

Figure 4.2. Endoscopic mucosal resection.

Source: https://www.gastromedicine.com.au/images/endoscopic-mucosal-resection-img.jpg.

4.1. Anatomy of the Upper Gastrointestinal Tract

Learning Outcome

1. Describe the components of the upper GI tract
2. Focus on functions of each component of upper gastrointestinal (GI) surgery
3. Learn about common diseases affecting the upper GI tract

The upper GI tract comprises various essential anatomical structures that work together to facilitate digestion. The esophagus, a muscular tube connecting the pharynx and stomach, plays a crucial role in propelling food down through peristalsis. Its anatomy is specifically designed for food passage, featuring a stratified squamous epithelium that provides protection from mechanical wear. Once the food is swallowed and passes through the esophagus, the stomach serves as both a reservoir and a blender, possessing the significant capacity to secrete strong digestive acids and enzymes that break down the food into a semiliquid consistency. The digestive system consists of regions—the fundus, body, and antrum—each playing its own special role in the digestion process. Identification of these anatomical structures is significant for surgeons, as their knowledge influences surgical technique and approach in upper gastrointestinal surgery, particularly in conditions where intervention is required, such as esophageal cancer or peptic ulcer disease. The duodenum, the initial portion of the small intestine, is further along the upper gastrointestinal tract where primary chemical digestion occurs. The duodenum is provided with chyme from the stomach, with bile from the liver, and digestive enzymes from the pancreas; hence, it has a crucial role to play in nutrient absorption. Its characteristic C shape accommodates the pancreas and bile duct comfortably, allowing digestive juices to be blended. Anatomically, the duodenum also has a vital role to play since it triggers signals to the pancreas to secrete additional enzymes and the liver to secrete bile for efficient digestion. Complications involving ulcers or obstruction of the duodenum can severely impact digestive function, which can be addressed through surgery that requires a comprehensive understanding of duodenal anatomy. It is essential for surgeons to allow for optimal outcomes in procedures such as duodenal resections or bypass surgeries, where the preservation of surrounding structures is paramount. The relationship between the anatomic structures of the upper GI tract and their functions is significant in the realm of surgery. For instance, surgical complications such as gastric bypass can lead to a range of postoperative disorders, including pancreatic exocrine insufficiency (PEI). This is a condition that arises from altered anatomy and is capable of precipitating significant clinical issues through overlapping signs with other gastric bypass outcomes, as claimed in recent research. Malabsorption and steatorrhea are present in patients, complicating diagnosis and treatment further. The necessity for specialized follow-up care and ongoing management, such as replacement therapy with pancreatic enzymes, supports the necessity to understand the anatomy of the upper GI tracts following surgery. Surgeons must navigate the intricacies of the upper gastrointestinal tract to prevent potential complications and provide comprehensive care to post-surgery patients, emphasizing the interrelatedness of anatomy and surgical outcome in upper gastrointestinal surgery (Figure 4.3).

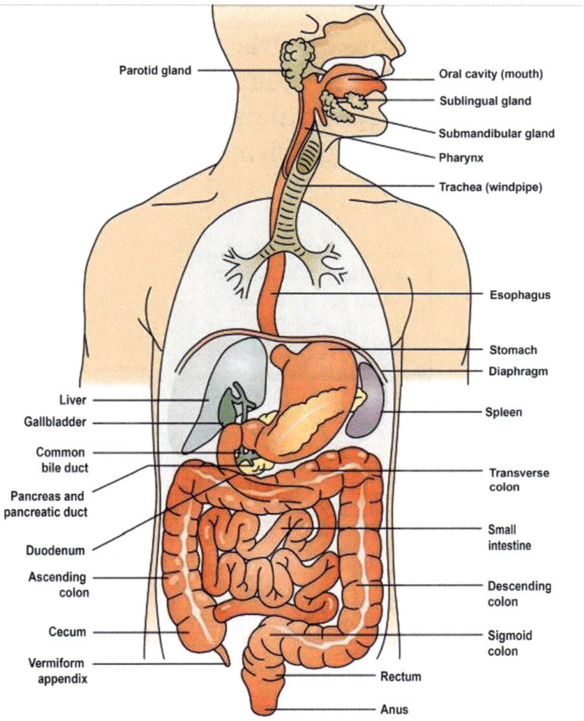

Figure 4.3. Anatomy of the upper gastrointestinal tract.

Source: https://img.brainkart.com/article/article-Anatomy-of-the-Gastr-eWX.jpg.

4.1.1. Components of the Upper GI Tract

The upper part of the GI tract comprises several vital components that play a role in digestion as well as overall gastrointestinal function. These include the esophagus, stomach, and the duodenum, which is the first portion of the small intestine. Each organ performs specific yet interconnected functions to perform effective food processing. The esophagus primarily serves as a food pipe, utilizing synchronized muscular contractions, known as peristalsis, to propel ingested material from the mouth to the stomach. Once food reaches the stomach, various physiological mechanisms begin, including the secretion of gastric acid and enzymes that initiate protein digestion. Understanding these factors is an essential part of healthcare for workers, particularly surgeons who perform upper gastrointestinal surgery, as variations in anatomical and functional characteristics would significantly influence surgical techniques and outcomes. The stomach is divided into several regions: the fundus, body, antrum, and pylorus, each of which plays a specific role in the digestion process. The fundus and body are primarily used for the storage and mixing of food, while the antrum is responsible for breaking food into small particles for chewing. Pylorus regulates the passage of digested food into the duodenum, reflecting the function played by these sections in correct digestive flow. Interference with any of these parts, such as obstructions and ulcers, may lead to serious complications requiring surgery. Upper GI surgical methods are constantly being refined, with innovations geared towards minimizing risk and enhancing recovery, so surgeons must understand the physiological nuances of the upper GI tract (Phillips et al., 2016).

Moreover, optimal upper gastrointestinal surgery often involves an interdisciplinary approach that combines several diagnostic modalities and surgical techniques for optimal patient outcomes. Gastrointestinal ultrasound (GIUS) has also been found to be a valuable method in this context, providing non-invasive access to the anatomy and function of the upper GI tract. Refining its use through development by an expert task force, the GIUS application provides a better understanding of esophageal, stomach, and duodenal conditions, facilitating improved preoperative assessment and postoperative monitoring (Calabrese et al., 2016). With cooperation between specialists and the application of advanced imaging, medical practitioners can enhance the accuracy of surgery and reduce the likelihood of complications, recognizing the importance of knowledge in upper GI anatomy for the conduct of upper GI surgery.

4.1.2. Role of Each Component

In upper GI surgery, several factors synergize to achieve successful outcomes during procedures. The equipment used in surgery, such as scalpels, forceps, and electrocautery units, all have different functions that are essential for precision during procedures like resections or anastomoses. Scalpels provide incisions with sharp edges that minimize tissue trauma, whereas forceps assist in retracting tissues to provide good exposure of the surgical area. Electrocautery devices, on the other hand, enable the accurate coagulation of blood vessels, thereby reducing intraoperative bleeding and enhancing surgical effectiveness. Proper selection and application of such devices are important, crucial because improper devices or techniques can lead to problems such as infection, postoperative delay of healing, or even intraoperative catastrophes.

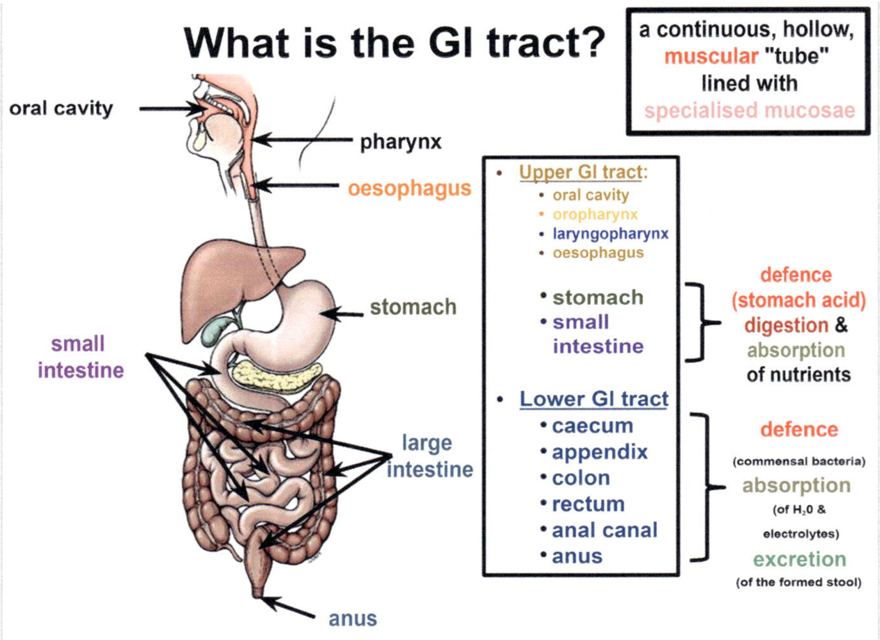

Figure 4.4. Diagram of upper GI tract.

Source: https://i.pinimg.com/originals/62/80/f1/6280f115c006e08d3905b0f59e871e5b.png.

Another fundamental component of upper GI surgery is the use of imaging and navigation technologies. These technologies, including endoscopic equipment and advanced imaging modalities, provide real-time visualization of the GI tract, allowing surgeons to make well-informed decisions during procedures. Highly sophisticated imaging systems can provide vital information regarding the anatomy and pathology of the gastrointestinal tract, enabling surgeons to better navigate complex regions without damaging surrounding tissues. For example, the invention of capsule endoscopy, a non-surgical imaging modality that uses small cameras to photograph along the GI tract, represents a giant leap in diagnostic capacity. Integration of these technologies into surgical procedures increases precision and might assist in improving patient outcomes by making procedures possible with greater accuracy and fewer complications.

The role of postoperative care in upper GI surgery cannot be overstated, highlighting the importance of employing a multidisciplinary approach to patient management. Factors like pain management, nutrition, and careful observation play key roles in promoting recovery and preventing complications. For instance, nutrition after surgery is important due to the altered digestive process following surgery, which can be enhanced by specific diet modification steps required to ensure proper healing and recovery. Furthermore, effective pain management programs promote patient comfort and facilitate early mobilization, significantly influencing the recovery phase. Regular screening for complications, such as leaks or infections, allows any issues to be addressed simultaneously, thereby reducing the risk of an extended hospital stay or reoperation. All these factors, combined, work towards optimizing the overall effectiveness of upper GI surgical interventions, highlighting the need for an integrated strategy in patient care (Figure 4.4).

4.1.3. Common Diseases Affecting the Upper GI Tract

The upper gastrointestinal tract is susceptible to a range of diseases that can have a significant impact on patients' health. Esophageal varices are one of the most frequent causes of upper GI bleeding, which is primarily due to portal hypertension in cases of liver disease. A significant study validated that 51.3% of upper GI bleeding was attributed to esophageal varices, highlighting their clinical importance and the need for treatment at the earliest opportunity to prevent life-threatening bleeding (Elghuel et al., 2012). Bleeding varices are typically treated with endoscopic interventions, though severe cases can be treated with surgery to stop further risk and harm. Awareness of the considerable morbidity and mortality for this condition highlights the value of early diagnosis and timely referral for surgery in the context of upper GI surgery. Peptic ulcer disease is also a common disease of the upper GI tract, which has symptoms ranging from mild distress to severe complications such as perforation or severe bleeding. 25.0% of the causes of upper GI bleeding can be attributed to peptic ulcers, and as a condition, it bears a severe burden of upper GI disorders (Elghuel et al., 2012).

Furthermore, the incidence of H. pylori infection in patients diagnosed with gastritis, as reported in a study, indicates a direct relationship between this pathogen and the production of ulcers. Specifically, the study observed that 53% of patients with gastritis were positive for H. pylori. This connection highlights the importance of targeted treatment approaches that address both the ulcer and the accompanying bacterial infection. Complicated ulcers resistant to drugs or in cases of perforation may require surgical intervention, necessitating a cautious approach by medical practitioners. The prevalence of gastritis and esophagitis also explains standard inflammatory processes in the upper GI tract, since gastritis is identified in 47.9% of results. Symptoms that arise with these conditions often cause significant discomfort, leading patients to seek endoscopic assessment and treatment. In addition to focused medical interventions, surgery may be considered for malignant or chronic conditions that develop following chronic inflammation. The incorporation of surgical intervention can thus be a vital factor in addressing not only complications arising due to long-standing gastritis and esophagitis but also their underlying causes. With the increased recognition of these common upper GI conditions, a comprehensive understanding of their relevance to surgical management remains crucial for optimizing the outcomes of upper gastrointestinal surgery.

Test Your Knowledge

1. What are the three parts of the duodenum?
2. Which sphincter controls the passage of food from the esophagus to the stomach?

4.2. Indications for Upper Gastrointestinal Surgery

Learning Outcome

1. Explain the Benign conditions requiring surgery
2. Define the malignant conditions and cancer treatment
3. Discuss the emergency situations necessitating surgical intervention

Upper GI surgery encompasses a range of procedures designed to address various severe diseases that affect the stomach, esophagus, and duodenum. Upper GI bleeding is one of the primary causes for surgery, as it is a complication of conditions such as peptic ulcers or esophageal varices. Specifically, there is enough evidence that the highest incidence of cases of upper GI bleeding is because of esophageal varices in patients with a pre-existing liver disease, as noted in studies that report morbidity and mortality of the condition (Elghuel et al., 2012). Surgery, including emergency surgery, may be necessary in instances of bleeding unresponsive to conservative treatment or if patients develop signs of shock or increased comorbidities. Thus, identification of the need for surgery is crucial to maximize patient benefit and minimize complications. Malignancy is another key indication for upper GI surgery. Reoperation by surgery is warranted in patients with upper GI cancer because it remains one of the most effective ways to achieve long-term survival. The development of signs such as obstructive dysphagia, gastric outlet obstruction, or weight loss may point to the need for surgical evaluation and treatment (Elghuel et al., 2012). In addition, the requirement for surgical intervention is typically heightened when the tumors invade surrounding structures or cause gastrointestinal obstruction. Clinical assessment and imaging procedures guide decision-making towards the importance of timely surgery to enhance the prognosis and quality of life for patients with these very aggressive diseases. Of particular interest, anticoagulation control during upper gastrointestinal surgery is an added challenge, particularly in patients requiring emergency surgery. Previous studies confirm the efficacy of idarucizumab in reversing the anticoagulant effect of drugs like dabigatran, a necessary action for patients with intractable gastrointestinal bleeding. Rapid normalization of hemostasis in these cases ensures readiness for surgery, highlighting the intersection of pharmacotherapy and surgical readiness. Additionally, understanding the bleeding resolution and surgical readiness timeline is essential to ensure optimal outcomes with this patient group. Therefore, the application of multidisciplinary strategies with medical and surgical expertise is vital while navigating the confounded landscape of indications for upper GI surgery (Figure 4.5).

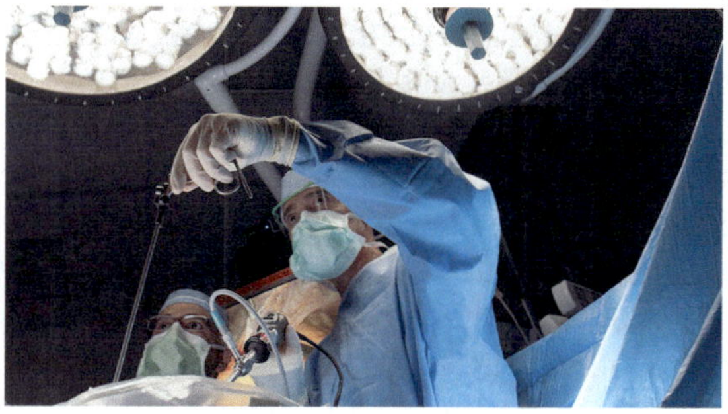

Figure 4.5. Indications for upper gastrointestinal surgery.

Source: https://clevelandcliniclondon.uk/-/scassets/images/org/locations/london/specialties/ddsi/upper-gastrointestinal.jpg.

4.2.1. Benign Conditions Requiring Surgery

Therapy of benign pathology of the upper GI tract is often surgical when the symptoms are unmanageable or at risk of progressing into serious complications. Pathologies such as gastric ulcers, benign tumors in the form of adenomas, and esophageal strictures are liable to produce significant morbidity if left untreated. Varying surgical methods are used based on the specific diagnosis, from laparoscopic resection to endoscopy. For instance, strictures can be treated effectively using endoscopic methods to dilate and excise occluding lesions. Conservative management is well responded to in a large majority of patients, but surgery cannot be avoided to ensure quality of life and prevent complications like perforation or the evolution of malignancy in certain benign lesions; hence, surgical expertise is a priceless component of disease management. Esophageal strictures, usually secondary to chronic gastroesophageal reflux disease (GERD) or from previous surgery, are a benign lesion that needs surgical correction. Endoscopic dilatation of a stricture can be performed and has become less painful, taking less time for the patient to recover in the hospital. Surgery, however, may be required if strictures recur or are refractory to treatment. Surgical management comprises esophagectomy or surgical reconstruction of the esophagus, which may lead to improved swallowing and symptom relief. Interestingly, complication rates for these procedures, including those associated with endoscopy, require meticulous preoperative planning and assessment. Recognition of potential adverse effects enhances the readiness of surgical teams and yields optimal patient outcomes in upper gastrointestinal surgery, underscoring the importance of meticulous technique and thorough postoperative care (Abbas et al., 2013).

In addition to strictures of the esophagus, other benign lesions, such as pancreatic lesions, are also indicated for surgery and treatment. Pancreatic cysts, for example, may be asymptomatic but carry the potential for malignant change. Operations, nonetheless, can be called for based on size, symptomatology, and potential risk factors. Cholecystitis or gallstones, gallbladder disease, also generally need to be surgically removed for relief of symptoms and avoidance of acute complications. Patients with complex presentations, such as in acute cholecystitis, can be managed with laparoscopic cholecystectomy to avoid the risks of open surgery. The emphasis on meticulous surgical technique and early intervention highlights the breadth of benign disorders treated through upper GI surgery, encouraging an active patient management approach that encompasses both short-term and long-term health outcomes (Aabakken et al., 2017).

4.2.2. Malignant Conditions and Cancer Treatment

Care of malignant conditions in the upper GI tract presents unique challenges, particularly when surgery is required. Laparotomy remains a standard of surgical practice for tumor resection in this region, but it is more than mere surgical intervention. Chronic pain following surgery is a frequent occurrence in patients, and a rate of prevalence has been found in research as 18% four years post-surgery. This neuropathic disorder has a significant influence on the quality of life of patients, with decreased functioning and more symptoms regardless of cancer status or age. The intersection between surgical outcome and cancer treatment necessitates that preoperative planning and postoperative management be considered comprehensively to avoid such chronic pain, in which multidisciplinary teams play a crucial role in patient outcomes, particularly in contexts of upper GI surgery (Bruce et al., 2006). Furthermore, diagnosis and treatment of malignancies, such as neuroendocrine tumors or small bowel lymphomas, also complicate upper GI surgical interventions. With nontraumatic small intestine perforation tending to appear as acute surgical emergencies in most cases, diagnosis is only made at laparotomy in a good proportion. Due to the rarity of small bowel malignancies and their nonspecific nature, early and accurate diagnosis remains replete with challenges. For conditions such as T-cell lymphoma, surgery must be combined with adjuvant therapy because surgery alone will not adequately address the systemic nature of the condition (Banu et al., 2016).

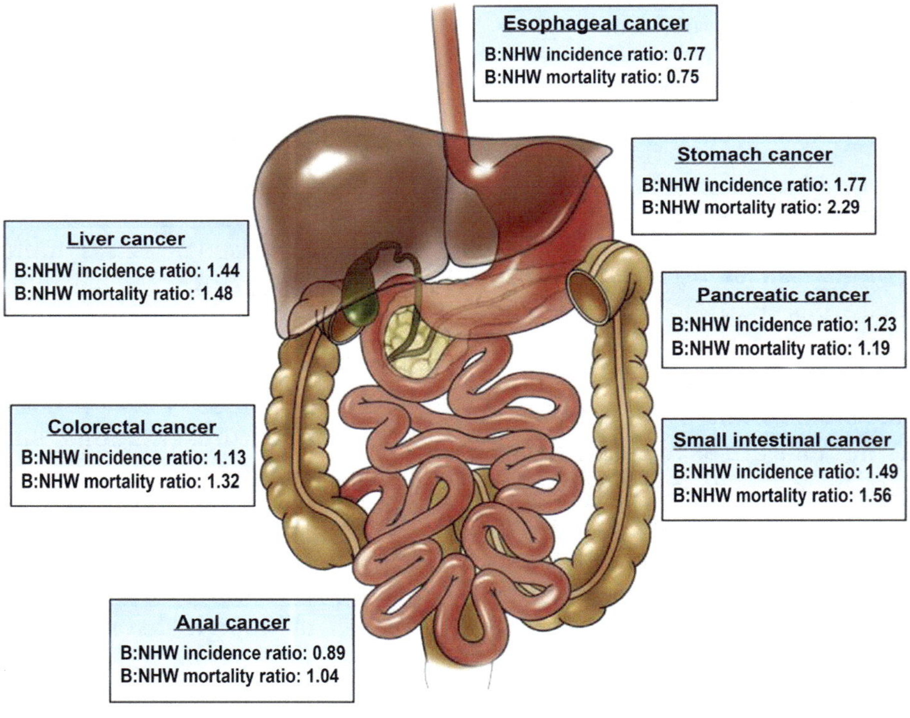

Figure 4.6. Malignant conditions and cancer treatment for upper gastrointestinal surgery.

Source: https://gastroenterologyinstituteofnashik.com/wp-content/uploads/2020/03/1-s2.0-S0016508517360304-gr1.jpg.

Therefore, while surgical procedures such as segmental enterectomy may be definitive immediate salvagers, long-term success is to a large extent contingent upon prolonged cancer treatment regimens following preliminary intervention (Banu et al., 2016). Ultimately, the setting of malignant disease and treatment in upper GI surgery underscores the need for ongoing innovation and research in surgical techniques and postoperative management. Understanding of the psychological and physical burden on patients, specifically about chronic pain and functional impairment, paves the way for improved protocols that enhance recovery and quality of life after surgery. With improved utilization of data on surgical outcomes and patient experience by surgeons, they are in a position to craft entire treatment plans that not only address tumor killing but also the entire welfare of patients undergoing the complexity of cancer therapy. This is a crucial aspect of surgical oncology improvement, aiming not only to enable patients to survive but also to lead a quality life worth living (Bruce et al., 2006; Banu et al., 2016) (Figure 4.6).

4.2.3. Emergency Situations Necessitating Surgical Intervention

In the domain of upper GI surgery, the normal course of events is one of emergency presentation necessitating the immediate performance of surgery. The primary reason for this emergent surgery is life-threatening situations like a massive GI bleed, possibly due to any one of several conditions, for example, peptic ulcers or tumors. Timely identification of the location of such bleeding is important because delay can significantly worsen the patient's prognosis. Procedures such as esophagogastroduodenoscopy (EGD) are commonly employed in diagnosing and managing upper GI bleeding, but in cases of uncontrolled hemorrhage, surgical treatment must be seriously considered.

The gravity of the case highlights the importance of rapid assessment and treatment so that patients can receive adequate surgical treatment early enough to avoid complications or death due to prolonged hemorrhagic periods. Additionally, patients treated with anticoagulants present unique challenges in emergency situations, particularly among those requiring upper GI surgical interventions. In situations where a patient is experiencing a significant bleeding event with anticoagulants like dabigatran, reversal of the drug becomes the number one priority immediately. Idarucizumab is a reversal antidote agent that is used particularly to reverse dabigatran's anticoagulant effect. Clinical trials have shown that this agent can rapidly reverse anticoagulation in emergency cases, thereby making surgery safer when administered as necessary. The effectiveness of intravenous idarucizumab 5 g in the therapy for hemostasis is emphasized by studies that have shown that it achieved immediate and total reversal in the majority of subjects.

Therefore, such knowledge and practice of medical interventions have implications that are significant for surgical outcomes as well as overall patient survival in emergency conditions (Pollack et al., 2016). Moreover, some indications for the surgery in children and adolescents with upper gastrointestinal emergencies are worth high consideration. Diseases such as corrosive ingestions and gastrointestinal tract obstruction necessitate immediate evaluation and potential surgical intervention. Pediatric guidelines mandate the necessity of achieving diagnostic endoscopies to ascertain the extent of damage and immediate foreign body extraction when necessary. Identifying such emergencies is crucial, as they can lead to potentially fatal complications if left untreated. Surgical procedures also target not only the alleviation of immediate hazards to the patient's life but also guarantee a safe recovery by preventing long-term issues such as stricture formation or sepsis. Thus, early intervention in children emphasizes the critical value of upper gastrointestinal surgery in emergencies (Aabakken et al., 2017).

Test Your Knowledge

1. When is surgery indicated for gastroesophageal reflux disease (GERD)?
2. What are the surgical indications for peptic ulcer disease?

4.3. Types of Upper Gastrointestinal Surgical Procedures

Learning Outcome

1. Explain the esophagectomy
2. Define the gastrectomy
3. Describe the fundoplication

Upper GI surgery encompasses a broad variety of interventions whose primary aim is to address disorders involving the esophagus, stomach, and the proximal portion of the small intestine. The most common is perhaps esophagectomy, in which part or the whole of the esophagus is removed surgically and is usually used in conditions such as esophageal cancer or severe dysplasia. The technique used may range from open to minimally invasive laparoscopic, based on the case and patients' overall condition. A procedure frequently performed is fundoplication for gastroesophageal reflux disease (GERD) in which the upper part of the stomach is wrapped around the esophagus to prevent it from refluxing. All these procedures are linked to their respective hazards and benefits; hence, a proper choice of patient and preoperative assessment are necessary to gain the optimum benefit. Gastric surgery also plays a crucial role in the management of upper gastrointestinal ailments, particularly those complicated by gastric tumors or benign diseases leading to obstruction or severe gastritis. Partial or total gastrectomy, for instance, is performed in gastric cancer. This surgical procedure not only aims to excise cancerous tissue but also addresses concomitant complications such as obstruction, perforation, or profuse bleeding. The indication of resection techniques is often represented by complications after less invasive methods for intervention, such as biliary-enteric interventions, in which enteric perforations can result in severe morbidity, as demonstrated in postoperative complications studies (Koep et al., 1979).

An appropriate indication for surgery, as well as an aggressive diagnostic approach, becomes imperative to reduce risks and enhance patient survival. Furthermore, surgical control of gastric cancer is crucial, particularly where the rates of incidence are high, as evidenced in retrospective studies outlining the treatment experience of specific populations (Chalya et al., 2012). Surgical procedures may include gastrojejunostomy, which is typically reserved for palliation in patients with advanced disease. With nearly a quarter of patients presenting for surgical management of gastric cancer developing postoperative complications, with considerable mortality, surgical management must be combined with satisfactory oncological management to achieve acceptable results. Late diagnosis of gastric cancer requires greater awareness and effective screening strategies, particularly in resource-limited settings where health inequalities have a profound impact on detection and control. It is therefore critical to understand the scope of surgery to improve outcomes in upper GI surgery (Figure 4.7).

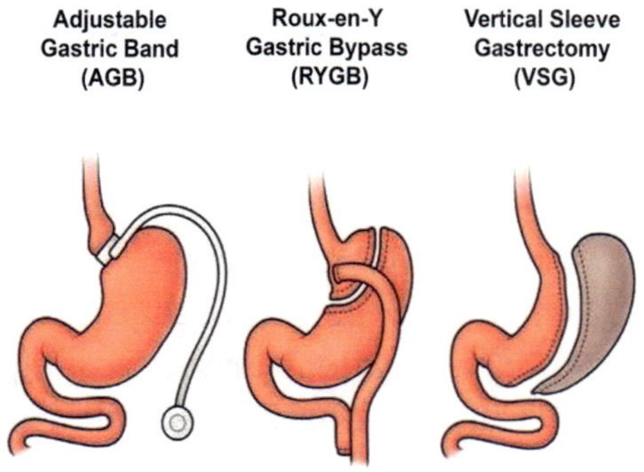

Figure 4.7. Types of upper gastrointestinal surgical procedures.

Source: https://livertransplantindia.net/wp-content/uploads/2021/04/Gastrointestinal-surgery-infographics.jpg.

4.3.1. Esophagectomy

Esophagectomy, the surgical removal of the esophagus, is a significant therapeutic option for various esophageal diseases, particularly esophageal carcinoma. The procedure involves the resection of the affected section of the esophagus, the surrounding lymph nodes, and, in most cases, the reconstruction of the esophagus using a segment of the stomach or intestine. Such a challenging operation is typically necessary due to the late presentation of the disease, when other, less complex modalities are insufficient. Given the complexities involved, such as navigating through critical anatomy and preventing postoperative complications, esophagectomy is a procedure that needs high levels of surgical expertise and multidisciplinary patient care. Whether or not to have this surgery underscores the need for complete preoperative assessment and counseling of the patient regarding intervention risk and pathways of recovery.

Postoperative complications following esophagectomy are the primary determinant of outcome in patients undergoing this procedure, and anastomotic leak is the most crucial issue. These leaks occur at the site where the remaining esophagus is anastomosed, typically resulting in severe morbidity. Literature shows that modifiable risk factors such as smoking and malnutrition have a significant impact on the rate of leaks as well as overall recovery. Preoperative optimization of patients should be achieved by recommendations that include nutritional support and cessation programs of smoking, potentially decreasing complication rates. Additionally, maneuvers designed to reduce ischemia and optimize operative time have been emphasized in the literature. By implementing such mechanisms and adhering to best practices, clinical teams can significantly enhance procedural success as well as optimize postoperative care for patients undergoing esophagectomy, thereby making it an essential part of upper gastrointestinal surgery (Philllips et al., 2016).

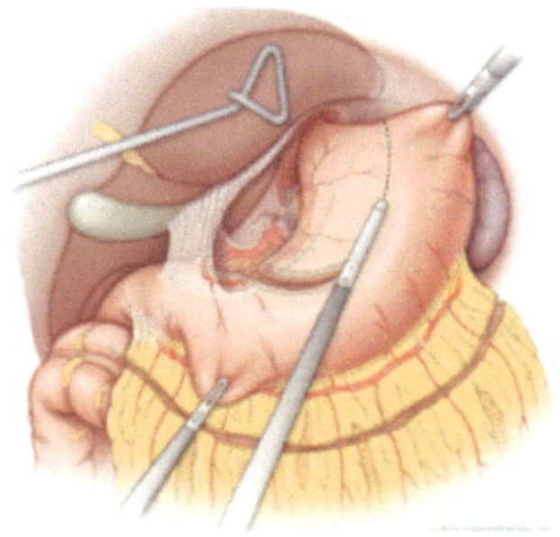

Figure 4.8. Minimally invasive esophagectomy.

Source: https://stanfordhealthcare.org/content/dam/SHC/treatments/v/images/vats-esophagectomy-neo-esophagus.jpg.

The outcome following esophagectomy is highly variable, depending on various factors, including stage at presentation of the tumor and patient health status. Even though the operation could be curative for the localized esophageal cancer, survival in patients depends on rigorous compliance with follow-up and postoperative care. Research also identified early detection and intervention strategies to improve outcomes following esophagectomy, suggesting an organized approach to treating esophageal disease. Additional investigation into minimally invasive techniques, that is, video-assisted thoracoscopic surgery (VATS), also identifies many perceived benefits, such as reduced hospital stays and quicker recovery. As this field of upper gastrointestinal surgery evolves, it will be crucial to remain sensitive to the nuances of esophagectomy and implications (Bou-Antoun et al., 2013) (Figure 4.8).

4.3.2. Gastrectomy

Gastrectomy, essential surgical procedure encompassing partial or total gastrectomy, occupies an important place in the branch of surgery that deals with the upper gastrointestinal tract. The intervention is highly indicated in patients with malignant conditions, such as gastric cancer, and severe benign pathologies that impair the function and/or integrity of the gastrointestinal tract. Improvements in surgical techniques, particularly the advent of minimally invasive techniques such as robot-assisted gastrectomy, have enabled enhanced patient outcomes. With the use of advanced technology and expertise, surgeons can perform complex surgeries with enhanced precision and decreased postoperative morbidity, suggesting a tendency towards a more patient-centered approach in surgical therapy (Cirocchi et al., 2017). The implications of gastrectomy are extensive beyond intraoperative and early postoperative outcomes, profoundly affecting long-term health and nutritional status. Patients postoperatively will often experience dramatic alterations in their physiology following gastric tissue removal, which can lead to complications of malabsorption and vitamin deficiency. Those patients can also require lifetime dietary adjustments to accommodate their altered digestive abilities, underscoring the need for comprehensive preoperative counseling and postoperative management programs. Surgeons and clinic staff must ensure that patients are well-prepared for such changes, as holistic care is imperative in the postoperative phase of gastrectomy (Beekley et al., 2018).

Follow-up of gastrectomy patients is also important for the long term to treat possible complications that may arise. Acute care surgeons must also be knowledgeable about the types of complications arising from gastric surgery, such as post-bariatric-related issues, nutritional deficiency, and anatomic alterations that influence management priorities. Patients become older and develop unrelated intra-abdominal disease with advancing age, so a reasonable degree of knowledge regarding their prior surgeries is needed to differentiate between anticipated surgical complications and emergent pathology. Therefore, an interdisciplinary process combining surgical expertise with ongoing nutrition and psychological care is paramount for achieving long-term success and maintaining quality of life in gastrectomy patients (Beekley et al., 2018).

4.3.3. Fundoplication

Fundoplication is a standard surgical procedure created to correct gastroesophageal reflux disease (GERD) through the fortification of the lower esophageal sphincter. Involves the folding of the stomach's fundus over the esophagus, fundoplication aims to create a new valve mechanism that prevents the reflux of stomach contents. Chronic GERD patients often present with severe symptoms and complications, such as esophagitis and Barrett's esophagus, that can lead to esophageal cancer. Fundoplication not only alleviates these symptoms but also corrects the underlying anatomical defects that cause GERD. Its effectiveness is supplemented by a marked reduction in both symptoms and the need for ongoing pharmacologic therapy, marking its importance in upper GI surgery. The fundoplication referral typically follows a careful evaluation, which includes endoscopy and 24-hour pH studies. Surgical intervention will generally be limited to those patients who are medically non-responsive or have complications of reflux. Open or laparoscopic methods can be used in fundoplication, with the latter being more frequently employed due to its less invasive nature and improved recovery times. One of the most significant things to consider are the types of fundoplication operations that are available, such as the Nissen, Toupet, and Dor procedures, with varying indications and benefits. The Nissen fundoplication, for instance, is the most popular of the variations and is generally associated with excellent outcomes in symptom relief and improvement in quality of life, solidifying its status as one of the foundations of treatment management for GERD in upper GI surgery. Although fundoplication has many benefits, several risks and complications require careful patient selection and experience on the part of the surgeon. Dysphagia, bloating, and retention of gas are common postoperative complications, which are typically related to the altered anatomy and physiology of the esophagus and stomach following surgery. The recurrence of reflux symptoms is also a significant concern in patients requiring revisional surgery. Present studies reveal that even though recurrence rates in fundoplication are reasonably low, they are more in individuals with a history of repair of hiatal hernia. Also, technological advancements in the form of materials used for surgery and the techniques themselves, such as the use of mesh in hiatus hernia repair, can influence the long-term outcome of fundoplication (Boachie et al., 2013; Aly et al., 2015). Overall, ongoing research and innovations in surgical techniques will continue to enhance the application of fundoplication in the effective management of GERD (Figure 4.9).

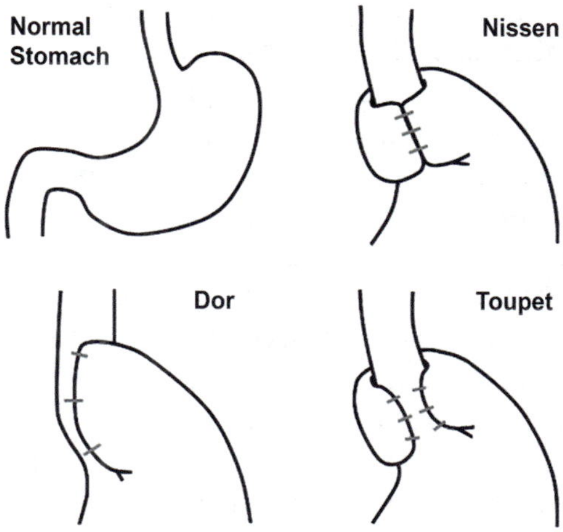

Figure 4.9. Fundoplication.

Source: https://operativereview.com/wp-content/uploads/2022/11/Fundoplications.jpg.

Test Your Knowledge

1. What is the primary purpose of a Nissen fundoplication?
2. Which part of the stomach is removed during a subtotal gastrectomy?

4.4. Preoperative Assessment and Preparation

Learning Outcome

1. Identify the patient evaluation and history
2. Define the diagnostic imaging and tests
3. Describe the preoperative counseling and consent

Preoperative assessment and preparation are crucial to achieving the best results in upper gastrointestinal surgery. This mandatory procedure involves a thorough analysis of the patient's medical history, physical condition, and reasons for surgery. Nutritional status, history of comorbidities, and obesity are some of the key parameters that identify operability. Malnutrition, in particular, has been indicated to increase postoperative complications like anastomotic leaks, and therefore, preoperative nutritional therapy is essential. Modifiable risk factors, according to recent evidence, need to be managed; for example, five to seven days of immune-modifying dietary support is recommended in malnourished patients (Philllips et al., 2016). This thorough assessment not only aids in tailoring the surgical procedure but also enhances general patient safety and recovery protocols, which are crucial in gastrointestinal surgery. In addition to evaluating physical health and nutrition, preoperative psychological assessment is equally important. Patients having upper gastrointestinal surgery can become anxious due to waiting for surgery and concerns over the risks. These psychological stressors can lead to postoperative complications in the recovery process. Having healthcare professionals provide counseling, education, and support can make a significant difference in preventing these problems, ultimately leading to better surgical outcomes. Screening for psychiatric comorbid conditions, such as depression, can also identify those who might need additional support, fostering holistic preoperative care since obesity is another significant intraoperative risk factor (Agius et al., 2014), actively dealing with these psychological factors in addition to physical evaluation gives priority to improved surgical outcomes and experiences. Preoperative preparation process, including side planning, also involves meticulous planning for intraoperative and postoperative complications. Surgeons and anesthesiologists work closely together to ensure that all variables, including medications, allergies, and anesthetic histories, are meticulously scrutinized.

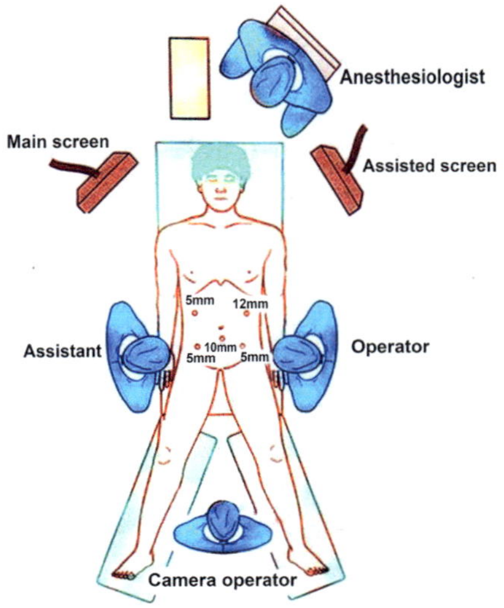

Figure 4.10. Preoperative preparation: the position of the patient, surgeon, screen, and trocar.

Source: https://www.researchgate.net/publication/336569594/figure/fig1/AS:814495635079180@1571202300213/Preoperative-preparation-the-position-of-patient-surgeon-screen-and-trocar.png.

Furthermore, higher-order imaging and diagnostic tests may be necessary to optimize surgical planning, especially in complex cases. Reducing operating time and technical difficulty is essential since these factors have a significant bearing on complications like anastomotic leakage (Philllips et al., 2016). Therefore, another critical component of preoperative preparation is practical preoperative order communication to patients. This includes fasting regimens, medication changes, and explanation regarding the surgical process itself, so that patients are correctly informed and set for the surgical experience ahead. This high level of preparation not only reduces risk but also empowers patients, causing them to have an active approach to their surgical expertise (Figure 4.10).

4.4.1. Patient Evaluation and History

An extremely important aspect of GI surgery at an advanced level involves meticulous patient evaluation and detailed history-taking. This is done not only to ensure proper diagnosis of conditions to be operated upon but also to build an effective treatment plan. The evaluation typically starts with surgeons beginning with an entire review of the patient's medical history, especially for symptoms such as abdominal pain, dysphagia, and gastrointestinal bleeding. Individuals with foreboding symptoms, such as melena or hematemesis, are more likely to require emergent assessment, as these signs may signal a serious underlying disease. Secondly, being aware of the prior gastrointestinal illnesses of a patient—or realizing risk factors, such as chronic alcohol abuse or use of non-steroidal anti-inflammatory drugs—is better able to anticipate complications and tailor prevention in operative treatment (Elghuel et al., 2012). In upper GI surgery, though, special attention is reserved for the impact of obesity on surgical outcomes. Given the ballooning rates of obesity across the globe, as debated in recent literature, the interlinkage between obesity and increased risk for surgery justifies a more careful patient evaluation beyond bare minimum history-taking (Agius et al., 2014). Obese patients not only have a heightened incidence of diseasediseases like type 2 diabetes and hypertension, like reflux disease, but also comorbid diseases, like type 2 diabetes and hypertension, which may complicate the surgery and postoperative recovery. Therefore, health-related complications and body mass index (BMI) consideration become mandatory because they determine preoperative risk stratification and postoperative care. Thus, thorough patient assessment can significantly enhance the preparedness of surgical teams to produce the best outcomes. Lastly, patient history needs to incorporate psychosocial factors, which are now more widely recognized as key determinants in treatment outcomes and recovery. Psychological testing may uncover how mental health can affect coping and compliance with post-op instructions. For instance, patients with a history of depression or anxiety may present unique challenges to recovery from upper GI surgery. Clinicians generally employ validated screeners during evaluation to identify such issues and then might intervene or refer to mental health professionals as indicated. By integrating psychosocial elements into patient evaluation, healthcare providers can gain a more informed understanding of the patient's overall health condition, which in turn allows for more tailored and effective surgical care (Elghuel et al., 2012).

4.4.2. Diagnostic Imaging and Tests

Diagnostic imaging holds a top spot in preoperative patient evaluation for upper gastrointestinal surgery. Various modalities, including ultrasound, CT, and MRI, provide valuable information about the anatomy of and pathology within the gastrointestinal tract. These modalities are required to diagnose tumors, gauge their size and location, and assess the encasement of surrounding structures, highlighting the importance of this information in planning surgery. For instance, CT scans are particularly effective at detecting the presence of masses, lymphadenopathy, or vascular invasion, which are crucial in determining the resectability of neoplasms. Thus, proper utilization of diagnostic imaging modalities is of paramount importance to maximize surgical outcomes and minimize intraoperative complications. Biochemical investigations complement diagnostic imaging by providing information on the functional status of gastrointestinal lesions and their associated endocrine disturbances. For example, elevated serum markers are indicative of neuroendocrine tumors and potentially may require a tailored surgical intervention. In this instance, the integration of laboratory studies with imaging tests enables a better understanding of the patient's status, making the creation of individualized surgical plans more straightforward. The complexity of such cases, particularly with pancreatic neuroendocrine neoplasms, underscores the importance of an interprofessional process to ensure that each aspect of diagnosis and treatment is thoroughly evaluated. In this case, physicians collaborate within specialties to interpret test results and make informed choices about the most appropriate surgical interventions needed to address specific characteristics of the tumor and patient needs (Almar et al., 2019). Furthermore, the advanced technology of diagnostic examinations necessitates an organized system to effectively supervise the interdisciplinary nature of upper gastrointestinal surgery. The interface of advanced imaging technology and particular biochemical assays enhances clinicians' abilities for diagnosis and disease management, such as pancreatic neuroendocrine neoplasms that have special challenges due to their uncommon biological behavior and requirement for therapy. By doing so, the establishment of pathways for diagnostic imaging and management can have a profoundly positive impact on patient outcomes. Having these procedures carried out in a well-organized system enables healthcare professionals to manage the complexities of surgical oncology better and deliver care that is correct and individually customized (Caplin et al., 2017). Such a systematic process is crucial for optimizing patient pathways and increasing overall success rates for surgery in the upper gastrointestinal sector (Figure 4.11).

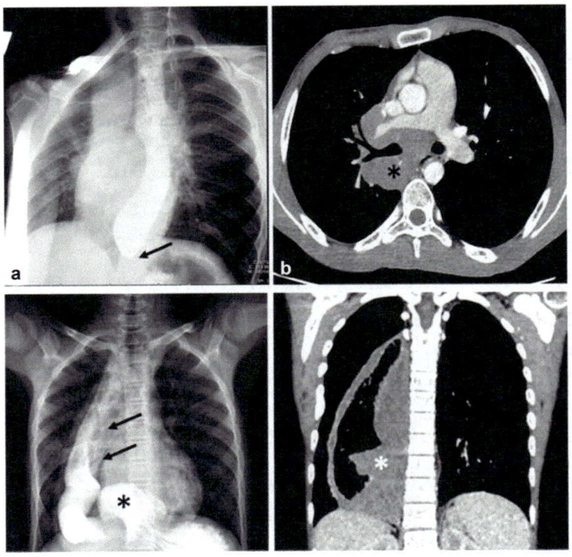

Figure 4.11. Diagnostic imaging and tests.

Source: https://media.springernature.com/lw685/springer-static/image/art%3A10.1186%2Fs43159-020-00061-9/MediaObjects/43159_2020_61_Fig7_HTML.png.

4.4.3. Preoperative Counseling and Consent

Preoperative counseling is an essential component of the process leading up to upper gastrointestinal surgery, guiding patients through the complexity of their respective operations. The intent of this counseling is to provide comprehensive information about the surgery, including risks, benefits, and expected outcomes. Open communication enables doctors to dispel any misinformation while managing the emotional aspects of surgery, ultimately fostering a supportive environment. Effective counseling enhances informed consent, as patients are better equipped to understand their choices. Additionally, it enhances compliance with preoperative guidelines, which are crucial in minimizing surgical complications. This multidimensional process not only enhances focus on informed decision-making but also harmonizes patient expectations with clinical reality, thereby improving overall satisfaction and post-surgical outcomes (Al-Haddad et al., 2014). The informed consent process is embedded in good medical ethics, allowing patients to become autonomous individuals in making decisions about their medical treatment. In upper GI surgery, the consent process must include not only the single procedure but also potential complications that may arise, such as infection, bleeding, and risks associated with anesthesia. Clear exposition of the factors is essential, as it empowers patients who will ultimately be presented with life-altering consequences. Involving family members in the conversation can also be beneficial for understanding, allowing for a more holistic decision-making process. Consent must be considered an evolving conversation rather than a procedure, and patients must be enabled to feel cared for and engaged throughout their surgical journey. This procedure is a sign of the healthcare practitioners' compliance with ethical practice and patient-focused care (N/A, 2021).

In addition, preoperative counseling holds importance that extends beyond the surgery itself to encompass the psychosocial determinants, which have a significant potential to affect the patient's outcome. These can be anxiety, depression, and inadequate social support that will determine recovery trajectories and the success of postoperative treatment. As such, it is essential to include mental health screening in counseling intervention. These assessments can help identify which patients will benefit from additional psychological care, thereby enhancing their general surgical readiness and recovery. Furthermore, lifestyle modification discussions, such as diet and exercise, should be integrated to strengthen long-term postoperative health outcomes. Ultimately, the holistic practice of preoperative counseling and consent not only informs patients but also empowers them with coping strategies to proceed with their surgery with confidence (Al-Haddad et al., 2014).

Test Your Knowledge

1. Why is assessing nutritional status important before major gastrointestinal surgery?
2. What preoperative tests are essential for evaluating cardiac risk in surgical patients?

4.5. Surgical Techniques and Approaches

Learning Outcome

1. Describe the open surgery vs. laparoscopic surgery
2. Define the robotic-assisted surgery
3. Discuss the innovations in surgical techniques

Among the techniques of minimally invasive upper gastrointestinal surgery, the choice of operative technique has a significant impact on patient outcomes and procedure success. Open surgical methods were once the gold standard of care, offering direct access to lesions and facilitating tumor excision. The evolution of new minimally invasive methods, however, has brought a significant change to surgical technique, most specifically with the advent of laparoscopy. These laparoscopic approaches not only diminish trauma associated with more extensive incisions but also extend times of recovery, minimize postoperative pain, and diminish the incidence of complications such as wound infection. As surgical technology advances, the application of laparoscopy to upper GI surgery is increasingly becoming a common trend, together with a growing understanding of both procedural effectiveness and patient safety. The surgical management of gastrointestinal stromal tumors (GISTs) exemplifies the necessity for careful surgical techniques in specific clinical circumstances. GISTs, though relatively rare, have the potential to cause severe complications such as gastrointestinal hemorrhage or intestinal obstruction due to their random occurrence along the gastrointestinal tract. Those at the Treitz level are especially problematic due to their atypical locations, often not identified with standard diagnostic imaging modalities. The optimal management of GISTs remains surgical resection for curative purposes, despite the challenges associated with preoperative diagnosis. As emphasized in recent studies, the use of non-invasive imaging techniques, such as ultrasound and computed tomography, can aid in preoperative planning and define appropriate surgical management in these patients, resulting in better outcomes and reducing the likelihood of recurrence (Georgescu et al., 2016). In addition, the incorporation of advanced technologies in upper gastrointestinal tract surgery is radically altering the prelude to surgical techniques and strategies. The past two decades have been characterized by a striking transition towards laparoscopic surgery, which has shown superior outcomes compared to conventional open techniques in most gastrointestinal operations. Importantly, this method promotes faster recovery, reduced postoperative pain, and lower hospital stays (Berloco et al., 2012). In liver transplant, however, synchronization of laparoscopic procedures with donor surgeries has also been equally promising in improving survival in patients with end-stage liver disease. Such advances not only reflect technological advancements but also a consistent determination within the surgical community to develop methodologies that ensure patient safety while achieving optimal therapeutic outcomes in upper GI surgery. The continuous evolution of surgical techniques underscores the need to adapt to newer methods that enhance patient care and surgical outcomes (Figure 4.12).

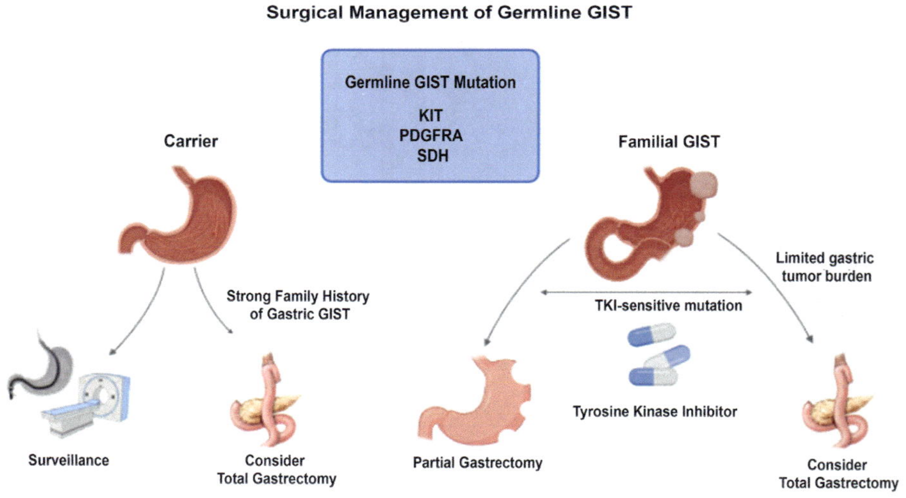

Figure 4.12. Surgical management of germline gastrointestinal stromal tumor.

Source: https://media.springernature.com/lw685/springer-static/image/art%3A10.1245%2Fs10434-023-13519-y/MediaObjects/10434_2023_13519_Figa_HTML.png.

4.5.1. Open Surgery Versus Laparoscopic Surgery

The evolution of surgical techniques in the field of upper gastrointestinal surgery has increasingly inclined patients towards laparoscopic procedures compared to open procedures. The reason for this is that there are numerous advantages associated with laparoscopic surgery, including the development of smaller incisions that lead to reduced postoperative discomfort, shorter durations of hospital stay, and fewer instances of complications like wound infection. The minimally invasive technique of laparoscopic surgery results in quicker rehabilitation for patients, thereby reducing the length of hospital stay—a polar opposite of prolonged recovery commonly associated with open surgery. With this, several procedures that were done initially with open surgery are now being done routinely under laparoscopy, with this proving to be a revolution in the field of upper gastrointestinal interventions (Berloco et al., 2012). When it comes to individual surgical conditions, the choice between laparoscopic and open approaches is particularly significant. A case in point would be with gastrointestinal stromal tumors (GISTs), where the dominant management paradigm continues to focus on complete surgical resection with uninvolved margins. As laparoscopic resections become more popular, controversy surrounding their effectiveness compared to open resections continues to hold merit. Retrospective analyses demonstrate that laparoscopic surgery has favorable outcomes, including decreased operation time and a comparable hospital stay for the patient, highlighting the importance of meticulous operative evaluation of tumor size and location. As intimidating as the case is with GISTs, laparoscopy is a viable option, demonstrating that patients' needs are being addressed through surgical progress (Alecu et al., 2019). However, the advantages of laparoscopic surgery will not always outweigh those of open techniques in every case. Physicians will need to consider variables such as patient health, pathology size and location, and their own experience when determining the optimal surgical method. Open surgery remains a viable alternative, especially in complex situations where direct visualization and access to internal structures are critical. Furthermore, as laparoscopic outcomes continue to improve, there will inevitably be instances where open surgery can provide better access or improved control over complications. Hence, an in-depth understanding of both modalities, alongside evolving developments, is essential to optimizing patient outcomes in upper gastrointestinal surgery and preserving a patient- and clinically individualized strategy.

4.5.2. Robotic-Assisted Surgery

In recent years, robotic surgery has emerged as a significant advance in the field of upper gastrointestinal surgery, particularly while undertaking procedures like total gastrectomy. Robotic technology enables surgeons to achieve improved precision and control, particularly for intricate procedures that require delicate maneuvers. For instance, a study of patients undergoing total gastrectomy through the robotic method indicated that the technique not only minimized the estimated blood loss to 126.55 ± 73 mL on average but also maintained the percentage of R0 resections at 100%, that is, successful tumor resection with no cancerous margins. Furthermore, the implementation of tailored approaches, such as the Parisi Technique, has been successful in improving surgical outcomes, with an illustration of how advanced robotics can be used to supplement patient care (Cirocchi et al., 2017).

In addition, the transition from open to robotic-assisted operations earns its place within broader trends in surgical practice that aim for minimally invasive approaches. Robotic systems, which enable the use of smaller incisions, provide essential advantages over traditional methods, including reduced pain during the postoperative period and shorter recovery times. Robotic surgery has other benefits that can lower the rate of complications, such as wound infections, and permit quicker hospital discharges. Since laparoscopy already greatly revolutionized most surgical specialties, robotic approaches are the following line in minimally invasive surgery, most significantly so in cases of upper gastrointestinal disease, which most commonly feature problems of dissection with complicated anatomy (Berloco et al., 2012).

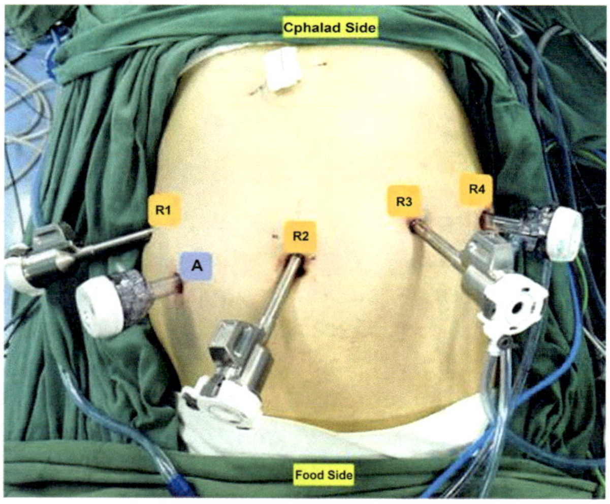

Figure 4.13. Robot-assisted laparoscopic combined with endoscopic partial gastrectomy (RALE-PG).

Source: https://www.frontiersin.org/files/Articles/1391387/fsurg-11-1391387-HTML/image_m/fsurg-11-1391387-g001.jpg.

Robotically assisted approaches will gradually replace upper gastrointestinal surgery in the future, driven by ongoing technological advancements and growing evidence of their effectiveness. As additional evidence accrues for the successful outcomes of robotic surgery, the surgical fraternity is not only bound to adopt these techniques but also to further optimize them in order to integrate them harmoniously. The synergy of optimized technology, surgeons' skills, and augmented surgical skills holds significant promise for improved patient safety and satisfaction. Hence, with robot-assisted surgery becoming more common, it has the potential not only to enhance individual surgical outcomes but also to redefine the paradigms of care within the field of upper gastrointestinal surgery (Figure 4.13).

4.5.3. Innovations in Surgical Techniques

Advances in surgical techniques have been spurred on significantly by technological advances focusing on efficiency and outcome for the patient, particularly in upper GI surgery. Studies indicate that one such advance has been the expansion of specialized surgical facilities, including ambulatory surgery centers and physician-owned specialty hospitals. Studies indicate these organizations aim to enhance the quality of services at the expense of lower costs; however, support for their competitive aim remains limited. According to recent systematic reviews, even when such advantages are present, they should be assessed in terms of their impact on traditional full-service general hospitals to ensure quality healthcare is widely accessible and fair to all patients (Annemans et al., 2013). This highlights the necessity for an equilibrium strategy in embracing innovation in operating rooms to ensure not only technological innovation, but also systemic integrity of health provision. Another significant innovation in upper GI surgery is the use of advanced endoscopic methods maximizing procedure effectiveness while minimizing patient discomfort. A recent publication introduced a new endoscope holding device that enables single-handed manipulation, facilitating easier surgical procedures. In controlled trials, this innovation was found to reduce manipulation times and surgeon ergonomic complaints by a considerable degree while enhancing their focus throughout procedures. The device effectively integrates an active zoom function with a passive holder, enabling the surgeon to maintain unhampered control of the endoscope, a crucial requirement in minimally invasive surgery (Bauwens et al., 2020). Such an integration of technologies not only simplifies surgery duration but also improves surgical precision, eventually leading to better patient recovery times and satisfaction. The trend toward minimally invasive surgery, more recently fueled by robotic and 3D imaging technology, is yet another revolutionary development in upper gastrointestinal surgery. Robotic systems have revolutionized the way surgeries are performed on complex anatomical structures by providing enhanced dexterity and precision compared to conventional techniques. With three-dimensional imaging, these technologies enhance visualization and anatomical awareness, which are crucial in navigating the complex upper gastrointestinal tract. As more and more surgeons adopt such instruments, there is growing evidence that supports lower complication rates as well as reduced hospital stays. Thus, the use of such cutting-edge techniques in routine practice is not only cost-effective but also eliminates variation in patient experience and outcomes, further affirming the importance of innovation in surgical procedures (Bauwens et al., 2020).

Test Your Knowledge

1. Define the robotic-assisted surgery
2. What is the difference between open and laparoscopic surgical approaches?
3. Which surgical layers must be carefully closed to prevent postoperative hernia?

4.6. Postoperative Care and Complications

Learning Outcome

1. Describe the immediate postoperative care
2. Define the common complications and their management for upper gastrointestinal surgery
3. Identify the long-term follow-up after upper gastrointestinal surgery

Postoperative care following upper gastrointestinal surgery is critical to minimizing complications and facilitating recovery. Effective pain management is a crucial consideration in such situations, particularly following procedures such as pancreatoduodenectomy. Epidural analgesia (EDA) is gaining favor among surgeons as an approach to pain management with the additional advantage of minimizing complications. Research has indicated that EDA patients experience significantly fewer wound disturbances, unplanned intubations, and pulmonary embolism. Additionally, EDA has been associated with lower pain scores in the initial days following surgery, lending credence to its role in recovery. This personalized approach to pain control, therefore, not only aims to improve patient comfort but most significantly reduces the risk of postoperative complications, thereby highlighting the pivotal role of directed postoperative therapeutic strategies in maximizing outcomes (Ceppa et al., 2019).

Surgical teams need to understand the diverse complications that can arise after upper gastrointestinal surgery. These complications may be early or late in the postoperative period and may be infection, delayed gastric emptying, or life-threatening issues such as pancreatitis and biliary obstructions. Surgeons should be vigilant in monitoring their patients for both general and surgery-specific complications.

For instance, in patients undergoing bariatric surgery, there are risks of bowel obstruction, leaks, or hernias due to the extensive anatomical reconstruction during surgery. Acute care surgeons should be familiar with the surgical procedure being performed and the typical post-bariatric surgical emergencies they can expect, thereby preparing them to overcome these complications as they occur (Beekley et al., 2018).

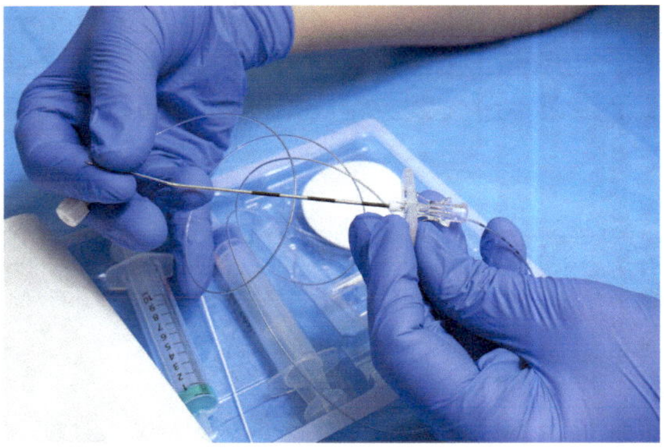

Figure 4.14. Epidural anesthesia (EA).

Source: https://anesthguide.com/wp-content/uploads/2023/05/EDA-set-kateter-genom-nal-demonstration.jpg.

Incorporating adequate postoperative care plans can significantly decrease the risk associated with upper gastrointestinal surgery. These guidelines should incorporate proper monitoring, early mobilization, and nutritional support, which are important in maximizing recovery. Additionally, educating the patient on possible complications and warning signs following surgery is highly significant for the immediate detection and intervention. Active interventions in postoperative care are effective in reducing readmission rates and enhancing patient satisfaction. For example, the treatment of complications such as infections or malnutrition early in the process can be employed to avoid extensive morbidity. By creating a culture of vigilant postoperative care, medical teams can significantly enhance the overall surgical process and outcomes for patients undergoing upper gastrointestinal procedures, ultimately resulting in improved long-term health outcomes (Ceppa et al., 2019) (Figure 4.14).

4.6.1. Immediate Postoperative Care

Following upper gastrointestinal surgery, early postoperative management is crucial in preventing complications and facilitating optimal recovery. This phase is initiated mainly in the post-anesthesia care unit (PACU), where careful observation of vital signs is maintained. The primary aim is to identify even subtle complications, such as bleeding, infection, or respiratory distress, as early as possible. During this phase, patients are generally conscious of requiring pain control, since optimal analgesia has a massive impact on outcome following recovery. Monitoring for the return of gastrointestinal function, including tolerance for oral intake and bowel sounds, is also included in this. Complications assessment and management watchfulness is required in optimizing postoperative trends, ultimately enhancing overall surgical outcomes (N/A, 2018). In conjunction with monitoring the patient's vital signs and pain control, education is a crucial component of immediate postoperative care. Healthcare providers must inform families and patients about the postoperative orders required and signs of complications, such as inappropriate discharge or pain in the operative area. Proper communication of diet advancement expectations, activity restrictions, and follow-up is essential for ensuring compliance and ultimately achieving successful results. Patient involvement can also ensure autonomy and reduce anxiety. Addressing these educational requirements allows healthcare practitioners to enable well-informed decision-making, which has also been found to improve patient satisfaction and outcomes following upper gastrointestinal surgery (Ndongo et al., 2010). Moreover, the psychological aspect of postoperative care cannot be overlooked. Anxiety and concern regarding the success of surgery may impede recovery; thus, reassurance and emotional support are key components of postoperative care. Establishing a rapport with hospital staff can help alleviate patients' anxieties and foster a healing environment. Empathic communication, active listening, and participation in a social support system can significantly contribute to the welfare of patients during the vulnerable early recovery phase. Furthermore, interdisciplinary care that incorporates nursing, nutrition, and mental health services can address the patient's total needs and facilitate the healing process during recovery time. All of these aspects highlight the importance of holistic care in postoperative rehabilitation following upper GI surgery (N/A, 2018) (Figure 4.15).

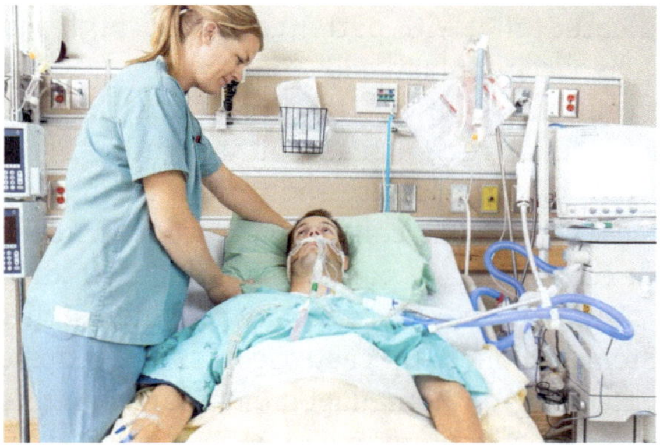

Figure 4.15. Post anesthesia.

Source: https://stabilityhealthcare.com/wp-content/uploads/2023/04/PACU-Nurse-2_158643701.jpg.

4.6.2. Common Complications and Their Management

Upper gastrointestinal surgery, although commonly required in the treatment of most pathological conditions, also has its fair share of complications that may significantly impact patient outcomes. One common complication experienced after the operation is gastrointestinal hemorrhage, which may result from several causes, such as anastomotic leak or erosion of the abutting organs. Clinically significant gastrointestinal hemorrhage has occurred in approximately 23% of involved patients in one series of 150 orthotopic hepatic transplants, with survival of only 15% for the patients who developed this complication (Koep et al., 1979). Appropriate management includes monitoring, imaging studies to localize the source of bleeding, and urgent surgery where necessary. The formation of a large peritoneal drainage is also required in cases of significant internal hemorrhage, to ensure proper fluid balance and prevent complications such as stagnant blood in the peritoneal cavity. Another common complication that must be managed in upper gastrointestinal surgery is enteric perforation, particularly following biliary-enteric surgery. Clinically, enteric perforations in 20 patients after such a procedure had a very low survival rate, and that indicates just how dangerous the complication is (Koep et al., 1979). It involves initial rapid detection of the perforation, typically necessitating reoperation to repair the defect and decontaminate the peritoneal cavity of bile and intestinal contents. The surgeons must be aggressive in diagnosis, employing imaging methods and even exploratory surgery to determine the extent of the injury. Prompt treatment is also crucial to avoid secondary ailments such as sepsis or disseminated peritonitis that can further exacerbate the patient's condition and reduce the survival rate significantly. With the increasing percentage of upper gastrointestinal procedures represented by bariatric surgery, surgeons must be especially sensitive to the complications involving deranged gastric anatomy. These occur either early or late in the postoperative course and range from leaks secondary to sleeve gastrectomy to obstructions created by internal hernias. Acute care surgeons must be aware of these potential complications while being cognizant of other common abdominal catastrophes, such as appendicitis or pancreatitis, that can occur regardless of previous surgery. Practical preoperative patient evaluation and postoperative monitoring are crucial in managing these complications. Additionally, a customized strategy that addresses the specific anatomical changes after surgery is crucial for maximizing patient results and reducing the risks associated with such procedures.

4.6.3. Long-Term Follow-Up and Lifestyle Changes

Long-term follow-up after upper gastrointestinal surgery is crucial in ensuring optimal patient outcomes, particularly in terms of lifestyle changes and health maintenance. Since morbid obesity is defined as a chronic condition that needs ongoing care, the role of a multidisciplinary team becomes relevant after surgery. Nutritional monitoring is typically required for patients to prevent complications, such as malnutrition, which can result from inadequate dietary changes following surgery. A thorough follow-up plan, with regular assessments of dietary intake and lifestyle modifications, can significantly impact weight maintenance and overall health. The development of complications such as pancreatic exocrine insufficiency (PEI) underlines the necessity of long-term medical follow-up. The condition can potentially arise from maldigestion and malabsorption, which can complicate the patient's overall recovery and quality of life, thus necessitating long-term follow-up (Arnelo et al., 2017). Moreover, the consequences of altered gastrointestinal anatomy following upper gastrointestinal surgery necessitate individualized lifestyle adjustments tailored to each patient's specific needs. For instance, those with gastric bypass operations are typically recommended a vitamin- and mineral-fortified diet while balancing protein intake simultaneously. This is not only to counteract nutrient deficiencies but also to ensure adequate digestion and nutrient assimilation. The dietary modifications must be followed by behavioral modifications that reinforce a healthy lifestyle, such as increased physical activity and regular follow-up visits. An adequate follow-up schedule can help detect and manage any nutritional challenges that arise, aiding patients in adapting successfully to a healthier lifestyle that is beneficial to long-term outcomes after surgery. Follow-up time tables of long-term also need to include screening for potential complications such as gastric cancer and type I gastric carcinoids in patients with atrophic gastritis (AG) disease. Studies have indicated that AG patients are at high risk of gastric neoplastic lesions, where frequent surveillance is of key importance in the early diagnosis of such diseases at an early stage of development. Evidence shows that the number of cases of gastric cancer and carcinoids every year conspicuously points to regular monitoring in the long term. Accordingly, the inclusion of systematic follow-up gastroscopies and biopsies in the long-term management plan facilitates early detection and management and, in the long term, enhances patient prognosis. To this end, doctors should emphasize the importance of adhering to follow-up recommendations to ensure optimal results and encourage long-term lifestyle changes that promote overall health management following surgery (Annibale et al., 2015).

Test Your Knowledge

1. What are the early signs of an anastomotic leak after gastric surgery?
2. How is postoperative ileus managed in upper GI surgical patients?

SUMMARY

By placing an emphasis on the key innovations and challenges of upper gastrointestinal surgery, it is evident that ongoing innovation and research are necessary to improve patient outcomes. The convergence of sophisticated technologies and advanced techniques has led to greater surgical precision, with the ability to reduce recovery times and complication rates associated with traditional open surgery. Moreover, the development of successful drainage techniques, such as EID and EVT, has been observed to yield positive results in managing complications, including anastomotic leaks that arise after oncologic procedures. Not only do these interventions point to high rates of closure, but also towards the trend of surgical practice moving away from invasive interventions (Jung et al., 2021). As more sophisticated surgical techniques are created, a parallel focus on patient and risk stratification will be vital to optimize results. Moreover, an understanding of the multi-factorial etiology of complications of upper gastrointestinal surgery can play a significant role in influencing clinical practices. Research indicates that the severity of blood loss, surgical procedure type, and patient comorbidities are essential in establishing mortality rates for nonvariceal upper gastrointestinal bleeding (верхних отделов et al., 2019). This highlights the importance for medical practitioners to monitor a holistic assessment strategy before and during surgery. By integrating risk stratification tools such as the Charlson comorbidity index and the Rockall scale, physicians can enhance preoperative planning and postoperative care, thereby decreasing adverse outcomes and overall patient harm. In conclusion, upper gastrointestinal surgery is an environment of constant change, characterized by technological development and increasing knowledge regarding patient care. The effective implementation of novel therapeutic techniques holds the promise of an illustrious future, marking a shift toward less invasive and more effective methods of surgery tailored to meet the diverse needs of the patient population. With research continuing to shed insight into the dynamics of surgery risks and patient outcomes, the healthcare community must embrace this knowledge. By embracing such a collaborative system, upper gastrointestinal surgery will not only progress but also enhance the quality of patient care, firmly establishing it as an integral part of surgical medicine.

The field of upper gastrointestinal surgery is characterized by significant technical advancements and postoperative care, particularly in the case of PD. A seminal study assessed the role of EDA in postoperative pain control in patients with PD undergoing surgery and revealed significant benefits associated with its use. Among 671 patients, outcomes indicated EDA-treated patients had lower rates of wound disruptions, unplanned intubations, and pulmonary complications compared with their non-EDA counterparts. The study highlights the importance of utilizing maximally effective pain control methods to enhance outcomes and reduce complications following primary operations. Furthermore, the association of EDA with lower pain scores in the early postoperative period suggests a potential benefit for EDA in daily care following PD, such that its implementation can become part of routine practice throughout upper gastrointestinal surgery to maximize postoperative outcomes. Another aspect of note of upper gastrointestinal surgery is the early detection of gastroesophageal cancer, which has a relatively poor prognosis due to late presentation. Evidence suggests that the patient interval, or the time it takes for patients to receive care after showing symptoms, plays a crucial role in determining outcomes for gastroesophageal malignancies. By identifying the variables that influence the delay, clinicians can tailor interventions to promote early diagnosis and treatment. The study identifies methodological limitations present in the existing cancer literature, including inconsistencies in definitions and a lack of qualitative findings related to patients' experiences. These variations hinder global statistical meta-analysis and necessitate greater patient awareness and education to allow for earlier clinical presentation, eventually improving survival rates among patients with gastroesophageal cancer. Implications of such data in clinical practice are necessary for the improvement of techniques in upper GI surgery. EDAs demonstrated effectiveness in patients with postoperative pain management and complication prevention is a compelling basis for their adoption as routine practice in surgery. Concurrently, removal of diagnostic delays for gastroesophageal cancer requires concerted action in patient education and awareness campaigns. This would significantly contribute to achieving optimal surgical outcomes through increased device implementation rates. With research development continuing, the combination of new methods of pain control, including EDA, with pre-emptiveness to reduce patient interval in the presentation of cancer demonstrates a multiplier approach crucial to enhancing the overall effectiveness of upper gastrointestinal operations.

KEY TERMS FROM THIS CHAPTER

- Achalasia
- Barrett's esophagus
- Esophageal cancer
- Esophagectomy
- Fundoplication
- Gastric cancer
- Gastroesophageal reflux disease (GERD)
- Anastomotic leak
- Dumping syndrome
- Esophageal perforation
- Feeding jejunostomy
- Gastrectomy
- Gastric outlet obstruction
- Gastrojejunostomy

CRITICAL THINKING QUESTIONS

1. **Which of the following is the most common surgical procedure for treating gastroesophageal reflux disease (GERD)?**
   a. Billroth II gastrectomy
   b. Nissen fundoplication
   c. Esophagectomy
   d. Pyloromyotomy
2. **Which type of hiatal hernia involves upward displacement of the gastroesophageal junction and part of the stomach into the thorax?**
   a. Type I (Sliding hernia)
   b. Type II (Paraesophageal hernia)
   c. Type III (Mixed hernia)
   d. Type IV (Complex hernia)
3. **Which of the following is the most specific investigation for diagnosing achalasia cardia?**
   a. Chest X-ray
   b. Barium swallow
   c. Upper GI endoscopy
   d. Esophageal manometry
4. **Dumping syndrome is most commonly seen after which surgical procedure?**
   a. Nissen fundoplication
   b. Total colectomy
   c. Partial gastrectomy (Billroth II)
   d. Cholecystectomy
5. **Which of the following is a poor prognostic factor in gastric carcinoma?**
   a. Tumor confined to mucosa
   b. Absence of lymph node metastasis
   c. Signet ring cell histology
   d. Early satiety as presenting symptom

Short Answer Questions

1. What are the indications for surgical intervention in patients with gastroesophageal reflux disease (GERD)?
2. Describe the main types of hiatal hernias and their clinical significance.
3. What is the pathophysiology of peptic ulcer disease?
4. Outline the classification and surgical options for gastric cancer based on TNM staging.
5. What are the complications of partial gastrectomy, and how is dumping syndrome managed?
6. Explain the role of laparoscopic Nissen fundoplication in the treatment of GERD.
7. How is achalasia cardia diagnosed and surgically treated?
8. Compare the surgical approaches for esophageal carcinoma.

Answers to Critical Thinking Questions

1. (b); 2. (a); 3. (d); 4. (c); 5. (c)

REFERENCES

1. Tringali, A., Thomson, M., Dumonceau, J., Tavares, M., Tabbers, M., Furlano, R., Spaander, M., Hassan, C., Tzvinikos, C., Ijsselstijn, H., Viala, J., Dall'Oglio, L., Benninga, M., Orel, R., Vandenplas, Y., Keil, R., Romano, C., Brownstone, E., Hlava, Š., . . . Zambelli, A. (2016). Pediatric gastrointestinal endoscopy: European Society of Gastrointestinal Endoscopy (ESGE) and European Society for Paediatric Gastroenterology Hepatology and Nutrition (ESPGHAN) Guideline Executive summary. *Endoscopy*, *49*(01), 83–91. https://doi.org/10.1055/s-0042-111002Abbas, M., Adler, D., Affi, A., Alexander, L., Caetano, A. C., Andriulli, A., Apel, D., et al. (2013). *Emergencies after endoscopic procedures.* https://core.ac.uk/download/55625568.pdf (accessed on 12th July 2025).
2. Agius, R. (2014). *An evaluation of the bariatric surgical patient.* https://core.ac.uk/download/46602470.pdf (accessed on 12th July 2025).
3. Alema, N. O., Ogwang, D. M., Okello, T. R., & Pecorella, I. (2016). *An evaluation of 605 endoscopic examinations in a rural setting, Lacor Hospital in Northern Uganda.* https://core.ac.uk/download/188828821.pdf (accessed on 12th July 2025).
4. Al-Haddad, M., Anand, B. S., Baron, T. H., Berg, D. E., Bhutani, M. S., Bottrell, T., Boyle, M., et al. (2014). *Clinical evaluation, imaging studies, indications for cytologic study, and preprocedural requirements for duct brushing studies and pancreatic FNA: The Papanicolaou Society of Cytopathology recommendations for pancreatic and biliary cytology.* https://deepblue.lib.umich.edu/bitstream/2027.42/106723/1/dc23095.pdf (accessed on 12th July 2025).
5. Allardice, G. M., Coubrough, S., Noone, A., Reilly, J., et al. (2008). *Results from the Scottish national HAI prevalence survey.* https://core.ac.uk/download/9023284.pdf (accessed on 12th July 2025).
6. Almalioglu, Y., Araujo, H., Ornek, E. P., Sitti, M., et al. (2018). *Magnetic-visual sensor fusion-based dense 3D reconstruction and localization for endoscopic capsule robots.* http://arxiv.org/abs/1803.01048 (accessed on 12th July 2025).
7. Almar, E., Arveux, P., Autelitano, M., Baldi, I., Bara, S., Barchielli, A., Benfatto, L., et al. (2019). *Treatment challenges in and outside a specialist network setting: Pancreatic neuroendocrine tumors.* https://core.ac.uk/download/287859188.pdf (accessed on 12th July 2025).
8. Aly, A., Devitt, P. G., Game, P. A., Gan, T. J., et al. (2015). *Laparoscopic repair of very large hiatus hernia with sutures versus absorbable mesh versus nonabsorbable mesh: A randomized controlled trial.* https://core.ac.uk/download/43335357.pdf (accessed on 12th July 2025).
9. Annemans, L., De Regge, M., Duyck, P., Gemmel, P., et al. (2013). *Physician-owned specialized facilities: Focused factories or destructive competition?: A systematic review.* https://core.ac.uk/download/55777137.pdf (accessed on 12th July 2025).
10. Annibale, B., Corleto, V. D., Di Giulio, E., Esposito, G., et al. (2015). *Occurrence of gastric cancer and carcinoids in atrophic gastritis during prospective long-term follow-up.* https://core.ac.uk/download/54520617.pdf (accessed on 12th July 2025).
11. Arebi, N., Saunders, B. P., & Surgical Procedures, Endoscopic. (2005). *Endoscopy: An evolving specialty.* https://core.ac.uk/download/46602009.pdf (accessed on 12th July 2025).
12. Arnelo, U., Haas, S. L., Löhr, J.-M., Martin, I., et al. (2017). *Pancreatic exocrine insufficiency after bariatric surgery.* https://core.ac.uk/download/188827229.pdf (accessed on 12th July 2025).

13. Banu, P., Constantin, V. D., Nistor, M. F., Popa, D., et al. (2016). *Perforated small intestine in a patient with T-cell lymphoma: A rare cause of peritonitis.* https://core.ac.uk/download/144552420.pdf (accessed on 12th July 2025).
14. Bauwens, K., Blanckaert, B., De Pauw, T., Dewaele, A., et al. (2020). *A novel hybrid 3D endoscope zooming and repositioning system: Design and feasibility study.* https://core.ac.uk/download/286549295.pdf (accessed on 12th July 2025).
15. Beekley, A., Davis, K. A., Johnson, D. C., Lim, R. B., et al. (2018). *Early and late complications of bariatric operation.* https://core.ac.uk/download/213444927.pdf (accessed on 12th July 2025).
16. Berloco, P. B., Di Laudo, M., Frattaroli, F. M., Guglielmo, S., et al. (2012). *Laparoscopy in liver transplantation: The future has arrived.* https://core.ac.uk/download/154948504.pdf (accessed on 12th July 2025).
17. Bernstein, R. A., Dubiel, R., Eikelboom, J. W., Glund, S., et al. (2017). *Idarucizumab for Dabigatran reversal – Full cohort analysis.* https://core.ac.uk/download/83049746.pdf (accessed on 12th July 2025).
18. Besecker, E. S., Cooper, T. K., Deiter, G. M., Holmes, J., et al. (2016). *Mesenteric vascular dysregulation and intestinal inflammation accompanies experimental spinal cord injury.* https://cupola.gettysburg.edu/cgi/viewcontent.cgi?article=1073&context=healthfac (accessed on 12th July 2025).
19. Boachie, C., Bojke, L., Campbell, M. K., Corbacho, B., et al. (2013). *Clinical and economic evaluation of laparoscopic surgery compared with medical management for gastro-oesophageal reflux disease: 5-year follow-up of multicenter randomized trial (the REFLUX trial).* https://core.ac.uk/download/11304053.pdf (accessed on 12th July 2025).
20. Bou-Antoun, S., Cromwell, D. A., Gurol-Urganci, I., Lim, T., et al. (2013). *Impact of Caesarean section on subsequent fertility: A systematic review and meta-analysis.*
21. Bruce, J., & Krukowski, Z. H. (2006). *Quality of life and chronic pain four years after gastrointestinal surgery.* https://core.ac.uk/download/177033.pdf (accessed on 12th July 2025).
22. Calabrese, E., Dietrich, C. F., Dirks, K., Gilja, O., et al. (2016). *EFSUMB recommendations and guidelines for gastrointestinal ultrasound – Part 1: Examination techniques and normal findings (short version).* https://core.ac.uk/download/74321243.pdf (accessed on 12th July 2025).
23. Caplin, M., Falconi, M., Fusai, G. K., Lykoudis, P., et al. (2017). *Treatment challenges in and outside a specialist network setting: Pancreatic neuroendocrine tumors.* https://core.ac.uk/download/168403284.pdf (accessed on 12th July 2025).
24. Ceppa, E. P., Colgate, C. L., Fennerty, M. L., House, M. G., et al. (2019). *Post-pancreatoduodenectomy outcomes and epidural analgesia: A 5-year single institution experience.* https://core.ac.uk/download/187423802.pdf (accessed on 12th July 2025).
25. Chalya, P. L., Jaka, H., Koy, M., Mabula, D., et al. (2012). *Gastric cancer at a university teaching hospital in Northwestern Tanzania: A retrospective review of 232 cases.* https://core.ac.uk/download/pdf/11307769.pdf (accessed on 12th July 2025).
26. Cirocchi, R., D'Andrea, V., Desiderio, J., Gemini, A., et al. (2017). *New totally intracorporeal reconstructive approach after robotic total gastrectomy: Technical details and short-term*

outcomes. https://core.ac.uk/download/98347731.pdf (accessed on 12th July 2025).

27. Dahiya, R., Dahms, S. E., Gleason, C. A., Lue, T. F., et al. (1999). *Bladder acellular matrix graft: In vivo functional properties of the regenerated rat bladder*. https://core.ac.uk/download/323074003.pdf (accessed on 12th July 2025).
28. Elghuel, A., Timraz, A., Olokoba, A. B., Kankaria, A. G., Liwa, A., Meaden, C., Zaltman, C., et al. (2012). *A fibreoptic endoscopic study of upper gastrointestinal bleeding at Bugando Medical Centre in Northwestern Tanzania: A retrospective review of 240 cases*. https://core.ac.uk/download/pdf/11307794.pdf (accessed on 12th July 2025).
29. Georgescu, L. C., Pătraşcu, T., Tobă, M. E., Ungureanu, A., et al. (2016). *Gastrointestinal stromal tumor (GIST) of the Treitz's angle – A very rare cause of high bowel obstruction*. https://core.ac.uk/download/144552989.pdf (accessed on 12th July 2025).
30. Jung, C., Hallit, R., Müller-Dornieden, A., Calmels, M., Goéré, D., Chaput, U., Camus, M., et al. (2021). Endoscopic internal drainage and low negative-pressure endoscopic vacuum therapy for anastomotic leaks after oncologic upper gastrointestinal surgery. *Endoscopy*. https://www.semanticscholar.org/paper/9626932bb46e861c96e5ceb4294843596f0c5e01 (accessed on 12th July 2025).
31. Khulusi, S., Lee, A., & Watson, R. (2017). *Which interval is most crucial to presentation and survival in gastroesophageal cancer: A systematic review*. https://core.ac.uk/download/151161832.pdf (accessed on 12th July 2025).
32. Koep, L. J., Starzl, T. E., & Weil, R. (1979). *Gastrointestinal complications of hepatic transplantation*. https://core.ac.uk/download/12203829.pdf (accessed on 12th July 2025).
33. Lorenz, W., & Rothmund, M. (1989). *Theoretical surgery: A new specialty in operative medicine*. https://core.ac.uk/download/11550720.pdf (accessed on 12th July 2025).
34. Ndongo, B. C., Mballa, G. A. E., Hyder, A. A., Juillard, C., et al. (2010). *Patterns of injury and violence in Yaoundé, Cameroon: An analysis of hospital data*. https://core.ac.uk/download/323075033.pdf (accessed on 12th July 2025).
35. Phillips, B. (2016). *Reducing gastrointestinal anastomotic leak rates: Review of challenges and solutions*. https://core.ac.uk/download/155271752.pdf (accessed on 12th July 2025).
36. Pollack, C. V. (2016). *Evidence supporting idarucizumab for the reversal of dabigatran*. https://core.ac.uk/download/213442189.pdf (accessed on 12th July 2025).

LIVER, PANCREATIC, AND BILIARY SURGERY

5

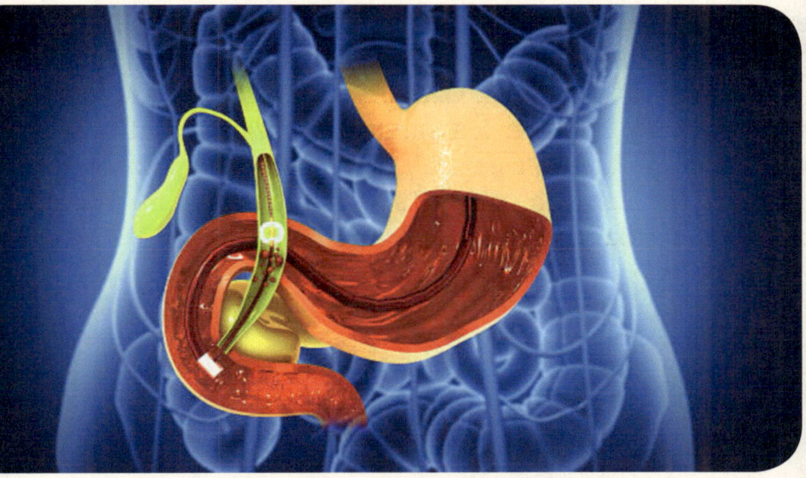

LEARNING OBJECTIVES

After studying this chapter, you will be able to:

1. Understand the anatomy and function of the liver
2. Explain the overview of pancreatic anatomy
3. Discuss the biliary system anatomy
4. Focus on indications for surgery in liver, pancreatic, and biliary surgery
5. Learn about surgical techniques in liver, pancreatic, and biliary surger
6. Evaluate the postoperative care in liver, pancreatic, and biliary surgery

Introduction

The science of pancreatic, liver, and biliary surgery forms the core of managing complex diseases of these organs. Pancreatic cancer, the third leading cause of cancer-related deaths, is a classic illustration of the necessity for new surgical techniques and treatment strategies. A lack of effective screening modalities also compounds the delicacy of early detection of pancreatic cancers. Thus the disease is often diagnosed late. This has profound consequences for patient outcomes and surgical interventions, since surgical removal is only possible in a minority of cases. Efforts have concentrated on maximizing early detection strategies, such as the examination of circulating tumor cells (CTCs), which can provide insightful genomic information regarding the type and behavior of a tumor (Pimienta et al., 2017). Thus, comprehension of the role of surgery in treating liver, pancreatic, and biliary diseases is essential to overcome such ongoing challenges. Surgical interventions in this context extend beyond tumor resection to encompass various means of addressing complications secondary to malignancies. In obstructive jaundice that commonly occurs with pancreatic cancer, early biliary drainage is essential. Endoscopic procedures are more likely to be applied due to their being less invasive; however, some conditions necessitate more surgical interventions. Open drainage surgery, for instance, may be inevitable in the instance of unresectable tumors. One should note the double bypass biliodigestive construction technique, which is especially beneficial to patients presenting with combined manifestations such as obstructive jaundice and gastric outlet obstruction. This highlights the need for surgical approaches to vary according to the diverse clinical presentations of pancreatic disorders, underscoring the importance of specialized surgical expertise. Additionally, the history of liver, pancreatic, and biliary surgery is ever-evolving, influenced by technological advances and our increasing understanding of disease processes. More recent methods, such as robotic and laparoscopic surgery, have improved recovery and reduced postoperative morbidity, and advances in imaging technologies are complementing planning pre-surgery. Furthermore, translation of liquid biopsies and CTCs analysis to clinical practice has the potential to enable personalized treatment regimens, facilitating improved results. With ongoing research, the future of biliary, pancreatic, and liver surgery is not only in enhanced surgical procedures but also in embracing an interdisciplinary mindset that incorporates oncological, radiological, and pathological expertise. The endgame, nonetheless, remains the same: to enhance survival rates and the overall quality of life for patients facing pancreatic and biliary pathology (Figure 5.1).

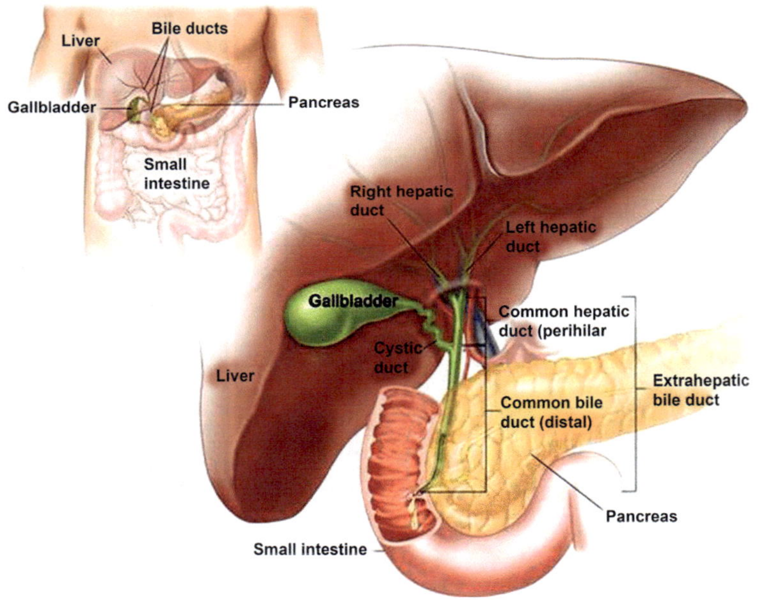

Figure 5.1. Hepato pancreato biliary surgery.

Source: https://thesurgicalclinics.com/wp-content/uploads/2021/03/hepato-pancreato-biliary-surgery.png.

Definition of Liver, Pancreatic, and Biliary Surgery

The surgical disciplines of liver, pancreatic, and biliary surgery encompass a range of procedures that address the management of disorders affecting the liver, pancreas, bile ducts, and gallbladder. The procedures are significant in the management of diseases such as cancers, traumatic injuries, and chronic inflammatory conditions. Liver surgery entails mainly procedures that include liver resections and transplantation, necessitated by liver tumors or end-stage liver disease. Pancreatic surgery, on the other hand, involves sophisticated techniques such as the Whipple procedure to resect tumors and maintain digestive tract integrity. Biliary surgery corrects disease or bile duct or gallbladder obstruction to enable bile to flow consistently from the liver into the intestine. All the above operations are components of the healing of serious gastrointestinal disease and improving the quality of life in patients. In addition, their definitions and categorizations are broad and complex, with implications for the clinical approach to patient care. A complex understanding of the anatomy and physiology of the organs is needed, as the success of surgery will significantly vary depending on the underlying condition, as well as the patients' health status. For instance, liver resection may be sufficient for a localized tumor growth, but fulminant liver disease may require advanced interventions such as transplantation. Each operative section requires specialized skills and planning to resolve the issues posed by vascular pedicles and biliary anatomy. With the increase in obesity-induced conditions and metabolic derangement syndromes, and rising incidence of malignancies in the liver and pancreas, the role of these branches of surgery will keep growing, highlighting the need for innovation and specialized training in these fields (Kyrou et al., 2010).

Apart from refining surgical techniques, continued research and innovation in liver, pancreatic, and biliary surgery are focused on minimizing complications and enhancing postoperative care. As surgical methods become progressively minimally invasive—that is, with the evolution of laparoscopic surgery—outcomes show dramatic improvements in recovery times and rates of patient morbidity. Furthermore, postoperative treatment—for example, nutritional supplementation and monitoring for postoperative complications such as infection or biliary fistulae—is an essential part of patient recovery, with profound effects on long-term success. The incorporation of multidisciplinary teams, including surgeons, oncologists, and gastroenterologists, reflects the contemporary approach to managing complex gastrointestinal diseases. With the evolving global health concerns, especially in regions most affected by diseases and surgical conditions, continuous emphasis on education and innovative surgical procedures in liver, pancreas, and biliary surgery remains paramount (Ndongo et al., 2010).

Relevance of the Surgical Procedures in Modern Medicine

The refinement of surgery in liver, pancreatic, and biliary surgery is a milestone in modern medicine with profound effects on patient outcomes. Minimally invasive techniques, particularly robot-assisted procedures, have emerged as essential tools in refining surgical precision, reducing patient morbidity, and shortening hospital stays. An agreement reached among surgical experts, notably at the ROBOT4HPB conference, is that robotics can expand the application of minimally invasive methods to further hepatobiliary procedures. This reflects a trend towards more sophisticated interventions that appreciate both the efficacy and safety of operations for enhancing overall health quality for patients with critical liver and pancreatic diseases (Hobeika et al., 2024). Thus, the combination of these technologies not only enhances surgical proficiency but also marks a broader trend within medical practice towards utilizing innovation to optimize and modernize patient care. In addition to technological innovation, the importance of surgery in the therapy of liver, pancreatic, and biliary illnesses cannot be overstated. These procedures are often life-saving when they concern cancers of these organs, which are presented as formidable challenges in oncology. Traditional techniques have created room for novel approaches that complement evolving therapies, including complementary therapies from traditional Chinese medicine (TCM). Research has revealed the clinical efficacy of specific TCM therapies, such as Huaier Granule and Huachansu, when used in conjunction with surgical techniques. Their potential to enhance patient outcomes underscores the worth of combined treatment modalities in modern medicine, particularly as subsequent evidence emerges to validate their therapeutic merit (Wu et al., 2024). Their coexistence highlights the need for ongoing research and adaptation to develop effective treatment modalities for complex diseases.

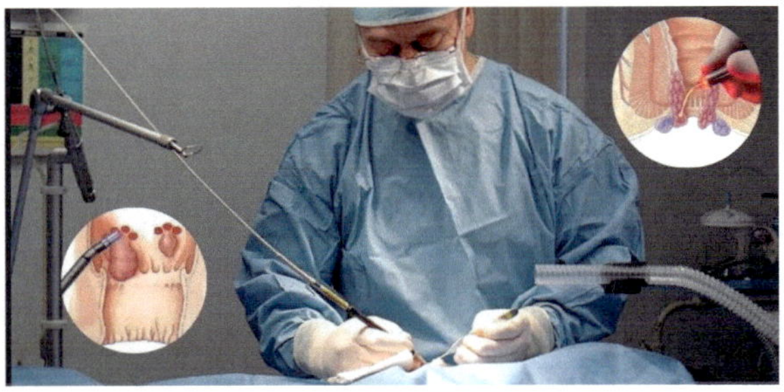

Figure 5.2. Modern surgeries.

Source: https://www.restoracare.in/wp-content/uploads/2022/03/laser-piles-surgery.jpg.

Further, the evolving nature of liver, pancreatic, and biliary surgery emphasizes the importance of special training and expertise among surgical professionals. As technologies begin to penetrate the surgical domain, the need for comprehensive training programs becomes increasingly greater. Robotic surgery, to take a case point, involves not only surgical skill but a close understanding of the associated technologies and attendant implications in patient care. The ROBOT4HPB consensus also emphasized the credentialing of this specialty to ensure that surgeons are adequately prepared to perform these advanced techniques safely (Hobeika et al., 2024). Professional development training and continuous learning equip surgeons with the necessary skills and data to manage the intricacies of these procedures, thereby enhancing patient outcomes and solidifying the role of surgical interventions as pillars of modern medicine (Figure 5.2).

5.1. Anatomy and Function of the Liver

Learning Outcome

1. Describe the structure of the liver and its lobe
2. Focus on functions of the liver in metabolism and detoxification
3. Define the common diseases affecting the liver

The liver, a crucial organ of the human body, is primarily responsible for numerous metabolic processes. Situated in the right upper quadrant region of the abdomen, the liver is a central organ for carbohydrate metabolism, protein synthesis, and fat storage. The intricate anatomy of the liver, with hepatic lobules composed of hepatocytes, enables it to perform these functions efficiently. Hepatocytes are specialized cells that assist in modulating glucose by storing excess form as glycogen. They also produce albumin and clotting factors, helpful in maintaining osmotic pressure and normal hemostasis, respectively. The liver detoxifies numerous metabolites and drugs, thus guarding the body against toxins. An understanding of liver function and anatomy is core to liver, pancreatic, and biliary surgery since impaired liver function will directly influence the success of surgery and patient recovery. One of the most essential functions of the liver is bile production, a chemical essential for digestion and fat absorption. Bile is secreted by the liver and stored in the gallbladder, where it is released into the small intestine as needed. This two-step storage-secretion system of bile is critical, as it facilitates the efficient emulsification of fat consumed, allowing for the easy absorption of fat-soluble vitamins A, D, E, and K. The liver also plays a significant role in maintaining homeostasis by regulating serum lipids, such as cholesterol and triglycerides. The anatomical relation of the liver to the biliary apparatus is significant in operative cases, especially for biliary disease or obstruction. Operation often needs a precise knowledge of these functions because complications can arise from disturbed bile flow during pancreas and liver procedures.

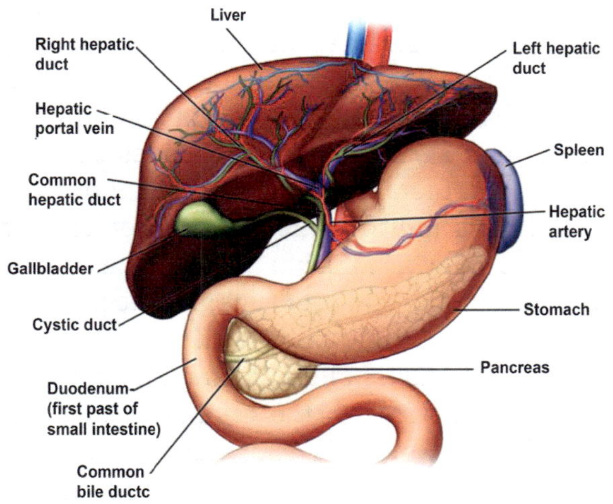

Figure 5.3. Liver: Anatomy and functions.

Source: https://www.hopkinsmedicine.org/-/media/images/health/1_-conditions/liver-gallbladder-and-pancreas/liver-anatomy.png.

Moreover, the liver's double blood supply from the hepatic artery and portal vein reinforces its sophisticated physiology. The hepatic artery delivers oxygenated blood, and the portal vein delivers blood rich in nutrients from the gastrointestinal tract, so the liver may metabolize nutrients absorbed and deliver them to systemic circulation only after they have been metabolized. This innovative arrangement is critical to the liver's function in metabolism since it allows effective conversion of substrates to a useful form while getting rid of waste products. For liver, pancreatic, and biliary surgery, knowledge of vascular anatomy is essential; vascular complications may be linked to significant postoperative morbidity. Preoperative planning must carefully consider the double blood supply to prevent complications in surgery involving the liver or immediately adjacent structures, as these can have a detrimental effect on recovery and liver function (N/A, 2009; Adams et al., 2017) (Figure 5.3).

5.1.1. Structure of the Liver and Its Lobes

The liver is a highly structured organ that has four major lobes: the right lobe, the left lobe, the caudate lobe, and the quadrate lobe. The largest of these is the right lobe, which accounts for approximately 60% of the liver's mass, with the left lobe being smaller and located medially to the right. The posterior and superior caudate lobes are supplied by the caudate artery, indicating their unique vascularization, which becomes crucial for surgical processes. The quadrate lobe, situated between the gallbladder and the round ligament, functions in bile storage and secretion. This separation of the liver into individual lobes is essential to understand the functionality and maintain the metabolic activities, like detoxification, protein synthesis, and biochemical production for digestion. In the lobular architecture of the liver, the structural framework gets subdivided into functional units known as liver lobules. They are hexagonally arranged units composed of hepatocytes, which are the primary functional cells and are involved in various metabolic activities. Each lobule is structured around a central vein and portal triads that consist of branches of the hepatic artery, portal vein, and bile ducts. This facilitates effective blood flow and secretion of bile. Inter-lobular communication through hepatic sinusoids enables blood flow, facilitating the transfer of nutrients and waste products. Surgically, the accurate understanding of these lobular structures is crucial for the success of liver resections and minimally invasive procedures aimed at treating pathological processes of liver function. The caudate lobes' distinctive vascularization and anatomical relationship with surrounding structures are also significant in hepatobiliary procedures. Studies indicate that the caudate artery plays a substantial role as it creates an essential blood supply to the lobe and limits of the hilar bile duct, which carries bile from the liver. The caudate artery is also classified into various types based on its structure, for instance, as independent branches or those with a common tract with other arteries. Understanding such vascular complexities as seen in radiological studies may contribute to enhancing surgical precision during surgeries involving liver segment resection or transplantation (Kenji et al., 2013). Given the complex function of the liver in digestion and metabolism, understanding its structural anatomy is priceless to surgeons involved in pancreatic, liver, and biliary surgery (N/A, 1989).

5.1.2. Functions of the Liver in Metabolism and Detoxification

The liver is an organ in the body that serves as a metabolic hub, carrying out a range of biochemical reactions vital for maintaining the body's homeostasis. Among its essential functions is the control of carbohydrate metabolism, where it stores surplus glucose as glycogen and, upon demand, regenerates glycogen to glucose for use in energy consumption. In addition, the liver plays a vital role in lipid metabolism by producing lipoproteins and cholesterol and facilitating the oxidation of fatty acids. All these processes of metabolism are significant since they ensure the availability of the body's constant supply of energy and adequate amounts of primary metabolites and, hence, overall health. The efficient functioning of these processes highlights the liver's involvement in metabolic activity and illustrates its adaptive role in equilibrating energy within the organism. Detoxification is a second key function of the liver, highlighting its capacity to filter and eliminate potentially toxic substances from the circulatory system. The process is essentially the transformation of toxins into forms which are less harmful and usable for excretion. One of such pathways is the cytochrome P450 enzyme system, a significant drug metabolizing system. Evidence indicates that conditions such as cholestasis significantly affect this process of detoxification by altering the expression of enzymes such as CYP3A1 and CYP3A2 in the cytochrome P450 system, demonstrating the liver's sensitivity to physiological conditions and enhancing its detoxifying ability under varying conditions (Albertoni et al., 2017). These changes can lead to a range of metabolic disturbances, indicative of the liver's multifunctional role not only in xenobiotic detoxification but also in regulating the pharmacokinetics of most drugs given to patients. Furthermore, the liver's role in incorporating bile acids into metabolic signaling illustrates its multifunctional role in the regulation of many metabolic pathways. Bile acids were traditionally recognized . Still, their role in lipid and glucose metabolism has recently been demonstrated through mechanisms involvingfor their role in aiding digestion. Still, their involvement in lipid and glucose metabolism has recently been demonstrated through mechanisms that involve receptors such as the farnesoid X receptor (FXR) (Adorini et al., 2018). This dual function positions bile acids as significant signaling molecules that act with gut microbiota, hence further controlling metabolic functions. The altered composition of bile acids is then able to change signaling pathways, illuminating the intricate relationship between liver function and overall metabolic health. Such awareness thus lends strong justification to the potential therapeutic targets in metabolic disorders, underscoring the liver's central role in detoxification and systemic metabolism (Figure 5.4).

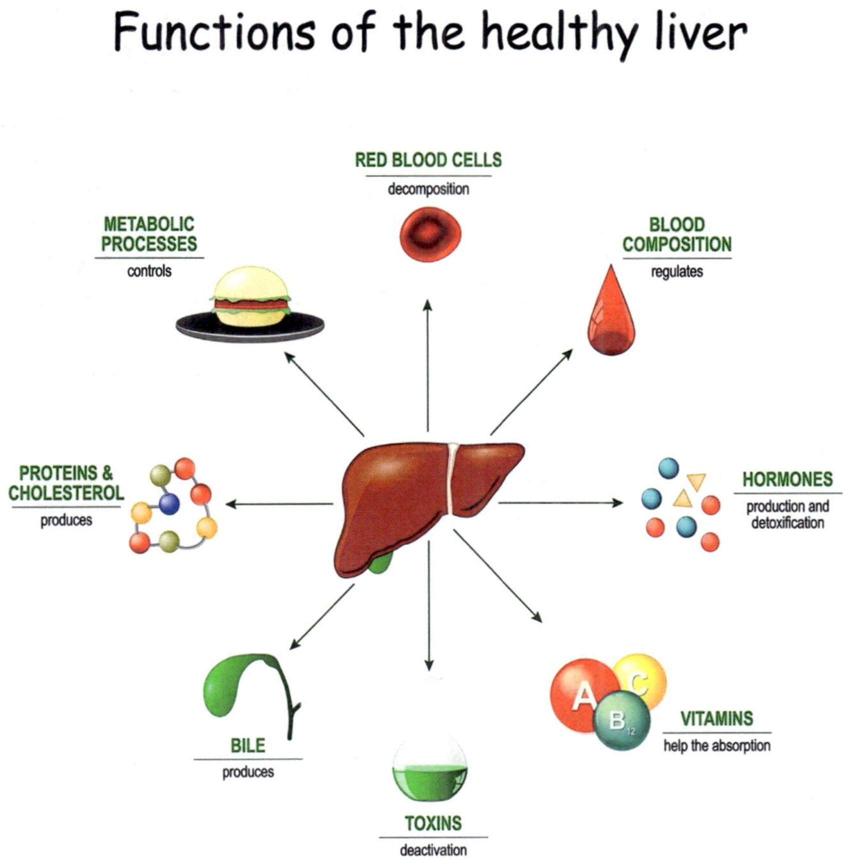

Figure 5.4. Functions of the liver in metabolism and detoxification.

Source: https://img1.wsimg.com/isteam/ip/0e230687-1eeb-45c5-bcb6-fc3853fdb103/Functions%20of%20the%20Liver.jpg/:/cr=t:0%25,l:0%25,w:100%25,h:100%25/rs=w:1280.

5.1.3. Common Diseases Affecting the Liver

The liver is an organ susceptible to numerous types of disease, each of which has the potential to impact overall wellness significantly. The most frequent liver disease is probably hepatitis, an inflammatory liver disease that could be caused by viral infections, alcohol misuse, or autoimmune disordersviral infections, alcohol misuse, or autoimmune disorders. Chronic hepatitis could lead to severe complications, such as cirrhosis or liver cancer, necessitating surgical interventions like liver transplantation. The importance of these conditions places emphasis on the early diagnosis and specialized surgical management, as proper treatment can dramatically improve patient outcomes, along with lessening the socioeconomic load on healthcare systems. With ongoing surgical innovations, a comprehensive understanding of the complexities of liver disease remains crucial in optimizing treatment protocols and determining the most effective surgical approaches for patients. Yet another predominant illness that affects the liver is fatty liver disease, and it will manifest in two major types: alcoholic and non-alcoholic fatty liver disease (NAFLD). NAFLD has emerged as a significant public health problem, especially with growing rates of obesity worldwide. NAFLD will progress to non-alcoholic steatohepatitis (NASH), and it entails liver cell inflammation and damage. Progression of NASH can eventually lead to cirrhosis and liver failure, and in such cases, consideration for liver transplantation is warranted. Management of fatty liver disease is usually best treated using multimodal therapy, such as lifestyle modification and potential surgery for severe cases, demonstrating the importance of interprofessional collaboration. Knowledge about the intricacies of NAFLD and NASH helps tailor effective prevention programs and surgical therapies that minimize damage to the liver. Cholestatic liver diseases, such as primary sclerosing cholangitis and primary biliary cholangitis, are also significant causes of liver dysfunction and are typified by blocked bile flow and chronic liver damage. They can lead to complications, including cirrhosis or increased risk of liver carcinoma, and thus are at the forefront of liver surgery discussions. There is a growing perception of the need for more sophisticated treatment modalities, such as the development of surgical procedures, such as liver transplantation, in patients with end-stage liver disease. Moreover, with the expanding horizon of knowledge regarding the pathology and evolution of cholestatic liver diseases, the introduction of new diagnostic strategies and therapeutic devices in a balanced approach becomes imperative to optimize patient results. The coordination of surgical specialists with the remainder of the medical system is crucial to addressing the challenges posed by these complex liver diseases and ensuring that patients receive integrated care that encompasses both medical and surgical management (Figure 5.5).

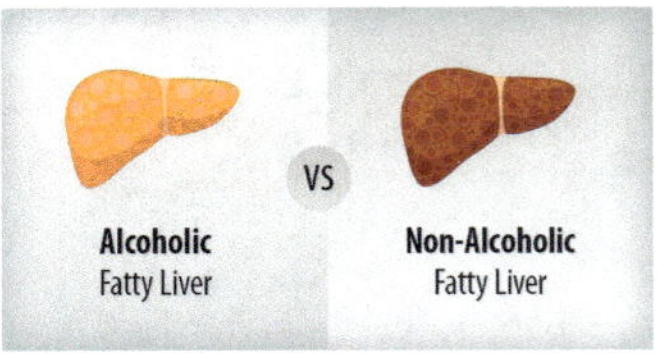

Figure 5.5. Alcoholic and non-alcoholic fatty liver disease (NAFLD).

Source: https://medicanorthbengalclinic.com/wp-content/uploads/2022/07/Fatty-Liver-Disease.jpg.

Test Your Knowledge

1. What are the main anatomical lobes of the liver?
2. Which liver function is essential for the detoxification of blood?

5.2. Overview of Pancreatic Anatomy

Learning Outcome

1. Explain the structure of the pancreas and its regions;
2. Define the role of the pancreas in digestion and hormone production;
2. Discuss the diseases and conditions affecting the pancreas.

The pancreas is a vital organ located in the retroperitoneal space, performing vital functions in both endocrine and exocrine activities. The pancreas is anatomically divided into four primary sections: the head, the neck, the body, and the tail. The head of the pancreas lies alongside the duodenum and is overlapped by the C curve of the intestinal loop, whereas the neck serves as a transitional area between the head and the body. The body of the pancreas lies horizontally and is situated above the large vessels or blood vessels of the abdominal cavity, or the tail extends to the left side up to the splenic hilum. This unique anatomy highlights the pancreas's function, which is not only to secrete digestive enzymes but also hormones such as insulin and glucagon, which play a critical role in glucose homeostasis in the body. The pancreas is primarily supplied with blood by branches of the celiac trunk and the superior mesenteric artery, ensuring a rich vascular plexus that is essential for its function. The body and tail are supplied by the splenic artery, and the pancreaticoduodenal artery is given off by the gastroduodenal artery to supply the head and neck. This rich blood supply not only maintains the pancreatic tissue but also facilitates the transport of hormones into the circulatory system. The pancreas is also closely associated with the biliary system; the common bile duct traverses its head to enter the duodenum. Knowledge of the complex vascular anatomy is crucial in operating on pancreatic disorders to prevent accidental damage to these vessels during surgery, which can cause serious complications and impact the outcome of operations such as pancreatectomy and pancreaticoduodenectomy. A greater interface between pancreatic anatomy and surgery is realized while discussing the treatment of tumors, including pancreatic cancer. Recent developments in ultrasound-guided thermal therapies hold promise for treating pancreatic tumors using novel methods, including intraductal and transgastric approaches. Studies have shown that these methods can successfully ablate tumors while sparing important nearby structures, such as large vessels and the duodenum, thereby reducing surgical risks. Patient-specific simulations, in particular, were found to have high ablation capability, hinting that meticulous planning could maximize treatment efficiency while protecting nearby organs (Adams et al., 2017). With increasingly sophisticated surgical methods, awareness of pancreatic anatomy is crucial for producing safe and beneficial interventions, especially in the context of virulent diseases like pancreatic cancer, where a rapid and precise surgical response is of prime importance (N/A, 2009) (Figure 5.6).

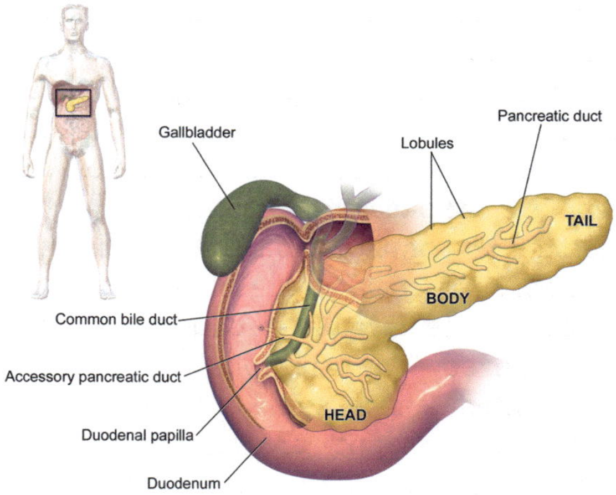

Figure 5.6. Pancreas anatomy.

Source: https://upload.wikimedia.org/wikipedia/commons/7/7e/Blausen_0699_PancreasAnatomy2.png.

5.2.1. Structure of the Pancreas and Its Regions

The pancreas is a vital organ located in the abdominal cavity, playing a crucial role in both digestive and endocrine functions. It is structurally separated into four major components: the head, neck, body, and tail. Its head lies in the duodenal curve, where it functions to secrete digestive enzymes, such as amylase and lipase, to aid in digesting carbohydrates and fats. The neck is transitional, merging smoothly with the body of the pancreas, which is the bulk of the pancreas. This anatomy is critical to organ function, as the enzymes that are released in the head are directed towards the duodenum. Knowledge of the anatomical arrangement of the pancreas is crucial during liver, pancreas, and biliary surgery, as it informs surgical management and techniques for preserving pancreatic function. Besides its specific locations, the pancreas also contains clusters of endocrine cells known as the islets of Langerhans, which play a crucial role in glucose metabolism. These islets secrete hormones like insulin and glucagon, which regulate blood sugar. The pancreatic body contains the majority of these islets and, therefore, contributes significantly to the pathophysiology of diabetes and other metabolic derangements. The intricate interaction between the endocrine and exocrine functions of the pancreas necessitates a thorough understanding of its anatomy, especially in the context of surgery, when the risk of mechanical damage to these hormone-producing cells must be minimized. The methods of pancreatic surgery, often laborious due to the organ's size and its close proximity to vital structures like the duodenum and large vessels, necessitate extensive preoperative imaging and planning. Surgical interventions involving the pancreas often require a thorough understanding of its blood supply and anatomical orientation. The pancreatic duct runs throughout its length, merging with the common bile duct at the ampulla of Vater before it enters the duodenum. This anatomical orientation is vital in the sense that it determines the techniques and methods applied in surgery. For instance, surgical resection of a pancreatic tumor, for example, in the setting of the Whipple procedure, requires careful dissection along these ducts to preserve integrity and ensure smooth postoperative drainage. Hence, the architectural nuances of the pancreas have a direct correlation with surgical complications and outcomes. As surgical techniques evolve, a comprehensive understanding of the pancreas's anatomy will remain at the forefront of advancing patient care in pancreatic, liver, and biliary surgery.

5.2.2. Role of the Pancreas in Digestion and Hormone Production

The pancreas plays a central role in the digestive process, functioning as both an exocrine and endocrine organ. Its double function enables it to secrete digestive enzymes, which play a key role in breaking down carbohydrates, proteins, and fats within the small intestine. The exocrine function of the pancreas secretes substances, including amylase, lipase, and proteases, into the duodenum, facilitating nutrient digestion. Apart from this, these enzymes are secreted in inactive forms to prevent autolysis of pancreatic tissue. When they reach the intestinal lumen, they become activated, allowing the digestion process to be initiated and nutrients to be absorbed effectively by the intestines. Understanding the pancreas's role in digestion is a must in diagnosing and treating digestive disorders-related conditions, which can practically influence a patient's overall health as well as nutritional status. In addition to its role in digestion, the pancreas plays a central role in hormonal regulation within the body. The endocrine function of the pancreas is composed of clusters of cells known as the islets of Langerhans, which secrete hormones such as insulin, glucagon, and somatostatin. Insulin plays a crucial role in glucose metabolism, facilitating the entry of glucose into cells and, consequently, lowering blood sugar levels. Conversely, glucagon increases blood glucose levels by causing the breakdown of glycogen in the liver. Somatostatin is a hormone that inhibits the release of insulin and glucagon, thereby facilitating homeostasis. There is a need to maintain balance among these hormones; abnormalities may lead to metabolic diseases, such as diabetes mellitus, highlighting the importance of pancreatic health in achieving endocrine balance and optimal metabolic function. The consequences of pancreatic dysfunction go beyond digestion and hormone secretion, calling for an integrative strategy towards surgical interventions. Conditions like pancreatic cancer, endocrine tumors, and pancreatitis may need surgery, especially when they interfere with the normal function of the pancreas. Effective treatment of endocrine tumors, for instance, requires an appropriate understanding of hormonal secretion and its pathologic effects because endocrine tumors may result in several hormonal syndromes or metabolic disturbances (Eijck et al., 2004). Surgical excision is the treatment of choice in local disease with curative potential. In the case of metastatic disease, however, an interdisciplinary approach using non-surgical methods is the preferred mode of management. This highlights the importance of interprofessional working among healthcare professionals to ensure patient outcomes are maximized and both endocrine and digestive functions can be restored or effectively controlled (Alvaro et al., 2015) (Figure 5.7).

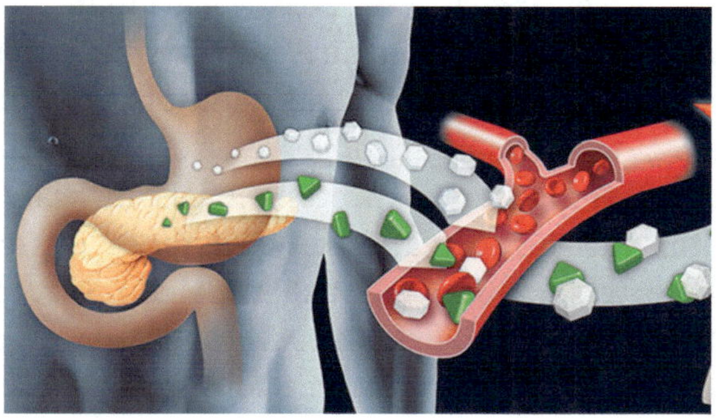

Figure 5.7. Two role of the pancreas in digestion.

Source: https://www.hopkinsmedicine.org/-/media/images/health/1_-conditions/liver-gallbladder-and-pancreas/pancreas-digestion-thumb.jpg.

5.2.3. Diseases and Conditions Affecting the Pancreas

The pancreas plays a significant role in digestion as well as glucose homeostasis and, therefore, is predisposed to a multitude of conditions and diseases. Pancreatitis, pancreatic cancer, and congenital anomalies are most likely to affect digestive as well as general health. Pancreatitis, an inflammation of the pancreas, can be caused by gallstones or alcohol consumption, presenting with either acute or chronic symptoms. Acute pancreatitis represents a severe inflammation of sudden onset, which must be treated urgently. In contrast, chronic pancreatitis is caused by prolonged damage that impairs digestion and can lead to diabetes mellitus when the gland develops a loss of function in insulin secretion. Awareness of the conditions is crucial for surgery that intends to relieve and control the complications of pancreatic disease symptomatically. Congenital pancreas diseases, while rare, provide testimony to the genetic complexity of pancreatic disease. Congenital dilatation of the bile duct, for example, is a familial disease that presents ominous difficulty as a consequence of bile stasis, which can lead to severe complications such as cholangitis and pancreatitis. Recent research has established that CDD is genetically heterogeneous, meaning that several mutations in several genes can lead to this disorder (Campbell et al., 2016). Identification of the underlying genetic factors is critical in diagnosis and formulation of early treatment. While research continues to uncover the genetic etiology of these congenital disorders, the latter increasingly underlines the necessity for tailor-made surgical methods capable of effectively overcoming the respective difficulties that they impose in patients who may be candidates for liver, pancreatic, or biliary surgery. Pancreatic malignancies are among the most virulent forms of cancer and vastly complicate the surgical approach and treatment prognosis. With an abysmally low five-year survival rate, due in the main to late presentation, pancreatic cancer has been the focus of attention for surgical oncologists (Ndongo et al., 2010). The intricacy of pancreatic anatomy, coupled with its proximity to key vascular structures, adds further challenge to the process of resection. Advances in surgical techniques such as the Whipple procedure, which removes the head of the pancreas along with portions of the bile duct and intestine, are intricate and highly dangerous. Imaging and minimally invasive medical technologies, and improved understanding of cancer biology, will be required to improve the outcomes of the surgery for patients with pancreatic cancers. Resolution of pancreatic disease complexity is crucial in developing comprehensive surgical strategies and enhancing patient outcomes.

Test Your Knowledge

1. What are the main parts of the pancreas?
2. Which duct drains pancreatic enzymes into the duodenum?

5.3. Biliary System Anatomy

Learning Outcome

1. Explain the components of the biliary system
2. Define the function of bile in digestion
3. Describe the common disorders of the biliary system

Understanding the anatomy of the biliary system is crucial in the context of liver, pancreatic, and biliary surgery, as it is central to the management of many hepatobiliary diseases. The biliary system contains different structures, including the gallbladder, bile ducts, and associated structures, to facilitate the storage and transport of bile from the liver to the duodenum. Hepatocytes secrete bile that is stored in minute bile canaliculi, which then merge to form larger ducts, eventually forming the right and left hepatic ducts. They merge to form the common hepatic duct, which ultimately merges with the cystic duct of the gallbladder to form the common bile duct.

This intricate network is essential for digestion and requires a comprehensive understanding to conduct surgery effectively, particularly in conditions such as gallstones and cholangitis. The pear-shaped gallbladder, located below the liver, plays a crucial role in storing and concentrating bile. It temporarily stores bile secreted by the liver and releases it into the duodenum during digestion, particularly after consuming fatty meals. The anatomy of the gallbladder comprises several critical features, including the fundus, body, and neck, with varying structural components influencing surgical intervention. Knowledge of its anatomical variants and its proximity to major vascular structures is crucial in minimizing complications that may arise during surgeries, such as cholecystectomy. In addition, growing recognition has been observed regarding the correlation between protein levels in biliary fluid and the formation of gallstones, which supports surgeons' interest in being aware of subtle pathological changes in the biliary tract that can affect the outcome of surgery (Abell et al., 1991).

Knowledge of the anatomy of the biliary system, in the practice of the operating room, not only makes operative maneuvers easier but also maximizes the diagnosis and treatment of disease of the biliary tract. Surgeons must contend with complex anatomical interactions, particularly when operating on pathologies that involve the pancreas, which shares significant anatomical relationships with the biliary apparatus. The ampulla of Vater, for instance, is the region where the common bile duct and pancreatic duct merge and discharge their contents into the duodenum. This is especially so in the case of diseases like pancreatic cancer or obstructive jaundice, as these have the potential to produce changes in the usual biliary drainage. An intimate knowledge of the anatomy of the bile ducts and familiarity with variations and pathophysiologic considerations become essential in developing sound treatment strategies and maximizing surgical procedures in bile duct conditions (N/A, 2009) (Figure 5.8).

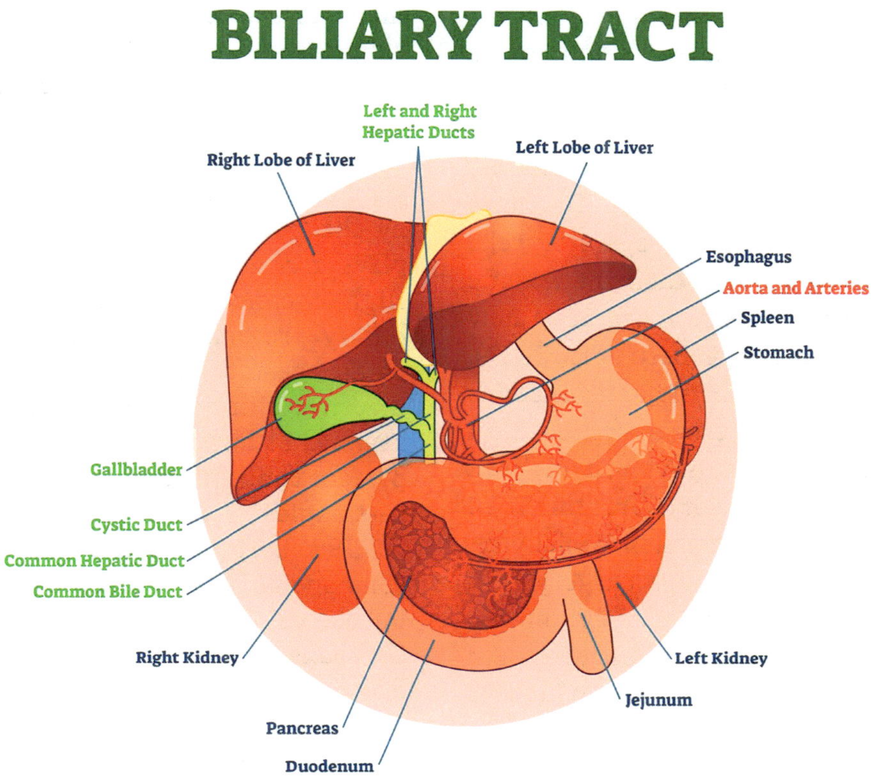

Figure 5.8. Biliary system anatomy.

Source: https://www.verywellhealth.com/thmb/fiHWPHtgHC1BfewDlPHoekUeNhQ=/1500x0/filters:no_upscale():max_bytes(150000):strip_icc()/GettyImages-930064116-83edb075ecfc48e0919dbd03b1235c63.jpg.

5.3.1. Components of the Biliary System

The biliary system comprises several key anatomical structures that play a crucial role in the processing and digestion of fats. The central structure of this system is the gallbladder, which is pear-shaped and receives and concentrates the bile. Bile is essential to emulsify the fats in the small intestine so that they can be digested and absorbed. The flow of bile is controlled by bile ducts, for example, the right and left hepatic ducts that unite to form the common hepatic duct. The plexus offers an adequate route of bile flow from the liver to the duodenum, particularly when one is eating. The intricate interaction of the elements demonstrates the biliary system's significance in gastrointestinal health and highlights its importance in surgical intervention correcting ailments such as cholestasis and gallstones.

The ampulla of Vater is another significant component of the biliary system, where the common bile duct meets the pancreatic duct before they both drain into the duodenum. This convergence facilitates the mixing of bile and pancreatic secretions, aiding the digestion process. The sphincter of Oddi controls bile and pancreatic secretion flow, preventing their retrograde movement into the ducts while maintaining the discharge of these enzymes into the small intestine. Dysfunction of this sphincter can cause biliary obstruction, which needs surgery to correct pathologies like pancreatitis or bile duct injury. Moreover, the biliary tree's complex architecture and stem/progenitor cell roles are gaining interest in terms of therapeutic potential. Research on human biliary tree stem/progenitor cells (hBTSCs) is directed towards their therapeutic application in liver cirrhosis, indicating a new frontier for future surgery (Aliberti et al., 2017). Understanding the components and functions of the biliary system is crucial for surgical experts, particularly those involved in liver, pancreas, and biliary surgery. Treatment of ailments such as biliary obstruction, cholangitis, and gallbladder disease through surgery calls for an in-depth understanding of the biliary system's anatomy. Surgical procedures aim to reestablish normal bile flow, which is crucial in preventing complications such as infection or pancreatitis. Moreover, advances in cryopreservation technologies for hBTSCs hold promise for regenerative approaches to biliary surgery. Those advances offer the possibility of generating cell banks with an accessible supply of stem cells for eventual use in treating hepatic and biliary diseases, thereby enhancing clinical outcomes (N/A, 2009). With further study, the understanding of biliary system components will continue to influence surgical methods and patient care.

5.3.2. Role of Bile in Digestion

The function of bile in digestion is diverse, with its primary role being to emulsify fats and facilitate the absorption of fats by the small intestine. Bile is secreted in the liver and stored within the gallbladder and is a mixture of bile salts, cholesterol, phospholipids, and bilirubin. Cholecystokinin is released, which leads to the release of bile by the gallbladder during digestion when fats are ingested through food. Bile salts act on lipids, reducing their surface tension and allowing pancreatic enzymes to hydrolyze them more effectively into fatty acids and monoglycerides. Fat must be emulsified for digestion to occur, which would otherwise remain as large, undigested globules, significantly hindering its absorption and use by the body. Secondly, the bile composition plays a crucial role in digestive homeostasis. Higher concentrations of cholesterol and biliary proteins have been implicated in the pathogenesis of gallstones, which can complicate digestive efficiency. Research indicates that in samples of bile with cholesterol crystals, total protein concentration is higher in comparison to samples of bile without crystals (Abell et al., 1991). This suggests that not only do the components of bile influence digestion, but their imbalances may also contribute to disease states like gallstones that can be surgically treated. Prevention of gallstone development relies on maintaining a delicate balance between the levels of bile components, highlighting the importance of effective liver function in supporting digestion and overall health. The clinical relevance of bile function extends into the fields of liver, pancreatic, and biliary surgery, particularly when one considers disease states such as liver disease and transplantation. Alcoholic liver disease is one such issue that causes complications complicating the bile's role with digestion as well as overall liver function and overall biliary system wellness. Studies show that treatment, such as liver transplant, can function in treating alcoholic liver disease complications—without a significant risk of future complications related to bile function after surgery (Andrea et al., 2001). What is known about how bile function impacts liver health and the associated surgical treatments for biliary diseases provides vital information regarding improving outcomes through surgeryas well as for , as well as enhancing the quality of life for patients. This complex relationship highlights the role of an effectively developed biliary system, not only in digestion but also in overall metabolic health (Figure 5.9).

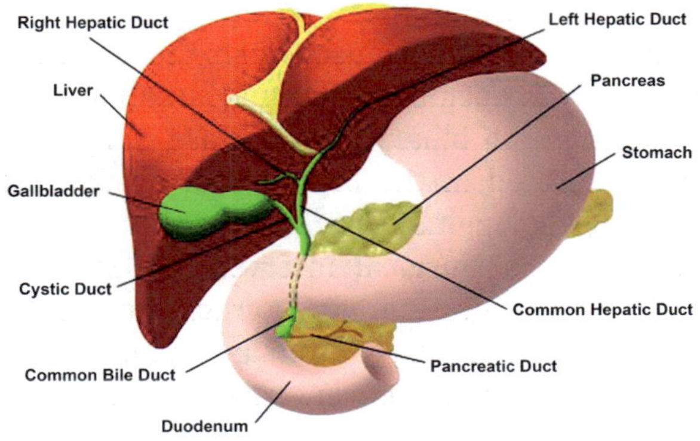

Figure 5.9. Major functions of bile.

Source: https://blogger.googleusercontent.com/img/b/R29vZ2xl/AVvXsEjaLPULdRJaISQsg1mPO5rgR95W5Mi6Q3cIHU-v8KyL_6Uo_NIve1qU73MLH_eYi4QBZpq-4oSEg9ZIaizBN_SNKuQjXD4kVeXe5gekCzItA2xRBHMuI95Q6cxp1SfgNwPZzLTfXLF4257-/?imgmax=800.

5.3.3. Common Disorders of the Biliary System

The biliary tree, comprising the gallbladder and bile ducts, is susceptible to numerous diseases that can have a profound impact on overall health. Gallstones, or cholelithiasis, due to the crystallization of bile components, are one of the most frequent conditions. They are commonly linked with signs like abdominal pain, jaundice, and nausea. Gallstone development can lead to complications such as acute cholecystitis, where the gallbladder is inflamed, or pancreatitis, in the event of a blockage of the pancreatic duct by a stone. With increasing incidence rates associated with obesity and diet, gallstone formation risk factors and pathogenesis must be known to plan preventive and therapeutic interventions in the framework of biliary surgery. Another major disorder that affects the biliary system is primary biliary cholangitis (PBC), an autoimmune disease characterized by the progressive destruction of intrahepatic and extrahepatic bile ducts. The condition is most frequently encountered in middle-aged women and, if left untreated, can lead to liver cirrhosis and cholestasis. Clinical symptoms are pruritus, fatigue, and right upper quadrant pain, which exacerbate the diagnosis and make therapeutic challenges greater. Treatment begins most often with ursodeoxycholic acid, which has been shown to improve the function of the liver and retard disease progression. PBC has also been described as having a potential genetic etiology in recent reports, with studies on environmental factors that precipitate its onset. Early detection and intensive treatment are therefore crucial in ensuring improved patient outcomes in PBC cases within liver and biliary surgery practice. Congenital biliary diseases, though rare, are also challenging to treat. Congenital bile duct dilatation (CDD) is a good case in point of an illness that can spiral into serious complications such as cholangitis, pancreatitis, and even hepatocellular carcinoma if not treated adequately. CDD occurs exclusively in children and is characterized by an aberrant dilatation of the bile ducts with bile retention, leading to injury of the liver. Current genetic studies have further emphasized the genetic heterogeneity of CDD, with the identification of mutations in genes associated with developmental disorders and cholangiocarcinomas, thereby establishing a complex relationship between the disease's etiology and genetics. The multiscalar nature of CDD further underscores the importance of early surgical management, as early intervention can significantly improve long-term outcomes and prevent major complications associated with this disease in biliary surgery (Campbell et al., 2016).

Test Your Knowledge

1. What are the main parts of the pancreas?
2. Which duct drains pancreatic enzymes into the duodenum?

5.4. Indications for Surgery

Learning Outcome

1. Describe the conditions requiring liver surgery
2. Define the reasons for pancreatic surgery
3. Discuss the biliary surgery indications

In the context of liver, pancreatic, and biliary surgery, the indications for surgery have undergone significant changes over the past few years. Surgery is usually indicated in the case of several conditions, such as tumors, congenital defects, and traumatic damage. For example, when dealing with malignant biliary tumors (MBTs), a multidisciplinary approach is essential due to the complexities involved in their management. Current practices also emphasize the importance of imaging in preoperative staging and follow-up, which in turn influences the decision-making process surrounding surgical intervention. By correlating high-level imaging techniques, clinicians can accurately measure tumor size and extent, which is an important consideration in planning for surgery and therapy (Cannavale et al., 2016). The accuracy at this level is vital to ensure maximal results and to individualize interventions according to the unique anatomical and pathologic features of every patient. Another critical area of surgical intervention pertains to hepatocellular carcinoma (HCC) and usually necessitates liver resection or transplantation. Tumor staging and liver function are crucial prognostic indicators of surgical candidacy. For a patient with cirrhosis, for instance, liver function tests must be well evaluated to decide whether surgery is possible. Laparoscopic techniques are increasingly being favored in this context, offering minimally invasive alternatives with the potential to simplify recovery time and reduce postoperative morbidity. The disruptive impact of laparoscopy can be best illustrated through procedures such as partial hepatectomy for HCC, where the benefits of smaller scars from the wounds include less pain and a shorter hospitalization duration (Berloco et al., 2012). Therefore, surgeons must weigh these factors judiciously in deciding on surgical treatment for liver tumors. In biliary tract disease, surgery is often indicated in the presence of obstructive jaundice, cholangitis, or gallstones with serious complications. Surgical intervention, such as biliary bypass or stenting, is crucial to the re-establishment of biliary drainage and symptom palliation. Such maneuvers are critical in the event of malignant obstruction, where surgical timing has a profound impact on overall survival. The incorporation of laparoscopic techniques has further optimized such therapeutic regimens, resulting in reduced morbidity and improved patient quality of life following surgery. Guidelinescontinue to direct surgical practice, with an emphasis placed on the necessity of modern clinical pathways that take into consideration new technology and therapies to maximize patient outcomes after biliary surgery (Cannavale et al., 2016) (Figure 5.10).

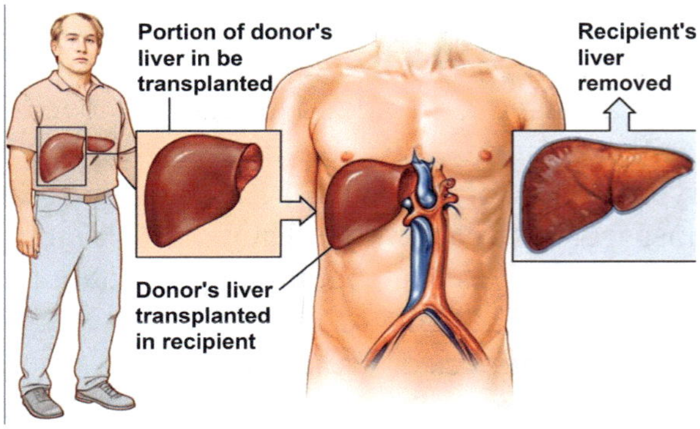

Figure 5.10. Liver transplant.

Source: https://ctshospitals.b-cdn.net/wp-content/uploads/2024/10/Liver-Transplant-Success-Rate-in-India-2-1024x671.webp.

5.4.1. Conditions Requiring Liver Surgery

The demand for liver surgery generally arises from several pathological conditions that compromise hepatic function and require remedial efforts. Among the leading indications for surgical treatment are liver tumors, comprising benign and malignant tumors. Benign tumors are composed of various types, including hemangiomas and focal nodular hyperplasia, among others. Malignant tumors are most significantly hepatocellular carcinoma. The natural history of these tumors can lead to significant morbidity and mortality, such that early surgical resection or, in complicated cases, liver transplantation becomes necessary. Outside of neoplastic processes, liver surgery is required regularly for complications of cirrhosis, including portal hypertension, where procedures such as transjugular intrahepatic portosystemic shunt (TIPS) can palliate symptoms and improve quality of life by reducing variceal bleeding. Cholestatic liver disease is also a condition with an emergent presentation in which an operation is warranted. Among these, bile duct obstruction is a critical problem requiring intervention in the form of surgery to restore bile drainage. Primary sclerosing cholangitis and cholangiocarcinoma can produce biliary stricture, resulting in increased intrahepatic pressure and subsequent liver damage if untreated. Surgical interventions may include bile duct exploration, stenting, or resection of the blocked biliary tract to decompress and prevent additional hepatocellular damage. Of particular interest has been the use of therapeutic agents, such as tauroursodeoxycholic acid (TUDCA), which has been extensively studied for its potential to alleviate symptoms of cholestatic liver injury. This may lead to more favorable surgical intervention outcomes in advanced stages of the disease (Bogaerts et al., 2017). Likewise, the surgical treatment is also needed for traumatic liver injuries. Both penetrating and blunt trauma wounds may lead to severe hemorrhage that necessitates immediate surgical management to tamponade bleeding and restore damaged hepatic tissue. Its management is based on the intensity of the injury and the stability of the patients' hemodynamics. Minor injuries could be treated conservatively, but severe laceration or avulsion of the liver could require resection or even limited hepatectomy. Knowledge of the injury's mechanism, as illustrated in studies that determine patterns of trauma, is essential for establishing proper treatment protocols. With changing patterns of trauma worldwide, the optimization of the surgical procedure and post-operative management continues to be important in improving the outcome in liver injury patients (Ndongo et al., 2010) (Figure 5.11).

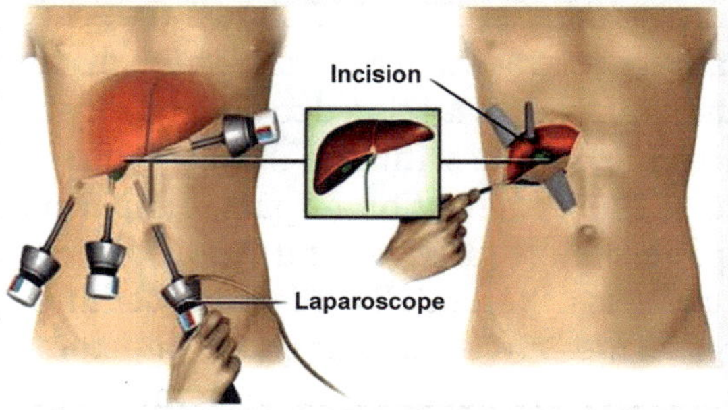

Figure 5.11. Laparoscopic-liver-surgery.

Source: https://obesitysurgeryindore.com/wp-content/uploads/2022/05/Laparoscopic-Liver-Surgery.png.

5.4.2. Reasons for Pancreatic Surgery

Surgical treatment of the pancreas is typically triggered by a variety of pathological processes impacting the organ's function and health. Among the primary indications for surgery is the formation of malignant tumors, with pancreatic adenocarcinoma. The aggressive malignancy is prone to presenting advanced-stage disease at diagnosis and, therefore, is an essential component of curative treatments. Surgical excision has a significant role in augmenting survival, particularly when the tumor is localized and has not invaded adjacent structures. Furthermore, tumor-related complications such as obstructive jaundice may lead to high morbidity, for which surgery is undertaken to alleviate symptoms and improve quality of life. Such procedures are carefully planned to remove the neoplasm and surrounding tissue, thereby giving patients a chance for prolonged survival and relief from symptoms. A second significant indication for pancreatic surgery is the management of benign conditions, such as chronic pancreatitis and pancreatic pseudocysts. Chronic pancreatitis, characterized by recurrent, irreversible harm to the pancreatic tissue with continued inflammation, generally results in disabling pain significantly impairing patients' quality of life. Research has shown that chronic pain, particularly when associated with disability or unemployment, is related to poor quality of life scores in patients with this illness (Abberbock et al., 2017). Alleviation of pain, enhancement of pancreatic drainage, and improvement of function can potentially be achieved through surgical measures, such as pancreatectomy or drainage of the pseudocyst. By removing such problematic symptoms through surgery, patients can develop a new sense of normalcy along with better overall health, pointing to the vital role of surgical interventions in managing non-malignant pancreatic disease.

Moreover, surgery may be indicated in cases with rare neoplasms, such as MAEC. The uncommon tumor is characterized by acinar cell and endocrine cell differentiation, and as such, is difficult to diagnose and treat. However, the initial treatment in patients with resectable disease will normally be surgery. De Both et al. (2017) state that, despite difficulty in making a firm diagnosis of MAEC, early surgical treatment can improve the prognosis, particularly after due evaluation of response to therapies like peptide receptor radionuclide therapy. The infrequency of the condition also underscores the specialized sophistication of pancreatic surgery, which may involve multidisciplinary therapies and individualized treatment protocols to effectively treat uncommon conditions. With ongoing improvements in surgical technique and diagnostic capabilities, the scope of pancreatic surgery is likely to expand, and with this, the effectiveness of treating both common and uncommon pancreatic conditions will become possible.

5.4.3. Biliary Surgery Indications

Biliary surgery indications are miscellaneous and mainly determined by the biliary tree's underlying pathology. Surgical treatment is commonly required in biliary obstruction, which may result from numerous different etiologies such as gallstones, strictures, tumors, or pancreatitis-related issues. Gallstone patients may present with either acute cholecystitis or recurrent episodes of biliary colic and commonly need laparoscopic cholecystectomy as a primary treatment. Additionally, malignant biliary tumors (MBTs) require prompt intervention, as they can lead to significant morbidity and mortality if not addressed adequately. The management of MBTs is intricate and shifts according to the localization and extent of the disease, indicating the need for a comprehensive evaluation by a multidisciplinary team to delineate the appropriate surgical approach and adjunctive therapies (Cannavale et al., 2016). Another critical factor in deciding the need for biliary surgery is the development of cholangitis, an infectious process secondary to bile duct obstruction of inflammation. The patient may present with jaundice, fever, and epigastric pain requiring immediate relief by decompression of the biliary tract. ERCP would typically be employed to decompress the obstruction; however, in cases where endoscopic maneuvers fail, surgical exploration may be necessary. Besides, conditions such as biliary atresia in pediatric patients often call for early action in life in the form of surgery to guarantee bile flow and prevent liver damage. The timing and nature of interventions are vital to optimizing surgical results and enhancing the quality of life for patients, especially among young populations with unique challenges (Cannavale et al., 2016).

During the past two decades, improvements in both minimally invasive techniques and equipment have revolutionized biliary surgical practice, enabling faster recovery rates and fewer complications. Laparoscopic procedures have dramatically changed surgical indications by providing treatment options previously unavailable through open surgery. The ability to perform laparoscopic cholecystectomy and other biliary operations with fewer incisions has subjected patients to less postoperative pain, fewer hospital days, and decreased surgical site infection rates. With indications for biliary surgery continuing to evolve, the use of laparoscopic methods is proving crucial, especially in the context of liver transplantation, where preoperative evaluation and preparation are vital for successful outcomes. Thus, continuous research and innovation will continue to define and expand the indications for biliary surgical interventions (Figure 5.12).

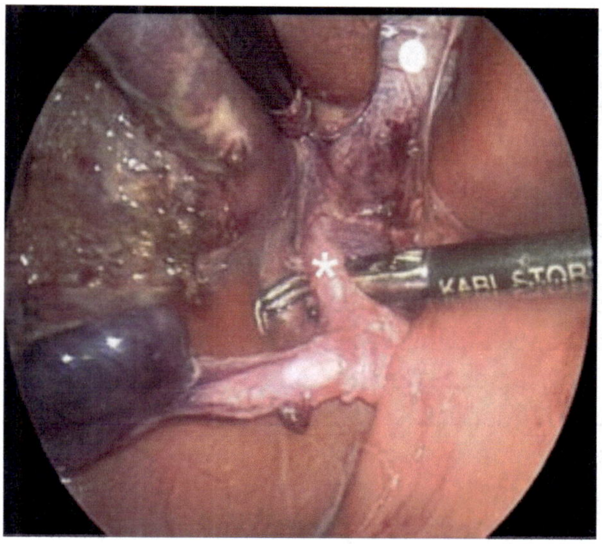

Figure 5.12. Biliary tract surgery.

Source: https://ars.els-cdn.com/content/image/1-s2.0-S0065310114000127-gr17.jpg.

Test Your Knowledge

1. What are the common surgical indications for hepatocellular carcinoma?
2. When is a Whipple procedure indicated for pancreatic tumors?

5.5. Surgical Techniques

Learning Outcome

1. Explain the open surgery vs. laparoscopic surgery of liver, pancreatic, and biliary procedures
2. Define the innovations in surgical techniques of liver, pancreatic, and biliary procedures
3. Describe the role of robotic surgery in liver, pancreatic, and biliary procedures

In liver, pancreatic, and biliary surgery, the choice of surgical approaches is paramount in the treatment of complex diseases such as malignancies, most importantly, pancreatic cancer. The intrinsic challenging character of pancreatic cancer, that is, difficult-to-identify metastatic behavior, dictates an individualized surgical approach. Re-excision of the tumor is usually the goal of surgery; however, very few patients are candidates for curative surgery due to the advanced stage of disease at presentation. As discussed in recent literature, tumor cells in circulation (CTCs) represent a new frontier for evaluating the genomic profile of tumors and thereby assisting in decision-making and prognosis in surgery. The integration of CTCs into preoperative assessment can render interventions more effective by enabling the evaluation of patients with a greater probability of benefiting from surgery and providing information regarding the residual burden of cancer after surgery, thus optimizing the long-term management of this refractory disease (Pimienta et al., 2017).

In cases where surgical resection is not feasible, alternative approaches are used to alleviate symptoms and enhance the quality of life for patients. Obstruction of the biliary tract, one of the common complications of advanced pancreatic cancer, needs adequate surgical drainage to relieve jaundice and its consequences. Among the various methods, endoscopic techniques have established themselves as the gold standard for biliary drainage, providing a less invasive approach with satisfactory outcomes. However, in cases where the tumor is found to be unresectable intraoperatively, open biliary drainage must be performed. Surgical operations, such as double bypass biliodigestive anastomoses, have shown promise in the management of both gastric outlet obstruction and obstructive jaundice, highlighting the versatility of surgical procedures in terms of intraoperative outcomes. These new surgical techniques are of importance in treating the sequential presentation of pancreatic malformations and ensuring optimal care for the patient. Moreover, innovative strides in surgery techniques continue to shape the practice of liver, pancreatic, and biliary surgery. Robotic-assisted techniques and minimally invasive laparoscopic surgical approaches have revolutionized traditional surgery with quicker recovery rates and reduced postoperative complications. Equally advanced surgical techniques enable surgeons to access the intricate anatomy of the pancreas and surrounding structures with greater precision, thereby improving outcomes during surgery. In addition, continued research on the use of liquid biopsies, particularly for CTC detection, also holds the potential to further optimize surgical planning by providing real-time feedback on tumor behavior and treatment outcome. Hence, as the field advances, the incorporation of new technologies and techniques will remain crucial in addressing the advanced challenges presented by liver, pancreatic, and biliary diseases, ultimately improving patient survival and quality of life (Figure 5.13).

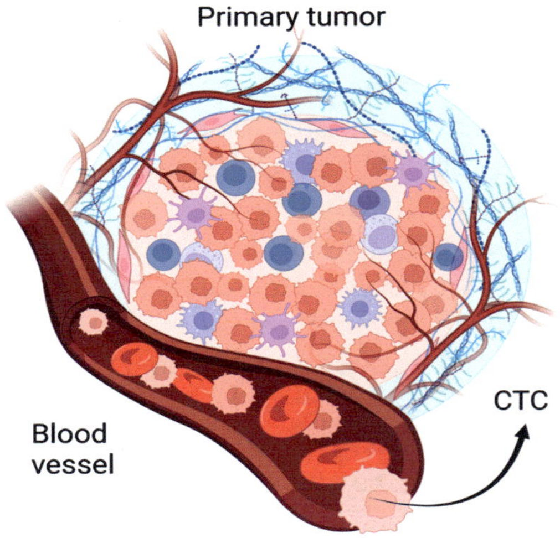

Figure 5.13. Circulating tumor cell.

Source: https://upload.wikimedia.org/wikipedia/commons/thumb/0/06/Circulating_tumor_cells_-_en.png/1200px-Circulating_tumor_cells_-_en.png.

5.5.1. Open Surgery Versus Laparoscopic Surgery

With the evolving trends of surgical procedures, open surgery versus laparoscopic surgery has been the primary concern, especially for liver, pancreatic, and biliary surgeries. Open surgery, which involves bigger incisions, produces greater postoperative pain and longer recovery times due to the extent of tissue damage incurred in the process. In contrast, laparoscopic surgery involves the use of minimally invasive methods that leverage the use of tiny cuts, which make surgeons perform intricate procedures with less physical toll on the patient. The innovation is key to organ-specific interventions, where accuracy and recovery rates serve as benchmarks of success. The trend toward minimally invasive methods is just part of an overall movement to enhance patient comfort and accelerate recovery, ultimately transforming patient care procedures in numerous surgical specialties, including those of the liver and biliary tracts. Laparoscopic methods have benefits far beyond patient comfort. Complications such as infections and hemorrhage, which are more common with open surgery because of increased exposure of tissues, are believed to be reduced by laparoscopic surgery. By making smaller incisions, patients lose less blood, resulting in shorter hospital stays and lower healthcare costs. In the case of liver transplantation, incorporation of laparoscopic techniques into standard practices has made tremendous leaps. Aside from easing donor surgeries, the combination also improves recipient outcomes, offering optimism to patients who have end-stage liver diseases the advancements in laparoscopy, a platform where innovation and improved clinical outcomes can blossom, confirming it as one of the pillars in present-day surgery, particularly for liver, pancreatic, and biliary surgery (Berloco et al., 2012).

The incorporation of laparoscopic techniques into more complex domains of surgery is accompanied by far-reaching implications for implementation and training. The relatively steep learning curve involved with laparoscopic surgery demands rigorous training procedures for surgeons to master the techniques that enable such procedures. While some believe that the inherent dangers of laparoscopic surgery will discourage its widespread adoption, particularly in regions with limited access to training and technology, the advantages still outweigh the disadvantages. Current studies indicate that the more experience the surgical teams accumulate, the less often complications occur. Additionally, technological advancements in tools such as advanced imaging systems and robot-assisted surgical platforms continue to enhance the performance of laparoscopic surgery. Thus, the open vs. laparoscopic controversy in liver, pancreatic, and biliary surgery situations not only continues but also underscores a paradigm shift toward revolutionary minimally invasive care, destined to transform surgical practices for generations to come (Ndongo et al., 2010).

5.5.2. Innovations in Surgical Techniques

The perioperative environment for liver, pancreas, and biliary surgery has undergone significant changes with the advent of novel surgical techniques that enhance precision and improve patient outcomes. Among the advances is the application of minimally invasive surgical procedures such as laparoscopic and robot-assisted surgeries. These procedures reduce patient morbidity and hospital stay by restricting tissue damage and shortening recovery periods. Laparoscopic methods allow for small incisions, which not only improve cosmetic results but also result in decreased postoperative pain. As documented in the literature, such developments are particularly valuable in the management of complex disease conditions, such as pancreatic cancer, where precise surgical intervention significantly impacts the patient's prognosis and quality of life (Agarwal et al., 2017). Developments in imaging technologies also provide these approaches with real-time, high-definition imaging of the operative field, facilitating more informed decision-making during procedures. Other areas of development include the advancement of advanced imaging and navigation systems that enhance the surgeon's capability to perform resections of greater complexity. Approaches such as intraoperative ultrasound and fluorescence imaging provide valuable information regarding tumor margins and vascular anatomy, making surgery more precise. These tools enable surgeons to make informed decisions regarding the extent of resection, based on more reliable information, and minimize injury to surrounding healthy tissue. Additionally, innovations in biliary reconstruction, including the use of biological grafts or tissue-engineered constructs, have been promising at reducing complications due to bile leaks and strictures. With ongoing research into these options, optimized surgical techniques have significantly improved liver and biliary disease treatment (Achtemiichuk et al., 2013), highlighting the crucial value of innovation in enhancing patient outcomes. Aside from technical innovation, ongoing research and interdisciplinary collaboration have led to the development of new methods for preoperative assessment and postoperative management. Recovery protocols, augmented with multidisciplinary advice from nutritionists, anesthesiologists, and rehabilitation experts, are now shaping the care pathways for surgical patients.

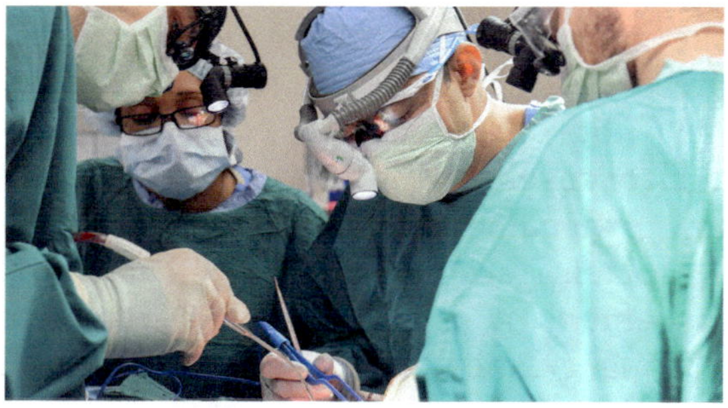

Figure 5.14. Hepatobiliary and pancreatic surgery.

Source: https://med.emory.edu/departments/surgery/_images/pancreatic-biliary-surg.jpg.

The emphasis placed on prehabilitation—preoperative physical conditioning and optimal nutrition optimization—tries to minimize complications and maximize recovery patterns. It is a comprehensive approach to ensure that patients are best prepared for surgery, giving them the maximum chances of recovery. As we see increased focus on patient-centered care in the practice of surgery, improvement in surgical techniques will also continue, along with better support mechanisms, to complement the overall treatment model required to treat liver, pancreatic, and biliary tract diseases that are complex in nature (Agarwal et al., 2017) (Figure 5.14).

5.5.3. Role of Robotic Surgery in Liver, Pancreatic, and Biliary Procedures

Robotic surgery has revolutionized the field of liver, pancreatic, and biliary procedures, providing surgeons with greater precision and control. The new technology capitalizes on robotic-assisted platforms, enabling minimally invasive strategies that are particularly beneficial in complex anatomical regions, such as the liver and pancreas. Robotic devices provide the surgeon with a three-dimensional view and greater maneuverability than traditional laparoscopic methods, which can facilitate the removal of tumors and reconstruction of biliary tracts. These advancements lead to improved surgical outcomes, including reduced blood loss and quicker postoperative recovery. The application of robotic surgery to these sensitive areas is thus not only a technological advance but also represents a new standard in the treatment of patients undergoing these complex surgeries, ultimately with the aim of enhancing their overall quality of life. Evidence has also pointed to the benefits of robotic surgery in oncologic environments, particularly in the treatment of liver and pancreatic cancer. Studies have shown that robotic methods can achieve lower rates of complications and shorter hospital stays than open surgery. Robotic tools offer fine control to dissect tissue delicately without damaging surrounding tissue, enabling more extensive removals of the tumor. Besides, with the progressive advancement of technology, its other capabilities, such as enhanced dexterity and visualization, allow surgeons to perform tasks that would otherwise be very difficult. This enhancement is crucial in enabling patients to undergo more advanced and effective treatments in line with ongoing efforts to achieve excellence in surgical procedures. Robotic-assisted surgery thus not only maximizes patient benefit but also sets a higher standard for what can be achieved in liver and pancreas surgery. Supplementing robotic techniques to biliary surgery has also opened the door to new possibilities for intervention in otherwise technically complex problems. For instance, robotic surgery is increasingly being employed to investigate and correct biliary obstruction with accurate targeting through the ductal systems, thereby reducing the risk of complications such as bile leaks. The advantages of reduced incision sizes result in less overall postoperative pain and reduced recovery periods, which are critical factors for patients. While robot-assisted surgery becomes increasingly mainstream as part of the surgical setup, its uses in liver, pancreatic, and biliary surgery are going to increase even further. The reassuring results surrounding robot-assisted surgery continue to stimulate research and clinical practice, suggesting that this technology will not only transform how surgeons work but also enhance training and skill acquisition for surgeons in the future. As robotic technologies continue to evolve, the future for robotic surgery as the building block for future treatment paradigms for hepatobiliary surgery looks optimistic.

Test Your Knowledge

1. What are the key steps involved in performing a hepatic lobectomy?
2. How is the bile duct reconstructed during a Whipple procedure?

5.6. Postoperative Care and Complications

Learning Outcome

1. Describe the common postoperative complications
2. Define the importance of monitoring and follow-up care of liver, pancreatic, and biliary surgeries
3. Identify the strategies for effective recovery of liver, pancreatic, and biliary surgery

Postoperative care after liver, pancreatic, and biliary surgery is central to decreasing complications and optimizing patient outcomes. Patients undergoing very lengthy surgeries can develop a variety of complications, ranging from infection to respiratory complications and pain control issues. Pain control is particularly crucial because inadequate pain control causes patient distress, delayed recovery, and increased risk of complications. Latest evidence shows that epidural analgesia (EDA) as part of postoperative care can reduce complications such as wound breaks and unplanned intubation. More specifically, it is evidence that EDA improves postoperative pain scores on the first critical days following the operation, which can potentially result in more rapid mobilization and recovery for patients undergoing complex surgery such as pancreatoduodenectomy (Ceppa et al., 2019). Therefore, the judicious use of pain-alleviation measures is an integral component of postoperative care. Besides alleviating pain, infection control during the postoperative phase is crucial in liver, pancreas, and biliary surgeries. SSIs can produce severe morbidity and prolong hospital stay, and therefore, complicate the course of recovery. Preventative methods must encompass careful wound care and appropriate application of prophylactic antibiotics. Studies have shown that patients who receive EDA experience a statistically significant reduction in the incidence of superficial wound infections, with an odds ratio indicating lower rates of future complications. This correlation underscores the importance of incorporating EDA into surgical patient postoperative management to enhance recovery and reduce infection rates (Ceppa et al., 2019). Postoperative aggressive monitoring, directed at potential complications and infection, can have a profound impact on patient outcomes. Postoperative care in general includes the treatment of potential pulmonary complications, which are common for patients after complicated abdominal surgery. Respiratory complications such as pneumonia and prolonged mechanical ventilation can cause significant delays in recovery and increase the duration of stay in the hospital. Steps to minimize these risks include early mobilization, respiratory therapy, and vigilant monitoring of respiratory function. Evidence suggests that patients under EDA may experience fewer pulmonary complications, as adequate analgesia can facilitate more effortless respiratory mechanics and encourage patients to actively engage in postoperative deep breathing exercises (Ceppa et al., 2019).

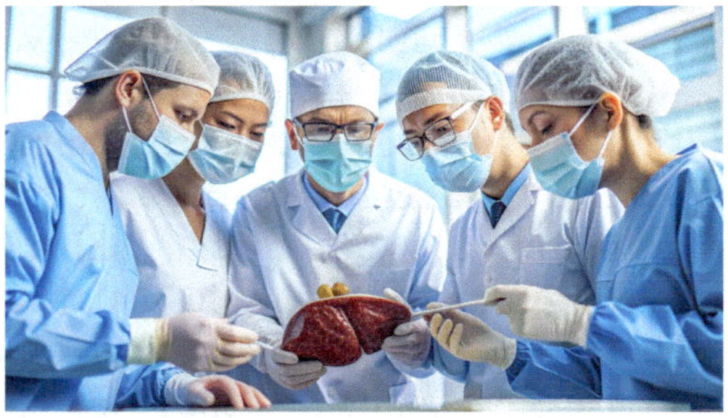

Figure 5.15. Postoperative care in liver, pancreatic, and biliary surgery.

Source: https://medwayhospitals.com/wp-content/uploads/2024/10/team-transplant-doctors-surgeons-evaluate-quality-health-donor-liver-transplantati-scaled.webp.

The multidisciplinary approach to postoperative care, particularly in liver, pancreatic, and biliary surgery, is ultimately aimed at minimizing complications and enhancing recovery, which reflects the complexity of patient surgical recovery and care (Figure 5.15).

5.6.1. Common Postoperative Complications

In the area of liver, pancreatic, and biliary surgery, many complications can arise from surgery, significantly impacting patient recovery and outcome. The most frequent complication is infection risk, manifesting in numerous different forms such as superficial wound infections or severe intra-abdominal abscesses. These are of great concern after major surgeries like pancreatoduodenectomy, given the broad range of operations and the manipulation of deeply located organs. According to studies, strategies such as the use of epidural analgesia can reduce infection rates and improve postoperative pain control, thereby providing a more favorable environment for healing in patients (Ceppa et al., 2019).

In addition, infection risk can be managed through proper surgical technique and careful postoperative monitoring, which remains a primary concern in avoiding these complications. Another urgent postoperative complication commonly observed in liver, pancreatic, and biliary surgery is the formation of pancreatic fistulas. These are instances when pancreatic juices leak from the site of resection or anastomosis and result in significant morbidity. Pancreatic fistulas may occur at highly variable rates based on the surgical procedure, and the patient's condition, the surgeon's skill level, and the patient's condition also have significant contributions to their occurrence. Their management usually involves prolonged hospitalization and may necessitate reintervention or drain placement, complicating patients' recovery. The classification and characterization of pancreatic fistula by the International Study Group on Pancreatic Fistula

(ISGPF) classification have provided valuable tools for clinicians in evaluating risk levels and potential treatment strategies, as well as forecasting the severity of postoperative complications (Ndongo et al., 2010). Aside from infections and pancreatic fistula, surgical patients become susceptible to respiratory complications that may range from atelectasis to pneumonia. Such complications are particularly significant in patients with extensive abdominal surgery because postoperative pain can compromise practical respiratory function and mobilization. Studies indicate that epidural analgesia not only enhances pain relief but also decreases respiratory complications, thereby promoting quicker recovery and improved patient outcomes (Ceppa et al., 2019). Encouragement of early ambulation and initiation of respiratory physiotherapy are two essential facets of postoperative care that can further reduce these risks. With the development of the field of liver, pancreatic, and biliary surgery, awareness of and management of usual postoperative complications are essential to optimize patient care and improve surgical success rates.

5.6.2. Importance of Monitoring and Follow-Up Care

The importance of close monitoring and aggressive follow-up treatment following liver, pancreatic, and biliary surgery cannot be overstressed. Successful surgery is often just the beginning of a patient's recovery process. Adequate follow-up management is essential to detect complications such as infections, biliary leak, or recurrent disease early, particularly in pancreatic cancer. The use of routine imaging and laboratory examinations can provide valuable information regarding a patient's health status, allowing issues to be identified and corrected early. This also minimizes the chances of late complications and enhances the overall quality of life for patients after surgery. For instance, patients having pancreatic surgery benefit significantly from structured follow-up, which significantly improves survival and treatment outcomes due to earlier detection. The last few years have seen advancements in tracking technologies, including the use of biomarkers and liquid biopsies, that have changed the climate of follow-up treatment. These are especially suited for the treatment of pancreatic cancer, where diagnosis is often delayed and existing treatment techniques tend to carry limited efficacy. Circulating tumor cells (CTCs), for example, capture rich information regarding tumor dynamics and can suggest the presence of residual disease or metastasis. By effectively identifying and characterizing CTCs, clinicians can potentially tailor other treatment regimens, thereby improving prognostic assessments and treatment outcomes.

The monitoring highlights the importance of adopting a proactive approach to post-operative patient care, demonstrating that surgery alone is insufficient without a functional mechanism for ongoing observation and intervention (Pimienta et al., 2017). Moreover, the psychological aspect of follow-up care should not be overlooked as the patients may develop anxiety and fear of recurrence following major surgical procedures. Following up regularly reduces such worries by providing reassurance to the patients and facilitating a therapeutic patient-provider relationship. The follow-up may also include support groups and education materials so that the patients can share experiences and coping strategies. Such an integrated approach not only takes care of the physical health of the patients but also ensures mental well-being, which is critical for healing. Appropriate monitoring and follow-up interventions are necessary for health staff to adopt as integral components of the surgical procedure, ultimately maximizing patient outcome and satisfaction (Ndongo et al., 2010) (Figure 5.16).

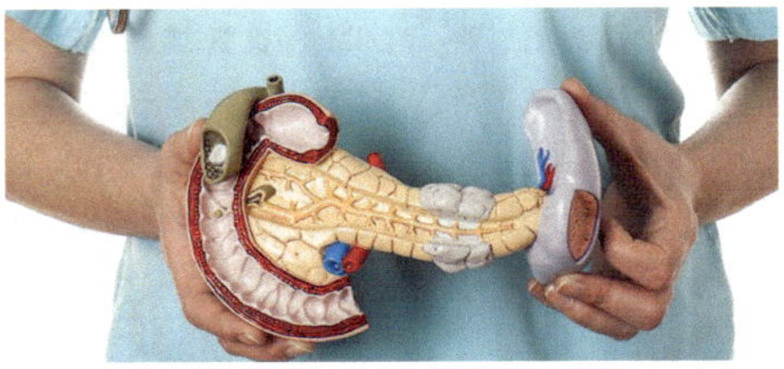

Figure 5.16. Laparoscopic pancreas surgery.

Source: https://www.neoalta.com/images/easyblog_articles/32/b2ap3_large_Why-opt-for-Laparoscopic-Pancreas-surgery.jpg.

5.6.3. Strategies for Effective Recovery

Effective recovery following liver, pancreatic, and biliary surgery hinges upon a multidisciplinary strategy with both preoperative and postoperative interventions. Preoperative optimization is key in minimizing complications and optimizing patient outcomes. This could include nutritional optimization, for example, advising patients to optimize their protein intake in an effort to support recovery following surgery. Additionally, the use of aggressive prehabilitation programs is likely to improve physical conditioning, which is beneficial as it offsets the physiological impact of surgery. Aggressive preoperative assessment and a carefully delineated recovery plan can significantly lower the risk for postoperative complications, such that the entire surgical experience becomes favorable for those having intricate liver and pancreatic surgery. Therefore, an integrated preoperative plan forms the basis for an uneventful postoperative course. Planned recovery postoperatively is equally significant and must be tackled on a multi-modal level according to individual patient requirements. Effective pain management, for instance, is vital to promote comfort and allow early mobilization, and this can serve to drastically reduce complications such as deep vein thrombosis and pulmonary embolism. Moreover, monitoring for signs of infection or complications like biliary leaks is also important, since early detection enhances the outcome of recovery. Nutrition is also essential in the postoperative setting, where re-establishment of nutrition through enteral feeding or parenteral nutrition can be necessary until patients regain normal gastrointestinal function. An interprofessional model of collaborative care, where multiple teams collaborate to uphold and treat the multicomponent needs of recovering patients, facilitates a reinforced transition towards well-being. The recent advancements in cell therapy indicate glimpses of revolutionary strategies for recovery, particularly in liver cancer treatment or cirrhosis management. Research on human biliary tree stem/progenitor cells (hBTSCs) suggests that employing cryopreservation techniques can optimize the clinical application of these cells. As established, hBTSCs that have been cryopreserved using a serum-free medium supplemented with dimethyl sulfoxide and human serum albumin exhibit comparable functional competency to freshly isolated cells and even yield greater albumin upon engraftment. This technology not only promotes patient-specified therapies but also aligns with the growing trend of personalized medicine throughout surgical recovery. Through the use of the most advanced cutting-edge biotherapeutic techniques, surgical teams can substantially enhance the quality of care, resulting in better recovery for patients undergoing liver, pancreatic, and biliary surgeries (N/A, 2009; Aliberti et al., 2017).

Test Your Knowledge

1. What are the warning signs of a postoperative bile leak?
2. How is pancreatic fistula managed after pancreatic surgery?

SUMMARY

With the advancement of liver, pancreatic, and biliary surgery, the afterword to this discussion illustrates the profound importance of technological advances in the area. Central to this development is the emergence of laparoscopic approaches, which have successfully transformed prevailing paradigms. The advent of minimally invasive methods not only enhances the recovery rate of patients but also reduces complications associated with traditional open surgery. By highlighting such advancements, it becomes increasingly clear that the addition of novel surgical techniques is pivotal to creating new standards of care and, therefore, significantly affecting patient outcomes. The astounding surgical outcomes with liver transplantation, particularly in the treatment of end-stage liver disease, further highlight the necessity of constant progress in surgical technology, primarily in laparoscopic surgery (Berloco et al., 2012). In addressing the need to incorporate technology, the intricate patient needs associated with liver, pancreatic, and biliary procedures must also be considered. Demographics influencing the outcome of surgery are recognized to enhance surgical practice and patient care. The injury patterns seen in patients requiring intervention of the liver or pancreas necessitate a broader approach to treatment plans that address both physiological and psychosocial aspects. For instance, trauma occurrence in regions where injury rates are high necessitates special pre-surgery assessment and post-operative follow-up to guarantee patient management in a holistic fashion. Ultimately, a broader vision will facilitate enhanced surgical planning and align healthcare providers with patients to achieve better overall health outcomes among targeted groups (Ndongo et al., 2010). In integrating the primary aspects of liver, pancreatic, and biliary surgery, it becomes clear that the future of this medical specialty depends on forward-looking research and reflective surgical practices. The interaction between new surgical techniques and patient-oriented practices will invariably dictate the course of surgical procedures in the years to come. As we approach the next level of advancements, continuing education and responses are crucial for healthcare professionals. An inculcation of new technology acceptance as well as patient safety and operation effectiveness will eventually translate into improved survival rates as well as quality of life for the patients. Such acceptance is warranted so that liver transplantation and pancreatic and biliary duct surgery can continually improve, ensuring that the practice remains current and effective in addressing the complex needs in this specialty (Berloco et al., 2012).

In liver, pancreatic, and biliary surgery, advances have significantly contributed to our understanding of regenerative mechanisms and postoperative management. Among the most debated points is the role of peribiliary glands (PBG) in biliary regeneration following severe cholangiopathy. It has been shown that PBG are crucial for the repair of the biliary epithelium, with cellular proliferation and differentiation following injury. A novel *ex vivo* model demonstrated that PBG cells can proliferate and mature, enabling the recovery of epithelial integrity in human bile ducts following extensive damage. This finding demonstrates the application of PBG-derived stem cells in therapy to enhance biliary duct healing mechanisms, which can be beneficial for patients undergoing relevant procedures (Carpino et al., 2019). Also significant is the study of pain care measures in the course of pancreatoduodenectomy, an advanced surgical procedure with postoperative complications and pain issues. There is evidence that the use of epidural analgesia (EDA) can safely prevent undesirable results of the procedure. Data collected from an extensive cohort analysis revealed that individuals who received EDA experienced significantly fewer complications, including wound disruption and pulmonary embolism, compared to those who did not receive this type of analgesia. EDA was also associated with improved pain scores in the first few days post-operation, demonstrating its effectiveness as a means of pain management. The findings highlight the importance of optimizing analgesic measures to enhance patient recovery in biliary and pancreatic surgical environments (Ceppa et al., 2019).

Ultimately, the application of these findings in clinical practice shows the ever-changing nature of liver, pancreatic, and biliary surgery. The results achieved through the study of PBG and EDA not only validate the necessity of new techniques in surgery recovery but also advocate for further research of regenerative techniques and pain reduction. As surgical procedures continue to evolve, it is essential that surgeons are well-informed about the latest advancements that can improve patient outcomes. This emerging body of evidence represents a paradigm shift toward a progressively interdisciplinary model, with surgical expertise augmented by regenerative medicine and enhanced postoperative care strategies, thereby paving the way for increasingly successful therapies for liver and biliary disease.

KEY TERMS FROM THIS CHAPTER

- Bile duct injury
- Biliary drainage
- Cholecystectomy
- Distal pancreatectomy
- Hepatectomy
- Insulinoma
- Liver transplantation
- Biliary atresia
- Cholangiocarcinoma
- Choledocholithiasis
- Gallbladder cancer
- Hepatocellular carcinoma (HCC)
- Liver abscess
- Pancreatic cancer

CRITICAL THINKING QUESTIONS

1. **Which of the following is the most common cause of obstructive jaundice?**
   a. Viral hepatitis
   b. Gallstones in the common bile duct (choledocholithiasis)
   c. Hemolytic anemia
   d. Liver metastasis
2. **Which of the following is a significant indication for performing a Whipple procedure (pancreaticoduodenectomy)?**
   a. Chronic pancreatitis
   b. Pancreatic pseudocyst
   c. Carcinoma of the head of pancreas
   d. Hepatocellular carcinoma
3. **A 45-year-old woman presents with right upper quadrant pain and fever. Ultrasound shows gallstones and a thickened gallbladder wall. What is the most likely diagnosis?**
   a. Acute pancreatitis
   b. Acute cholecystitis
   c. Hepatitis
   d. Liver abscess
4. **Which serum marker is most specific for hepatocellular carcinoma (HCC)?**
   a. CA 19-9
   b. CEA
   c. AFP (Alpha-fetoprotein)
   d. CA-125
5. **A pancreatic pseudocyst is best defined as:**
   a. A cyst lined by epithelium
   b. A non-inflammatory collection of fluid
   c. A fibrous-walled collection of pancreatic fluid lacking epithelial lining
   d. A neoplastic cystic lesion of the pancreas

Short Answer Questions

1. What are the common causes and indications for liver resection?
2. How is hepatocellular carcinoma (HCC) diagnosed and staged?
3. What is the difference between obstructive and non-obstructive jaundice, and how are they evaluated?
4. List the surgical options for treating gallstone disease and their indications.
5. Describe the clinical features and management of acute pancreatitis.
6. What is the Whipple procedure, and in which condition is it commonly performed?
7. What are the complications of laparoscopic cholecystectomy?
8. How is a pancreatic pseudocyst diagnosed, and when is surgical intervention indicated?

Answers to Critical Thinking Questions

1. (b); 2. (c); 3. (b); 4. (c); 5. (c)

REFERENCES

1. Machicado, J. D., Amann, S. T., Anderson, M. A., Abberbock, J., Sherman, S., Conwell, D. L., Cote, G. A., Singh, V. K., Lewis, M. D., Alkaade, S., Sandhu, B. S., Guda, N. M., Muniraj, T., Tang, G., Baillie, J., Brand, R. E., Gardner, T. B., Gelrud, A., Forsmark, C. E., . . . Yadav, D. (2017). Quality of Life in Chronic Pancreatitis is Determined by Constant Pain, Disability/Unemployment, Current Smoking, and Associated Co-Morbidities. *The American Journal of Gastroenterology, 112*(4), 633–642. https://doi.org/10.1038/ajg.2017.42Abell, C., von Ritter, C., Jüngst, D., Fiske, D., Gallinger, Z., et al. (1991). *Role of high total protein in gallbladder bile in the formation of cholesterol gallstones.* https://core.ac.uk/download/12167349.pdf (accessed on 12th July 2025).
2. Achtemiichuk, Y. T., Nahirnyak, V. M., Olijnyk, I. Y., Tsyhycalo, V., et al. (2013). *Development of the sphincteric apparatus of the extrahepatic bile ducts in the prenatal period of human ontogenesis.* https://core.ac.uk/download/144955075.pdf (accessed on 12th July 2025).
3. Adams, M. S., Diederich, C. J., Salgaonkar, V., Scott, D., et al. (2017). *Theoretical investigation of transgastric and intraductal approaches for ultrasound-based thermal therapy of the pancreas.* https://core.ac.uk/download/323063407.pdf (accessed on 12th July 2025).
4. Adorini, L., Aguilar, F., Ajouz, H., Al-Salami, M., Al-Salami, H., Alpert, E., Amaral, L., et al. (2018). *Pharmacological applications of bile acids and their derivatives in the treatment of metabolic syndrome.* https://core.ac.uk/download/195697333.pdf (accessed on 12th July 2025).
5. Agarwal, D. M., DeWitt, J., Eagleson, M., Easler, J. J., et al. (2017). *A multidisciplinary approach to pancreas cancer in 2016: A review.* https://core.ac.uk/download/129149165.pdf (accessed on 12th July 2025).
6. Albertoni, L., Baldo, V., Baldovin, T., Carrara, A., et al. (2017). *Pregnane X receptor and constitutive androstane receptor modulate differently CYP3A-mediated metabolism in early- and late-stage cholestasis.* https://core.ac.uk/download/141699970.pdf (accessed on 12th July 2025).
7. Aliberti, C., Alvaro, D., Bastianelli, C., Berloco, P. B., et al. (2017). *Cryopreservation protocol for human biliary tree stem/progenitors, hepatic and pancreatic precursors.* https://core.ac.uk/download/98348621.pdf (accessed on 12th July 2025).
8. Alvaro, D., Berloco, P. B., Cardinale, V., Carpino, G., et al. (2015). *Adult human biliary tree stem cells differentiate to β-pancreatic islet cells by treatment with a recombinant human Pdx1 peptide.* https://core.ac.uk/download/54525022.pdf (accessed on 12th July 2025).
9. Berloco, P. B., Di Laudo, M., Frattaroli, F. M., Guglielmo, S., et al. (2012). *Laparoscopy in liver transplantation: The future has arrived.* https://core.ac.uk/download/154948504.pdf (accessed on 12th July 2025).
10. Bogaerts, E., Colle, I., Devisscher, L., Geerts, A., et al. (2017). *Modulation of the unfolded protein response by tauroursodeoxycholic acid counteracts apoptotic cell death and fibrosis in a mouse model for secondary biliary liver fibrosis.* https://core.ac.uk/download/91389603.pdf (accessed on 12th July 2025).
11. Campbell, D., Cheng, G., Cherny, S. S., Chung, R., et al. (2016). *Genetic study of congenital bile-duct dilatation identifies de novo and inherited variants in functionally related genes.* https://core.ac.uk/download/77601212.pdf (accessed on 12th July 2025).

12. Cannavale, A., Catalano, C., Fanelli, F., Fiocca, F., et al. (2016). *Updated management of malignant biliary tract tumors: An illustrative review.* https://core.ac.uk/download/98341455.pdf (accessed on 12th July 2025).

13. Caplin, M., Falconi, M., Fusai, G. K., Lykoudis, A., et al. (2017). Treatment challenges in and outside a specialist network setting: Pancreatic neuroendocrine tumors. https://core.ac.uk/download/168403284.pdf (accessed on 12th July 2025).

14. Carpino, G., de Jong, I. E. M., Gaudio, E., Gouw, A. S. H., et al. (2019). Peribiliary glands are key in regeneration of the human biliary epithelium after severe bile duct injury. https://core.ac.uk/download/188829741.pdf (accessed on 12th July 2025).

15. Ceppa, E. P., Colgate, C. L., Fennerty, M. L., House, M. G., et al. (2019). Post-pancreatoduodenectomy outcomes and epidural analgesia: A 5-year single institution experience. https://core.ac.uk/download/187423802.pdf (accessed on 12th July 2025).

16. De Both, A., De Man, M., Geboes, K., Hoorens, A., et al. (2017). Treatment of a mixed acinar-endocrine carcinoma with uptake on 68Gallium-DOTATOC positron emission tomography-computed tomography: A case report. https://core.ac.uk/download/84594808.pdf (accessed on 12th July 2025).

17. DiMartini, A. M., Demetris, A. J., Jain, A., Balan, V., Bassendine, M., Becker, P., Belle, S., et al. (2001). *Liver transplantation for alcoholic cirrhosis: Long-term follow-up and impact of disease recurrence.* https://core.ac.uk/download/12205555.pdf (accessed on 12th July 2025).

18. Eisenmenger, W., Holle, G. E., Pradayrol, L., Riedel, F., et al. (1986). Diffuse somatostatin-immunoreactive D-cell hyperplasia in the stomach and duodenum. https://core.ac.uk/download/12167709.pdf (accessed on 12th July 2025).

19. Hobeika, C., Pfister, M., Geller, D., Tsung, A., Chan, A., Troisi, R. I., Rela, M., et al. (2024). Recommendations on robotic hepato-pancreato-biliary surgery. The Paris Jury-Based Consensus Conference. Annals of Surgery, 281, 136–153. https://www.semanticscholar.org/paper/4f988b3da5e938c61ed6bc7c0f01959fca6454f4 (accessed on 12th July 2025).

20. Ibukuro, K., Ohkohchi, N., Oshiro, Y., Sasaki, R., Takeguchi, T., et al. (2013). Analysis of the caudate artery with three-dimensional imaging. https://core.ac.uk/download/56654663.pdf (accessed on 12th July 2025).

21. Kyrou, I., & Weickert, M. O. (2010). Clinical problems caused by obesity. https://core.ac.uk/download/46324.pdf (accessed on 12th July 2025).

22. Ndongo, B. C., Mballa, G. A. E., Hyder, A. A., Juillard, C., et al. (2010). *Patterns of injury and violence in Yaoundé, Cameroon: An analysis of hospital data.* https://core.ac.uk/download/323075033.pdf (accessed on 12th July 2025).

23. Pimienta, M., Edderkaoui, M., Wang, R., Pandol, S., et al. (2017). The potential for circulating tumor cells in pancreatic cancer management. https://core.ac.uk/download/323077820.pdf (accessed on 12th July 2025).

24. van Eijck, C. H. J., de Herder, W. W., Krenning, E. P., Lamberts, S. W. J., et al. (2004). Considerations concerning a tailored, individualized therapeutic management of patients with (neuro) endocrine tumors of the gastrointestinal tract. https://core.ac.uk/download/18512572.pdf (accessed on 12th July 2025).

25. Wu, J., Tang, G., Cheng, C.-S., Yeerken, R., Chan, Y., Fu, Z., Zheng, Y., et al. (2024). Traditional Chinese medicine for the treatment of cancers of hepatobiliary system: From clinical evidence to drug discovery. Molecular Cancer, 23. https://www.semanticscholar.org/paper/b9ece98df36b71b2d588c895c1447eec521668a7 (accessed on 12th July 2025).

ABDOMINAL WALL SURGERY

6

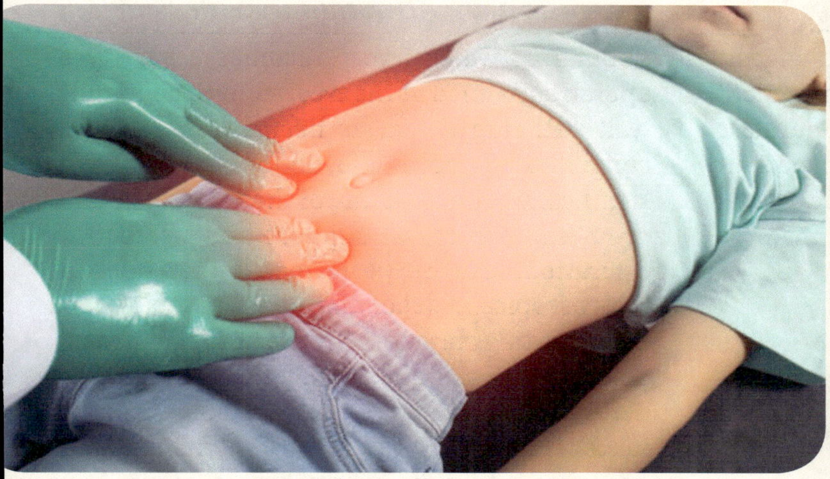

LEARNING OBJECTIVES

After studying this chapter, you will be able to:

1. Understand the anatomy of the abdominal wall
2. Explain the indications for surgery for the abdominal wall
3. Discuss the surgical techniques in the abdominal wall
4. Focus on risks and complications in abdominal wall surgery
5. Learn about advances in surgical technology
6. Evaluate the patient perspectives on abdominal wall surgery

Introduction

The field of abdominal wall surgery has seen significant advancements aimed at improving surgical techniques and patient recovery. Historically, abdominal wall surgery had been associated with prolonged recovery periods and significant postoperative pain due to the mobilization of the internal structures. In response, research has focused on the development of methods, such as the open posterior component separation (PCS) technique, to enhance surgical outcomes, particularly in the repair of complex hernias. PCS is noteworthy for its excellence in reducing recurrence rates and facilitating repairs at uncommon sites of hernia, thus expanding indications for surgery. With such techniques evolving, it becomes imperative to investigate their implications, particularly in relation to postoperative pain control and recovery patterns. The appreciation of the complexity of such surgical procedures provides the basis for research into their efficacy and limitations within contemporary practice. Postoperative pain control is an essential determinant of improving overall outcome in abdominal wall surgery.

Traditional analgesic techniques, including systemic opioids, have been widely used, but can also be linked to side effects and prolonged recovery. Recent studies, including the use of thoracic epidural analgesia (TEA), attempt to assess alternative interventions that can help improve faster recovery. Literature shows that TEA administration can lead to earlier recovery of bowel function, something that impacts the postoperative course and hospital stay duration of patients significantly. Sellers et al. (2017 shed light on a study of whether TEA is on par with systemic opioids in terms of analgesic efficacy following open PCS. Proper management of pain helps surgeons avoid postoperative complications and ensure maximum patient satisfaction, thereby transforming the model of abdominal surgery recovery.

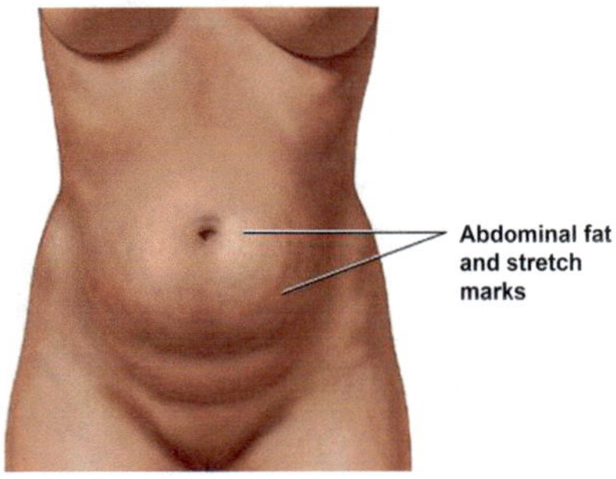

Figure 6.1. Abdominal wall surgery.

Source: https://ssl.adam.com/graphics/images/en/19108.jpg.

The integration of new technologies also plays a crucial role in optimizing abdominal wall surgery, with a synergistic combination of surgical precision and patient comfort. For instance, new technologies such as one-hand controlled endoscope positioning devices optimize surgical dexterity without requesting cognitive load from the surgeon. Bauwens et al. (2020) show how these devices encourage a more ergonomic style, minimizing the physical strain on the surgeon without losing control over intricate surgical movements. This innovation has a significant impact on the operational process, resulting in smoother procedures and reduced operative times, as well as improved patient safety. With advancements in abdominal wall surgery, the interplay between improved techniques and enhanced pain management strategies underscores the need for continuous evaluation of clinical outcomes, ensuring that such innovations serve to improve patient care (Figure 6.1).

Definition of Abdominal Wall Surgery

Abdominal wall surgery includes a variety of operations aimed at the treatment of abdominal wall pathology, such as hernias, trauma, and congenital defects. The abdominal wall is a significant outer covering of the internal organs, providing structural support and protection. Operations can be performed either open or laparoscopically, depending on the pathology and the operating surgeon's preference. The primary objectives of the operations are to correct the defects, remove pain, and reestablish normal function and aesthetics of the abdominal region. Advances in minimally invasive techniques have led to reduced rehabilitation times, decreased postoperative discomfort, and reduced scarring, making abdominal wall surgery an integral component of modern surgery. Moreover, the abdominal wall surgery is not only limited to hernia repair but also plays a vital role in managing complications of abdominal trauma or infection. For instance, procedures such as decompressive laparotomies may lead to open abdomen treatment, particularly if there is intense intra-abdominal hypertension. Such conditions should be well managed because they prevent further complications and enhance patient outcomes. More recent approaches, such as negative pressure therapy, demonstrate the value of an altered surgical method that accommodates individual patient needs and personal situations. These new developments are indicative of the dynamic nature of abdominal wall surgery and its capacity to keep pace with advancements in medical technology and surgical technique understanding (Bjorck et al., 2015). Furthermore, the definition and scope of abdominal wall surgery can also include cosmetic procedures aimed at enhancing the cosmetic appearance of the abdominal region. This area has gained increased interest with the evolution of minimally invasive techniques, where repairs are not only functionally restoring but also consider patients' self-concept and quality of life. As practitioners gain a deeper understanding of the holistic treatment context, the overlaps between reconstructive and aesthetic procedures become key to surgical planning. Specifically, experiences and dialogue in abdominal wall surgery contribute to the goal of lower complication rates and enhanced recovery pathways, thereby providing integrated care to patients who undergo such procedures (Athanasiou et al., 2015). Through its multidimensional definition, abdominal wall surgery reflects the evolution in surgical technique, confirming the extent of its magnitude beyond mere mechanical fixations.

Importance of the Abdominal Wall to Overall Health

The abdominal wall is a critical protective barrier, both guarding significant organs and allowing general body function. Composed of several layers of fascia and muscles, the abdominal wall plays a crucial role in maintaining intra-abdominal pressure. Such pressure supports bodily functions like digestion and respiration. The integrity of the abdominal wall directly affects these processes; any compromise or loss, whether due to surgery or injury, can lead to severe complications. For example, operations that incise the abdominal wall must consider potential risks like hernias and intra-abdominal infections, which would arise if the structure of the walls were breached. Without an intact abdominal wall, an individual is destined to experience more risks of morbidity related to complications that lie outside the area where surgery is conducted, making its role in overall health well-established. In addition, the relevance of the abdominal wall extends to posture and core stability. The abdominal muscles not only provide biomechanical function but also help with spinal balance and alignment. When these are affected, as often occurs after abdominal surgery, patients can experience impairments in physical function and quality of life. Rehabilitation following surgery tends to emphasize the importance of strengthening these muscles to restore core stability and normal function, highlighting the interdependence of abdominal health and overall well-being. Current research highlights the connection between the proper functioning of the abdominal wall and physical function, underscoring the need for surgical intervention that is planned with this structure's protection in mind. The consequences of successful rehabilitation are vast, from mobility to avoiding complications associated with long-standing conditions associated with compromised abdominal support. Additionally, understanding potential challenges that might arise post-operatively is essential in optimizing patient outcomes. Surgeons must walk the tightrope of a complete surgical cure as opposed to maintaining abdominal wall integrity to avoid such complications as bowel perforation and hernia formation. Evidence from surgical studies reveals that complications can significantly prolong recovery and stay in hospital, highlighting the value of meticulous surgical techniques. Efforts to improve surgical practice, such as those guided by damage control (DC) principles, reflect the flexibility and evolution of techniques in abdominal surgery and a heightened emphasis on the role of the abdominal walls in overall well-being. The accomplishment of surgical operations depends on an extensive knowledge of the function of the abdominal wall, ultimately striving to promote patient recovery and long-term health outcomes when faced with surgical complications (Chalya et al., 2012; Ball et al., 2017) (Figure 6.2).

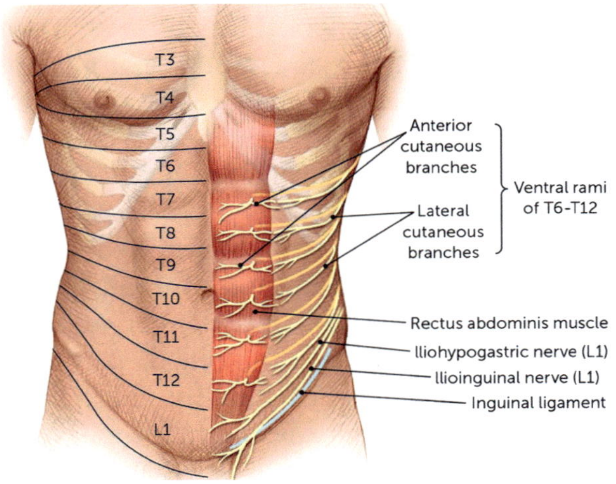

Figure 6.2. Abdominal-wall-nerves.

Source: https://www.central-health.com/wp-content/uploads/abdominal-wall-nerves.jpg.

6.1. Anatomy of the Abdominal Wall

Learning Outcome

1. Describe the layers of the abdominal wall
2. Focus on the abdominal wall comprises several key muscle groups
3. State the role of fascia and connective tissue

Abdominal wall anatomy plays a crucial role in understanding the intricacies of abdominal wall surgery. Functionally, the abdominal wall contains several layers, such as the skin, subcutaneous tissue, muscular layers, and peritoneum. The muscles primarily involved are the rectus abdominis, external oblique, internal oblique, and transversus abdominis, each contributing structural support and motion. These muscles are responsible for core stability and covering of the abdominal viscera. Understanding the relationships between the anatomy in this region, particularly during surgery, is necessary because it guarantees that the surgeon can carry out the procedure safely and does not harm structures that are around the surgical field. Additionally, the presence of blood vessels and nerves in these layers should also be considered, as maintaining the integrity of these structures is crucial to recovery and post-surgical functionality. Moreover, anatomical differences have a significant influence on the outcome of surgery, and therefore it is essential that surgeons possess a thorough knowledge of patient anatomy. For instance, the site and direction of large arteries and veins, such as the aorta and inferior vena cava, can vary, which could have implications on surgical interventions and methods used during the repair of abdominal walls. For this purpose, the anatomy serves not only as a reference point but also as a potential site for complications during the operation.

The awareness of such a variation is particularly important in terms of laparoscopic techniques that rely on minimizing tissue trauma and preserving function. Surgical innovation, including the development of minimally invasive surgery, underscores the importance of continually evolving anatomy to improve post-surgical and patient care outcomes (Bhogal et al., 2011). Specific anatomical landmarks are also critical to the successful implementation of some surgical procedures, including hernia repair and abdominal wall reconstruction. Surgeons must decide on the most desirable site for incisions, which in most instances is a compromise between function and cosmetic outcome. The omentum, with its rich vascular supply, has become a topic of interest in recent years as a potential option for reconstruction surgeries due to its stable anatomy and ability to provide soft tissue coverage (Chu et al., 2018). The ability to understand and manage such anatomical structures is essential for gaining favorable results in surgical reconstruction. Lastly, a comprehensive understanding of abdominal wall anatomy not only aids in the conduct of surgical procedures but also further enhances patient safety and optimizes long-term recovery, thereby augmenting the level of surgical excellence in abdominal wall surgery (Figure 6.3).

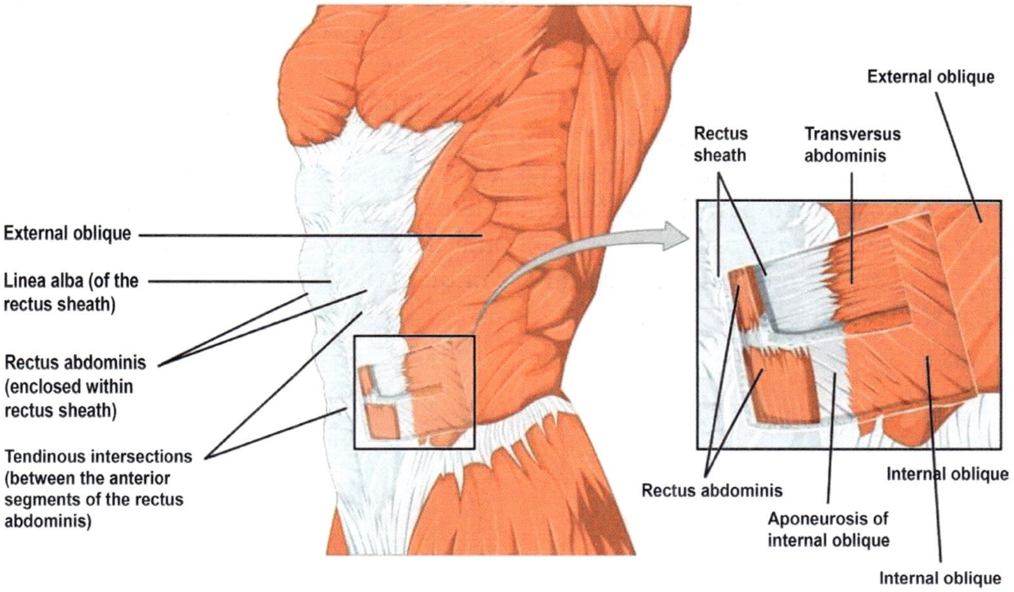

Figure 6.3. Anatomy of the abdominal wall.

Source: https://teachmeanatomy.info/wp-content/uploads/Muscles-of-the-Anterolateral-Abdominal-Wall-1024x604.jpg.

6.1.1. Layers of the Abdominal Wall

Through finding the intricacies of surgery on the abdominal wall, one must consider the layers that comprise the abdominal wall itself. The abdominal wall is composed of numerous layers, each serving a vital role in maintaining its structural integrity. The very first layer that one sees, the skin, protects from exterior trauma and contains sensory receptors. Beneath the skin lies the subcutaneous tissue, which varies in thickness and composition between individuals, yet serves as a cushioning and insulation. Opposing these layers is the fascia, an important connective tissue that encapsulates the abdominal muscles, allowing internal organs to be held snugly in place. Understanding these layers and their roles is crucial for surgeons, as any surgery in the area requires a detailed understanding of how these layers function and interact within the overall dynamics of the abdominal wall. With advanced techniques in surgery, abdominal wall defect repair necessitates an advanced level of understanding of the anatomical layers involved. The three most superficial layers of muscle—transversus abdominis, internal oblique, and external oblique—are all crucial for maintaining abdominal pressure and protecting internal organs. These layers of muscle are significant in surgery, where the tissues must be carefully negotiated and reconstructed in an effort to achieve a successful repair. New surgical technologies, such as laparoscopic procedures, have provided us with further insights into interactions with muscle and the importance of preserving it intact. Therefore, the surgeons must be skilled not only in how they approach such layers but also in how they stabilize them so that function is regained and complications are minimized. Layering of the muscular layer provides a channel for successful surgical treatment without impairing the functioning and aesthetic purposes of the abdominal wall. Post-operative evaluation of the abdominal wall layered anatomy is essential in assessing the magnitude of surgical outcomes. By using aids such as ultrasonography and computed tomography, physicians can visualize the various sonographic appearances of the abdominal wall post-surgery. The techniques enable the identification of complications, such as recurrence, which may occur following meticulous incisional hernia repair. Understanding the process of repairing involves understanding the anatomy of these layers and how they must be reconstructed successfully, a point highlighted in the literature on three-layered anatomical hernia reconstruction (Aguirre et al., 2009). Furthermore, postoperative treatment is necessary for any complications, since improper healing of any of these layers can lead to functional disability or cosmetic deformity in patients, emphasizing the need for meticulous surgical techniques that respect the delicate architecture of the abdominal wall (Figure 6.4).

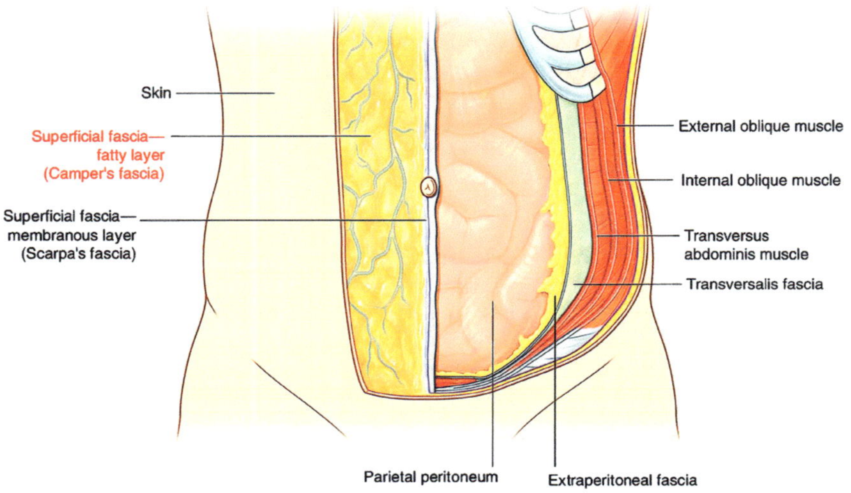

Figure 6.4. Layers of the abdominal wall.

Source: https://beldholm.com.au/wp-content/uploads/2024/10/image-52.png.

6.1.2. Key Muscles Involved

The abdominal wall comprises a series of significant muscle groups that provide structural support and allow for motion in various directions. The rectus abdominis, external obliques, internal obliques, and transversus abdominis form the core of this musculature, each contributing to the overall function of the abdominal wall. The rectus abdominis, commonly referred to as the "six-pack" muscle, provides longitudinal support and plays a crucial role in spinal flexion. The external obliques, on either side of the abdomen, assist with trunk rotation and lateral flexion and protect internal contents. They must be best treated in the surgery of the abdominal wall because injury or compromise of their integrity can significantly influence postoperative recovery and functional results. In modern surgical techniques, knowledge of the role of the transversus abdominis muscle has become essential, especially in methods used in hernia repair and abdominal wall reconstruction. This inner layer of deep muscles serves as a natural corset, giving intra-abdominal pressure and stability to the core. Techniques such as the transversus abdominis plane (TAP) block have emerged as successful adjuvants in laparoscopic surgery, significantly reducing the administration of anesthetics and enhancing postoperative pain management (Jiang et al., 2018). By stimulating the muscle during procedures, surgeons can optimize recovery by keeping the muscle functional and preventing surgery complications caused by weak core stability. The interaction of these muscles is intricately interwoven, serving to highlight the importance of precise surgical techniques that acknowledge their functions in both stability and movement.

Lastly, the interrelations between the abdominal wall muscles are further complicated by the presence of structures, such as the linea alba and fascia, which are composed of connective tissue and function to provide points of muscular attachment and general structural support. These tissues merge with the muscles mentioned above to facilitate coordinated tasks that are essential in activities such as bending and twisting. Additionally, modern recommendations incorporate new techniques, including myofascial release and laparoscopic techniques for hernia fixation, which emphasize the preservation of muscles (Bain et al., 2019). With the evolution of abdominal wall surgery, a complete understanding of these workhorse muscles will remain paramount in tailoring operative techniques to maximize healing with the fewest complications. This focus not only optimizes surgical outcomes but also addresses the rapidly growing tendency toward minimally invasive techniques for restoring functional tissue integrity economically.

6.1.3. Role of Fascial and Connective Tissue

The function of connective tissue and fascia in abdominal wall surgery is essential, as these layers not only provide support but also play critical roles in healing and preventing complications, such as incisional hernias. Fascia is a layer of superficial connective tissue that envelops organs and muscles, providing a stabilizing function while allowing for movement and structural support. Under abdominal wall surgery, the anatomy of the fascia, including its formation and function, aids the surgeon in making informed incision placement choices and in selecting effective closure techniques. Increasing knowledge of fascial planes may lead to improved results, particularly in high-risk patients with many incisional hernias, such as those who are obese and those undergoing laparotomy (Kleinrensink et al., 2013). Maintaining the fascia gently during surgery can also reduce the risk of complications related to wound healing and facilitate better postoperative outcomes. Connective tissue, comprising collagen and elastin fibers, helps maintain the structural framework of the abdominal wall. The mechanical properties of connective tissue allow for both flexibility and strength, which are crucial during the healing process after surgery. After surgery, integrity of this connective framework becomes the center of attention, particularly in surgeries in which mesh repair is employed to stabilize the abdominal wall to prevent hernia formation. Studies have shown that mesh materials interact with the surrounding connective tissue, forming scar tissue that incorporates the mesh into the abdominal wall with success (Alves et al., 2017). This incorporation is vital because good incorporation is responsible for the general stability and solidity of the treated site, thereby minimizing the frequency of complications such as hernias and improving optimal postoperative recovery. Additionally, the vascular supply of fascia and connective tissues greatly dictates surgical outcomes. A well-vascularized zone promotes good healing and nutrient delivery, which is essential in the abdominal wall because surgical trauma can compromise the blood supply. Research has established parallels between human and rat anatomy regarding the vascular supply to the abdominal wall; therefore, understanding blood flow patterns can inform surgical planning and execution (Alves et al., 2017). Increased awareness of vascularization in fascia can help surgeons make informed decisions regarding operations such as mesh repair. Optimal blood supply to the fascia and underlying tissues minimizes potential complications and promotes better healing after abdominal wall surgery (Kleinrensink et al., 2013). Such a combined comprehension of fascia and connective tissue is crucial in formulating surgical procedures and improving patient care (Figure 6.5).

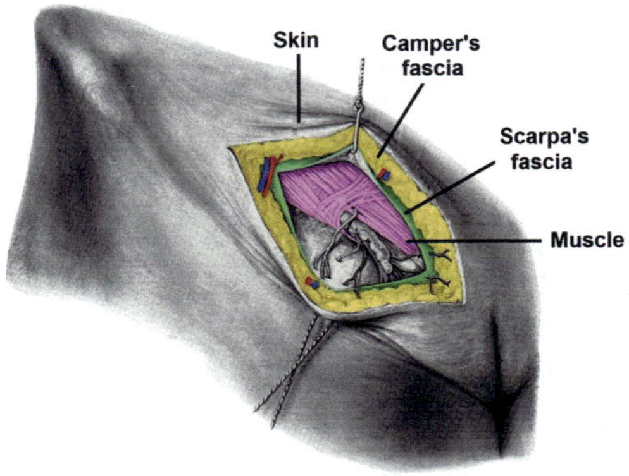

Figure 6.5. Layers of the anterolateral abdominal wall fascia muscle.

Source: https://teachmeanatomy.info/wp-content/uploads/Layers-of-the-Anterolateral-Abdominal-Wall-Fascia-Muscle-1024x800.jpg.

Test Your Knowledge

1. What are the layers of the anterior abdominal wall from superficial to deep?
2. Which muscle forms the main component of the rectus sheath?

6.2. Indications for Surgery

Learning Outcome

1. Explain the hernias and their types
2. Define the trauma and injury to the abdominal wall
3. Discuss the tumors and other pathological conditions

The decision to proceed with surgical repair of abdominal wall disease is primarily determined by pathophysiology and severity of symptoms. Hernias, for example, typically pose a clear-cut indication for surgery when they become painful, incarcerated, or strangulated. This emergency arises due to the risk of compromised blood supply to the affected tissue, which can lead to severe sequelae, including necrosis. In addition, specific operative indications are graded according to the size of hernias; once a defect in the abdominal wall exceeds a particular size, incarceration has an excellent likelihood of developing. Thus, prompt surgical treatment, apart from alleviating pain, also removes potentially dangerous conditions, underscoring the importance of early surgical intervention for such ailments. During abdominal wall surgery, preoperative assessment is key to guaranteeing optimal surgical results. of the patient's overall health status, particularly in high-risk groups, is essential in determining whether a patient is suitable for surgery. Patients with comorbid conditions such as cardiovascular, renal, or pulmonary diseases should be thoroughly assessed to prevent perioperative complications. According to research, personalized perioperative cardiac management is crucial for surgery success and safety. Such evaluation more often than not leads to preoperative treatments or adjustments, which enable patients to withstand the surgical stressors. Proper pre-operative assessment thus paves the way for safer abdominal wall-related surgical interventions and provides a ground for postoperative recovery (Poldermans et al., 2009). Furthermore, advances in surgical techniques have a significant influence on indications for surgery, particularly between the traditional open and minimally invasive surgery fields. Advances in technology, such as laparoscopic procedures, have led to more indications for surgery with reduced incisions, resulting in fewer postoperative complications and shorter recovery times. The development of procedures, particularly those for managing conditions like aortic aneurysms, notes a shift from more risky open procedures to less traumatic and safer options (Bhogal et al., 2011). In the continued advancement of surgical skills, indications for intervention will likely follow suit, underscoring the need for new practices in improving patient outcomes. This adaptation highlights the work of surgical evolution not only as a response to clinical needs but also as a proactive approach to enhancing the quality of abdominal wall surgery (Figure 6.6).

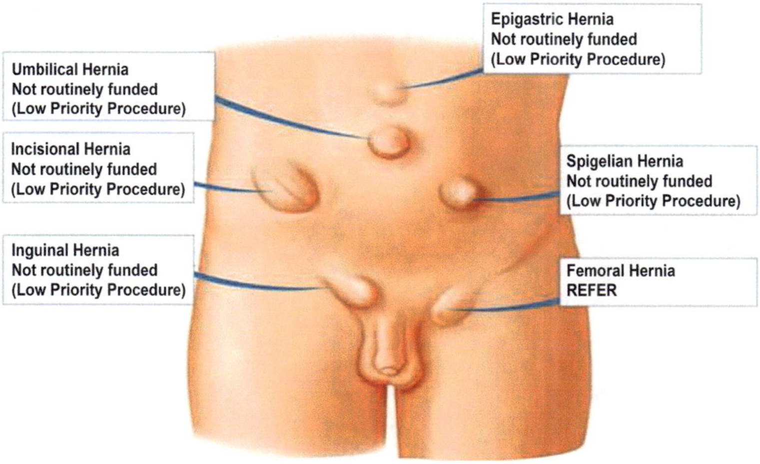

Figure 6.6. Surgical treatment of abdominal wall hernia.

Source: https://www.blueblisshospital.com/Images/GI_surgery_procedures_13.jpg.

6.2.1. Hernias and Their Types

An understanding of hernias and their various types is relevant in the context of abdominal wall surgery. Hernias occur when tissue or an organ protrudes through an abnormal opening in the fascia of the abdominal wall, giving rise to various forms depending on their location and nature. The inguinal hernia is the most frequent one, and it occurs primarily in the groin area and is much more prevalent in men due to anatomical reasons. Under this category, consumptive data indicate that inguinal hernias come in indirect and direct types, with the indirect type being the more frequent occurrence. These types are crucial in selecting appropriate surgical measures, as each has specific challenges and implications for patient recovery. In general, a comprehensive understanding of these types is essential for efficiently shaping surgical measures. The second principal category of hernias includes ventral and incisional hernias, which are typically caused by weakness in the abdominal wall. These hernias usually follow prior operations, where integrity to the abdominal wall is lost through incisions. Repair of such hernias is of paramount importance, given that they are associated with significant morbidity and complications, including recurrence. The advent of new surgical techniques, such as laparoscopic procedures, has become trendy with their minimally invasive nature, which enhances recovery time and reduces postoperative pain. The International Endohernia Society guidelines emphasize the need for regular updates on surgical techniques, as techniques evolve to ensure best practices in herniorrhaphy (Bain et al., 2019). Thus, staying current with the most recent events is instrumental in enhancing surgeons' patient outcomes. Furthermore, certain risk factors, such as obesity, age, and lifestyle choices, contribute to the development and recurrence of hernias. One here is the increasing rate of incisional hernias due to a surge in abdominal operations worldwide. Evidence suggests that patients with these hernias present late, resulting in increased rates of complications and a greater need for early intervention (Kingsnorth et al., 2012). For example, literature has shown that the use of elective surgical procedures, compared to emergency interventions, is associated with significantly improved outcomes. Beyond this, knowledge of patient demographics and presentation symptoms can be hugely influential in determining surgical approaches. Through a comprehensive assessment of these variables, surgeons can optimize repair strategies, thereby limiting complications and promoting long-term success in abdominal wall surgery (Figure 6.7).

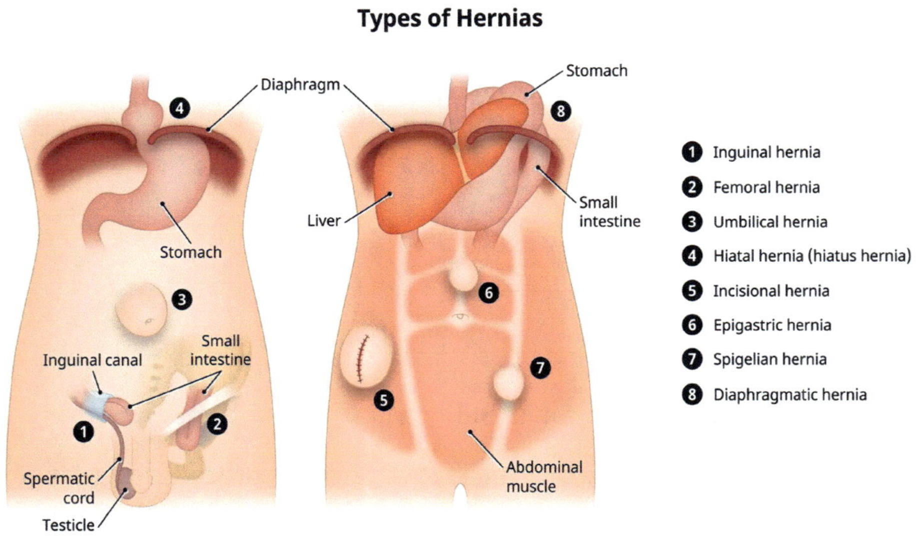

Figure 6.7. Hernia surgery.

Source: https://cdn-assets-eu.frontify.com/s3/frontify-enterprise-files-eu/eyJwYXRoIjoiaWhoLWhlYWx0aGNhcmUtYmVyaGFkXC9maWxlXC9hSkpHQ0ZZQ1JjcjljeGlnaGZDbi5qcGcifQ:ihh-healthcare-berhad:porTaSi9romUO7NpJP3fLMq6C-QIwfySnCXhfRpC0k0?format=webp.

6.2.2. Trauma and Injury to the Abdominal Wall

The abdominal wall serves as a significant barrier to internal structures and a support device in overall trunk function and stability. Trauma and injury in this area can pose a significant challenge to surgical management. Blunt trauma, penetrating trauma, or surgical complications are the primary etiologies of such trauma, resulting in musculature and fascia disruptions of the abdomen.

The challenges of these injuries extend beyond tissue injury, as they also cause metabolic derangements, infection, and intra-abdominal compartment syndrome. Ongoing assessment of the severity of injury and aggressive intervention are essential. The best result often necessitates a multidisciplinary intervention involving trauma surgeons, intensivists, and rehabilitation physicians to deal with both surgical and postoperative convalescence, which reflects the level of sophistication involved in best abdominal wall repair. Advances in techniques in trauma care have emphasized the importance of damage control principles that enable the immediate management of severe abdominal wall trauma. Development of damage control (DC) surgery has revolutionized traumatic abdominal injury management with a protocol-based measure for dealing with complex cases where conventional methods do not produce desirable results. Through the application of abbreviated laparotomy and expedited conservative surgical procedures, surgeons are in a better position to treat lethal injuries while reducing long-term exposure to surgical interventions, opening the door to stable patient status. Furthermore, the incorporation of DC surgery with prophylactic open abdomen techniques has been discovered to have promise in preventing secondary complications, such as intra-abdominal hypertension. This advancement in surgical technique not only demonstrates an enhanced understanding of trauma physiology but also marks a trend towards patient-centered care strategies that prioritize early intervention and optimal recovery pathways (Ball et al., 2017). Trauma and injury care strategies for the abdominal wall involve a firm understanding of varied surgical approaches for the purpose of optimizing recovery results. Negative pressure wound therapy is an example of processes that have emerged as essential adjuncts to surgery, facilitating enhanced healing of complicated wounds while managing infection risk. Treatment goals include maintaining fluid balance, preventing further injury, and optimizing closure of the abdominal cavity. Current studies emphasize the utility of intra-abdominal pressure measurement as a guide to surgery, particularly in open abdomen treatment protocols. The classification of open abdomen injuries has also evolved to enable enhanced comparison of surgical procedures and results among different patient groups. Surmounting these challenges ensures that surgical teams remain capable of delivering high-quality trauma care, especially in light of the ongoing advancements in surgical innovation and patient management (Bjorck et al., 2015).

6.2.3. Tumors and Other Pathologic Conditions

The abdominal wall serves as a significant barrier to protect internal organs while imparting structural stability and mobility. Yet, it may be ruptured by numerous pathological processes, including tumors and traumatic injuries. Tumors may arise from several cellular lineages, either as benign or malignant tumors. In abdominal wall surgery, tumors not only make surgery complicated but also stress the necessity of thorough preoperative assessments. The surgeons must assess the extent of tumor involvement in the surrounding tissues and plan the operation accordingly. Sarcomas or metastasizing tumors can lead to highly altered anatomy, and hence, safe and effective surgical procedures are required to achieve patient outcomes. Such interventions are generally extremely complex and require multidisciplinary teams, emphasizing the need for both oncological and surgical expertise to achieve optimal outcomes. In abdominal wall surgery, one particular problem is that of non-traumatic perforation of the small intestine, which often originates from underlying pathology like malignancies. Tumors, particularly lymphomas, are a significant challenge, since the nonspecific presentation makes diagnosis tough until surgery becomes inevitable. The pathological conditions may lead to perforation, which must be addressed urgently to prevent major complications like peritonitis. Surgical treatment generally includes resection of the affected segment of bowel and, in some cases, an anastomosis. As suggested in the literature, with the acute problems addressed by surgery, the general prognosis remains heavily influenced by the underlying status of the system, maintaining the necessity of an overall treatment plan with adjuvant therapies for the effective treatment of malignancies (Banu et al., 2016).

Treatment of abdominal wall tumors goes beyond surgery and includes continuous follow-up for recurrence and metastasis. After primary surgery management, patients typically undergo follow-up examinations to ensure proper disease control. The data on prevalence among abdominal tumor burden reveal rising rates, particularly in regions with potential access disparities and shortages in preventive care, as well as healthcare. As implied by evidence, the outcome of such tumors is supplemented by associated injuries, especially in developing nations where trauma and cancer are prevalent (Ndongo et al., 2010). This necessitates having integrated healthcare practices that encompass not only primary surgical care but also long-term oncological follow-up. A multidisciplinary approach guarantees patients receive holistic treatment, improving overall outcomes by addressing both the surgical and medical components of the disorder (Figure 6.8).

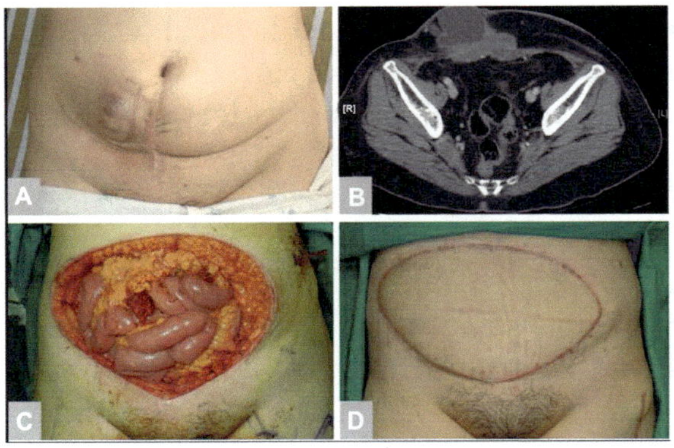

Figure 6.8. Tumors and other pathological conditions.

Source: https://www.researchgate.net/publication/331478975/figure/fig4/AS:732350128353283@1551617285580/Case-3-A-59-year-old-patient-with-a-malignant-transformation-of-abdominal-wall.png.

Test Your Knowledge

1. What are the common indications for surgical repair of an inguinal hernia?
2. When is surgical intervention necessary for abdominal wall trauma?

6.3. Surgical Techniques

Learning Outcome

1. Explain the open surgery vs. laparoscopic surgery for the abdominal wall
2. Define the robotic-assisted surgery of abdominal wall surgery
3. Describe the postoperative care and recovery for the abdominal wall

Surgical techniques in the surgery of the abdominal wall have also seen widespread advancements, further enhancing the results of patients with complex procedures. One of the aspects of this advancement is the introduction of damage control surgery (DC), which recognizes the need for immediate stabilization in severely injured trauma patients. The operations in DC are aimed at short laparotomy and conservation surgery techniques through the facilitation of immediate hemorrhage and contamination control without extending the invasive process in the patient. This approach is essential in cases where recovery and resuscitation must be accorded the highest priority, particularly in the trauma care model. By giving utmost priority to controlling immediately life-threatening injuries in the first instance, surgeons can avert complications, hence improving patient survival rates and allowing subsequent surgeries once the patient has been stabilized. With growth in this specialty, it is essential to understand and implement proper surgery techniques to maximize outcomes in patients. Along with damage control surgery, open abdomen care has also seen remarkable developments. Management of the open abdomen with appropriate therapy involves a combination of different innovations that are focused on rapid closure and reducing complications. Contemporary methods are directed toward maintaining fluid balance and facilitating early abdominal wall closure. Among the most effective tools has been the employment of abdominal negative pressure therapy, which not only dresses the abdominal contents but also allows for fascial edge approximation. The deployment of this modality is highly correlated with higher closure rates, demonstrating its effectiveness in the operating room. Routinely, intra-abdominal pressure monitoring is a key measure in the direction of surgical management, thus highlighting the importance of vigilant monitoring of changing patient status. Progress of this nature highlights seminal advances in intra-abdominal hypertension and management-specific surgical methods relevant to abdominal wall surgery. The progressive character of surgical procedures is also reflected in the unabated challenges involving intra-abdominal hypertension and management.

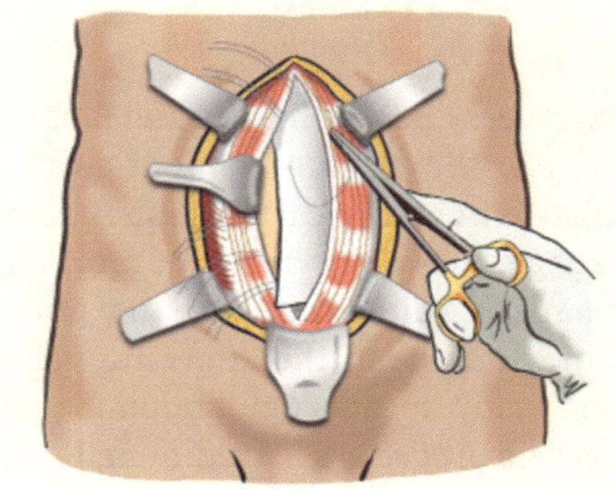

Figure 6.9. Surgical techniques in abdominal wall surgery.

Source: https://lh3.googleusercontent.com/proxy/mGXMDQzSvDTs24adsg6O7QGLwMiHXnUb_jE65j9HabejiEzepyJdC38Spf7E-9GW2J0Ed0db_F-YNQNvS1WI7RxUcUSd4cHG0xzp_ig-rskkCNKisdvXu4zFjCk2HCLnP0tAa16igLhU1ww.

Prophylactic treatments, such as the open abdomen technique, arose as a result of complications such as abdominal compartment syndrome arising from damage control laparotomy. As history indicates, such techniques represent an innovative step from an evolving understanding of trauma treatment and patient physiology, moving past outdated tactics to more suitable alternatives. The creation of a novel classification system for open abdomen is remarkable because it provides a systematic approach to measuring the efficacy of various strategies and closures. Through facilitating a common knowledge in the realm of surgery, these developments enable surgeons to individualize their approaches in line with the individual patient presentation and trauma patterns, emphasizing the dynamic nature of surgical techniques in current abdominal wall surgery (Bjorck et al., 2015; Ball et al., 2017) (Figure 6.9).

6.3.1. Open Surgery Versus Laparoscopic Surgery

The controversy between open and laparoscopic surgery for the repair of abdominal walls intensified as new surgical techniques developed. Open surgery, under which bigger cuts are performed to gain access to the abdominal cavity, has long been the conventional way of repairing many hernias and abdominal repairs. However, the procedure is traditionally followed by more extended recuperation and more postoperative pain. In contrast, laparoscopic surgery involves small incisions, facilitated by specialized instruments and cameras, which can decrease tissue damage and shorten healing time. Implications of such differences are most important to patients, as shorter hospital stays and reduced pain can maximize overall outcomes and patient satisfaction. Existing evidence suggests that laparoscopic surgery has advantages in certain instances. For instance, a comparative study of laparoscopic transabdominal preperitoneal (TAPP) and open repair of an obturator hernia revealed significantly shorter hospital stay durations and lower postoperative inflammation in the laparoscopic group (Sun et al., 2025). More specifically, patients who received laparoscopic repair had a median hospitalization of seven days compared to 13 days for the open repair group. Also noteworthy is that the laparoscopic intervention resulted in less blood loss, which could potentially lead to a quicker recovery and fewer complications, suggesting its possible benefit in specific instances. Such evidence suggests that while open surgery remains an appropriate choice, laparoscopic techniques are potential alternatives that can lead to improved patient outcomes.

Another extremely significant area of contrast is postoperative pain and recovery figures between the two surgical approaches. A laparoscopic intraperitoneal onlay mesh (IPOM) repair was compared with an open Rives–Stoppa repair, revealing that patients in the laparoscopic group had lower pain scores at various time points following surgery (Havrylov et al., 2024). Patient pain was significantly less after IPOM compared with the open repair, indicating a significant advantage for laparoscopic techniques. Furthermore, the operating time was significantly shorter for the laparoscopic group, indicating a more straightforward surgical process. These findings cumulatively corroborate the claim that laparoscopic surgery is capable of providing both pain relief and operational efficiency, and that might be an arguably favored choice in addressing abdominal wall issues.

6.3.2. Robotic Surgery

Surgical techniques have developed significantly, particularly with the adoption of robot-assisted surgery as a component of abdominal wall surgery. The new technique enhances the precision of surgery using robotic systems, which help surgeons perform complex procedures with improved visualization and control. One of the most critical applications of robotic-assisted surgery is in abdominal wall hernia repair, where open repair has historically grappled with recovery and post-op issues. The advent of laparoscopic approaches and robot-assistance, however, has made minimal invasiveness more desirable for hernia repair. These robot platforms can navigate through the intricate structure of the abdominal wall, achieving higher dexterity and enabling finer movements that are challenging to achieve through conventional means. As research continues to develop in the area, the effect of these innovations on patient recovery time and success is coming to the forefront. Internationally, guidelines have been established to harmonize robotic-assisted procedures for the surgical treatment of the abdominal wall. As highlighted by the International Endohernia Society, these guidelines are an aggregation of best practices and have been created as new evidence and procedures appear. Continued update, such as major updates regarding robotics and other minimally invasive techniques, testifies to the evolving nature of surgical practice. The revised guidelines are informed by recent advances, such as the release of the transversus muscle and the application of Botulinum toxin (Botox) in hernia repair, which are gaining popularity due to their potential to enhance surgical results. Thus, their addition to the surgical armamentarium is not a matter of optional sophistication but a crucial measure for augmenting patient care and optimizing recovery stages in abdominal wall surgery (Bain et al., 2019). Apart from that, pitting robotic-assisted techniques against standard methods has created a paradigm shift in managing abdominal surgeries, particularly urinary diversions. While the majority of robotic-assisted radical cystectomies still employ extracorporeal urinary diversion, the development of intracorporeal urinary diversion marks the growing flexibility of the robotic system in urological surgery. Both procedures have some advantages; yet, as reported recently, robotic intracorporeal urinary diversion has been found to actually reduce discomfort from bowel exposure and shorten postoperative recovery time (Balbay et al., 2016). This has raised a continued dispute that requires more research to verify the long-term outcomes of robotic techniques across numerous surgical specialties. The precision and versatility of robotic surgery not only enhance existing techniques but also leave room for potential future innovations in abdominal wall surgery, positioning surgeons to offer new solutions to challenging surgical issues (Figure 6.10).

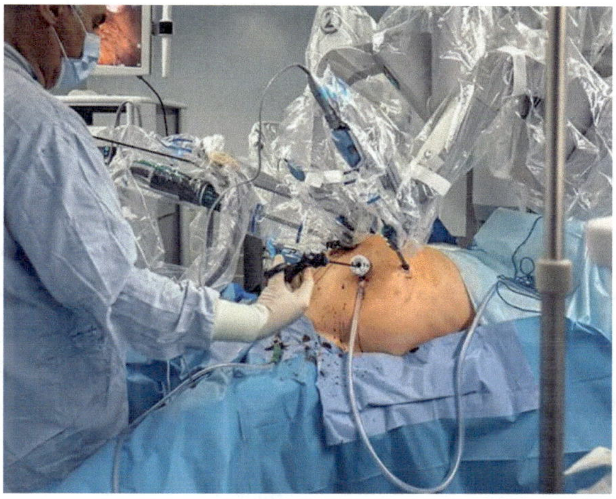

Figure 6.10. Robotic surgery in abdominal wall.

Source: https://www.apexhospitals.com/_next/image?url=https%3A%2F%2Fbed.apexhospitals.com%2Fuploads%2FHernia_repair_f20f77bc55.jpg&w=1200&q=75.

6.3.3. Postoperative Care and Recovery

Effective postoperative care is crucial to achieving enhanced recovery outcomes in patients undergoing abdominal wall surgery. Adequate pain control is directly responsible for recovery, and studies have concluded that interventions such as epidural analgesia (EDA) have very favorable outcomes for patients. Minimizing pain not only alleviates pain but also decreases the occurrence of complications such as wound dehiscence and unplanned intubation. For instance, EDA patients exhibited a significantly lower incidence of pulmonary embolism and septicaemia compared to their counterparts without this form of pain management. Consequently, the incorporation of EDA into postoperative treatments can result in shorter hospital stays, lower rates of dependency on mechanical ventilation, and improved overall recovery parameters after abdominal surgical procedures (Ceppa et al., 2019). In addition to pain management, programs of postoperative recovery should incorporate evidence-based programs that limit the incidence of potential complications. An example of such a program that has been demonstrated to restrict respiratory complications following surgery is the COUGH bundle. This systematic approach encompasses the use of early mobilization, deep breathing, and patient education in determining the incidence of pneumonia and respiratory distress. The application of the COUGH bundle has proven very promising, particularly for patients at risk of surgery. From studies, compliance with the protocol has been observed, resulting in a considerable decrease in hospital-acquired pneumonia and unplanned reintubations, which justifies its application to comprehensive postoperative care (Hilton-Christie et al., 2020). The inclusion of these in the postoperative care protocol not only enhances patient safety but also enhances return to functional health at a faster pace. A further crossroads is found between pain management and preventive measures, which emphasizes the importance of a multidisciplinary approach to postoperative recovery. Collaboration among surgical teams, nurses, and rehabilitation specialists can lead to more coordinated care pathways for patients. Following abdominal wall surgery, management of both the short-term postoperative needs—such as the management of pain with modalities such as EDA—and the introduction of preventive interventions like the COUGH bundle optimizes the recovery potential best. This integrative framework is essential in reducing the occurrence of adverse events and optimizing recovery outcomes, ultimately ensuring increased patient satisfaction and decreasing healthcare costs. Having a culture of awareness and adherence to these practices is crucial for achieving improved clinical outcomes in abdominal wall surgery and other similar operations (Ceppa et al., 2019; Hilton-Christie et al., 2020).

Test Your Knowledge

1. What is the difference between open and laparoscopic hernia repair techniques?
2. How is mesh placement performed during abdominal wall reconstruction?

6.4. Risks and Complications

Learning Outcome

1. Identify the common surgical risks of abdominal wall surgery
2. Define the specific complications related to abdominal wall surgery
3. Describe the long-term effects of abdominal wall surgery

The technical complexities involved in abdominal wall surgery are underscored by the list of risks and complications that can significantly impact patient outcomes. Among the most common complications is wound infection, which can happen due to diverse factors ranging from the type of surgery done to patients' intrinsic medical conditions. Comorbid patients, for instance, obesity or diabetes, carry higher risks due to an impaired healing process. These patients are likely to experience prolonged hospital stays and incur additional medical costs, making optimal preoperative assessment and postoperative care essential. Furthermore, infection prevention methods, such as the administration of prophylactic antibiotics and the use of aseptic techniques, are essential in reducing these risks and achieving the overall success of the procedure. Another major complication caused by surgery of the abdominal wall is the recurrence of the hernia. This issue can have a high incidence rate, particularly in hernia repair operations, where operative technique and mesh selection are significant variables. Various reports have indicated that the application of proper materials and techniques, specifically laparoscopic or robotic-assisted techniques, can yield lower recurrence rates than traditional open techniques. Additionally, patient factors such as tissue integrity and age must be considered when evaluating risk; older patients may have an increased risk of recurrence due to reduced collagen synthesis and decreased tissue elasticity. Thus, meticulous attention to the surgical plan and postoperative care is needed to avert recurrence and achieve optimal long-term outcome. Complications of abdominal wall surgery can extend to include early physical health issues as well as overall patient quality and recuperation. Pain after surgery is frequent and, in some patients, can be chronic, resulting in functional impairment and adversely impacting quality of life. Proper pain management techniques, including the use of multimodal analgesia, have been demonstrated through research to play a crucial role in promoting patient satisfaction and facilitating a more rapid recovery. Also, psychological complications such as depression and anxiety may arise due to complications or prolonged recovery times. These are considerations because good, integrated care plans with physical and mental support will ultimately influence the outcome of surgery. This approach is critical due to the high-risk interaction of complications and risks of abdominal wall surgery, with a stress on proper preoperative counseling and postoperative follow-up (Figure 6.11).

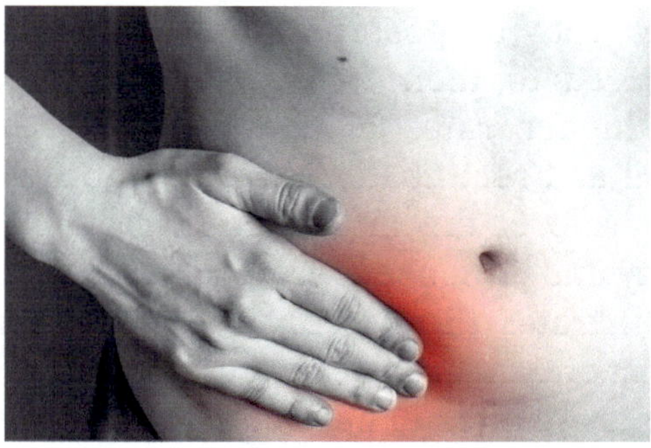

Figure 6.11. Risks and complications in the abdominal wall.

Source: https://texasherniaspecialists.com/wp-content/uploads/2023/01/AdobeStock_246204762-1-1024x684.jpeg.

6.4.1. Common Surgical Risks

Surgical procedures, including abdominal wall surgery, inherently come with a variety of risks that significantly influence the outcome of patients. Some of these risks include complications such as infection, bleeding, and allergic reactions to anesthesia. The risk of infection is high for the operation site, and this may occur due to inadequate sterilization protocols or breakdown of postoperative care. Bleeding is also excessive during surgery, and it can lead to transfusion and extended recovery times. Anesthesia is also not free from risk factors, ranging from mild side effects to fatal complications, particularly among individuals who have a pre-existing medical condition. Such risks must be detected and managed to limit the frequency of adverse events, thereby allowing both patients and medical practitioners to approach the complex nature of surgical interventions with a well-informed understanding of potential complications (Moldovan et al., 2016). Obesity subsequently ranks among the crucial determinants of risk during surgery, particularly abdominal wall surgery. Obese patients have a higher risk of complications, including infection of the wound and delay in healing. It has been observed that obese patients show a higher rate of postoperative complications compared to their non-obese counterparts, with higher rates of complications in the wound and reintubation (Hakala et al., 1990). Furthermore, the interrelationship between obesity and prolonged recovery periods starkly demonstrates the necessity for preoperative assessment tailored to these patients. These patients are often in need of a more aggressive response to pre-surgical care, with attention focused on weight control interventions that can reduce complications and promote better perioperative and postoperative results. Therefore, targeting obesity as a modifiable risk factor is a key factor in maximizing the safety and efficacy of abdominal wall surgery. In addition to obesity, additional comorbidities significantly contribute to the overall risks of abdominal wall surgery. Diabetes, cardiovascular conditions, and pulmonary disease can also increase surgical risks as well as complicate recovery from surgery afterwards. For instance, patients with diabetes are at greater risk for infection and wound healing problems, further complicating their course through surgery. The literature presented here emphasizes the need for correct patient selection and preoperative management tailored to mitigate such risks in the proper manner (Moldovan et al., 2016). Further, appropriate postoperative care and observation become crucial in comorbid patients to allow timely intervention at the first indication of complications. A multidisciplinary approach, with surgeons, anesthesiologists, and primary care doctors, is beneficial in the care of at-risk patient populations, which in turn seeks to enhance surgical outcomes and minimize the incidence of common surgical hazards associated with abdominal wall surgery.

6.4.2. Complications Related to the Surgery of the Abdominal Wall

Abdominal wall operation, as common as it is for diseases such as hernias, comes with a very specific set of complications to which clinicians need to be prepared to respond. Surgical site infection (SSI) is perhaps the most frequent complication and can lengthen recovery time and have a detrimental effect on the patient's outcome. In keeping with evidence, SSI risk may be heightened in diabetes or obesity comorbidities that impair healing of wounds and predispose the patient to infection. Effective prophylaxis through proper administration of antibiotic and meticulous surgical technique is paramount in eliminating this risk. The high rate of SSI indicates the need for highly skilled surgical teams with specialized training in performing abdominal wall operations because their competency can lead to better patient outcomes through reducing the rate of surgery complications like SSI and optimizing the quality of surgery care.

Another severe complication of abdominal wall surgery is hernia recurrence, particularly following the repair of an inguinal hernia. It has been suggested in research that specialized surgical units for abdominal wall surgery have a significant impact on recurrence rates. For example, a retrospective cohort study found that the recurrence rate among patients treated in specialized units was 3%, compared to 15% in non-specialized units (López Cano et al., 2023; Gonçalves et al., 2023). This dramatic variance can be attributed to a multidimensional mix of factors intervening between the surgeon's experience and the application of standardized evidence-based methods tailored to a specific hernia repair. The solution to the problems of recurrent hernia not only necessitates surgical competence but also knowledge of the patient's own risk factors, thereby emphasizing the value of a multidisciplinary team approach to the management of abdominal wall surgery complications. Surgical chronic pain is yet another complication that can occur in patients undergoing abdominal wall surgery in the form of chronic postoperative inguinal pain. It can have disastrous effects on the quality of life of a patient and lead to permanent disability. Mechanisms of pain postoperatively are multifactorial, with nerve injury, scarring, and the body's response to the surgery by inflammation. The incidence of chronic pain may vary; however, evidence suggests that patients treated in specialty abdominal wall surgery units experience fewer chronic pain cases compared to their counterparts in general surgery wards (López Cano et al., 2023; Gonçalves et al., 2023). Hence, the focus on specialized surgical instruction, postoperative treatment, and early intervention practices becomes critical in averting chronic pain and facilitating maximum recovery after abdominal wall surgery (Figure 6.12).

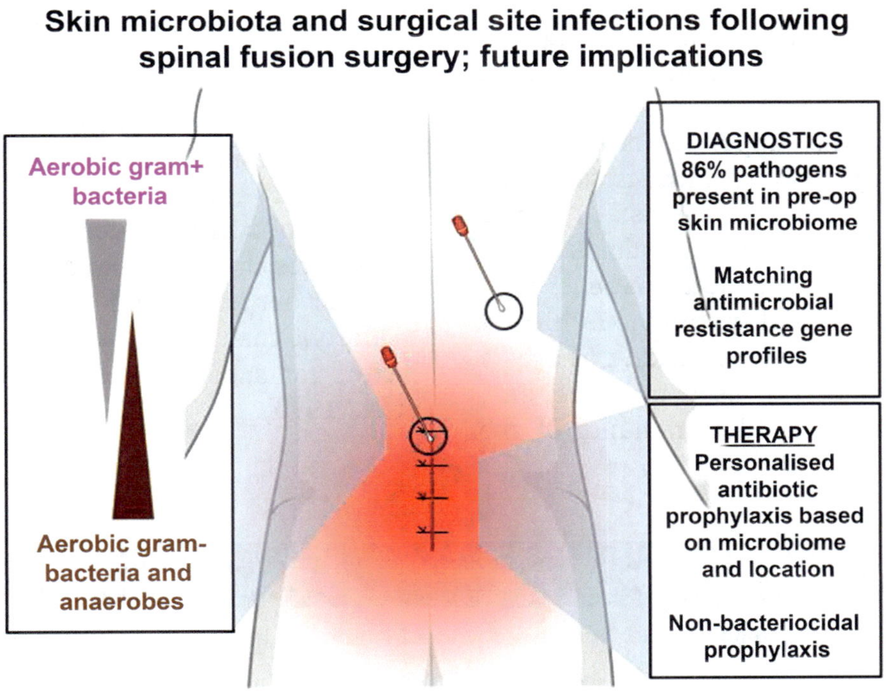

Figure 6.12. Surgical site infection (SSI) in the abdominal wall.

Source: https://www.bjsacademy.com/admin/backend/storage/app/articles/BJS/BJSA/surgical-science/ss012/12_03.jpg.

6.4.3. Long-Term Effects and Considerations

The long-term effects of surgery on the abdominal wall encompass various outcomes that can have a profound impact on a patient's quality of life. Complications from the procedure can persist beyond the postoperative period, affecting physical health and overall well-being. Notably, patients are often left with the complaint of discomfort or pain in the area of operation, which can disrupt normal daily function and cause an enhanced perception of limited mobility. Chronic pain syndromes are possible in some patients and emphasize the need for a total approach to pain management with an emphasis on ending the underlying causes of pain. Moreover, illnesses such as obesity have been observed to aggravate postoperative complications; in a study, for instance, it was observed that obese patients had higher rates of morbidity and mortality compared to their non-obese counterparts, emphasizing the utmost importance of preoperative assessment and interventions for risk reduction (Hakala et al., 1990). Another important factor in the long-term management of patients following abdominal wall surgery is the risk of hernia recurrence. Recurrence rates for abdominal wall hernias can be unacceptable in patients with certain risk factors such as previous history of surgery, advanced age, or obesity. The type of surgery and material used for abdominal wall repair are crucial determinants of the likelihood of hernia recurrence. There has been improvement in minimally invasive interventions that have offered new alternatives for reducing complications of traditional open surgery, since smaller cuts and faster healing accompany them. The long-term impacts of innovative materials such as synthetic meshes, however, remain an area of research (Bhogal et al., 2011). These are important factors to consider in determining optimal patient outcomes and how surgical techniques can be improved in the future. Patient education and postoperative care are two extremely critical factors involved in managing the long-term effects of abdominal wall surgery. Patients must be given proper instructions regarding limitations of activity, complications, and follow-up visits. These are significant in facilitating the involvement of patients in recovery and ultimately toward the success of long-term outcomes. Psychosocial care may also be necessary to address emotional and psychological problems that might be part of the recovery process from surgery. Integrating psychological resources into treatment, along with medical care, can help alleviate conditions such as depression or anxiety that might arise during surgery. Making sure the patient knows his or her long-term management plan encourages the patient to take a proactive role in his or her health and underscores the value of lifestyle changes, especially in those with risk factors for subsequent complications (Hakala et al., 1990).

Test Your Knowledge

1. What are the common complications associated with mesh hernia repair?
2. How can surgical site infections be prevented after abdominal wall surgery?

6.5. Advances in Surgical Technology

Learning Outcome

1. Describe the innovations in surgical instruments of abdominal wall surgery
2. Define the role of imaging technology in planning surgery
3. Discuss the future trends in abdominal wall surgery

Over the past few decades, advances in surgical technology have significantly expanded the scope of abdominal wall surgery, resulting in more precise and effective operations. Most notably, the incorporation of minimally invasive techniques has changed traditional procedures, allowing surgeons to perform complex procedures through smaller incisions. This shift reduces postoperative pain and scarring in patients, as well as postoperative times, leading to quicker returns to normal activities. The use of robotic-assisted surgical systems is one such example of this advancement, as it grants surgeons greater dexterity and a three-dimensional perspective of the operating site. These advancements enable complex maneuvers that are not easily performed through conventional laparoscopic methods, ultimately leading to improved surgical outcomes and enhanced patient satisfaction. Additionally, bioinspired material development has shown promising potential in augmenting surgical procedures in the abdominal cavity. Researchers have been investigating surface adhesion characteristics that enable small, portable devices to travel with ease through the tissue lining. Such devices, to be utilized during insufflated abdomen procedures, must benefit from advanced adhesion characteristics if they are to perform optimally. In addition to introducing state-of-the-art instrumentation for abdominal wall surgery, this new technology emphasizes the importance of biocompatibility and safety in surgical use. By the application of nature-based solutions to facilitate wet adhesion, the operating field can also experience further advancements that enhance the operating skills of surgeons and overall procedural safety, as in the research toward bioengineering principles in surgical technology (Gaskell et al., 2009). The future of surgical development is also observed in the evolution of method improvements for treating complex abdominal pathology, such as aortic aneurysms. Aortic aneurysm repair has a rich history that serves as a useful case study, illustrating the key leadership of surgical trailblazers who have guided preoperative techniques into the contemporary period. This innovation demonstrates the move from classical open surgery to the advent of minimally invasive techniques, reducing the risk of the procedure and enabling improved recovery in patients. The expanded application of such methods in surgery of the abdominal wall is essential, since they illustrate the possibility for complications to be reduced while patient results are optimized. As technology advances, the surgical team is better equipped to address the challenges posed by various abdominal disorders, demonstrating how ongoing improvements in surgical technology continually enhance and improve patient care (Bhogal et al., 2011) (Figure 6.13).

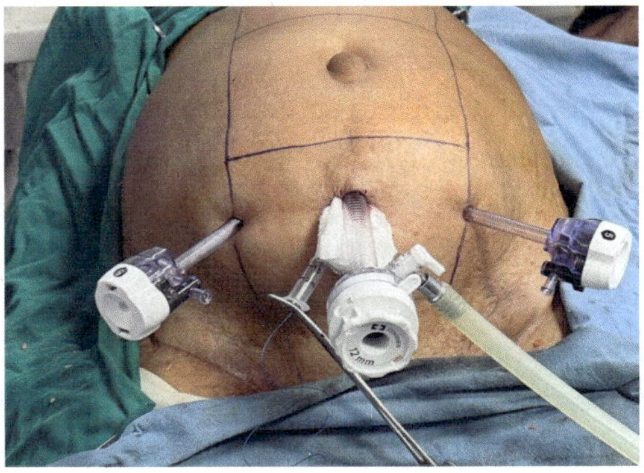

Figure 6.13. Advances in surgical technology for abdominal wall surgery.

Source: https://media.springernature.com/full/springer-static/image/art%3A10.1038%2Fs41598-024-78398-z/MediaObjects/41598_2024_78398_Fig1_HTML.jpg.

6.5.1. Innovations in Surgical Instruments

The surgical instrument field is constantly evolving, particularly in the case of abdominal wall surgery, where emerging technologies are significantly enhancing procedural effectiveness and patient outcomes. One such critical innovation is the development of sophisticated endoscope positioners that offer greater manipulation flexibility in the course of minimally invasive procedures. This technology provides relief from the task load of dealing with traditional rigid endoscopes, thereby improving the surgeon's dexterity and the accuracy of the procedure. As explained in recent studies, the addition of an active zoom capability to passive endoscope holders has led to improved ergonomics and reduced operating time through easy manipulation. These advancements create an even more intuitive operating environment, allowing surgeons to focus on their work rather than the ongoing management of instrument logistics (Bauwens et al., 2020).

In addition to revolutionary endoscopic technology, abdominal wall surgery has been significantly improved by advancements in laparoscopic surgical instruments. These instruments, including advanced graspers, needle holders, and customized suturing devices, are designed to render intricate procedures less invasive, thereby reducing recovery periods and postoperative problems. A survey of the practices within laparoscopic surgery indicates a strong trend away from conventional open approaches to these more recent methods. For instance, certain laparoscopic technologies have been demonstrated to offer equal or superior outcomes with far less patient trauma. Furthermore, the creation of multifunctional tools enables surgeons to perform multiple tasks without changing instruments, thereby optimizing the surgical process and enhancing the efficacy of procedures (Moldovan et al., 2016). The integration of technology and surgical instrument design is transforming the standard of care in abdominal wall surgery. The introduction of computer-based systems and robotically facilitated platforms has also transformed the art of surgery, enabling unprecedented precision and finesse during surgery. Not only do these technologies augment the surgeon's skill, but they also provide an unmatched vehicle for surgical training and mentorship. Robotic-assisted surgeries have been shown to improve patient outcomes while also reducing the learning curve for new surgeons. As these innovations expand, they are part of an ongoing effort to innovate surgical techniques, improve patient safety, and advance the capabilities of abdominal wall surgery (Moldovan et al., 2016; Bauwens et al., 2020).

6.5.2. The Role of Imaging Technology in Planning Surgery

The application of imaging technology plays a crucial role in planning abdominal wall surgery, significantly enhancing the accuracy and outcome of surgical interventions. Advanced imaging modalities, such as magnetic resonance imaging (MRI) and computed tomography (CT), facilitate a detailed assessment of the anatomy and pathology of patients. These technologies provide accurate information about the spatial relationships between the chief structures, such that the surgeons can devise a meticulous surgical plan according to the patient's needs. Apart from this, imaging allows for pre-surgical evaluation, ascertaining the extent of the disease and any potential complications, which in turn impacts the surgery. By viewing the anatomy in three-dimensional space, surgeons can more accurately anticipate potential difficulties that may arise during surgery, leading to improved preparation and potentially better patient outcomes. In addition to visualizing anatomical structures, advanced imaging capabilities enable the examination of tumor biology and the margins of resection. For instance, enhanced imaging capabilities enable surgeons to identify malignancies with spiculated borders or multifocality that would otherwise remain unseen, as observed in studies on the relevance of R1 resections during pelvic exenteration surgeries (Brown et al., 2018). Enhanced identification of such complexities enhances the ability of surgical teams to make informed choices, prompting the exercise of extreme caution when preparing for additional resections as necessary.

Therefore, a tight reading of imaging information can lead to improved management of tumors, and in turn, lower rates of local recurrence and increased survival. The interdisciplinary collaboration of pathologists, surgeons, and radiologists is crucial in refining surgical strategies, and imaging technology is a valuable tool in facilitating this transdisciplinary communication. Furthermore, the advent of new imaging systems, including minimally invasive modalities, has transformed surgery. Contemporary equipment, such as one-handed operated endoscopes with three-dimensional imaging capabilities, provides surgeons with improved hand dexterity and precision in the operating theater (Bauwens et al., 2020). The new technology not only simplifies the process but also maximizes the ergonomics of surgery, minimizing the risks of fatigue and discomfort for the surgical team. Lastly, imaging technology plays a part in addition to pre-operative planning, as it also contributes to determining the performance of the surgical procedure itself. By providing the best possible visualization of surgery, these technologies contribute to more effective interventions and the potential for shortened recovery times, emphasizing the central position imaging now occupies in the development of abdominal wall surgery (Figure 6.14).

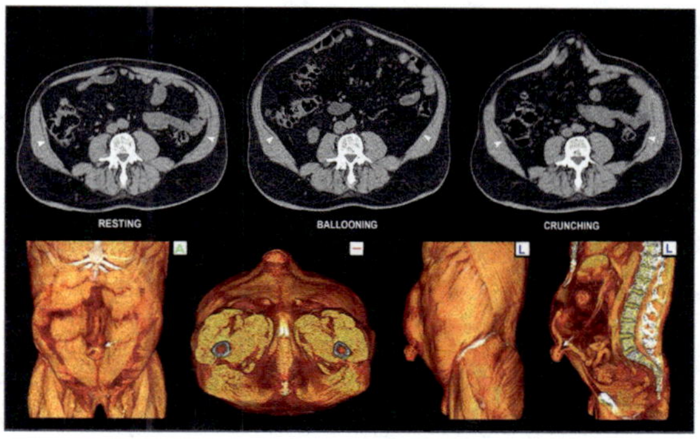

Figure 6.14. Imaging technology planning surgery in the abdominal wall.

Source: https://www.frontiersin.org/files/Articles/799277/fsurg-09-799277-HTML/image_m/fsurg-09-799277-g009.jpg.

6.5.3. Future Trends in Abdominal Wall Surgery

As abdominal wall surgery advances, advancements in minimally invasive procedures are shaping the future of the field. Laparoscopic and robot-assisted surgeries are increasingly becoming favored by surgeons due to the ability to minimize the size of the incision, reduce postoperative pain, and reduce recovery time. Future trends indicate an increased use of these techniques, driven by advancing technology and the provision of appropriate training for surgeons. In addition, the integration of newer imaging technologies, such as intraoperative ultrasound and augmented reality, holds the promise of further increasing surgical precision. These technologies, in addition to offering highly accurate delineation of anatomical structures, enable real-time assessment of intraoperative outcomes. As these technical advances become integrated into surgical practice, the future of abdominal wall surgery will soon lie in achieving maximal patient outcomes through less invasive intervention methods. The second significant trend is the personalization of surgical procedures with patient-specific modeling and simulation. Personalized medicine will revolutionize surgical planning by leveraging the use of computational fluid dynamics (CFD) and high-end imaging to create customized surgical paths for the patient. For instance, the upcoming years may witness an increase in the application of CFD in assessing hemodynamic alterations, such as in the case of coarctation of the aorta, where mechanical factors are crucial in predicting recovery after surgery. The ability to simulate the procedure and its consequences prior to surgery being conducted may assist in providing improved decision-making and higher predictability in surgery success. Therefore, regarding abdominal wall surgery that takes place in the future, a more selective intervention approach will be employed, depending on the patient-specific mechanical and biological characteristics of each case.

Furthermore, an enhanced emphasis on assessing long-term outcomes associated with different surgical techniques will be instrumental in redefining current practices in abdominal wall surgery. Evidence related to long-term morbidity from conventional versus minimally invasive surgery will inform best practice and support clinical guidance. Prospective and retrospective investigations will provide hints on complications, functional outcomes, and patient satisfaction across a range of patient groups. As recognized by studies evaluating pathological changes in vascular morphology in patients with aortic coarctation (Chan et al., 2011; Dholakia et al., 2012), understanding the underlying biomechanics and hemodynamics is crucial for prognosis. To this end, future abdominal wall surgery trends will no longer focus solely on immediate surgical success but also take into consideration the overall and long-term patient health trend after surgery, paving the way for better surgical skills and patient care.

Test Your Knowledge

1. How has robotic-assisted surgery improved outcomes in complex hernia repairs?
2. What role do biosynthetic meshes play in modern abdominal wall reconstruction?

6.6. Patient Perspectives

Learning Outcome

1. Describe the preoperative considerations and education on abdominal wall surgery
2. Define the psychological impact of abdominal wall surgery
3. Identify the patient satisfaction with abdominal wall surgery

Patient perception of abdominal wall surgery is essential in establishing the overall impact of such procedures. Hernia patients or those with abdominal wall defects usually experience a complex process of considering surgical options, risks, and convalescence. It is daunting when thinking about possible extreme lifestyle adjustments or surgical complications. Respecting the diverse needs of patients, from pain management to psychological well-being, is crucial for healthcare providers to create a caring environment. Placing patients at the center stage may allow surgeons to help allay fears, with understandable information about surgeries, for example, minimally invasive procedures that have emerged as non-threatening alternatives to traditional interventions. This step toward openness can enhance the patient's experience, for to understand the intricacies of their treatment instills a feeling of trust and collaboration within the healthcare relationship.

Effective communication in the patient-surgeon relationship is crucial. Patients place value on customized information that is tailored to the specific condition of the patient, surgical method, and post-operative expectations. Furthermore, patient education on potential emotional and physical adaptations following surgery is crucial to their recovery process. Incorporating education on management of post-operative pain and recognizing warning signs of complications could enable the patient to become an active participant in their recovery process. Investments in intensive pre-operative instruction seminars can not only render the procedures better comprehensible but also instill a greater sense of security in the patient experience.

This active practice of patient education perfectly underscores that successful surgical results not only rely on technical skill, but also on congruence between surgical aims and patient expectations. Patient impressions also comprise the evaluation of long-term results of abdominal wall surgery. Feedback regarding post-operative quality of life, functional recovery, and satisfaction is necessary to facilitate continuous improvement in surgical procedures. Health facilities that actively seek and learn from patient experiences are able to refine their surgical procedures, thereby improving standards of care. Reflective practice can lead to innovation in surgical techniques and models of post-operative care that are attuned to patient concerns. For instance, recent studies are focusing on the consideration of psychological issues like anxiety and body image issues, which influence recovery and long-term satisfaction (Bhogal et al., 2011). These dimensions can be addressed to mitigate the emotional effects that may arise from surgical intervention. Generally, perception from the patient as a core part of surgical practice helps to cultivate a comprehensive, responsive, and holistic healthcare environment (Figure 6.15).

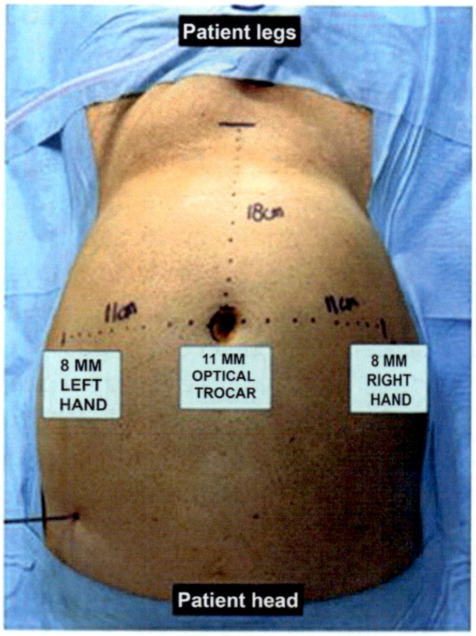

Figure 6.15. Patient perspectives on abdominal wall surgery.

Source: https://www.frontierspartnerships.org/files/myhome%20article%20library/13880/13880_Thumb_400.jpg.

6.6.1. Preoperative Considerations and Education

Preoperative conditions are crucial to a patient's abdominal wall surgery in order to optimize the patient's result. They consist of a thorough analysis of the patient's medical history, physical condition, and risk factors that may influence the surgery and the postoperative course. The surgeons are required to evaluate if the patient has comorbidities, the nutritional level, and previous abdominal surgeries, which would impact the complexity of the procedure. Additionally, the patient's lifestyle and expectations need to be understood when creating a tailored surgical plan that meets their unique circumstances. Appropriate education on the surgical procedure also needs to be part of this preoperative process so that patients are properly informed and ready psychologically for surgery, thus enhancing a feeling of autonomy and reducing anxiety toward surgery. Patient education is a cornerstone of the preoperative protocol for abdominal wall operations. Full explanation of the operative risks and benefits forms the foundation of informed consent and demystifies the surgical experience for the patient. Patient education for potential complications, such as infection or recurrence of hernia, is also valuable since it engages participation in their own health. Furthermore, discussing postoperative expectations, including recovery times and levels of activity, prepares patients for the procedure. As surgical methods continue to evolve, for example, through minimally invasive techniques and advances in hernia repair, informing patients about developments in care can more effectively educate and allay fears about the treatment process. Educating patients not only prepares them but also inspires them to adhere to postoperative instructions. In recent decades, the worth of standardized protocols in laparoscopic surgery has become increasingly evident, a sign of progress in managing abdominal wall hernias. The International Endohernia Society (IEHS) has developed and continues to update guidelines that provide a framework for surgical practice, emphasizing the importance of adhering to evidence-based practices (Bain et al., 2019). This commitment to continuous education and refinement ensures that surgical techniques are grounded in the most current research, thus optimizing patient safety and improving outcomes. Including these guidelines within preoperative education allows medical professionals to reassure patients of the quality and reliability of the operation. Furthermore, the inclusion of novel diagnostic and surgical methods such as robotic-assisted repair methods within these guidelines reflects the dynamic nature of surgical practice, whereby surgeons and patients alike must stay current in an ever-evolving specialty (Burity et al., 2014). This holistic focus on preoperative issues fosters a culture of cooperation and shared decision-making that ultimately benefits patients undergoing abdominal wall surgery.

6.6.2. Psychological Impact of Operation

Abdominal wall repair is highly psychologically affecting to a patient, and thus it is crucial to be aware of the mental health condition as well as the physical. Increased anxiety and depression are typically noted in the postoperative period immediately after the surgery and are significant predictors of overall recovery. Research indicates that the degree of pre-surgical anxiety is related to post-operative anxiety on the second day following surgery, suggesting the persistence of psychological distress following surgical procedures. This observation emphasizes the need for pre-surgical psychological assessment and intervention in an effort to better prepare patients for the emotional distress they are soon to experience. Since these psychology-related problems might have adverse impacts on pain experiences and rehabilitation processes, their position should be acknowledged when creating comprehensive post-surgical care procedures (Abiodun et al., 2005).

Furthermore, the psychological impact of surgery encompasses not only transient emotional responses but also may cause permanent shifts in mental status. Patients who undergo abdominal wall surgery often have difficulty with preoccupation regarding recovery and returning to regular activity, which can manifest as increased anxiety and depressive symptoms. In surgeries for conditions such as endometriosis, in which pain is experienced in the abdominal-pelvic area, long-term mental health problems may develop despite successful surgery. Although surgery, like laparoscopic excision, is meant to alleviate physical symptoms, underestimation of the psychological effect may result in incomplete recovery. Therefore, healthcare providers should place greater emphasis on mental health care, enabling patients to be presented with coping strategies that address both physical and psychological factors during recovery (Andronache et al., 2018).

Ultimately, having an integrated plan for addressing the psychological impact of surgery is crucial for enhancing patient outcomes. With multidisciplinary teams comprised of surgeons, mental health professionals, and pain management doctors, holistic treatment can be provided during recovery. That also includes coverage for nutritional advice, particularly for patients undergoing endometriosis surgery, as dietary changes can improve physical function and overall well-being. With the investigation of the multidimensional aspects of recovery, healthcare professionals can better support patients in managing anxiety, depression, and chronic pain, thereby improving quality of life post-surgery. The recognition of psychological mechanisms as part of the recovery process highlights the need for ongoing research and support to implement effective interventions tailored to individual patient experiences (Abiodun et al., 2005; Andronache et al., 2018).

6.6.3. Patient Satisfaction and Outcomes

In abdominal wall surgery, patient satisfaction is a critical determinant of surgical success since it not only represents clinical outcomes but also the overall experience of the patient during the postoperative period. With the increased emphasis on shared decision-making between surgeons and patients, patient satisfaction becomes crucial in ensuring that surgical goals are aligned with those of the patient. Patient satisfaction is closely associated with outcomes such as pain control and the success of herniorraphies, thus also influencing not only perceived quality of care but also long-term adherence to follow-up appointments. If patients are satisfied that they are informed and involved in their surgical procedure, they will report greater levels of satisfaction and better functional outcomes, which again highlights the impact of patient-centered approaches in abdominal wall surgery. Evaluating the effectiveness of varying surgical techniques in terms of patient satisfaction demonstrates meaningful trends. For instance, studies have compared the effectiveness of the Parietex (TM) Composite Ventral Patch in open ventral primary hernia repairs, yielding impressive results. Cumulative hernia recurrence was as low as 3% at two years, accompanied by a remarkable 99% of patients being satisfied with the outcome of their procedure at follow-up (Berrevoet et al., 2019). These numbers not only indicate the technical success of the operation but also reflect the improvement in quality of life that patients have experienced. This synergy between low recurrence and high rates of satisfaction indicates the need for ongoing efforts to optimize surgery methods that aim for patient-centered outcomes.

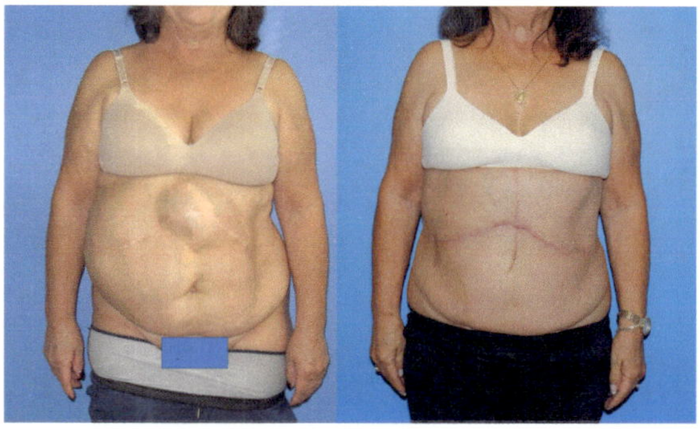

Figure 6.16. Patient satisfaction with abdominal wall surgery.

Source: https://drbriandickinson.com/wp-content/gallery/abdominal-wall-reconstruction-hernia-repair/abdominal_wall_recon_and_hernia_repair_orange_county.png.

Furthermore, analysis of surgical satisfaction dynamics also applies to the nature of the reconstructive procedures experienced in abdominal wall surgery. The evolution of strategy through various techniques is representative of patient preferences and the impact of surgical outcomes on broader recovery pathways. National data-based findings indicate that certain reconstructive surgeries, including latissimus flap surgeries, are declining; however, this decline is offset by an increase in autologous free flap reconstructions and patient satisfaction within this group (Athanasiou et al., 2015). These trends signal not only the evolving paradigms of surgical practice but also the growing recognition of patient needs and outcomes. Ultimately, establishing a culture that prioritizes patient satisfaction not only optimizes the surgical process but also enables the development of best practices in abdominal wall surgery (Figure 6.16).

Test Your Knowledge

1. How does postoperative pain management affect patient satisfaction after hernia repair
2. What role does cosmetic outcome play in patient satisfaction following abdominal wall surgery

SUMMARY

In abdominal wall surgery, one must identify the importance of specialized operating units in optimizing the outcome of patients, particularly in recurrent inguinal hernia repair. Studies have indicated that patients who underwent surgery by specialized abdominal wall surgery units had statistically significantly lower recurrence compared to those treated in non-specialized institutions. Specifically, studies suggest a reduction rate of recurrence from 15% to 3% among patients who have been operated on with specialized units, demonstrating just how important a role specialty care and surgical skill play in ensuring the highest levels of success with these surgeries (Gonçalves et al., 2023). This evidence suggests that the establishment of specialized units is not only an option but also an imperative step towards surgical procedures, with increased long-term rates of success and patient satisfaction. Furthermore, postoperative pain management and patient satisfaction are essential indicators that indicate successful outcomes in abdominal wall surgery. The use of certain materials and techniques, such as the Parietex Composite Ventral Patch (PCO-VP), has been proven highly beneficial in controlling recurrence rates and reducing postoperative pain. In a multicenter series of 126 patients, the two-year follow-up showed an incredibly low recurrence rate of 3%, testifying to the efficacy of this form of surgery in treating primary hernias. Moreover, the significantly decreased pain scores post-treatment also attest to the utility of technique optimization and material selection in achieving normal patient activity and quality of life outcomes (Berrevoet et al., 2019). These findings further support the notion that modern-day abdominal wall surgery, when performed with expert knowledge and advanced materials, can lead to significantly improved patient outcomes. Generally, the future of abdominal wall surgery is a two-legged column that is supported by specialization and innovation. Moving forward, it is necessary to prioritize special care in establishing specialized surgical units and adhering to advanced surgical procedures. Such factors are not only associated with reduced recurrence rates and greater safety but also with excellent long-term patient satisfaction. By prioritizing specialized care and embracing new materials and methods, the surgical community can address the multifaceted issues presented by conditions such as hernias and enhance the quality of treatment offered to patients. Continued research and implementation will be necessary as we strive to improve surgical outcomes in this critical and life-threatening area of medicine.

In the field of abdominal wall surgery, several significant advances in the management of diseases such as small abdominal aortic aneurysms (AAAs) and inguinal disruptions have emerged as areas of paramount interest. The contemporary approach to managing AAAs is centered on the importance of ongoing monitoring for small aneurysms, which are believed to be 3.0–5.4 cm in size. Evidence suggests that these asymptomatic conditions warrant follow-up until they are considered for surgical exploration at 5.5 cm. The surveillance is prompted by patient-specific factors, such as personal growth and the risk of rupture, which have been thoroughly studied and documented in extensive literature, offering invaluable guidelines to medical practitioners. These findings not only guide the timing of surgery but also underscore the importance of personalized patient care (Bown et al., 2013).

Another primary emphasis in abdominal wall surgery is the awareness of sports-related groin injuries, and more specifically, the occurrence of inguinal disruption (ID). A multidisciplinary consensus on this disorder attests to the necessity of a specific system of classification, differentiating it from so-called hernias, which are nonexistent in this case. Experts have suggested an amended management strategy that is primarily based on physiotherapy as the first-line treatment, reserving surgery for cases with complications. The emphasis on rehabilitation and reinforcement of musculature around the inguinal canal is key to achieving positive outcomes, reiterating that the use of multiple healthcare professionals to practice a multidisciplinary approach leads to better management of such conditions (Beaux et al., 2013).

The use of surveillance and multidisciplinary models of management in abdominal wall surgery highlights the need to shift clinical trends toward patient-centered practices. While research continues to shed light on the complexities of conditions like small AAA and inguinal disruption, it is increasingly clear that generic approaches may not suffice. Tailored treatments based on individual patient risk profiles and a qualitative, well-informed understanding of their condition are essential. This dynamic practice not only enhances the efficacy of surgical intervention but also aligns with contemporary health economics, holding the potential for cost-effective approaches to care maximization with optimized patient outcomes and utilization of healthcare resources (Bown et al., 2013; Beaux et al., 2013).

KEY TERMS FROM THIS CHAPTER

- Abdominal wall reconstruction
- Component separation technique
- Femoral hernia
- Herniorrhaphy
- Inguinal hernia
- Mesh repair
- Open hernia repair
- Chronic groin pain
- Epigastric hernia
- Hernioplasty
- Incisional hernia
- Laparoscopic hernia repair
- Obstructed hernia
- Recurrence rate

CRITICAL THINKING QUESTIONS

1. **Which of the following best differentiates a direct inguinal hernia from an indirect inguinal hernia?**
   a. Contents of the hernia sac
   b. Age of the patient
   c. Location relative to the inferior epigastric vessels
   d. Presence of pain
2. **Which of the following is the most common type of abdominal wall hernia?**
   a. Incisional hernia
   b. Umbilical hernia
   c. Inguinal hernia
   d. Epigastric hernia
3. **In Lichtenstein hernioplasty, what material is commonly used to reinforce the posterior wall of the inguinal canal?**
   a. Absorbable suture
   b. Stainless steel mesh
   c. Polypropylene mesh
   d. Silk suture
4. **Which of the following is a known risk factor for incisional hernia?**
   a. Obesity
   b. Early ambulation
   c. Supine positioning
   d. Low protein diet only
5. **Which hernia is more likely to become strangulated due to its narrow neck?**
   a. Direct inguinal hernia
   b. Femoral hernia
   c. Umbilical hernia in children
   d. Spigelian hernia

Short Answer Questions

1. What are the anatomical boundaries of the inguinal canal?
2. Differentiate between direct and indirect inguinal hernias based on their anatomical location.
3. What are the common risk factors for incisional hernia development?
4. What is the role of mesh in hernia repair, and what are the common types used?
5. Describe the clinical features and complications of a strangulated hernia.
6. What is the difference between open and laparoscopic hernia repair in terms of recovery and recurrence?
7. What are the indications for surgical repair of an umbilical hernia in adults?
8. Describe the key steps involved in a tension-free Lichtenstein hernioplasty.

Answers to Critical Thinking Questions

1. (c); 2. (c); 3. (c); 4. (a); 5. (b)

REFERENCES

1. Carr, E. C., Thomas, V. N., & Wilson-Barnet, J. (2004). Patient experiences of anxiety, depression and acute pain after surgery: a longitudinal perspective. *International Journal of Nursing Studies, 42*(5), 521–530. https://doi.org/10.1016/j.ijnurstu.2004.09.014Aguirre, M., Burger, M., Cassar, K., Deitch, E. A., den Hartog, D., Harrison, R., Ishida, H., et al. (2009). *Pre-, intra-, and postoperative sonography of the abdominal wall in patients with incisional hernias repaired via a three-layered operative suture method.* https://core.ac.uk/download/18510570.pdf (accessed on 12th July 2025).
2. Alves, S., Casal, D., Goyri-O'Neill, J., Iria, I., et al. (2017). *Blood supply to the integument of the abdomen of the rat: A surgical perspective.* https://core.ac.uk/download/129539752.pdf (accessed on 12th July 2025).
3. Andronache, L. F., Badiu, C. D., Grigorean, V. T., Mandu, I., et al. (2018). *Abdominal-pelvic pain in female patients with endometriosis – A review of the literature.* https://core.ac.uk/download/216809646.pdf (accessed on 12th July 2025).
4. Athanasiou, T., Aylin, P., Bottle, A., Darzi, A., et al. (2015). *Trends in immediate postmastectomy breast reconstruction in the United Kingdom.* https://core.ac.uk/download/77002746.pdf (accessed on 12th July 2025).
5. Bain, K., Bansal, V. K., Berrevoet, F., Bingener-Casey, J., et al. (2019). *Update of guidelines for laparoscopic treatment of ventral and incisional abdominal wall hernias (International Endohernia Society (IEHS)): Part B.* https://core.ac.uk/download/287940207.pdf (accessed on 12th July 2025).
6. Balbay, M. D., Canda, A. E., Catto, J. W., Dal Moro, F., et al. (2016). *Robotic intracorporeal urinary diversion: Practical review of current surgical techniques.* https://core.ac.uk/download/80153933.pdf (accessed on 12th July 2025).
7. Ball, C. G., Fabian, T. C., Feliciano, D. V., Ivatury, R. R., et al. (2017). *History of the innovation of damage control for management of trauma patients: 1902–2016.* https://core.ac.uk/download/84402892.pdf (accessed on 12th July 2025).
8. Banu, P., Constantin, V. D., Nistor, M. F., Popa, F., et al. (2016). *Perforated small intestine in a patient with T-cell lymphoma; a rare cause of peritonitis.* https://core.ac.uk/download/144552420.pdf (accessed on 12th July 2025).
9. Bauwens, K., Blanckaert, B., De Pauw, T., Dewaele, A., et al. (2020). *A novel hybrid 3D endoscope zooming and repositioning system: Design and feasibility study.* https://core.ac.uk/download/286549295.pdf (accessed on 12th July 2025).
10. Berrevoet, F., Doerhoff, C., Hopson, S., Jørgensen, L. N., et al. (2019). *Open ventral hernia repair with a composite ventral patch: Final results of a multicenter prospective study.* https://core.ac.uk/download/287940211.pdf (accessed on 12th July 2025).
11. Bhogal, R. H., & Downing, R. (2011). *The evolution of aortic aneurysm repair: Past lessons and future directions.* https://core.ac.uk/download/pdf/1631327.pdf (accessed on 12th July 2025).
12. Bilounga Ndongo, C., Etoundi Mballa, G. A., Hyder, A. A., Juillard, C., et al. (2010). *Patterns of injury and violence in Yaoundé, Cameroon: An analysis of hospital data.* https://core.ac.uk/download/323075033.pdf (accessed on 12th July 2025).

13. Bjorck, M., De Waele, J., Kaplan, M., Sibaja, P., et al. (2015). *How to deal with an open abdomen?* https://core.ac.uk/download/55742465.pdf (accessed on 12th July 2025).
14. Blugerman, G., D'Angelo, J. A., Habbema, L., Lisborg, P. H., et al. (2011). *Application of the liposuction techniques and principles in specific body areas and pathologies.* https://core.ac.uk/download/17179833.pdf (accessed on 12th July 2025).
15. Bown, M. J., Brown, L. C., Buxton, M. J., Glover, M. J., et al. (2013). *Systematic review and meta-analysis of the growth and rupture rates of small abdominal aortic aneurysms: Implications for surveillance intervals and their cost-effectiveness.* https://core.ac.uk/download/17192941.pdf (accessed on 12th July 2025).
16. Burity, J., Belo da Fonte, I., & Melo, P. B. (2014). *Radiological Society of North America (RSNA) 3D printing Special Interest Group (SIG): Guidelines for medical 3D printing and appropriateness for clinical scenarios.* https://core.ac.uk/download/212867900.pdf (accessed on 12th July 2025).
17. Ceppa, E. P., Colgate, C. L., Fennerty, M. L., House, M. G., et al. (2019). Post-pancreatoduodenectomy outcomes and epidural analgesia: A 5-year single institution experience. https://core.ac.uk/download/187423802.pdf (accessed on 12th July 2025).
18. Chalya, P. L., Chandika, A. B., Gilyoma, J. M., Kihunrwa, A., et al. (2012). Bowel perforation secondary to illegally induced abortion: A tertiary hospital experience in Tanzania. https://core.ac.uk/download/pdf/16666657.pdf (accessed on 12th July 2025).
19. Chan, F. P., Ellwein, L. M., Feinstein, J. A., Figueroa, C. A., et al. (2011). Computational simulations for aortic coarctation: Representative results from a sampling of patients. https://core.ac.uk/download/213089513.pdf (accessed on 12th July 2025).
20. Chu, M. W., Cook, J. A., Sasor, S. E., Tholpady, S. S., et al. (2018). Omental vascularized lymph node flap: A radiographic analysis. https://core.ac.uk/download/188008363.pdf (accessed on 12th July 2025).
21. de Beaux, A., Kingsnorth, A. N., Sheen, A. J., Åkermark, C., Stephenson, B. M., Beatty, D., Brennan, P. A., et al. (2013). *'Treatment of the Sportsman's groin': British Hernia Society's 2014 position statement based on the Manchester Consensus Conference.* https://core.ac.uk/download/9362135.pdf (accessed on 12th July 2025).
22. Dholakia, R. J., Eddinger, T. J., Jensen, E. S., LaDisa, J. F., et al. (2012). A coupled experimental and computational approach to quantify deleterious hemodynamics, vascular alterations, and mechanisms of long-term morbidity in response to aortic coarctation. https://core.ac.uk/download/213078816.pdf (accessed on 12th July 2025).
23. Gaskell, P. H., Jayne, D., Liskiewicz, T., Morina, A., et al. (2009). Providing adhesion for a miniature mobile intra-abdominal device based on biomimetic principles. https://core.ac.uk/download/50802.pdf (accessed on 12th July 2025).
24. Gonçalves, R., Lopez-Cano, M., Martínez-López, M., et al. (2023). Elective recurrent inguinal hernia repair: Value of an abdominal wall surgery unit. https://core.ac.uk/download/588850638.pdf (accessed on 12th July 2025).
25. Hakala, T. R., Holley, J. L., Lopatin, W. B., Shapiro, R., et al. (1990). Obesity as a risk factor following cadaveric renal transplantation. https://core.ac.uk/download/12204507.pdf (accessed on 12th July 2025).

26. Havrylov, H. O., Shulyarenko, O. V., Yosypenko, M. O. (2024). Comparison of laparoscopic intraperitoneal onlay mesh repair (IPOM plus) vs open Rives–Stoppa (RS) repair for ventral and incisional hernia. Acta Medica Lituanica, 31, 288–293. https://www.semanticscholar.org/paper/f5ab48d0c5aac2c4bbfff4b6cbef156e85bb8885 (accessed on 12th July 2025).

27. Hilton-Christie, S., Livie, J., Livie, V. (2020). Improving the use of the 'COUGH' bundle in Surgical High Dependency Unit, Ninewells Hospital, Dundee. https://core.ac.uk/download/323303779.pdf (accessed on 12th July 2025).

28. Jiang, M.-R., Li, T., Liu, G.-G., Liu, F., et al. (2018). Transversus abdominis plane block reduces remifentanil and propofol consumption, evaluated by closed-loop titration guided by bispectral index. https://core.ac.uk/download/323067899.pdf (accessed on 12th July 2025).

29. Kingsnorth, A. N., Adesunkanmi, A. R., Schutz, C., Maggiore, D., Watkin, D., Lewis, D. C., Crawford, D. L., et al. (2012). *Surgical management of inguinal hernias at Bugando Medical Centre in Northwestern Tanzania: Our experiences in a resource-limited setting.* https://core.ac.uk/download/pdf/11307796.pdf (accessed on 12th July 2025).

30. Kleinrensink, G. J., Eker, H. H., Nieuwenhuizen, J., Lange, J. F., Jeekel, J., Timmermans, L., et al. (2013). A double-blind randomized controlled trial comparing primary suture closure with mesh-augmented closure to reduce incisional hernia incidence. https://core.ac.uk/download/43290901.pdf (accessed on 12th July 2025).

31. López Cano, M., Martínez-López, M., Martínez-López, P., Rodrigues-Gonçalves, R., et al. (2023). Elective recurrent inguinal hernia repair: Value of an abdominal wall surgery unit. https://core.ac.uk/download/590285473.pdf (accessed on 12th July 2025).

32. Moldovan, C. A., Moldovan, D., Ungureanu, D. F., Ungurianu, D., et al. (2016). A retrospective surgical experience regarding open and laparoscopic procedures of the hepatic hydatid cyst with an up-to-date complete review of the literature and a focus on original Romanian techniques. https://core.ac.uk/download/144552988.pdf (accessed on 12th July 2025).

33. Poldermans, D., Bax, J. J., Boersma, E., De Hert, S., Eeckhout, E., Fowkes, G., Gorenek, B., et al. (2009). Guidelines for pre-operative cardiac risk assessment and perioperative cardiac management in non-cardiac surgery: The Task Force of the European Society of Cardiology (ESC) and endorsed by the European Society of Anesthesiology (ESA). https://core.ac.uk/download/55798032.pdf (accessed on 12th July 2025).

34. Sellers, A. (2017). Benefits of thoracic epidural analgesia in patients undergoing an open posterior component separation for abdominal herniorrhaphy. https://open.bu.edu/bitstream/2144/23993/5/Sellers_bu_0017N_12887.pdf (accessed on 12th July 2025).

35. Sun, Z., Tang, L., Wu, Z.-y., Hu, G., Xu, M. (2025). Retrospective comparison of laparoscopic and open surgery for obturator hernia: A single-center experience. European Journal of Medical Research, 30. https://www.semanticscholar.org/paper/a12dc7f06512d1cdd536cf2d1520b7b2ab89611b (accessed on 12th July 2025).

UROLOGY SURGERY

7

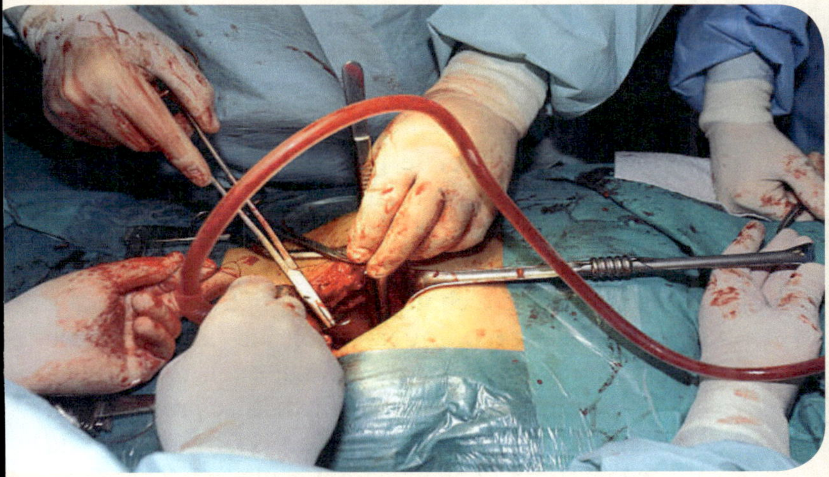

LEARNING OBJECTIVES

After studying this chapter, you will be able to:

1. Understand the types of urology surgery
2. Explain the indications for urology surgery
3. Discuss the preoperative for urology surgery
4. Focus on surgical techniques and procedures in urology
5. Learn about postoperative care in urology surgery
6. Evaluate the advances in urology surgery

Introduction

The urologic surgery specialty is a diverse set of procedures committed to the urinary tract and the male reproductive system, an example of the additional sophistication and complexity of surgeries in contemporary medicine. As a and significant branch of urology, this specialty has grown significantly in the past few decades, with advances in technology, surgery, and patient management. With the complexity of urological pathology, such as prostate cancer, urinary incontinence, and kidney stones, a detailed understanding of surgical techniques is crucial for clinicians. Additionally, the integration of minimally invasive technologies has significantly improved the quality of care, providing patients with the option of a speedy recovery and enhanced postoperative outcomes. This innovation necessitates constant reassessment of best practices to deliver optimum patient results in the urological surgery unit. It is essential for both practitioners and patients to be aware of the history of urology surgery and its present-day practice. The rise of specialty centers and ambulatory surgical centers has nurtured a trend towards specialized care patterns that are more efficient and accessible. Recent studies have taken this phenomenon into account, referencing the physician-owned specialty facility as a potential disruptive innovation in the healthcare system. However, as the research suggests, the opening of these specialist surgical centers should be monitored closely to measure their impact on full-service general hospitals.

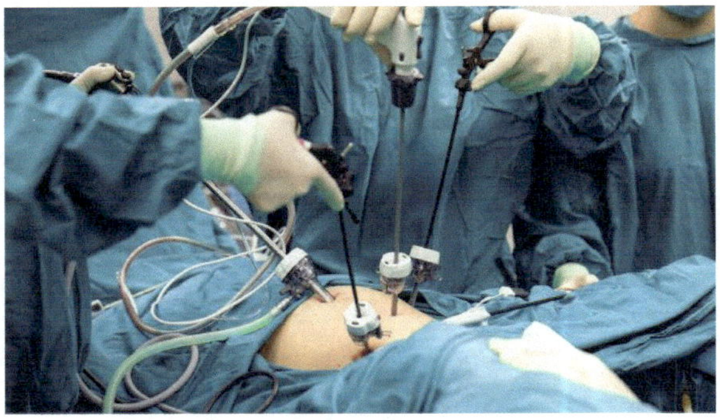

Figure 7.1. Urology surgery.

Source: https://www.actionhospital.in/public/uploads/blog/Laparoscopic-Urology.jpg.

The significance of these changes extends not only to surgical practices but also to broader healthcare delivery structures, and as such, a comprehensive review is necessary to examine how such specialist practices intersect with patient care in general. In reviewing the multifaceted process of urology surgery, it is apparent that multidisciplinary management is essential in handling the diverse range of urological disorders encountered by patients. Coordination between urologists, radiologists, oncologists, and nurses optimizes the effectiveness of surgical intervention as well as patient management in an integral fashion. Furthermore, a greater emphasis on evidence-based practice, as well as outcome evaluation, highlights the need for continuous research into the efficacy of various surgical methods. By examining published findings and analyzing patient experiences, practitioners can enhance their skills and contribute to the knowledge base regarding best practices in urology procedures. Ultimately, cultivating a substantial body of experience in the specialty is not merely an intellectual exercise; it is a doorway to enhanced patient outcomes and ongoing improvement in the quality of care for urologic procedures (Figure 7.1).

Definition of Urology Surgery

Urology surgery encompasses a specialized branch of surgical practice concerned with the management of diseases affecting the urinary tract and male reproductive system. Urology is a critical field of surgery involved in managing kidney, ureters, bladder, urethra, and allied male reproductive organs' conditions, such as prostate and testes. Urologists deploy a variety of operative techniques, ranging from minimally invasive techniques, such as laparoscopic techniques, to the traditional open techniques, depending on the individual disease presentation and patient condition. Additionally, urology is characterized by its complex interplay between surgical practice and medical technological progress, resulting in the development of new treatment modalities that enhance patient care and outcomes. One of the most essential features of urology surgery involves the treatment of localized prostate cancer. This is a prevalent disease that needs to be treated with caution-based surgery as per the needs of individual patients. Urologists have to undergo extensive treatments like radical prostatectomy and active surveillance based on the patient's overall health, cancer stage, and potential long-term consequences. One recent experiment developed a Core Outcome Set (COS) that acknowledges important measures for evaluating interventions for localized prostate cancer. The COS prioritizes quality of life, urinary function, and disease recurrence, all of which are crucial in evaluating the success of surgical interventions (Abel et al., 2017). Urology surgery is therefore central to both the physical and psychological well-being of patients living with prostate cancer. Furthermore, urologic surgery is often oriented by advancing clinical guidelines and grading mechanisms that enhance the accuracy of diagnosis and therapeutic interventions. The recent revision of the renal injury grading system by the American Association for the Surgery of Trauma (AAST) reflects advances in imaging technology, particularly computed tomography. These revisions aim to provide clarity to the care of high-grade renal trauma (HGRT) by offering improved definitions and classifications (Allen et al., 2020). Such advancements not only contribute to greater readiness for surgery but also to making more informed decisions regarding non-operative management options. With the improvement in the urology surgery specialty, there is a need for surgeons to be updated with guidelines and procedures that ensure the best results and the safety of patients in their surgical experience.

Importance of Urology in Healthcare

The relevance of urology in medicine cannot be overstated, as it encompasses a wide range of disorders that affect the urinary tract and male reproductive system. The specialty is not only crucial in the management of conditions such as urinary incontinence, bladder carcinoma, and prostate disease, but also because it forms part of the diagnostic process for systemic diseases. For instance, urologic conditions are often signs of broader systemic illnesses such as diabetes or cardiovascular disease, and therefore permit early interventions. Furthermore, the urology specialty employs advanced technologies and methods, such as minimally invasive procedures, which can greatly improve patient outcomes as well as quality of life. This aspect of urology highlights its core role in an interdisciplinary healthcare system, as urologists collaborate closely with other experts to provide integrated patient care, thereby emphasizing the relevance of urology within the broader healthcare landscape (Kazimierczak et al., 2015).

Furthermore, innovation in urology surgery, particularly through robotic-assisted surgery, underscores the advancement of this specialty. Techniques such as robot-assisted radical cystectomy, for example, have attracted attention because they promise to advance the precision of surgery and reduce postoperative complications. Complications arising from these procedures have been described as being worldwide; however, a critical examination reveals that they are predominantly low-grade and therefore offer scope for improvement in surgical practice. Management of surgical complications and minimization of techniques not only guarantee better patient outcomes but also lead to decreased healthcare expenses, resulting from shorter hospital stays and fewer interventions. The constant evolution and modification of urological surgical methods underscore the need for ongoing training and education in the field, reaffirming the importance of maintaining high standards in urology practice (Ahmad et al., 2017). Beyond surgical advancements, urology's contribution to public health initiatives is essential. Urologists play a crucial role in educating patients and the general public about preventive measures, early detection, and treatment options for urological diseases. These preventive strategies are essential for controlling the prevalence and burden of urinary stones and prostate cancer, both of which can become detrimental to health once developed. Through the promotion of awareness and understanding, urology is a key player in ensuring health equity and the accessibility of basic healthcare services. The incorporation of urology into general health programs further indicates its indispensable position in the healthcare program. With urologists continually staying ahead of the curve in treatment modalities and patient education, the field's impact on overall health outcomes will become increasingly compelling, underscoring the essential importance of urology to contemporary healthcare issues (Kazimierczak et al., 2015) (Figure 7.2).

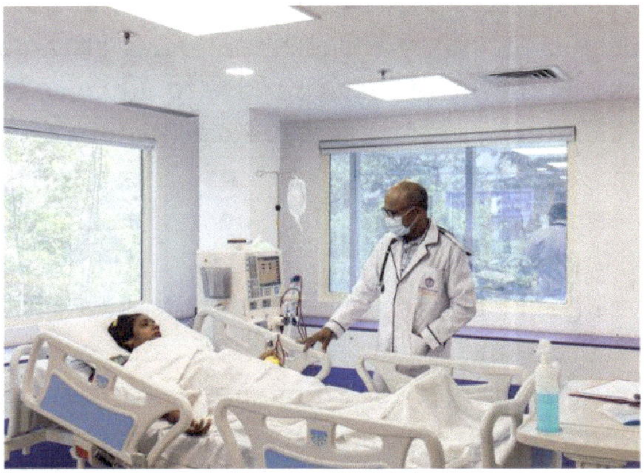

Figure 7.2. Urology in healthcare.

Source: https://www.epitomehospitals.com/wp-content/uploads/2024/05/Best-Urology-Hospital-NCR.jpg.

Overview of Common Urological Conditions

In urology, several conditions are benign but need surgical intervention. Among them, urinary tract infections (UTIs) stand out due to their prevalence, particularly in women. With antimicrobial resistance increasing, UTIs have become even harder to manage, triggering the pursuit of alternative management. Emerging evidence suggests the potential of nutraceuticals, such as D-mannose and N-acetylcysteine (NAC). These drugs can inhibit UTIs by preventing multiple pathogenic processes, such as inhibition of bacterial adhesion to urothelium and biofilm destruction. These findings suggest that clinical practice should be modified to incorporate alternative therapies alongside traditional antibiotic therapy to combat these infections more effectively (Rawashdah et al., 2017). An understanding of these trends is valuable to urologists as they tailor treatment protocols to patients at risk for recurrent UTIs following surgery or diagnostic procedures. Nocturia, which is represented by multiple voidings at night, is a true dilemma for both patient and physician alike, and it has a huge effect on quality of life. Nocturia is often concomitant with diminished bladder capacity, producing increased nocturnal urine volume (NUV) and interfering with restful sleep. Effective nocturia management usually involves identifying contributing causes that range from bladder dysfunction to conditions such as heart failure. Existing research emphasizes that targeted therapies aimed at reducing nocturnal urine output have a significant effect on maximizing bladder capacity in affected patients (Burgio et al., 2019). In the case of urologists, such facts not only provide guidelines for treatment but also highlight the importance of thoroughly evaluating patients during consultations. With the application of evidence-based practices, urologists can maximize patient outcomes and enable a higher quality of life for those afflicted with this pervasive yet disruptive disease. Another pervasive urologic disease is benign prostatic hyperplasia (BPH), most prevalent in older men. BPH is characterized by the growth of the prostate, which can lead to obstruction of urine and other conditions, such as retention of urine and increased risk of urinary tract infection. With increasing age, the incidence of BPH seems to rise, and thus it has emerged as a severe public health issue. Surgical treatments like transurethral resection of the prostate (TURP) and less invasive interventions are now mainstays of symptomatic BPH treatment. Though medications may initially be effective, surgery may then become a consideration when pharmacologic management fails to provide relief. Additionally, advancements in surgical techniques and the use of robotics-assisted surgery have improved recovery time and patient outcomes. Familiarity with the landscape of BPH and management of the condition is required by urologists, as they coordinate treatment for a population significantly affected by this condition.

7.1. Types of Urology Surgery

Learning Outcome

1. Describe the open surgery of urology surgery
2. Focus on laparoscopic surgery of urology surgery
3. Learn the robotic-assisted urology surgery

Urological surgery encompasses various procedures that are focused on diagnosing, treating, and managing conditions of the urinary tract and male reproductive organs. One of the most common urological procedures is cystectomy, which is the removal of the bladder. It is generally advised to patients with bladder cancer or severe bladder dysfunction. Following a cystectomy, patients may require reconstructive surgeries, such as the creation of a new bladder through the utilization of intestinal tissue, which enhances their quality of life and urinary function. Other surgeries, such as nephrectomy, partial or complete kidney removal, address several kidney diseases, such as tumors or kidney disease. Because these procedures are complicated and variable, understanding specific indications and outcomes is crucial to health care professionals handling urology. Another important category of urology surgery includes endourological procedures, which are minimally invasive operations performed with instruments passed through the urinary tract. Ureteroscopy, for example, is employed to remove kidney stones or correct ureteral stricture. The operation helps minimize patient recuperation time by providing highly effective correction of urological disorders. Over the past decade, technological advancements have also encouraged the development of robotic-assisted surgeries, enhancing accuracy and dexterity in procedures such as prostatectomy. Robotics enables the use of smaller incisions, resulting in less postoperative pain and shorter hospital stays. The addition of new surgical techniques marks a shift in the direction of minimally invasive procedures as a cornerstone in modern urological practice. Lastly, the branch of surgery in urology is applied in reconstructive surgery aimed at addressing congenital deformities, trauma, or other functional impairments of the urinary and reproductive tracts. Some of these procedures include penile reconstruction and bladder augmentation, aimed at restoring both form and function, as well as improving the overall quality of life for the patient. Beyond this, the emphasis on multidisciplinary treatment, especially for complex situations, is on coordinating care among urologists, oncologists, and other specialists. Cooperative agreements in this way offer holistic treatment plans that do more than treat short-term surgical outcomes, but instead long-term health and wellness. As advancements continue to rise in urology surgery, it is essential to stay updated on new and evidence-based methods to provide the best patient care (Rawashdah et al., 2017; Kazemier et al., 2025) (Figure 7.3).

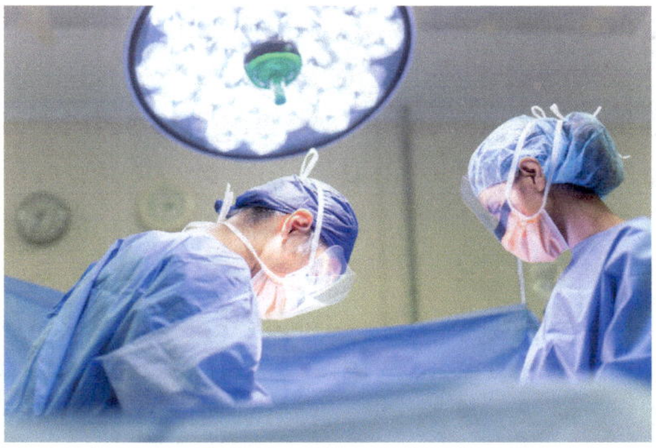

Figure 7.3. Urology procedures.

Source: https://urologicalsolutions.com.au/wp-content/uploads/2023/07/WEB-RES-72.jpg.

7.1.1. Open Surgery

Open surgery remains a fundamental urologic method of direct access to the target organ during operation. The process of such an approach is likely to vary significantly from minimally invasive methods, offering special advantages to some complex urological illnesses. For instance, procedures such as radical prostatectomy and nephrectomy can be performed with satisfactory accuracy, in which structures can be better seen and handled compared to laparoscopic surgery. The open technique is particularly valuable in the case of extensive disease involvement, when complete excision is most desirable. Moreover, the palpation associated with the open technique is more appreciative of tissue planes, which may enhance the success of surgery and reduce the incidence of complications. Therefore, while technical innovation in the areas of robotics and laparoscopy is significant, the role of open surgery in urology remains fundamental for treating rare patient populations and complex diseases. Advances in urologic surgical methods have highlighted the limitations and advantages of open surgery through comparative outcomes.

For instance, robotic-assisted surgery has advanced the precision and reduced invasiveness of surgery, as illustrated by prostate cancer treatment by radical prostatectomy. In urologic practice, the da Vinci surgical system has revolutionized the approach surgeons use for such challenging cases, offering the potential for enhanced dexterity and vision. However, reports indicate that open approaches can potentially yield better oncological results due to the surgeon's direct visualization and fine motor control during key phases of the operation. Furthermore, as mechanical techniques become more prevalent, it is essential to compare their performance with traditional open operation methods in a balanced manner, because subsequent research findings suggest that the same long-term oncologic outcomes are required for patients undergoing either of these techniques (Costa et al., 2013). Aside from well-established techniques, other surgical techniques have been developed to optimize the benefits of open techniques in the urologic practice. One is the development of minimally invasive surgery, where a single incision is employed for a variety of urological procedures, such as nephrectomy and ureterolithotomy. These techniques achieve their effects by minimizing postoperative pain and shortening the duration of recovery, without compromising direct visualization of the surgical field.

The use of high-technology equipment, such as the JakoscopeTM, whose powerful fiberoptic light source provides more intense illumination, demonstrates increased visibility without compromising the advantages of direct access. As noted, outcomes of these minimal access techniques postoperatively show the same levels of pain and morbidity as when undergoing traditional laparoscopic surgery, thereby expanding the line of options available to surgeons and patients (Frang et al., 2011). The ongoing evolution of open and innovative minimally invasive techniques reaffirms the dynamic position of urology surgery in responding to complex clinical needs.

7.1.2. Laparoscopic Surgery

Laparoscopy has emerged as the cornerstone of urological procedures, offering numerous advantages over open surgery. Laparoscopy is a less invasive procedure with tiny incisions and unique instruments that allow surgical operations using a camera for enhanced visualization. This process significantly reduces postoperative discomfort, leading to shorter recovery times, reduced hospital stays, and improved patient satisfaction. The application of laparoscopic methods in urological surgeries like nephrectomies and prostatectomies has been a prime example of the efficacy of the technique in handling complex conditions like prostate cancer and kidney stones.

The evolution of laparoscopic instruments and technology also enhances the precision and of these surgeries, lending further weight to their adoption in mainstream urological practice (Close et al., 2013). The technological progress in laparoscopic surgery has also given rise to robotic-assisted surgery, which further optimizes the advantages of minimal invasiveness. Robotic equipment provides surgeons with greater dexterity and a 3D view, significantly enhancing the manipulation of delicate tissues during prostatectomy and cystectomy. Experiments have shown that robot-assisted laparoscopic surgery results in fewer complications and shorter recovery times compared to the traditional method, validating its growing popularity among health professionals. In a critical evaluation of robot-assisted radical cystectomy complications, it was found that while complications are common, most cases are of low grade. This enhances the demand for using stringent safety protocols that can potentially reduce the risks of surgical complications associated with both robotic and conventional laparoscopic surgeries (Ahmad et al., 2017).

While beneficial, the implementation of laparoscopic procedures in urology has its own limitations. The surgeons must undergo specialized training in order to master skills that promise success in minimally invasive surgery. Furthermore, the purchase cost and maintenance of laparoscopic equipment can be a financial burden for some healthcare centers. Compounding these issues, the learning curve difficulties of laparoscopic surgery may potentially influence patient outcomes in the early stages of adoption. While laparoscopic techniques are expected to become the standard of care for urology, as the field continues to mature and more surgeons become proficient, current adoption rates remain the limiting factor. Through an emphasis on ongoing learning and the sharing of best practices between practitioners, the optimization of surgical outcomes and enhancement of patient safety are critical in the event of laparoscopic urology surgery (Close et al., 2013) (Figure 7.4).

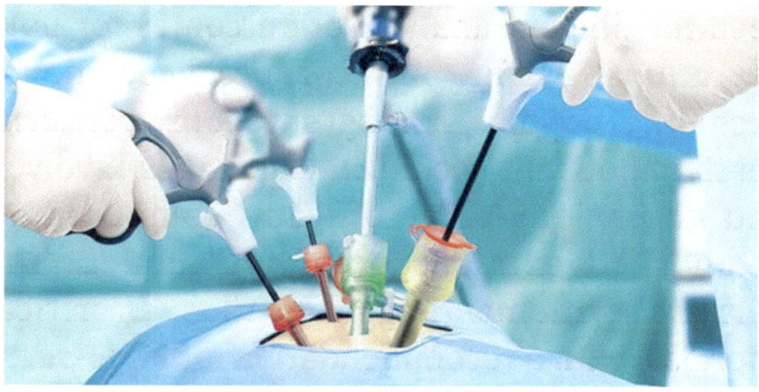

Figure 7.4. Urology laparoscopy surgery.

Source: https://www.yashodahealthcare.com/uploadedfiles/gallery/1603191148_uro-laparoscopy.jpg.

7.1.3. Robotic-Assisted Surgery

The addition of robotic-assisted surgery to urologic procedures, particularly in radical cystectomies, represents a significant advancement in surgical practice. The modality offers greater precision and control, with lesser trauma to the surrounding tissues and quicker recovery in patients. Robotic systems have revolutionized traditional surgical practices, enabling surgeons to perform complex procedures using minimally invasive techniques. Enhanced visualization and instrumentation provided via robotic platforms would allow surgeons to dissect significant anatomical structures better, eventually leading to improved functional results following surgery. These advantages are, however, open to rigorous scrutiny in relation to postoperative complications and overall efficiency versus established methods, ultimately calling for ongoing evaluation and refinement of robotic surgical technique. A timely subject of interest among robotic-assisted surgery is the intracorporeal versus extracorporeal controversy regarding urinary diversion following robotic radical cystectomy (RARC). Intracorporeal urinary diversion has gained popularity due to its purported benefits, including decreased bowel exposure and potentially fewer complications. Recent articles emphasize the need for diligent analysis of outcomes for both operations. Despite intracorporeal techniques becoming popular among surgeons, concerns persist about the technical challenges involved and their long-term efficacy compared to established extracorporeal techniques. The current evidence suggests that a critical appraisal with a recommendation for large-scale, long-term trials to determine the superiority of robotic intracorporeal urinary diversion and its use in modern urological surgical practice (Balbay et al., 2016). Evaluation of postoperative outcomes following robot-assisted procedures is essential since it highlights the safety and effectiveness of the procedures. One study of 134 patients with robot-assisted radical cystectomy indicated high rates of morbidity, where overall rates of complications were consistently high for both surgeries for urinary diversion. Interestingly, while most complications were low-graded, significant major complications were also prevalent. Concerns were raised about the learning curve associated with robotic techniques and whether it would impact surgical training (Ahmad et al., 2017). These results emphasize that despite all the technology, surgical technique and experience remain key to restricting complications. Meeting these challenges through more advanced training and protocolized approaches could heighten patient outcomes and reaffirm the role of robotic-assisted surgery in the field of urology.

Test Your Knowledge

1. What is the primary indication for performing a transurethral resection of the prostate (TURP)?
2. Which urological conditions are commonly treated with laparoscopic nephrectomy?

7.2. Indications for Urology Surgery

Learning Outcome

1. Explain kidney stones
2. Define prostate cancer
3. Discuss urinary incontinence

Urologic operations encompass a wide range of procedures with clear indications that significantly contribute to patient welfare. High on the list of interests is surgical removal of urinary tract obstructions, for instance, caused by kidney stones or tumors. Obstructions can become extremely complicated if not promptly alleviated. Ureteroscopic procedures, particularly ureteroscopic lithotripsy, have become a significant option for treating large renal calculi. This technique has undergone remarkable technological evolution, and urologists can now address stones previously deemed too large to be successfully treated. Using flexible ureteroscopes and advanced lithotripters, success in eliminating larger stones has been higher, rendering this technique a core part of urological practice, particularly for stones larger than 2 cm (Bagley et al., 2012). Besides, treatment of benign prostatic hyperplasia (BPH) frequently involves surgery, especially if medical treatment fails. BPH can cause annoying urinary symptoms, impairing the quality of life of the majority of men. Operations such as transurethral resection of the prostate (TURP) and newer procedures such as laser therapy can correct these symptoms by reducing prostatic tissue. Choice of the procedure is typically preceded by factors such as prostate size and patient health status. Furthermore, minimally invasive procedures are increasingly preferred since they usually result in shorter post procedure recovery and pain. With changing clinical practice, procedures are continually being optimized to allow for individualized treatment with maximum outcomes and minimal complications (Bagley et al., 2012). The urological procedures' indications also include the treatment of conditions such as malignancies in the urinary tract. Surgical interventions are essential in the care of cancer of the kidney, bladder, and prostate, with early removal of malignant tissue leading to improved survival. Nephrectomy or radical prostatectomy are the typical indications for localized disease, with advanced disease requiring multimodal treatment using a combination of surgery and adjuvant therapy. Notably, advanced innovations such as robot-assisted surgeries have transformed the treatment profile to achieve greater precision and lower recovery rates. In all cases, the surgical technique is governed by the type of tumor, stage, and general condition of the patient. This level of care in adhering to patient-specific factors is essential for decision-making regarding surgical interventions, making them both indicated and justified for effective cancer management (Frang et al., 2011) (Figure 7.5).

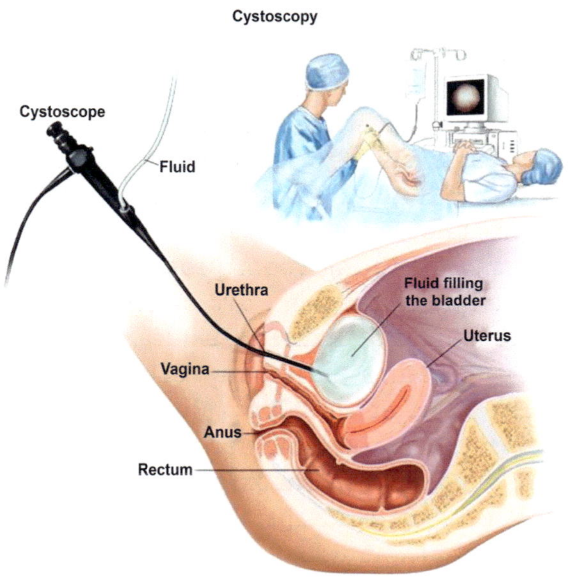

Figure 7.5. Cystoscopy-urethrocystoscopy.

Source: https://dreminozbek.com/wp-content/uploads/2024/08/Sistoskopi-Uretrosistoskopi-Nedir-Nicin-Kimlere-Yapilir-1024x1010.jpg.

7.2.1. Kidney Stones

The prevalence of kidney stones has seen a significant rise, warranting increased attention towards improving surgical outcomes in urology. Kidney stones, or nephrolithiasis, are created when minerals and salts precipitate in concentrated urine and solidify within the kidneys, leading to pain and complications if left untreated. Several minimally invasive techniques, including ureteroscopy and shockwave lithotripsy, have emerged as effective treatment modalities for the treatment of stones. This enhancement in accessible interventions coincides with increased efforts in research aimed at improving surgical methods, particularly in pediatric cases, where kidney stone occurrence has also been on the rise. Interestingly, a systematic review revealed a higher number of publications outlining interventions for pediatric stone disease, indicating the significance of advancing surgical procedures in urology (Aboumarzouk et al., 2017). Kidney stone treatment is mostly based on various factors, including stone size, location, and the patient's general health. ESWL remains a standard first-line treatment in most patients. It is a non-invasive procedure employing high-energy shock waves to shatter stones into tiny pieces, allowing for their excretion through the ureters. There is some evidence to suggest that as the size of the stone increases, the effectiveness of ESWL can be reduced, particularly for stones larger than 30 mm, where alternatives would be favored. This is a significant distinction, as it has been demonstrated that residual fragments can have a substantial impact on patient outcomes. Clinically significant residual fragments may cause recurrence and require further intervention, and therefore, the importance of residual fragments is highly pertinent in planning treatment (Chaussy et al., 2001).

In urology surgery, the management of kidney stones continues to evolve, characterized by the introduction of new techniques and technological advancements. Of these procedures, percutaneous nephrolithotomy (PCNL) has taken center stage, most notably for larger and more complex calculi. The past decade has witnessed a fivefold increase in literature about PCNL, pointing to its success as a minimally invasive intervention with higher patient recovery rates and outcomes. This shift towards these minimally invasive interventions is testimony to the field's commitment to offering safer, less traumatic alternatives for patients. As the prevalence of kidney stones rises, with most cases occurring in younger generations, ongoing study and development in urological interventions will be paramount to advancing patient care and outcomes in urology surgery (Aboumarzouk et al., 2017) (Figure 7.6).

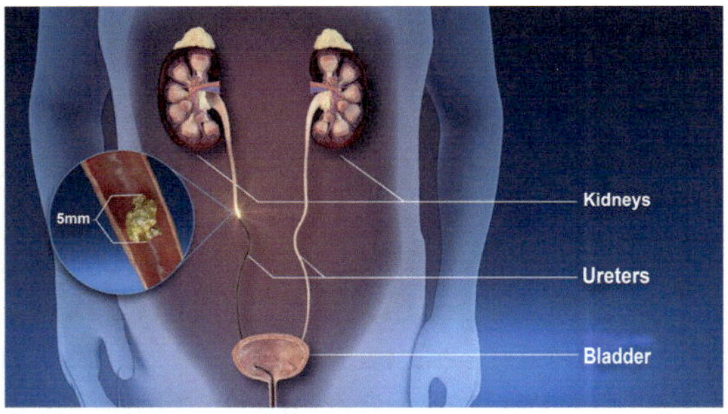

Figure 7.6. Kidney stones treatment.

Source: https://www.drvamsikrishna.com/wp-content/uploads/2019/04/Screen-Shot-2021-01-14-at-11.04.16-PM-1024x575.png.

7.2.2. Prostate Cancer

The treatment of prostate cancer has advanced considerably, making it imperative to have a thorough grasp of the effectiveness of treatment in different interventions. Among the challenges that clinicians and researchers in urology surgery face is the disparity in outcome measures and reporting standards in clinical trials. An initiative to counter this challenge has been the development of a core outcome set (COS), whose primary purpose is to harmonize the outcomes regarded as essential in assessing treatment efficacy in localized prostate cancer. This COS was established through systematic reviews and qualitative interviews with patients and healthcare professionals, before agreeing on 19 core outcomes that should be measured in clinical trials. They are both generic indicators of overall health, such as quality of life and disease recurrence, as well as intervention-specific outcomes, including postoperative complications and treatment failure. Thus, they offer more reliability to trial outcomes and ultimately influence clinical practice (Abel et al., 2017). With the addition of new technology and approaches to the urology surgery practice, the universe of prostate cancer treatment is growing increasingly sophisticated. Advances in computer-assisted medical intervention (CAMI) and robotic systems have significantly transformed surgical operations, promoting minimally invasive approaches that reduce morbidity and enhance patient recovery. For instance, laparoscopy and other tumor-killing techniques, such as high-intensity focused ultrasound (HIFU) and cryoablation, have gained widespread acceptance due to their accuracy and improved outcomes. Imaging modalities also enhance the potential of surgeons to navigate through soft tissues with comfort, bypassing complex anatomical complexities associated with prostate cancer. These technologies not only make operating room procedures more efficient but also enable urologists to tailor their techniques to fit diverse clinical scenarios, thereby elevating the quality of care in the specialty (Bart et al., 2006). Multidisciplinary strategies need to be combined to treat prostate cancer successfully. Ongoing communication among urology specialists, oncologists, and radiologists facilitates a personalized treatment regimen tailored to each patient's specific needs. The use of standardized outcome measures, as per the COS, ensures that everyone is on the same page when it comes to their treatment objectives, ultimately enhancing the survival and quality of life for patients. Furthermore, the integration of improved diagnostic techniques implies that recurrence of prostate cancer can be identified at an early stage, with a higher likelihood of curative treatments. With ongoing research refining treatment strategies and discovering new technologies, urology surgery practice will, in the not-so-distant future, be able to offer more specific and effective compelling management methods for prostate cancer, delivering better outcomes for patients (Figure 7.7).

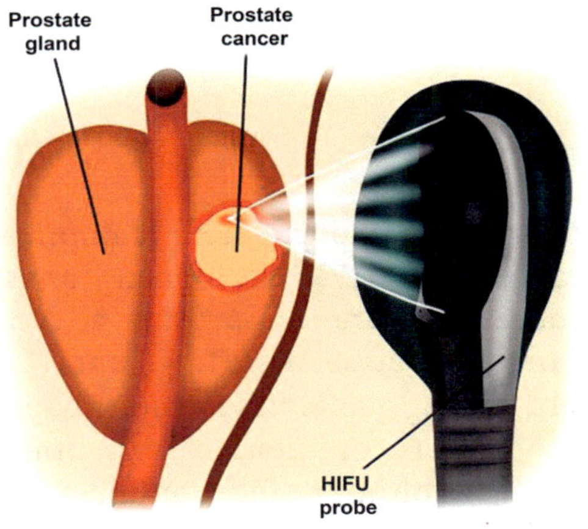

Figure 7.7. High intensity focused ultrasound (HIFU) for prostate cancer.

Source: https://storage.airomedical.com/images/ckfinder/blog-treatment-guides/cl2rcybur00040hs62fadel4b.jpg.

7.2.3. Urinary Incontinence

Urinary incontinence is a serious health condition, particularly for women, because it can significantly impact quality of life. Epidemiological studies demonstrate a strong association between obesity and urinary incontinence and quantify excess weight as a significant risk factor. Specifically, with each 5-unit increase in body mass index (BMI), the relative risk of developing urinary incontinence increases by 20%-70%. This dose-response effect highlights the need for intervention in weight control. Furthermore, stress incontinence occurs most frequently among obese women; the influence of body weight on symptoms and processes of urinary control is emphasized. Because of its high prevalence rates, obesity therapy by both surgical and non-surgical weight-loss interventions has emerged as a critical strategy in the care and treatment of urinary incontinence and has provided significant gains in patient outcomes (Subak et al., 2011).

Urinary incontinence in urology surgery is generally treated using multiple surgical techniques designed to enhance bladder function while preserving pelvic floor support. All these operations, such as the mid-urethral sling operations and autologous fascial sling operations, have gained wide acceptance since they are the least invasive and highly successful. The interventions also remove the psychological trauma and distress brought about by incontinence, and patients can regain confidence and normalcy in their lives. Nonetheless, physicians need to assess each patient's requirements based on the nature and severity of the incontinence, as well as any comorbidities. Adequate preoperative counseling and information about potential risks, advantages, as well as postoperative management are necessary to achieve optimal results from the procedure. Recent studies have shown that successful surgery can transform the quality of life in most patients, lowering the social stigma of urinary incontinence (Bodean et al., 2018). Despite progress made in the treatment of urinary incontinence with surgical methods, some attention must also be given to the overall impact of cancer treatments on pelvic floor health. Gynecologic cancers and their treatment—surgery, radiation, and chemotherapy—each may contribute significantly to urinary incontinence and other pelvic floor dysfunction. While cancer cure still constitutes the prime focus of therapy, the effects on pelvic floor health cannot be overstated.

Survivors frequently complain of problems with urinary dysfunction, which are still inadequately addressed in the framework of oncological rehabilitation. The increasing population of cancer survivors mandates a re-evaluation of follow-up management protocols after treatment to ensure detection and optimal management of pelvic floor dysfunction. Setting up follow-up counseling for these symptoms is imperative to enhance the quality of life among cancer survivors, highlighting the interconnectedness of oncology and urology in patient care (Bodean et al., 2018).

Test Your Knowledge

1. When is surgical intervention recommended for kidney stones?
2. What are the surgical indications for benign prostatic hyperplasia (BPH)?

7.3. Preoperative Considerations

Learning Outcome

1. Explain the patient evaluation and diagnosis for urology surgery
2. Define the risks and benefits of urology surgery
3. Describe the preparation and consent process of urology surgery

Effective preoperative planning is crucial to the success of urological surgery, particularly in optimizing patient outcomes and preventing complications. A systematic approach to assessing a patient's health can detect impending risks and enable individualized measures that optimize surgical safety. Key considerations include a detailed history of any prior surgeries, comorbidities such as diabetes or hypertension, and current medication regimens. These can highlight risks that will necessitate changes in the anesthesia or surgical technique. Detecting patients at higher risk for complications, for instance, can initiate preoperative treatments or additional monitoring during surgery, thereby improving overall outcomes and patient satisfaction. Knowledge of the patient's baseline status is most critical, as it directly influences postoperative recovery and complications (Ahmad et al., 2017). Additionally, anesthetic considerations are important, a sensitive equilibrium between safety and patient comfort. Fasting guidelines for the preoperative period are recommendations aimed at preventing aspiration and optimizing gastric content preparation before surgery. However, evidence suggests that prolonged fasting is a predictor of serious adverse reactions, such as dehydration and electrolyte imbalances, which can compromise the patient's condition on surgery day (Herbst et al., 2016). Studies have shown that adherence to contemporary fasting guidelines can reverse such risks, attesting to the importance of proper patient education regarding fasting expectations. Additionally, titrating fasting protocols to meet specific patient needs might also enhance the aggregate patient experience and safety. Proper anesthetic planning, such as the use of appropriate agents based on patients' health status and estimated surgical duration, contributes to reducing postoperative complications as well as enhancing recovery profiles. The psychological aspect of preoperative care cannot be overlooked, as anxiety and stress can have a significant effect on surgical outcomes. Good communication between healthcare providers and patients is essential to dispel fears and psychologically prepare them for the operation. Patient education about the urological surgical experience and realistic expectations can induce a sense of control and reduce anxiety levels. Preoperative counseling, therefore, becomes a core part of the preparation of the patient, creating a rapport and trust relationship between the patient and the operating team. The preoperative period must involve considerations of potential risks and postoperative recovery plans, clearly outlining a course of action before proceeding. Through both psychological and physiological means, urology clinics can offer a more cohesive form of patient care, leading to more straightforward surgical practices and improved recovery (Ahmad et al., 2017).

7.3.1. Evaluation of Patient and Diagnosis

The process of patient assessment and diagnosis is a crucial step in effective urology surgery, and it, in turn, determines the outcome of the treatment. A comprehensive history and general examination typically initiates proper evaluation. Clinicians document data regarding the patient's symptoms, duration of the illness, and severity, as well as family history and past medical conditions. Such comprehensiveness is relevant because it enables the physician to identify risk factors pertinent to urological disorders. For example, in the case of patients with kidney cancer, age, gender, and prior health status can heavily influence prognosis and treatment decisions.

The predictive modeling of kidney cancer recurrence highlights the importance of preoperative factors in predicting outcomes following surgery (Soyupak et al., 2012). This preliminary phase of assessment ultimately determines the selection of appropriate diagnostic tests and intervention measures. Diagnostic imaging and laboratory studies are crucial components of the urology patient evaluation, providing key information that complements clinical data. Methods such as ultrasound, computed tomography (CT), and magnetic resonance imaging (MRI) are routinely used to image the urinary tract and detect abnormalities, including tumors or obstructions. These modality tests are not only used to detect conditions but also to stage cancers and ascertain the degree of disease spread, thereby directing surgery. Lab tests such as urinalysis and serum creatinine are all valuable in providing information about renal function and intrinsic renal pathology. Multidisciplinary care, as demonstrated by the development of a Small Renal Mass Center, enables concurrent decision-making regarding diagnosis and treatment streams tailored to individual patient needs (Brown et al., 2016). This model highlights the importance of an environment of teamwork for optimizing patient outcomes. Translating diagnostic data requires consideration of each patient's unique situation, including comorbidities and specific circumstances. Integrated diagnoses, considering both radiological and clinical findings, enable healthcare teams to develop customized treatment plans in accordance with optimal practice guidelines. For instance, the interaction of patient variables—age and estimated glomerular filtration rate—with treatment choice highlights the complex decision-making process involved in treating small renal masses. In cases where patients are found to have high comorbidity scores or with some renal function disorders, active surveillance may be deemed to be more preferable, rather than imminent surgery. Thus, integration of diverse data points not only facilitates educated decision-making but also enhances the quality of care delivered in urology surgery. A customized strategy ultimately ensures that treatment modalities align with patients' health profiles and personal decisions, fostering increased commitment and compliance with recommended plans (Figure 7.8).

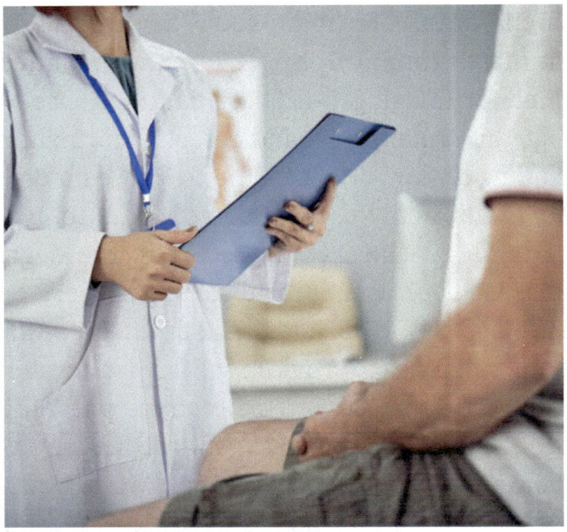

Figure 7.8. Urology diagnostic tools for precision.

Source: https://www.dssimage.com/wp-content/uploads/2025/04/urology.png.

7.3.2. Risks and Benefits of Surgery

The domain of surgery, and that of urology in particular, is a complex field of risk and reward that must be tread cautiously. Operations may offer unambiguous solutions to many urologic ailments, ranging from benign prostatic hypertrophy to bladder malignancies. The potential for relief of symptoms or removal of pathological tissue often far outweighs the inherent risk of the operation itself. However, surgical complications like infection, bleeding, and anesthesia complications can be a significant problem, especially in high-risk populations. The determination of risks becomes increasingly significant as the patient population shifts toward the elderly, who may have other comorbidities that complicate surgery. The quantification of a patient's frailty is particularly significant when estimating the risks of urological surgery. Studies of elderly surgical patients point to the value of evaluating frailty as a predictor of postoperative complications. For instance, a study incorporating the Edmonton Frail Scale showed that patients classified as frail experienced greater numbers of complications after surgery, supporting the need for individualized pre-operative evaluations to determine individual risk better. This assessment is crucial in that it can potentially be used to inform surgical decisions and patient counseling in a way that positions risk in relation to the potential of surgery. Finally, the ability to stratify patients based on these assessments can lead to improved outcomes and more patient safety for urological procedures (Barbieri et al., 2017). On the other hand, successful surgical interventions can have enormous dividends, particularly in enhancing patients' quality of life.

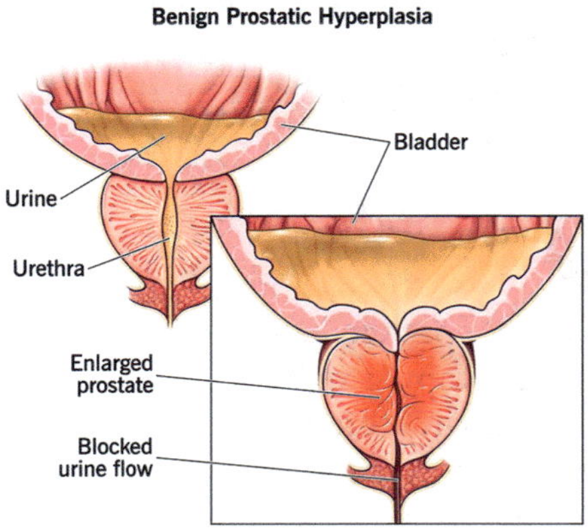

Figure 7.9. Benign prostatic hyperplasia (BPH).

Source: https://my.clevelandclinic.org/-/scassets/images/org/health/articles/9100-benign-prostatic-hyperplasia.

For instance, laparoscopic adrenal-sparing pheochromocytoma surgery has proven to have a profound capacity to normalize physiological function without a lifetime of steroid replacement, and that is certainly remarkable for its safety and efficacy in children with complex medical backgrounds such as von Hippel-Lindau disease. Such progressions not only sustain the treatment of acute medical conditions but also contribute to patient welfare in the long run and reduce healthcare expenditure associated with chronic disease management. The implications of surgery, therefore, cannot be overlooked;

however, the potential rewards in terms of patient outcomes and quality of life are equally significant, leading to a more comprehensive assessment of both parameters before making decisions (Bartsch et al., 2000) (Figure 7.9).

7.3.3. Preparation and Consent Process

Preparation and consent are key stages of the urology surgery process, as they have a direct impact on patient safety and outcomes of surgical treatment. Preparation is a step that involves a thorough preoperative assessment, during which several factors are considered, including the patient's medical history, comorbidities, and procedure type. This allows the surgical team to predict potential complications and intervene accordingly, tailored to each patient's needs. Moreover, operating teams typically collaborate with anesthetic and nursing staff to ensure that equipment preparedness and patient positioning are among the areas addressed. The preparatory process, with its multiple dimensions, provides an environment for an effective surgical experience, which is especially critical in urology surgery due to the need for accuracy, as well as precise handling of anatomy. Concurrent with preparation, obtaining informed consent is both an ethical and legal obligation that ensures patient autonomy during surgery. The process of consent should be clear, comprehensive, and understandable to enable patients to make informed decisions about their treatment. Surgeons should provide specific information about the procedure, including risks, benefits, alternatives, and prognosis. Greeting patients into a conversation, listening to what they have to say, and allowing them to ask questions strengthens their understanding and belief in the procedure. It not only respects patient autonomy but also fosters a collaborative working environment among patients and healthcare workers. In urological surgery, where patients may be emotional, establishing a free flow of communication through informed consent is essential in building confidence and giving patients the sense that they are important. Lastly, the consent process serves as a critical checkpoint before surgery. It provides a formal mechanism for reaffirming the patient's understanding of the treatment plan after extensive preoperative discussion. The process is crucial in preventing litigation risks and promoting adherence to medical standards. Moreover, it typically involves verifying the patient's identity, the surgical site, and the procedure being performed to help prevent mistakes. Such multi-layered consent is part of broader healthcare guidelines aimed at enhancing patient safety. In a clinical case in which the worst can happen, as is the case of robot-assisted kidney transplant with multi-vessel grafts (Alcaraz et al., 2018), a robust preparation and consent process is even more crucial in coping with the complexity of urology procedures and ensuring optimum patient outcome.

Test Your Knowledge

1. What imaging modalities are commonly used to diagnose urinary tract obstructions?
2. How is prostate enlargement assessed during clinical evaluation?

7.4. Surgical Techniques and Procedures

Learning Outcome

1. Identify the cystoscopy
2. Define the nephrectomy
3. Describe the ureteroscopy

The landscape of urological surgical practice has undergone significant changes due to technological advancements and increased awareness of minimally invasive surgery. The traditional open surgery involving big incisions and prolonged recovery times has, to a large extent, been substituted by laparoscopic methods that involve less pain during recovery and quicker recovery. One such innovation is single-incision laparoscopic surgery, where advanced instrumentation is used to facilitate complex procedures through minimal access. The Jakoscope™, an advanced fiber-optic device with high intensity, enables surgeons to perform multiple urological procedures, such as nephrectomies and ureterolithotomies, with greater visibility and precision. This technique not only reduces the size of the incision but also offers comparable morbidity results with standard laparoscopic techniques, highlighting the role of innovative surgical techniques in contemporary urology (Frang et al., 2011). In pediatric urology, the increasing prevalence of kidney stone diseases necessitates the development of innovative surgical practices for younger patients. A systematic review over the last couple of years has reported a considerable increase in publications regarding various interventions in pediatric kidney stone disease (KSD). Techniques such as ureteroscopy (URS), percutaneous nephrolithotomy (PCNL), and shockwave lithotripsy (SWL) have received significant attention in the literature, testifying to the evolution of intervention techniques that have successfully advanced in terms of complexity and application. For instance, articles on PCNL have doubled fivefold, reflecting a particular trend towards minimally invasive techniques emphasizing patient protection and healing (Aboumarzouk et al., 2017). This trend of growth reflects the evolving dynamics of pediatric urology as medical practitioners adapt to new technologies and refine surgical practices for improved patient outcomes. Furthermore, the advent of minimally invasive urological procedures marks a growing trend toward patient-focused surgery. Not only do the techniques focus on minimizing scars and post-surgery pain, but also on optimizing the efficiency of surgery and the time spent in the hospital. Among the procedures mentioned above, other developments include robotic operations that advance precision to an even higher level during complex interventions. The advances in technologies used in combination with traditional methods offer surgeons a toolkit that can be developed to meet the individual needs of each patient. As a result, contemporary urological practice is experiencing improved patient satisfaction rates and notably reduced recovery times, which verifies the role of these new technologies in the field of urological surgery (Frang et al., 2011) (Figure 7.10).

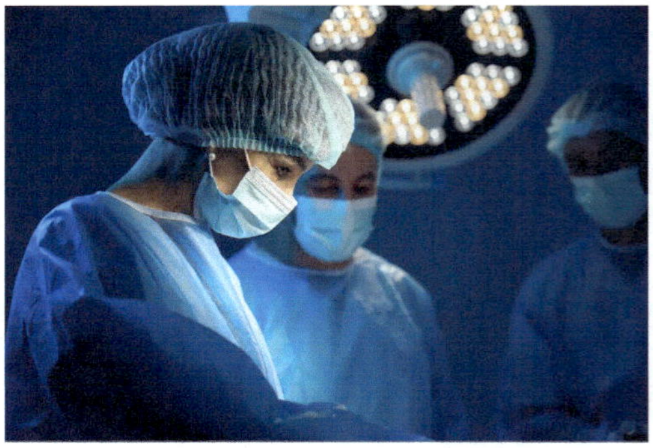

Figure 7.10. Surgical techniques in urology.

Source: https://b3378418.smushcdn.com/3378418/wp-content/uploads/2024/10/surgery-procedures.jpg?lossy=2&strip=1&webp=1.

7.4.1. Cystoscopy

Cystoscopy is a valuable diagnostic and therapeutic urologic intervention that involves direct visualization of the bladder and urethra by utilizing a cystoscope. This minimally invasive treatment has emerged as a cornerstone in the treatment of several urological conditions, with the potential for real-time visualization and simultaneous treatment. With the introduction of the cystoscope through the urethra, urologists can visualize strictures, stones, and tumors that other imaging modalities cannot visualize. Furthermore, cystoscopy is significantly utilized in the evaluation of lower urinary tract symptoms as it offers improved diagnostic accuracy. The procedure is possible on an outpatient basis, enhancing patient convenience and reducing the reliance on more invasive operative techniques. Cystoscopy is flexible as it also carries therapeutic roles, particularly in the repair of conditions like ureteroceles. A notable study demonstrated the effectiveness of cystoscopic-guided laser ablation of ureteroceles in canine patients, highlighting the technique's flexibility. The process involved careful treatment to bypass the ureter blockage, enabling effective treatment of patients presenting with concomitant urinary issues. Surprisingly, postoperative outcomes showed significant improvements, including symptom resolution of issues such as incontinence and pollakiuria, in treated animals. This not only emphasizes the efficacy of cystoscopy for treating challenging cases but also opens up space for its application in veterinary and human medicine (MH et al., 2019).

Recent advances in surgical practice further enhance the applicability of cystoscopy in urology. For instance, improvements in minimal access technology enable cystoscopic procedures to be performed with smaller incision sizes, thereby facilitating quicker recovery and lower morbidity rates compared to traditional laparoscopic procedures. The use of specially designed equipment, such as the Jakoscope™, allows for direct access without video-optical support, thereby making the procedure more effective. This technological innovation holds the promise of significantly benefiting patients by minimizing postoperative pain without sacrificing procedural effectiveness in all cases from nephrectomy to ureterolithotomy. Advances such as these underscore the continued leadership of cystoscopy in urologic surgery, enhancing patient outcomes and procedural efficiency (Frang et al., 2011) (Figure 7.11).

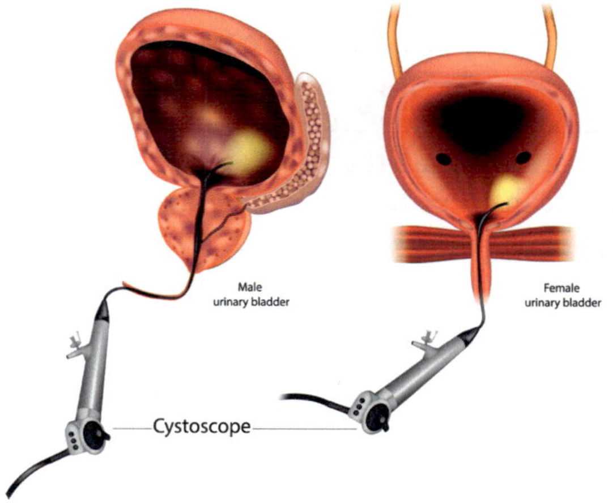

Figure 7.11. Cystoscopy.

Source: https://www.upnt.com/wp-content/uploads/2025/04/shutterstock_2146297883-1-scaled.jpg.

7.4.2. Nephrectomy

Nephrectomy, or surgical removal of a kidney, is a very significant urologic intervention with uses in the treatment of renal tumors, chronic kidney disease, and trauma. Nephrectomy is performed using various approaches, including open, laparoscopic, and robotic, each with its own advantages and disadvantages. The approach to be employed often depends on the nature of the condition being treated, the patient's overall health, and the surgeon's skill. For instance, while open nephrectomy provides direct access and allows for complex resections, laparoscopic nephrectomy diminishes incisional pain and stimulates quicker recovery rates. The evolution of surgery in nephrectomy confirms the ongoing progress of urologic surgery, showing not only improved outcomes for patients but also a trend towards increasingly minimally invasive interventions. Postoperative management of nephrectomy patients is equally crucial, with careful monitoring potentially diminishing complications and enhancing recovery. Hemorrhage, infection, and organ failure are among the most common postoperative complications that typically necessitate close observation and intervention. ERAS protocols have been applied more frequently to enhance recovery via multimodal analgesia, early mobilization, and volume optimization. Studies have shown that these types of strategies can significantly reduce the duration of hospital stays and improve overall patient satisfaction. Interestingly, the addition of robotic-assisted techniques, although still in its early stages, has proven promising in reducing complications and optimizing functional outcomes after nephrectomy surgery, suggesting that further research and clinical practice innovation are necessary to optimize surgical success (Canfield et al., 2012). As nephrectomy improves, so too will the implications for kidney transplantation. The lessons learned from nephrectomy procedures are applicable in kidney transplantation, particularly with regard to donor choice and surgical reconstruction of multicompartment grafts. Research on robot-assisted kidney transplant (RAKT) with multivessel grafts has highlighted the technical feasibility and favorable outcomes of the procedure, pointing to the potential of the method to expand the donor population and improve graft viability. The careful analysis of intraoperative and early postoperative complications in such studies has been crucial to refining surgical procedures and optimizing patient outcomes (Alcaraz et al., 2018). This acknowledgment highlights the interconnectedness of nephrectomy and transplantation protocols, underscoring the importance of ongoing communication among members of the urologic surgical community to optimize patient care (Figure 7.12).

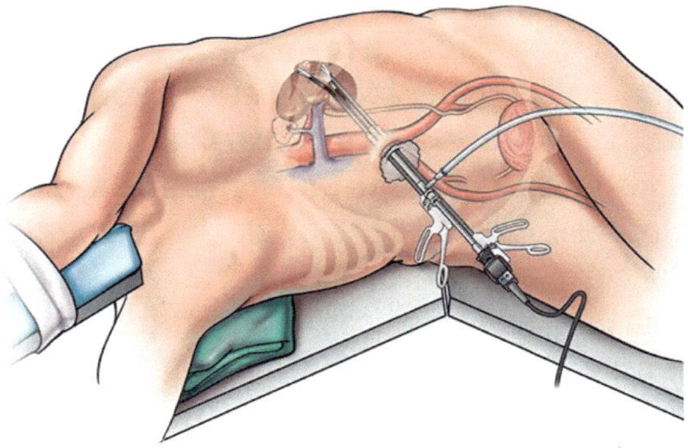

Figure 7.12. Nephrectomy.

Source: https://irenehealth.in/wp-content/uploads/2022/02/NEPHRECTOMY-LAP.webp.

7.4.3. Ureteroscopy

Ureteroscopy has emerged as a crucial device in urology surgery, particularly in the diagnosis and treatment of ureteral and renal stones. It is a minimally invasive procedure wherein the ureteroscope is passed through the urethra and bladder into the kidneys and ureters. With it, physicians can visualize and intervene directly in cases of urinary tract obstruction or calculi. As an alternative to conventional open surgery, ureteroscopy offers several advantages, including a shorter recovery time, reduced scarring, and the capability to effectively treat stones of varying sizes. Increasing evidence of kidney stone disease (KSD) in children and adults points to the importance of ureteroscopy in contemporary practice, and for this reason it is a widespread topic in modern medical literature on the progress of urological therapy (Aboumarzouk et al., 2017).

Recent research has highlighted significant advancements in ureteroscopy, particularly in managing large renal stones, which were previously challenging to treat. Innovations in flexible ureteroscope design and improved accessory instrumentation, such as laser lithotripsy equipment, have revolutionized the treatment of large stone burdens. The evidence suggests that innovation has enabled the effective treatment of stones greater than 2 cm, which previously required more invasive methods, such as PCNL (Bagley et al., 2012). Evidence suggests that ureteroscopy is capable of achieving high success rates, even in the presence of large stones, making it possible to treat a greater number of patients while establishing it as a first-line treatment in most situations. Thus, the practice of surgery continues to move in the direction of prioritizing effective, less invasive stone treatment. Furthermore, the efficacy and safety of ureteroscopy are demonstrated by its established success rates and low complication rates. After reviewing various studies, it is observed that the overall success rate in ureteroscopy is more than 90%, with nearly all patients requiring only one or two interventions to become stone-free. In addition, the rate of complications is very low, with most of them being minor and transient, thereby improving the technique's practicability and safety profile (Bagley et al., 2012). With the revolution of urology surgery, ureteroscopy is at the forefront not only because of its high success rate but also due to its adherence to the rising trend of less invasive surgical procedures. Thus, not only does ureteroscopy enhance patient care, but it is also the cornerstone of the new history of urologic surgical procedures.

Test Your Knowledge

1. What are the key steps in performing a laparoscopic nephrectomy?
2. How is a ureteral stent placed during endoscopic urologic surgery?

7.5. Postoperative Care

Learning Outcome

1. Describe the recovery process for urological surgery
2. Define the management of complications of urology surgery
3. Discuss the follow-up appointments for urology surgery

Postoperative management following urological operations is critical for a better recovery and the prevention of complications. Patients undergo various changes postoperatively, which require careful observation and management. The primary objectives of postoperative management are to control pain, prevent infection, and facilitate early mobilization. Appropriate pain control strategies, such as multimodal analgesia, not only enhance patient comfort but also enable earlier mobilization and improved outcomes. Appropriate postoperative assessment is also crucial in the early detection of symptoms of complications such as UTIs or catheter-associated infection, prevalent among the urologic population. Research has shown that postoperative UTIs underscore the significance of heightened surveillance during the postoperative course to detect and respond to potential problems early (Close et al., 2013). The role of antibiotic prophylaxis in preventing postoperative infections is significant, particularly in urologic surgery. Evidence detects varying patterns and efficacy of antibiotic delivery perioperatively, which have profound implications for patient outcomes (Ranjan et al., 2024). Poor or improper delivery of antibiotics can contribute to the development of resistant microbial strains, which complicate postoperative recovery and necessitate prolonged antibiotic treatment.

Evidence from research indicates that despite a significant percentage of patients receiving preoperative prophylaxis, a substantial percentage of patients develop surgical site infections. This highlights a key gap in current practices and underscores the need to implement evidence-based guidelines for targeted antibiotic therapies that consider the specific needs and risk factors of individual patients. These targeted steps can not only lower the incidence of UTIs but also enhance antimicrobial stewardship in health care settings (Ranjan et al., 2024).

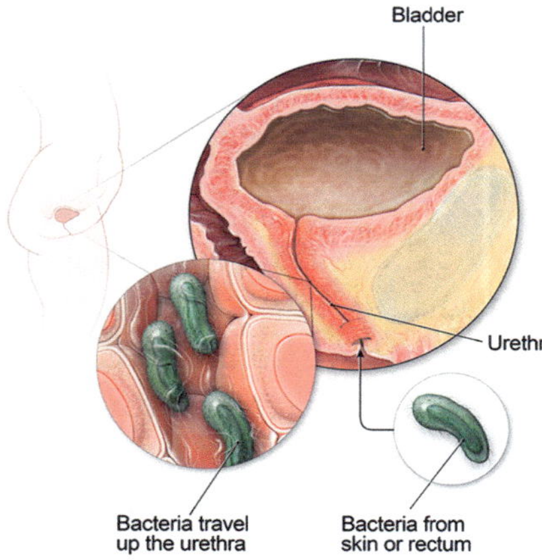

Figure 7.13. Urinary tract infections (UTIs).

Source: https://www.cdc.gov/uti/media/images/uti.jpg.

Moreover, patient education in postoperative care is necessary to facilitate recovery and prevent complications. Education of the patient regarding signs of infection, adherence to medication regimens prescribed by a healthcare provider, and lifestyle modifications can significantly enhance the postoperative course. Effective utilization of communication skills is essential to ensure that patients understand discharge orders and follow-up care requirements.

Active participation of patients in the recovery process not only empowers them but also instills confidence in both patients and health professionals to work together, resulting in improved postoperative adherence. Follow-up sessions combined with educational materials can be vital in detecting early complications and facilitating a smooth return to normal life, thereby promoting improvement in recovery after urological procedures (Close et al., 2013) (Figure 7.13).

7.5.1. Recovery Process

The recovery period following urological surgery is a crucial component that has a direct influence on patient outcomes and quality of life. Following surgery, patients typically undergo a multifaceted recovery process that involves physical recovery, adaptation to emotional factors, and ongoing evaluation of urological function. The variability in recovery experiences is due to numerous factors, including the type of surgery, the patient's pre-existing health status, and the presence of potential complications. For instance, patients who are operated for cancer of the prostate will experience certain postoperative side effects, such as sexual dysfunction and incontinence of urine, which play a significant role in determining their emotional status and quality of life. Thus, recovery should not only encompass medical interventions but even psychological management and rehabilitation explicitly to cope with these problems. A successful core outcome set (COS) is essential to standardizing the recovery process of urological surgery patients. Given the focus in recent research, developing a COS for localized prostate cancer addressing a spectrum of outcomes, such as urinary function, quality of life, and treatment success, brings into perspective the importance of standardized and measurable recovery outcomes. Such standardization facilitates improved communication among providers and reduces patients' ability to understand what they can expect in their recovery. In addition, through the identification and prioritization of key outcomes—such as the need for salvage therapy and perioperative complication rate—healthcare providers can enhance patient-centered care. This structured approach ensures that all aspects important to recovery are monitored and addressed, thereby contributing to a more favorable environment for patients to recover from their surgery (Abel et al., 2017).

Cooperation among clinicians, patients, and supporting organizations is crucial for achieving an optimal recovery process in urology surgery. Organizational initiatives by institutions such as UCAN Cancer Charity and Macmillan Cancer Charity have been pivotal in developing rehabilitation programs that consider patient engagement and education (Canfield et al., 2012). Such programs provide support systems and materials that enable the patient to manage post-operative problems effectively. For instance, patients can utilize instructional materials that provide expected recovery phases and strategies for managing typical complications. Additionally, open communication between patients and their teams can enhance the recovery support network. Outcomes are significantly improved when the recovery process is viewed in a more holistic manner, encompassing physical recovery, emotional recovery, and community support, thereby paving the way for enhanced long-term health following urologic surgery.

7.5.2. Management of Complications

In urologic surgery, complication management is a vital factor that needs careful attention and planning. Surgical interventions, such as those involving the removal of urinary tract stones, have made significant strides with the advent of minimally invasive techniques. As evidenced by recent developments, procedures such as percutaneous nephrolithotomy (PCNL) and extracorporeal shock wave lithotripsy (ESWL) have revolutionized the treatment protocol, substantially reducing the need for classical open surgery. A Maltese study at St. Luke's Hospital revealed a remarkable 90% success rate with no mortality for the initial 50 PCNs performed, underscoring the efficacy and safety of such novel procedures. However, urologists must remain vigilant in regulating potential complications during these procedures to ensure maximum patient protection and operating success (Cutajar et al., 1989). Moreover, complication management extends beyond the operating room to postoperative care, where vigilance is required to identify and correct problems early. Complications can vary along a continuum from mild to severe and can range from infections, hemorrhage, and organ injury. Systematic postoperative monitoring of the patient is required for the early identification of complications. For instance, pediatric circumcision complications have been thoroughly studied, where the median rate of any complication is found at 1.5%, and severe adverse events at the rate of approximately 2%. These statistics indicate the necessity for strict protocols to manage potential complications, particularly if circumcision is being performed by inexperienced clinicians or outside of sterile environments. Continuous education and adherence to stringent standards of best practice are of paramount importance in minimizing the risks inherent in surgical procedures (Halperin et al., 2010). Formulating a risk reduction strategy is an integral factor in the successful management of complications in urology surgery. Risk reduction strategies, such as improved training of practitioners and the availability of clean instrumentation, are essential in minimizing the risk inherent in surgical procedures. With the advancing field, evidence-based practices can be integrated to a great extent, minimizing complications.

Interdisciplinary collaboration among healthcare professionals can also enhance patient outcomes by fostering an integrated system of care. Data- and outcomes-based continuous quality improvement programs can also rationalize surgery practices in urology. Lastly, a bold strategy in complication management will not only boost the safety of surgery but will also promote an excellence culture in patient care in urology (Cutajar et al., 1989; Halperin et al., 2010) (Figure 7.14).

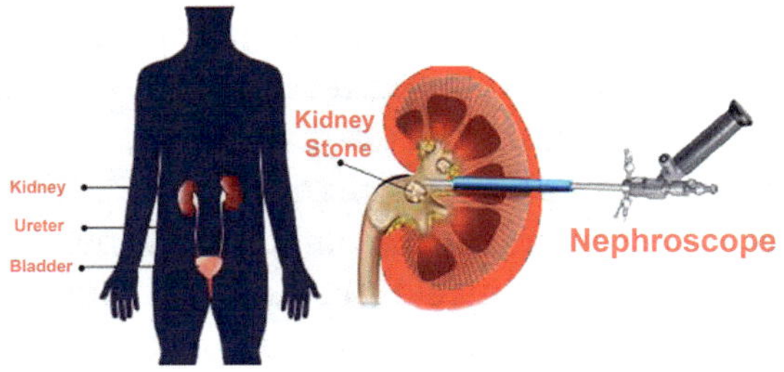

Figure 7.14. PCNL (percutaneous nephrolithotomy) in surgery.

Source: https://www.aasthakidneyhospital.com/wp-content/uploads/2020/06/PCNL-percutaneous-nephrolithotomy.jpg.

7.5.3. Follow-Up Appointments

Follow-up visits are a crucial component of treating patients who have undergone surgery for urological disorders, as they provide valuable opportunities to monitor recovery and assess the response to therapy. Follow-up visits also facilitate open communication between patients and healthcare personnel, allowing any postoperative problems or issues to be addressed. Follow-up visits also enable the detection of early signs of recurrence in conditions such as prostate or bladder cancer. Through these consultations, healthcare providers are able to track patients' progress, adjust treatment plans as necessary, and ensure that patients adhere to prescribed therapy regimens. In this way, follow-up visits are not routine visits, but an integral part of integrated care, ensuring the maximization of patient outcomes and satisfaction, and fostering a continuing relationship between the patient and the healthcare team. The effectiveness of follow-up visits in urologic surgery can be significantly augmented through the adoption of organized care policies. For instance, guidelines for patient management who are receiving Radium-223 treatment have placed high emphasis on coordinated communication and planning among multidisciplinary teams. (Carrió et al., 2017) Care models such as this ensure that all members of the team are well informed about the patient's current level of treatment and recovery.

Through streamlined follow-up scheduling and content, urologists can more accurately quantify essential factors such as pain, urinary function, and quality of life. This structured approach not only increases the likelihood of identifying any complications early on but also enables patient-centered care that responds to individual needs. When patients' concerns take center stage, they are more likely to comply with post-surgical follow-ups, resulting in improved health outcomes. Due to the new realities brought about by the recent challenges caused by the COVID-19 pandemic, follow-up appointments have also adapted to accommodate the new healthcare system realities. Due to historic pressure being placed on hospitals, operating departments were compelled to devise mechanisms of continuing patient care while minimizing risk exposure (Conte et al., 2020). This included reducing patient numbers, minimizing communication protocols, and having readily accessible personal protective gear. In the context of urology surgery, this has meant that follow-up appointments may potentially take place remotely or with reduced occupancy rates in clinics. Such adjustments support both providers and patients equally, without sacrificing the care that is needed. With advancing practice in medicine, particularly in the context of global health crises, the responsiveness and role of follow-up appointment systems for urological surgery will remain most crucial. This ensures that patients receive consistent, high-quality care, independent of extraneous variables.

Test Your Knowledge

1. How is urinary output monitored after major urologic surgery?
2. What are the common signs of postoperative urinary tract infection?

7.6. Advances in Urology Surgery

Learning Outcome

1. Describe the technological innovations in urology surgery
2. Define the minimally invasive techniques of urology surgery
3. Identify the future trends in urological surgery

Substantial advances in urology surgery have transformed the treatment and management of the majority of urological conditions. An example of such an advancement is the development of minimally invasive surgery, which has dramatically improved patient outcomes with less postoperative pain and shorter recovery times. For instance, minimally invasive methods such as ureteroscopy, shockwave lithotripsy, and percutaneous nephrolithotomy have become extremely popular due to their efficiency with lower rates of complications. A systematic review of treatment interventions for pediatric kidney stones reveals that the number of publications on such procedures has increased exponentially over a 16-year span, accompanied by growing interest and the evolution of surgical techniques. Specifically, the rise in publications of minimally invasive procedures reflects a shift in surgical practice aimed at having a lesser impact on patients, a trend supported by the literature (Aboumarzouk et al., 2017). Robotically assisted surgical techniques are another breakthrough innovation, particularly in the field of urologic oncology. The introduction of the da Vinci Surgical System in 2000 marked a significant advancement in surgical procedures for complex operations, such as radical prostatectomies. Robotic assistance was initially minimal, and fewer than 2.5% of surgeons utilized this technology. However, by 2013, robotic assistance for radical prostatectomies burst as the predominant approach, with an approximate 85% market share. This abrupt increase is reflective of growing confidence among urologic surgeons in robot-assisted surgery, which is more precise, offers improved visualization, and results in less blood loss compared to open techniques. As a result, urology surgery has undergone significant advancements with the advent of robotics, ushering in a new era of high-tech surgical procedures (Chang et al., 2017). The impact of these advancements in urology surgery extends beyond refining procedural techniques; they influence overall patient care and resident education. With the further acquisition of skills in minimally invasive and robotic surgery, surgeons also receive more intensive training, underscoring the importance of continuous education in surgery. The increase in the application of these new modalities reflects improved patient evaluation processes, preoperative planning, and postoperative care, which ultimately translate to improved Clinical outcomes. Moreover, ongoing work and scrutiny of the published literature yield robust evidence for a sustained body of knowledge that continuously educates practice and innovation in urological surgery. The trajectory of these advancements testifies to the dynamic character of the field and its responsiveness to new technology, manifesting intense devotion to maximizing patient care through surgical excellence (Aboumarzouk et al., 2017) (Figure 7.15).

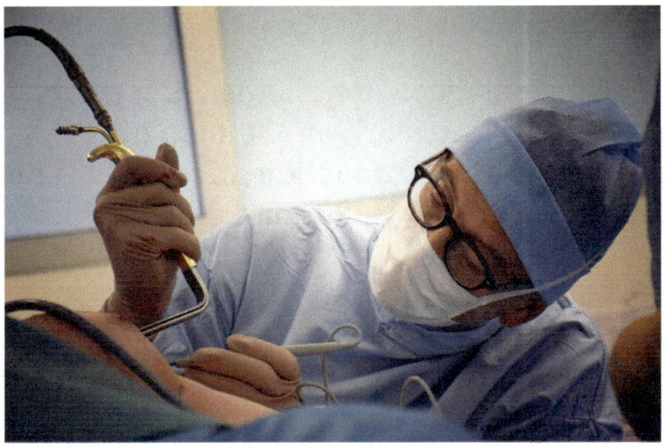

Figure 7.15. Advances-in-urological-surgery.

Source: https://brianrichardsonal.com/wp-content/uploads/2025/02/advances-in-urological-surgery-key-innovations-in-patient-care-scaled.jpg.

7.6.1. Technological Innovations

The integration of technology in urology surgery has revolutionized patient care and clinical outcomes, particularly in the management of complex urological disorders. Advances in medical imaging, such as 3D ultrasound and magnetic resonance imaging (MRI), have enhanced the preoperative assessment of tumors, allowing for more accurate staging and treatment planning. These technologies enable surgeons to visualize anatomical structures with unprecedented detail, permitting the precision necessary for minimally invasive surgery. These advances not only minimize trauma to surrounding tissues but also make it possible to achieve shorter recovery periods for patients. The benefits of these technologies extend not only to diagnosis but also to intraoperative navigation systems that guide surgical instruments with increased accuracy. Consequently, advancements in imaging and navigation technology are significantly altering the prospects of urology surgery, optimizing patient results through precision medicine. In the context of minimally invasive surgery, robotic technology has transformed traditional urological surgery, offering surgeons improved dexterity and control. Robotic procedures, such as prostatectomies and nephrectomies, have gained prominence as they minimize surgical trauma while enabling the manipulation of tissues with accuracy. The application of robotic technology, such as the da Vinci Surgical System, has proven to have certain advantages over open surgery, including reduced blood loss, shorter hospital stay, and improved postoperative recovery. In addition, robotic systems also tend to feature advanced optics and imaging, which provide improved visualization and contribute to enhanced surgical performance. As noted in recent literature, robotic-assisted techniques represent a central innovation in urology that provides surgeons with the ability to achieve better oncological outcomes while maintaining patient safety and health. This transition highlights the substantial impact of technological innovation on the practice of urological surgery. Endoscopic treatments have emerged as a revolution in the management of urological malignancies, especially for conditions such as upper tract urothelial carcinoma (UTUC). Traditional therapies, although they work, are expensive and induce notable morbidity. Advances in endoscopic technology over the past few years have ushered in the era of kidney-sparing therapy. Techniques such as flexible ureteroscopy with advanced laser technology allow precise tumor destruction with renal preservation. Based on various documented studies, these minimally invasive surgeries not only reduce complications associated with open surgery but also serve as effective alternatives for low-risk tumors, thereby improving the quality of life for patients. Challenges still persist, particularly regarding recurrence rates that require close monitoring. The ongoing evolution of endoscopic treatments promises a brighter future in urology surgery, with an emphasis on personalized treatment strategies and the importance of technological progress in surgery (Annemans et al., 2013; Andrade et al., 2025) (Figure 7.16).

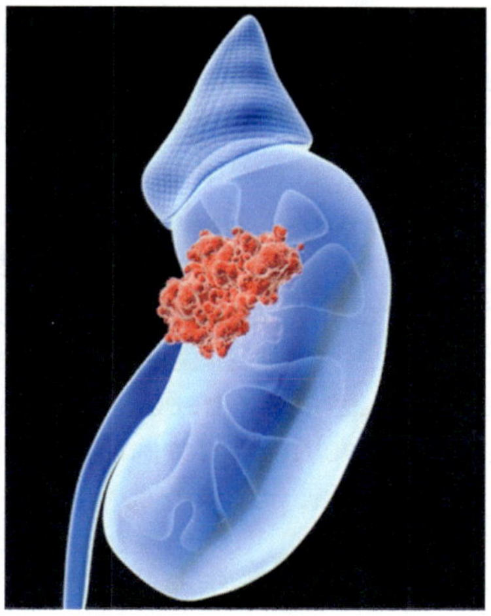

Figure 7.16. Upper tract urothelial cancer.

Source: https://www.hopkinsmedicine.org/-/media/greenberg-bladder-cancer-institute/images/utuc.jpg.

7.6.2. Minimally Invasive Techniques

Minimally invasive techniques have revolutionized the practice of urological surgery, yielding improved outcomes for patients in the recovery phase and ultimately in the results. Minimally invasive techniques, which include more minor cuts and less trauma to the surrounding structures, minimize postoperative complications and pain, with shorter recovery times. Percutaneous nephrolithotomy (PCNL) and extracorporeal shock wave lithotripsy (ESWL) are excellent examples of technological advancements in traditional surgical methods. The advent of PCN has revolutionized urinary tract calculi management, rendering open surgery nearly obsolete. With a 90% success rate and no mortality associated with early use, PCN is a shining example of the successful incorporation of minimally invasive techniques into urology, dramatically improving patient care and operative effectiveness (Cutajar et al., 1989). A new option to conventional laparoscopic techniques has emerged, bringing yet another battery of minimally invasive urological techniques to the table. This new technique is a minimally invasive method that entails the use of a single skin incision, 3–6 cm long, with direct visualization of the operative site. The employment of sophisticated instruments, such as the Jakoscope™, ensures superb visualization and maneuverability, allowing surgeons to achieve various urological procedures with ease. Procedures like nephrectomy, ureterolithotomy, and prostatic adenomectomy benefit from this approach because it combines direct access with minimal invasiveness. Compared to laparoscopic techniques, this approach has yielded the same levels of postoperative pain and morbidity while providing a fast option that ensures patient comfort and ease of procedure (Frang et al., 2011).

The increasing application of minimally invasive techniques in urological surgery indicates a paradigm shift toward improved patient outcomes. As technology continues to evolve, the scope for new applications in this field appears unlimited. Minimally invasive procedures have specific advantages, both in reducing physical trauma and addressing the longer-term facets of surgical operations, for example, scarring and convalescence. By integrating effective pain control regimes and advanced surgical equipment, urologists can provide safer, more effective care that addresses the demands and expectations of patients today. With rigorous clinical outcomes and continually advancing technological capabilities, minimally invasive techniques are poised to transform urologic surgery into an era of enhanced patient satisfaction and experience.

7.6.3. Future Trends in Urological Surgery

As technology improves, urologic surgery is poised to undergo a dramatic change. One of the most promising trends, certainly one of the most hyped, is the increasing use of robotic assistance in surgery. Ever since its inception with the da Vinci Surgical System, robotic assistance has gained firm traction among urologists. Not only does robotic surgery enhance precision, but it also lessens recovery time and complications from surgery. Numbers confirm this pattern: the proportion of robot-assisted radical prostatectomies increased from 22% to 85% across the decade, indicative of a trend toward increasingly sophisticated methods in urology surgery (Chang et al., 2017). The future will likely see greater innovation in robotic technology, the inclusion of artificial intelligence to assist intraoperative decision-making, and an improvement in patient outcomes. Minimally invasive surgical interventions are yet another major trend shaping the future of urological surgery. Improvements in procedures such as laser lithotripsy, ureteroscopy, and percutaneous nephrolithotomy (PCNL) have dramatically changed urinary stone management. Not only do these interventions reduce recovery times compared to open operations, but they also minimize the resulting morbidity, hence offering a better choice for patients (Katkar et al., 2023). Advances in imaging technology and instrumentation have refined the effectiveness of these procedures, allowing urologists to treat a broader range of urological ailments with greater precision. As more advanced and readily available equipment becomes available, even further integration of such minimally invasive methods is likely to prompt urologists to rethink how they approach conducting surgical procedures. Back to the future, the broad direction in urologic surgery is toward patient-centered care, exemplified by the incorporation of personalized medicine. This direction represents an evolving understanding of patient-specific traits and desires, driving the need for individualized treatment regimens tailored to address distinct needs. Future advancements in genomics and biomarker identification will also aid in the development of targeted therapies, enhancing the success of surgery and improving patients' quality of life. However, this revolution does not happen without hurdles; cost considerations, access, and the complexity of integrating these advancements must be surmounted for broader acceptance. As urology becomes increasingly utilitarian with technological advancements, it will be essential that patient-centricity remains a cornerstone of the future of urologic surgery (Katkar et al., 2023) (Figure 7.17).

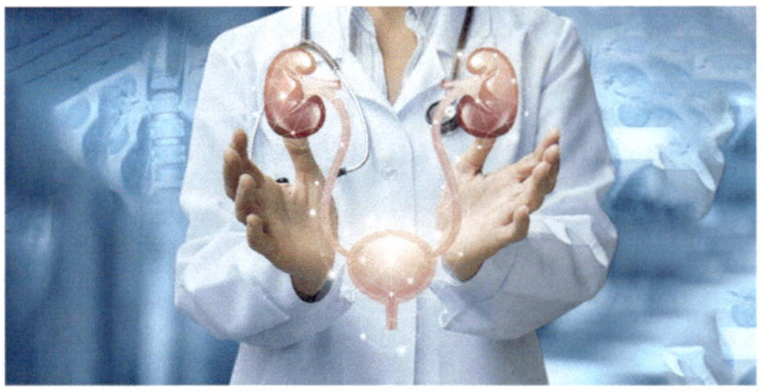

Figure 7.17. Trends in urological surgery.

Source: https://www.hjhospitals.org / blogimage/ L3d8Fi4eiSayFjd7 wnJ81slnEE4p G3y6xvn 56O0Z.jpeg.

Test Your Knowledge

1. How has robotic-assisted surgery improved outcomes in prostate cancer treatment?
2. What is the role of laser technology in managing kidney and bladder stones?

SUMMARY

The urology surgery practice itself continues to evolve with advancements in technology, surgical techniques, and improved understanding of the urological pathologies. The addition of minimally invasive approaches, including robotic-assisted surgery, has revolutionized treatment modalities, allowing for quicker recovery and improved outcomes for patients. As observed in ongoing clinical trials evaluating neoadjuvant therapy for muscle-invasive bladder cancer, the surgical model is shifting toward increased patient-centered care, considering both efficacy and quality of life. Results from studies indicate that the technical proficiency and precision offered by these technological advancements significantly contribute to the success of urologic surgery. Thus, such advancements bring into focus the need for continuous training and ongoing education among urologists in order to successfully harness these new means. Moreover, the relationship between preoperative factors and the outcomes of urology surgery remains a topic of considerable interest. Preoperative factors such as CIS status at initial TURBT have not been found to have a significant effect on patients' pathological reactions to neoadjuvant chemotherapy. In a multicenter study of 1213 patients, CIS appearance during TURBT did not correlate with overall survival results, suggesting that other factors may have a greater influence on patient prognosis. The result compels surgeons to consider a broader set of clinical predictors beyond traditional markers, ultimately leading to a more advanced method of treatment planning in urologic oncology (Takayanagi et al., 2018). Lastly, the frequent updating of injury grading systems in urology, especially kidney trauma, demonstrates the specialty's readiness to adapt to new evidence and practice standards. The recent change to the 2018 AAST grading of renal injuries highlights the importance of accurate classification of injuries in the outcome of clinical conditions. Though it offers more subtle anatomical variations than its predecessor, evidence finds that this new system is not significantly superior to the 1989 version in terms of predicting bleeding interventions. This illustrates the need for continuously assessing increasingly evolving standards and techniques for their usefulness and clinical significance (Allen et al., 2020). Thus, the conclusion of this excursion into urology surgery is more of a beginning point than a terminal one for ongoing inquiry and progress in the area, with the consequence that surgical practice refines itself in tandem with changing evidence and patient needs.

In urological surgery, it is essential to know all the treatments for localized prostate cancer. Since there are numerous treatments, a consensus is needed on optimal outcomes to enhance clinical effectiveness. A successful study aimed at developing a core outcome set (COS) in effectiveness trials in localized prostate cancer. This also involved a systematic review and qualitative input from prostate cancer patients and healthcare providers, highlighting the importance of incorporating patient feedback into clinical studies. The following COS reports 19 key outcomes, including survival metrics and complications such as urinary incontinence and sexual function. Such standardization facilitates the determination of effective therapies and better communication among providers, possibly maximizing therapeutic strategies in varied environments (Abel et al., 2017). Apart from prostate cancer, kidney transplant innovation in the techniques used is another critical area in urology surgery. The introduction of robot-assisted surgical methods has revolutionized the field, particularly for complex cases, such as GMVs with multiple vessels. One such recent study investigated the feasibility and outcomes of robot-assisted kidney transplantation (RAKT) using grafts from living donors, an observation that is invaluable to surgical practice. Results indicated that RAKT with GMVs yielded excellent early postoperative results without severe complications, disproving earlier assumptions regarding the danger of complex vascular anastomoses. Furthermore, this chapter suggests that proper use of innovative techniques is not just a matter of technological skills but also a thorough understanding of anatomical variations specific to patients (Alcaraz et al., 2018). As a whole, these studies demonstrate the importance of continuous innovation and standardization in urology surgery. By setting detailed standards through COS for prostate cancer clinical trials, as well as examining newer surgical techniques such as RAKT for complex kidney transplantations, the specialty reaffirms its commitment to optimal patient care. The inclusion of patient outcomes in the COS promotes a more holistic approach to treatment, while the examination of minimally invasive surgical methods illustrates a trend toward less invasive, yet effective, urologic interventions. These key points highlight the importance of ongoing research and adoption of urology surgery, ultimately causing practitioners to achieve improved results for their patients and, more significantly, how to address the nuances of present medical procedures (Abel et al., 2017; Alcaraz et al., 2018).

KEY TERMS FROM THIS CHAPTER

- Benign prostatic hyperplasia (BPH)
- Cystectomy
- Lithotripsy
- Nephrectomy
- PCNL (Percutaneous Nephrolithotomy)
- Prostatectomy
- Renal cell carcinoma
- Bladder cancer
- Hypospadias repair
- Neobladder reconstruction
- Orchiectomy
- Phimosis
- Pyeloplasty
- Testicular torsion

CRITICAL THINKING QUESTIONS

1. **Which of the following is the most common type of kidney stone?**
   a. Uric acid
   b. Cystine
   c. Struvite
   d. Calcium oxalate
2. **Which of the following is a classic indication for transurethral resection of the prostate (TURP)?**
   a. Renal artery stenosis
   b. Bladder cancer
   c. Recurrent urinary retention due to BPH
   d. Erectile dysfunction
3. **A 25-year-old male presents with sudden, severe testicular pain and an absent cremasteric reflex. The most likely diagnosis is:**
   a. Epididymitis
   b. Testicular torsion
   c. Varicocele
   d. Hydrocele
4. **Which tumor marker is most commonly elevated in testicular germ cell tumors?**
   a. CA-125
   b. AFP and β-HCG
   c. PSA
   d. CEA
5. **In the TNM staging of bladder cancer, T2 disease indicates:**
   a. Tumor confined to the mucosa
   b. Tumor invades the lamina propria
   c. Tumor invades muscularis propria
   d. Tumor invades adjacent organs

Short Answer Questions

1. What are the indications for surgical management of benign prostatic hyperplasia (BPH)?
2. Describe the evaluation and surgical options for a patient presenting with renal calculi.
3. What are the common complications following transurethral resection of the prostate (TURP)?
4. Explain the staging and surgical management of renal cell carcinoma.
5. What are the principles and indications of percutaneous nephrolithotomy (PCNL)?
6. Describe the clinical features and surgical treatment of testicular torsion.
7. What are the surgical approaches for managing urethral strictures?
8. How is bladder cancer diagnosed and managed surgically at different stages?
9. What is the role of ureteroscopy in urologic stone disease?
10 Differentiate between open, laparoscopic, and robotic-assisted approaches in urologic surgeries.

Answers to Critical Thinking Questions

1. (d); 2. (c); 3. (b); 4. (b); 5. (c)

REFERENCES

1. MacLennan, S., Williamson, P. R., Bekema, H., Campbell, M., Ramsay, C., N'Dow, J., MacLennan, S., Vale, L., Dahm, P., Mottet, N., & Lam, T. (2017). A core outcome set for localised prostate cancer effectiveness trials. *BJU International, 120*(5B). https://doi.org/10.1111/bju.13854Aboumarzouk, O., Giusti, G., Jones, P., Pietropaolo, A., et al. (2017). *Trends of intervention for pediatric stone disease over the last two decades (2000–2015): A systematic review of literature.* https://core.ac.uk/download/151208757.pdf (accessed on 12th July 2025).
2. Ahmad, I., Briggs, T. P., Hines, J., Kelly, J. D., et al. (2017). *In-depth critical analysis of complications following robot-assisted radical cystectomy with intracorporeal urinary diversion.* https://core.ac.uk/download/96881684.pdf (accessed on 12th July 2025).
3. Al Rawashdah, S., Al Salhi, Y., Carbone, A., Coppola, M., et al. (2017). *Prospective study to compare antibiosis versus the association of N-acetylcysteine, D-mannose and morinda citrifolia fruit extract in preventing urinary tract infections in patients submitted to urodynamic investigation.* https://core.ac.uk/download/98337961.pdf (accessed on 12th July 2025).
4. Alcaraz, A., Breda, A., Campi, R., Decaestecker, K., et al. (2018). *Robot-assisted kidney transplantation with regional hypothermia using grafts with multiple vessels after extracorporeal vascular reconstruction: Results from the European Association of Urology Robotic Urology Section Working Group.*
5. Allen, L., Anderson, R. E., Askari, R., Baradaran, H. R., et al. (2020). *The American Association for the Surgery of Trauma renal injury grading scale: Implications of the 2018 revisions for injury reclassification and predicting bleeding interventions.* https://core.ac.uk/download/287623169.pdf (accessed on 12th July 2025).
6. Andrade, L. C. B. A., Costa, I. D. S. D., Filho, F. S. M., Filho, G. A. D., et al. (2025). *Technological advances and the evolution of endoscopic procedures in the treatment of upper urinary tract tumors: Clinical impact and future perspectives.* https://core.ac.uk/download/654540037.pdf (accessed on 12th July 2025).
7. Annemans, L., De Regge, M., Duyck, P., Gemmel, P., et al. (2013). *Physician-owned specialized facilities: Focused factories or destructive competition?: A systematic review.* https://core.ac.uk/download/55777137.pdf (accessed on 12th July 2025).
8. Ather, M. H., Ettinger, S., Hoffman, S., Martin, R. A., McLoughlin, M. A., Ross, L. A., Scott, R. C., et al. (2019). *Endoscopic laser-ablation for the treatment of orthotopic and ectopic ureteroceles in dogs: 13 cases (2008–2017).* https://core.ac.uk/download/213444929.pdf (accessed on 12th July 2025).
9. Bagley, D. H., Healy, K. A., Kleinmann, N. (2012). *Ureteroscopic treatment of larger renal calculi (>2 cm).* https://core.ac.uk/download/213441651.pdf (accessed on 12th July 2025).
10. Balbay, M. D., Canda, A. E., Catto, J. W., Dal Moro, F., et al. (2016). *Robotic intracorporeal urinary diversion: Practical review of current surgical techniques.* https://core.ac.uk/download/80153933.pdf (accessed on 12th July 2025).
11. Barbieri, L., Dal Moro, F., Morlacco, A., Motterle, G., et al. (2017). *Frailty and elderly in urology: Is there an impact on post-operative complications?* https://core.ac.uk/download/129592620.pdf (accessed on 12th July 2025).

12. Bart, S., Baumann, M., Berkelman, P., Bolla, M., et al. (2006). *Medical image computing and computer-aided medical interventions applied to soft tissues. Work in progress in urology.* http://arxiv.org/abs/0712.2100 (accessed on 12th July 2025).

13. Bartsch, G., Elsner, R., Janetschek, G., Neumann, H. P., et al. (2000). *Laparoscopic partial adrenalectomy for bilateral pheochromocytomas in a boy with von Hippel-Lindau disease.* https://core.ac.uk/download/16432643.pdf (accessed on 12th July 2025).

14. Bodean, O. M., Cirstoiu, M., Diaconu, C. C., Marcu, D., et al. (2018). *Pelvic floor disorders in gynecological malignancies: An overlooked problem?* https://core.ac.uk/download/216808110.pdf (accessed on 12th July 2025).

15. Bottoni, F., Chang, S., Figueroa, M. S., Gaudric, A., et al. (2020). *Optical coherence tomography-based consensus definition for lamellar macular hole.* https://core.ac.uk/download/288432554.pdf (accessed on 12th July 2025).

16. Brown, D., Calvaresi, A., Gomella, L. G., Lallas, C. D., et al. (2016). *Clinical influences in the multidisciplinary management of small renal masses at a tertiary referral center.* https://core.ac.uk/download/83049484.pdf (accessed on 12th July 2025).

17. Burgio, K., Cohn, J. A., Davies, B., De Guchtenaere, A., Epstein, J. I., Feldstein, L. R., Friedman, B., et al. (2019). *Etiology of nocturia response in men with diminished bladder capacity.* https://core.ac.uk/download/286086651.pdf (accessed on 12th July 2025).

18. Canfield, S. E., Dahm, P., Griffiths, T. R., Leyshon, G., Hilvano-Cabungcal, D., et al. (2012). *Systematic review of perioperative and quality-of-life outcomes following surgical management of localized renal cancer.* https://core.ac.uk/download/9630469.pdf (accessed on 12th July 2025).

19. Carrió, I., De Vincentis, G., Du, Y., Fanti, S., et al. (2017). *Practical recommendations for radium-223 treatment of metastatic castration-resistant prostate cancer.* https://core.ac.uk/download/98347228.pdf (accessed on 12th July 2025).

20. Chang, S. L., Cheung, H., Chung, B. I., Del Giudice, F., et al. (2017). *Adoption of robotic assisted partial nephrectomies: A population-based analysis of U.S. surgeons from 2004–2013.* https://core.ac.uk/download/153365981.pdf (accessed on 12th July 2025).

21. Chaussy, C., Rassweiler, J. J., Renner, C., Thüroff, S., et al. (2001). *Treatment of renal stones by extracorporeal shockwave lithotripsy: An update.* https://core.ac.uk/download/16432642.pdf (accessed on 12th July 2025).

22. Close, A., Fraser, C., Gurung, T., Jia, X., et al. (2013). *Relative effectiveness of robot-assisted and standard laparoscopic prostatectomy as alternatives to open radical prostatectomy for treatment of localized prostate cancer: A systematic review and mixed treatment comparison meta-analysis.* https://core.ac.uk/download/19183823.pdf (accessed on 12th July 2025).

23. Conte, M. C., Lancaster, E. M., Pierce, L., Sammann, A., et al. (2020). *Rapid response of an academic surgical department to the COVID-19 pandemic: Implications for patients, surgeons, and the community.* https://core.ac.uk/download/323072299.pdf (accessed on 12th July 2025).

24. Costa, B., Palumbo, C., De Lorenzis, E., Gadda, F., Cozzi, G., Rosso, M., Talso, M., et al. (2013). *Robotics in uro-oncologic surgery.* https://core.ac.uk/download/80173448.pdf (accessed on 12th July 2025).

25. Cutajar, L. (1989). *New methods for the treatment of renal calculi: The St. Luke's Hospital experience*. https://core.ac.uk/download/46601744.pdf (accessed on 12th July 2025).
26. Frang, D., Jako, G. J., Repassy, D. L. (2011). *Minimal and direct access surgery in urology*. https://core.ac.uk/download/142040468.pdf (accessed on 12th July 2025).
27. Halperin, D., Larke, N., Schenker, I., Weiss, H. A., et al. (2010). *Complications of circumcision in male neonates, infants and children: A systematic review*. https://core.ac.uk/download/13097075.pdf (accessed on 12th July 2025).
28. Herbst, J.-A. M. E. (2016). *Preoperative fasting practices in adult elective surgery patients at Charlotte Maxeke Johannesburg Academic Hospital*. https://core.ac.uk/download/188774765.pdf (accessed on 12th July 2025).
29. Katkar, A. R., et al. (2023). *Innovations in minimally invasive techniques for urinary stone management*. https://core.ac.uk/download/596247504.pdf (accessed on 12th July 2025).
30. Kazemier, G., van Oostrum, J. M., Parlevliet, T., Wagelmans, A. P. M., et al. (2025). *A method for clustering surgical cases to allow master surgical scheduling*. https://core.ac.uk/download/pdf/6517196.pdf (accessed on 12th July 2025).
31. Kazimierczak, K. A., Skea, Z. C. (2015). *'I've used the word cancer but it's actually good news': Discursive performativity of cancer and the identity of urological cancer services*. https://core.ac.uk/download/42130404.pdf (accessed on 12th July 2025).
32. Soyupak, B., Gogus, C., Karabulut, E., Ozen, H., Turkeri, L., Yaycioglu, O., et al. (2012). *Patients with kidney cancer*. https://core.ac.uk/download/227071316.pdf (accessed on 12th July 2025).
33. Subak, L. L., Whitcomb, E. L. (2011). *Effect of weight loss on urinary incontinence in women*. https://core.ac.uk/download/323079415.pdf (accessed on 12th July 2025).
34. Takayanagi, A., Stephenson, A. J., Fairey, A. S., Thorpe, A., van Rhijn, B. W., Volkmer, B. G., Ercole, C. E., et al. (2018). *Concomitant CIS on TURBT does not impact oncological outcomes in patients treated with neoadjuvant or induction chemotherapy followed by radical cystectomy*. https://core.ac.uk/download/287581814.pdf (accessed on 12th July 2025).

PAEDIATRIC SURGERY

8

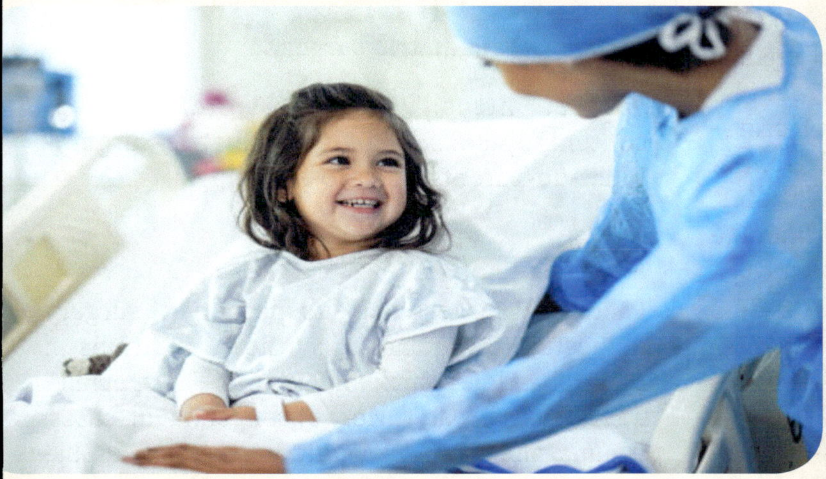

LEARNING OBJECTIVES

After studying this chapter, you will be able to:

1. Understand the historical background of pediatric surgery
2. Explain the standard pediatric surgical procedures
3. Discuss the surgical techniques and innovations of pediatric surgery
4. Focus on challenges in pediatric surgery
5. Learn about postoperative care in pediatric patients
6. Evaluate the future directions in pediatric surgery

Introduction

Pediatric surgery is a specialized branch of medical practice that focuses on the surgical needs of infants, children, and adolescents. Because pediatric patients are not simply small adults, their unique physiological and psychological characteristics necessitate personalized forms of surgical treatment. This is due to the numerous stages of growth that children experience, which can sometimes impact their ability to recover from surgical procedures and anesthetics. Moreover, the psychological and emotional management of surgery will differ to a considerable extent among young patients, requiring care and sensitivity during pre-operative and post-operative periods. Furthermore, the evolution of minimally invasive surgical techniques has transformed pediatric surgery, with faster recovery times and outcomes and fewer complications. It is essential to understand these factors, thus, to the healthcare workers involved in this field, so that they can give optimal care and enhance the level of children's surgical practice. Despite the intricacies inherent in pediatric surgery, there is a need to emphasize the importance of multidisciplinary cooperation among healthcare practitioners. Surgeons often collaborate with pediatricians, anesthetists, psychologists, and other professionals to create intensive treatment programs with an utmost emphasis on the general well-being of a child. Coordination in this manner enables every section of a child's physical, emotional, and social requirements to be addressed comprehensively. Education of health personnel in effective communication with children and their families is equally important to minimize anxiety and ensure cooperation when they undergo medical treatment. For instance, incorporating cross-cultural training into the medical school curriculum, as suggested by recent studies, can enable health professionals to manage multicultural patient backgrounds effectively, thereby becoming more effective in engaging patients and families from multicultural backgrounds (Joel et al., 2007). This combined approach not only improves surgical outcomes but also enhances the integration of the patient experience more effectively. As technology and surgery continue to advance, pediatric surgery is also poised to undergo transformation in the years to come. The application of new-generation technology, including robotic surgery and cutting-edge imaging technologies, promises exciting possibilities for enhanced precision and efficiency in operations. In addition, with growing awareness of the importance of mental well-being among society, the integration of psychological care with surgeries becomes more relevant. Teenage patients have anxiety and fear of undergoing surgery, and addressing these emotional components with structured psychological care can aid in recovery and improve surgical outcomes. Involvement in health management programs that meet these interdisciplinary needs can foster an even more conducive setting for young patients (Bonica et al., 2017). As practice evolves, continued investment in education, technology, and integrative care modalities will ensure that pediatric surgery remains attuned to the ever-evolving needs of children and families (Figure 8.1).

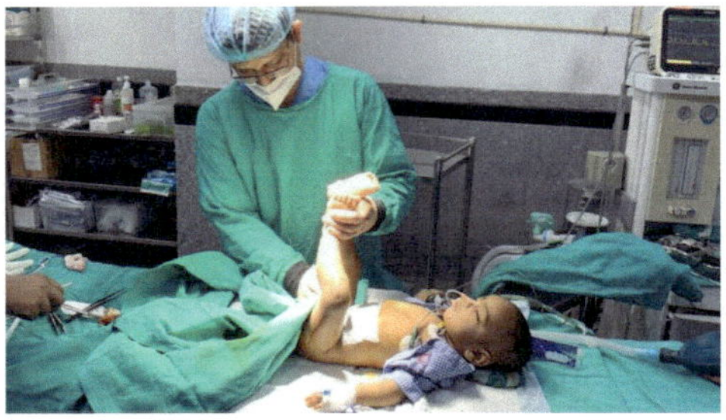

Figure 8.1. Pediatric surgery.

Source: https://sugunahospital.com/wp-content/uploads/2024/09/Pediatric-Surgery-What-do-parents-need-to-know.jpg.

Definition of Pediatric Surgery

Paediatric surgery is a subspecialty of surgery dedicated to the care of surgical conditions in children, adolescents, and infants. The specialty addresses a broad variety of congenital diseases, trauma, and acquired conditions that are curable by surgery. Pediatric surgery is distinct from adult surgery in that it takes into consideration the special physiological and developmental differences in children. These differences can affect not only surgical practice but also anesthesia, pain control, and postoperative care. Pediatric surgeons therefore undergo extensive training to adapt to these differences, ensuring balanced treatment that is specifically tailored to young patients. This specialized training thus has a ultimate impact on the overall results in younger patients, thereby reaffirming the necessity of specialized expertise in pediatric surgical practice. To balance the technical skill, pediatric surgery also emphasizes the role of multi-disciplinary care. Surgeons prefer working with pediatricians, anesthesiologists, and nurses to design customised management plans in accordance with the individual needs of the child's condition or disease. This collaboration is necessary to optimize surgical and postoperative management because young patients can have underlying complications due to their age or status. Surgical intervention not only addresses the immediate concern but also involves consideration of the child's long-term growth and development. As highlighted in current guidelines, communication with families is crucial throughout the entire surgical process, from preoperative counseling to postoperative follow-up, to ensure that parents and caregivers are well-informed and supportive of the treatment course (Akyol et al., 2019). Also, the field of pediatric surgery is continually evolving with advancements in technology and procedure. Procedures like minimally invasive surgery, including laparoscopic procedures, have spread more widely, with less recovery time and post-operative morbidity in the younger patient. Emerging technologies, including enhanced imaging capabilities and robotic-assisted procedures, have further defined the surgical profession, enabling more precise interventions. As these advances integrate into clinical practice, pediatric surgeons themselves must stay current with the latest research and evidence-based best practices to provide evidence-based care (Galliers et al., 2009). The complexity of surgery in vulnerable populations necessitates a relentless search for education and training in the profession to improve clinical outcomes and quality of life in children globally (Galliers et al., 2009) (Figure 8.2).

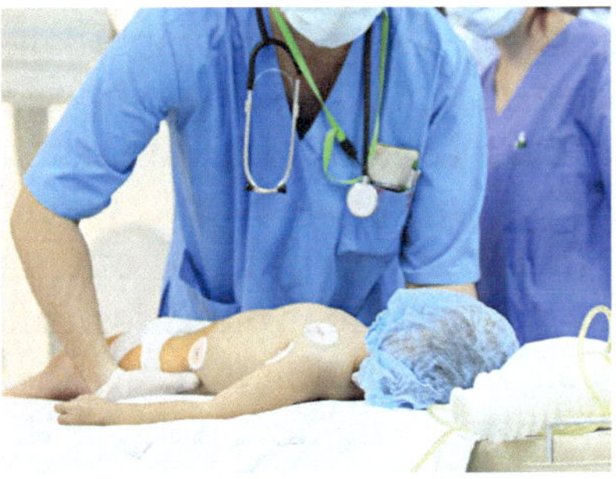

Figure 8.2. Paediatric surgery treatments.

Source: https://productimages.withfloats.com/serviceimages/actual/62d7c6d85834e77a5bf710e4Paediatric%20Surgery.

Importance of Specialization in Children

Specialization in pediatric care, particularly pediatric surgery, serves to bridge the anatomical and physiological differences between infants and adults. Children have unique medical needs due to their developing physiology, which cannot be adequately addressed by general practitioners. Pediatric surgeons are trained to diagnose and treat congenital abnormalities and surgical issues unique to this stage. For instance, pathologies like intussusception or congenital heart anomalies require skills that are more than usual operations. By working exclusively with pediatric patients, such surgeons gain more in-depth knowledge and develop specialized techniques that optimize surgical outcomes, minimize complications, and facilitate the highest rate of recovery for children. Therefore, the importance of specialization in pediatric surgery is highlighted by the severity of cases and the fragility of working with children (Galliers et al., 2009). Additionally, the change in healthcare policies also signifies a growing recognition of the necessity of specialization in pediatric service. Reforms to introduce experts into primary health care networks have sparked controversy among doctors regarding the competencies required to provide adequate treatment for pediatric patients. Critics argue that the widening of pediatricians' and other facial specialists' practice outside their specialization is contrary to the need for well-coordinated and complete care at this level, especially for children who require undivided attention to their developmental problems. While the purpose of these reforms may be to ease shortages of caregivers, there is a genuine concern that these reforms are not being mindful of the unique complexity of pediatric health (Kowalska-Bobko et al., 2016). Specialization ensures that the medical personnel possess the knowledge needed, but even the tacit knowledge of how to care, which is in alignment with the milestones of development. The focus on specialization in pediatrics ultimately means improved outcomes in pediatric surgery through enhanced training, research, and establishment of best practices for the child population. It enables comprehensive knowledge of common and rare childhood conditions, enhances surgical techniques, and encourages innovations in medical technology for children. Through engagement in ongoing education and research relevant to their field, pediatric surgeons are achieving considerable advances in pediatric surgical practice. These advances underscore the commitment to delivering the safest and most effective treatments for children, thereby reinforcing the value of specialization in pediatric surgery. Enhanced safety protocols, tailored surgical instrumentation, and targeted anesthetic practices are the outcomes of this specialty experience, ultimately reflected in better care for pediatric patients (Galliers et al., 2009).

8.1. Historical Background

Learning Outcome

1. Describe the evolution of pediatric surgery
2. Focus on the development of pediatric surgery
3. Learn about surgical techniques of pediatric surgery

Pediatric surgery has been significantly influenced by advances in neonatal care practices over the last few decades. The treatment of infants has, in general, witnessed its environment being changed, most prominently in the UK, where new techniques have been developed for more effectively saving the lives of vulnerable infants. Mechanical ventilation and total parenteral nutrition, for example, have been at the forefront of helping to keep prematurely born and critically ill infants alive. The establishment of neonatal intensive care units (NICUs) marked a watershed in this evolution, as specialized facilities provide individualized care necessary for the most fragile patients. Enhanced immediate care was the outcome of this specialized practice in neonatal medicine, and it paved the way for later developments in pediatric surgical interventions, demonstrating the interconnectedness of surgical practice and the evolution of neonatal medicine (N/A, 2001). In the 1970s and 1980s, new diagnostic techniques were developed that had a revolutionary impact on pediatric surgery. The establishment of non-surgical imaging modalities, such as ultrasound and magnetic resonance imaging, has revolutionized the diagnosis of congenital defects and the assessment of the need for surgical interventions in children. With these modalities, diseases in children were diagnosed earlier and classified more accurately, allowing for timely and informed decisions about surgical interventions. For instance, innovation in near-infrared spectroscopy has provided neurosurgeons with essential information about cerebral oxygenation and metabolic responses during surgery, resulting in improved patient safety rates. With post-surgical improvements and diagnostic advancements, the ability to perform minimally invasive surgery has risen, further reducing the complications of pediatric tic surgical procedures (Burgess et al., 2005). The application of these technological advances to the clinical setting has been instrumental in shaping the future of pediatric surgery and with the healthcare systems stepping up to include an interdisciplinary element in comprehensive care, the demand for multidisciplinary teams also increased. This collaboration among surgeons, neonatologists, radiologists, and specialists has resulted in improved patient outcomes and more effective treatment plans for children. As can be seen from the history of the national "Exemplar Programme" in the UK, as NHS Direct and general practice collaborated to enhance patient access and care, pediatric surgery has also adopted a similar model, driven by the need for interdisciplinary integration. Consequently, the developments in diagnosis and teamwork of the past have molded and developed the climate of pediatric surgery today (Burgess et al., 2005) (Figure 8.3).

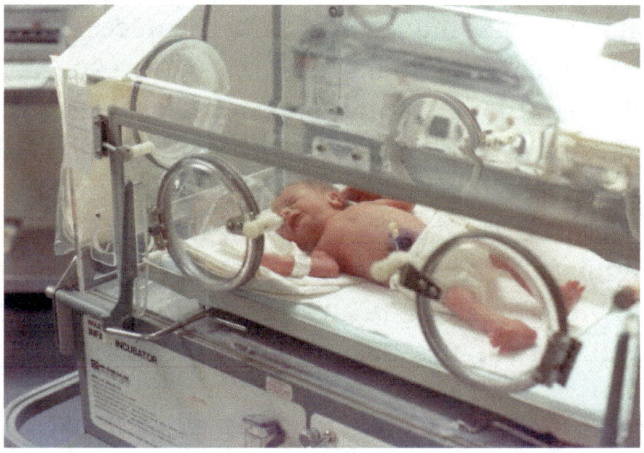

Figure 8.3. Neonatal intensive care unit.

Source: https://upload.wikimedia.org/wikipedia/commons/e/ee/Infant-Incubator-wBaby-1978-USA.jpg.

8.1.1. Evolution of Paediatric Surgery

Paediatric surgical progress is a fantastic journey from primitive procedures to highly advanced techniques tailor-made for the child. Earlier, surgery in infants and children was typically marred by a lack of appreciation for the unique physiological and developmental characteristics of the young patient. These operations, depending on the overall principles established for the adult, were partially successful and often accompanied by high mortality rates. However, through decades of relentless research and practice, the subspecialty has adopted advancements such as minimally invasive surgery and age-specific anesthesia regimens. The emphasis on customized surgical techniques has been crucial in reducing complications and improving long-term outcomes in young patients, demonstrating a commitment to quality improvement in children's surgical care (Isawumi et al., 2024). Furthermore, surgical technologies have led the way in creating pediatric surgery. Laparoscopic technology has revolutionized the nature of surgical procedures, enabling surgical procedures to be carried out with reduced intervention, which significantly reduces recovery time and postoperative discomfort for children. Such a transition towards minimally invasive surgery has also been facilitated by the advancement of imaging and robotic systems, which enhance accuracy and reduce reliance on extensive incisions. This innovation has also facilitated early intervention and diagnosis, allowing surgeons to treat complex congenital diseases more effectively. The ongoing utilization of sophisticated technology not only improves surgical results but also fosters a culture of innovation among practitioners in the field by encouraging continuous study aimed at enhancing the safety and well-being of pediatric patients (Gaskin et al., 2022). In addition, the historical context of pediatric surgery reflects broader societal changes and advances in medical science that have had a direct impact on standards of practice. Childrens health has been strongly advocated for and promoted, and stakeholders are increasingly aware of the specific psychological and physical issues surrounding the treatment of younger patients. This has resulted in increasingly stringent training programs for pediatric surgeons, with an emphasis on multidisciplinary practice and ensuring holistic care that extends beyond the theatre. With a focus on long-term health and quality of life, the growth of pediatric surgery is a testament to both the advancements in science and a commitment to addressing the complex needs of children in the surgical environment (Gaskin et al., 2022; Isawumi et al., 2024).

8.1.2. Key Figures in the Development of the Field

The development of pediatric surgery as a distinct specialty is largely due to visionary individuals who recognized the unique challenges presented by operating on children. One such early pioneer was Dr. Alfred Blalock, who in the mid-20th century significantly advanced the specialty by developing the

Blalock-Taussig shunt. This innovative procedure respected the demands of infants suffering from congenital heart disease, an emphasis on tailored surgical guidelines for younger patients. Not only did Blalock's contribution reinforce the success of surgery, but it also precipitated the establishment of pediatric surgical units in other hospitals. His efforts set an example of the kind of impact visionary clinicians can have on advancing medical procedures and improving the outlook for many children with severe congenital diseases. Apart from the efforts made by Dr. Blalock, other individuals also made special efforts to improve surgical techniques and bring pediatric surgery into a specialty of importance. Dr. Robert Lawson Tait, another renowned individual, was an expert in pediatric urology and demonstrated the importance of treating urological conditions in children. His innovative surgical practices, particularly in addressing conditions such as undescended testes and urinary tract abnormalities, shed light on the diversity of pediatric surgical needs. The collaboration of surgeons like Tait with pediatricians and anesthesiologists made possible the development of comprehensive care models that effectively addressed the multifaceted health issues of children. These advances contributed not just to the palette of surgical possibilities but also to the expansion of postoperative care protocols, making it possible to better understand the application of anesthesia in pediatric medicine. Pediatric surgery was also advanced by the creation of specialized training programs and societies of pediatric surgeons, stimulated in part by the efforts of leading figures within the field. These societies improved education, research, and dialogue among surgeons, with an emphasis on evidence-based practice and new surgical techniques. The activity of leading pediatric surgeons within academic centers has also emphasized the contribution of research to improving outcomes. For instance, congenital anomaly operations have been highly effective treatments, backing the argument that pediatric surgery is a necessary component of the healthcare of children. According to recent reports, the global health disease burden of congenital anomalies warrants the necessity for accessible pediatric surgical treatment, especially in low- and middle-income countries where the disease burden is most significant (Uba et al., 2014). Furthermore, dental students' need for structured information on surgical specialties aligns with the broader aim of enhancing knowledge among future professionals (Lee et al., 2018) (Figure 8.4).

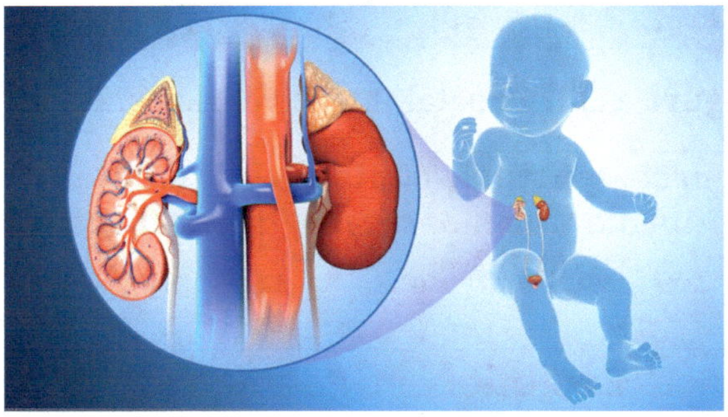

Figure 8.4. Pediatric urology.

Source: https://cdn.castleconnolly.com/dims4/default/818c247/2147483647/strip/true/crop/1000x563+0+0/resize/1200x675!/quality/90/?url=http%3A%2F%2Fcastle-connolly-brightspot.s3.us-east-1.amazonaws.com%2Fb9%2F4d%2F8fd1ac674c38ad6d6d2fa19d4d0b%2Fpillar-pediatric-urology-52-1200x675.jpg.

8.1.3. Milestones in Surgical Techniques

In children's surgery, advancements in surgical techniques have fundamentally redefined the management of a majority of conditions, particularly congenital defects. One such milestone is the application of minimally invasive surgical methods, which have been instrumental in reducing recovery times and postoperative morbidity among children. Traditionally, open surgeries contained intrinsic risks in the form of prolonged hospitalization and extensive physical injury. Advances in robotic and laparoscopic surgery have transformed the process, enabling surgeons to perform complex procedures with even greater precision and reduced scarring. Not only does this innovation cure physiological ailments, but it also significantly impacts the psychological well-being of adolescent patients and their families, who are likely to fear surgical interventions. Together, these developments illustrate a strong trend towards more patient-centered approaches in pediatric surgery, marking the way for better results and a more compassionate treatment for child surgical patients. Another milestone in innovations in pediatric surgical procedures is the development of standard protocols for managing congenital conditions, particularly those of congenital cataracts. As is the domain of more recent literature, pediatric cataracts remain a significant treatable cause of childhood blindness, affecting approximately 1 in 1000 to 2000 live births. Recent advances in germline genetics not only explain the genetic underpinnings of such cataracts but also inform treatment. Early surgery has been shown to significantly improve outcomes, particularly in individuals with a genetic etiology, such as those with crystallin mutations. However, the added risks of postoperative complications render careful consideration when determining the proper course. The integration of genetic information in preoperative diagnosis is therefore an essential aspect that has become a critical element in tailoring individual treatment protocols for the affected children (Audor et al., 2024).

Additionally, the introduction of multidisciplinary teams in pediatric surgery has been instrumental, and the quality of care to the child patient has been enhanced remarkably. These units usually consist of pediatric surgeons, geneticists, anesthesiologists, and nurses, all working together to provide the best surgical results and overall patient care. The combined expertise creates a multidisciplinary approach to complex cases, particularly those with congenital issues and conditions that require specialized treatment. Also, the emphasis on long-term follow-up care is part of pediatric surgical care itself nowadays, particularly in managing issues involving growth, development, and long-term complications that arise from primary interventions. Interweaving these disparate viewpoints not only enhances surgical accuracy and effectiveness but also facilitates a more unified experience for families navigating the complexities of pediatric surgery, ultimately affirming the significance of each milestone achieved in this evolving discipline (N/A, 1990).

Test Your Knowledge

1. When did pediatric surgery emerge as a distinct specialty from general surgery?
2. What significant advancement improved outcomes in neonatal surgery?

8.2. Common Pediatric Surgical Procedures

Learning Outcome

1. Explain appendectomy in children in pediatric surgery
2. Define the repair of congenital heart defects
3. Discuss hernia repair

With the most common pediatric surgical procedures in mind, the rising rate of pediatric kidney stone disease (KSD) cannot be ignored and has resulted in an increase in focused interventions. In a 16-year systematic review, researchers documented a significant increase in articles referring to techniques such as ureteroscopy (URS), shockwave lithotripsy (SWL), percutaneous nephrolithotomy (PCNL), open stone surgery, and laparoscopic stone surgery. The review detected an alarming trend in KSD practice, with increasing procedural documentation paralleling overall progress in minimally invasive practice. Specifically, the literature reveals almost double the number of published articles from the first period (2000–2007) to the second period (2008–2015), reflecting a greater focus on maximizing results and developing surgical techniques (Aboumarzouk et al., 2017). This reflects the need for healthcare providers to stay up-to-date on the most effective treatments for such conditions in children. Pediatric neurosurgery also illustrates the complexity of standard surgery in children. One recent study of a tertiary neuroscience center looked at morbidity and mortality as adverse events in pediatric patients over two years and showed a high incidence of adverse events. Among 549 procedures performed, 130 adverse events were reported, resulting in an estimated 23.7% rate of procedures with at least one adverse event. In addition, a considerable percentage of these operations, 14.8%, necessitated unplanned reoperations in the operating room, underscoring the inherent challenges of delivering safe and effective care in this subspecialty. These findings suggest that complications are an inherent and intrinsic aspect of pediatric neurosurgery, and therefore, ongoing monitoring and evaluation are necessary to improve the quality of care (Beez et al., 2017).

In a broader perspective of pediatric surgery, the extensive effect of rising adverse events is not limited to neurosurgery and KSD operations. With the advancement of surgical techniques, comprehensive information regarding potential complications has become increasingly important for pediatric surgeons. Continuing professional education driven by emerging research will be critical in addressing complications and delivering the best care. The adoption of new surgical approaches and evidence-based practices will be vital to minimizing risks and improving outcomes for patients. Therefore, medical practitioners must foster a culture of learning, collaboration, and open discussion for such routine operations, ultimately developing an adaptive approach to pediatric surgical management. As surgical complexity and diversity increase, monitoring surgical effectiveness and side effects will remain at the core of pediatric surgery practice (Figure 8.5).

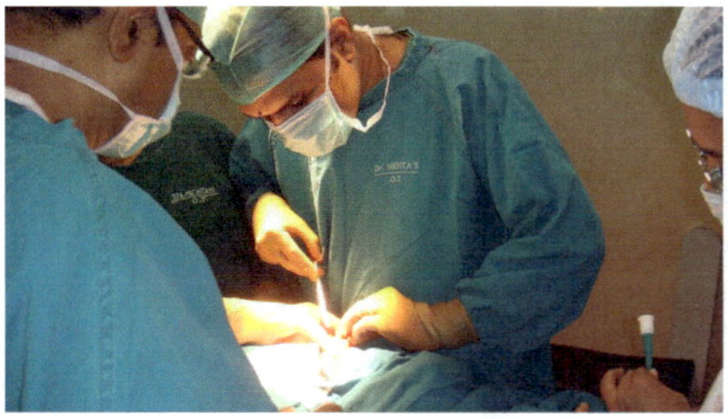

Figure 8.5. Pediatric surgical procedures.

Source: https://chennaichildsurgeon.com/wp-content/uploads/2020/10/dr-sankkarabarathi-paediatric-surgeon-chennai.jpg.

8.2.1. Appendectomy in Children

Among pediatric surgeries, appendectomy remains a crucial intervention due to the prevalence of acute appendicitis among children. Appendicitis is a surgical illness that is characterized by inflammation of the appendix and necessitates immediate medical and surgical intervention to prevent complications such as perforation or peritonitis. While it is the most common surgically emergent condition among children, available literature confirms a notable dearth of consensus regarding outcomes after appendectomy interventions. A recent study identified striking heterogeneity in the reported outcomes among various randomized controlled trials (RCTs) and systematic reviews (SRs) of treatments for appendicitis in children, observing that no core outcome set (COS) existed for patients in this group (Bhangu et al., 2015). Such heterogeneity not only complicates the clinical decision-making process but also hinders the ability to collate valuable evidence across studies, underscoring a compelling need for the use of standardized outcomes in future studies. Pain management after appendectomy is also a critical factor that should not be undermined. Relief from pain is vital during the overall recovery of children who have undergone surgery and plays a significant role in the quality of the surgical experience. There are proofs that inadequate pain control leads to increased anxiety and increased hospital stays, negatively influencing the child's recovery trajectory. The European Society for Paediatric Anesthesiology (ESPA) has created a Pain Management Ladder, a policy that seeks to enhance pain management practices in operating on children, such as those undergoing appendectomy (Adamek et al., 2018). Adhering to such formal pain management protocols ensures that kids receive adequate analgesic therapy, diminishes pain, and facilitates a smoother recovery process. Individualized pain management policies are of utmost importance, especially given the variations in available resources and medications across different healthcare facilities. Furthermore, postoperative management following an appendectomy involves the utilization of a multidisciplinary team protocol to improve outcomes among children. In view of the extremely high incidences of wound infections and intra-peritoneal abscess, intense monitoring and management are needed. While various studies have established risk factors for these complications, such as surgical technique and preoperative factors, standardization of postoperative care practice remains the most important. It is only a subset of RCTs that have directly assessed the primary outcomes, like those related to life impact and overall patient well-being, yet again increasing our understanding of the long-term significance of appendectomy in children, even more ambiguous (Bhangu et al., 2015). In the growing era of pediatric surgery, there is a need to develop comprehensive protocols and guidelines based on sound evidence. This will not only enhance patient treatment but also progress the body of knowledge regarding surgical intervention for pediatric appendicitis (Figure 8.6).

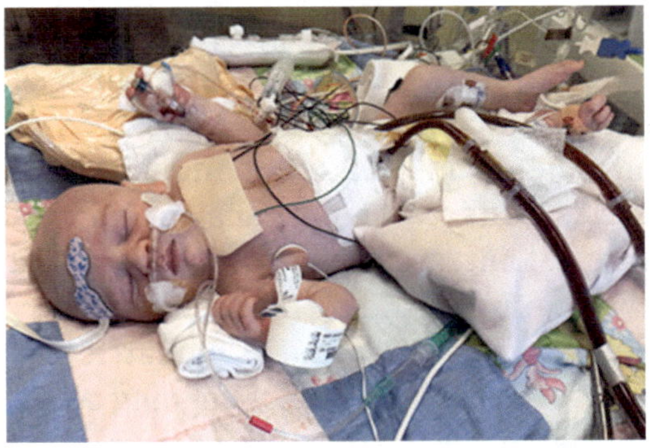

Figure 8.6. Congenital heart disease.

Source: https://www.actionlearningnetwork.org/wp-content/uploads/cmagBaker_CHD_400x267.png.

8.2.2. Repair of Congenital Heart Defects

The repair of congenital heart defects (CHDs) remains a pillar of pediatric surgery, correcting a variety of malformations that interfere with the normal anatomy and physiology of the heart. Such malformations, which occur at birth, can significantly impact the health and well-being of a child if left uncorrected. Operation is typically required to correct abnormalities such as septal defects, valvular abnormalities, and complex malformations that compromise hemodynamic stability. The final objectives of these operations are to restore normal circulation, prevent the risk of heart failure, and improve the quality of life. Mastery of these procedures not only demands a high level of expertise but also a general appreciation of the characteristically different anatomical and physiological difficulties presented by various types of CHDs, as these demand individualized techniques for maximum efficacy. The continued evolution of surgical techniques has led to increased success rates as well as decreased morbidity associated with the repair of congenital heart disease. For instance, minimally invasive procedures are being employed more and more to prevent trauma and enable fast recovery, particularly in complex conditions. Furthermore, the use of registries such as the Swiss Adult Congenital Heart Disease Registry (SACHER) provides greater insight into long-term outcomes and facilitates data-driven advancements in treatment modalities. Such registries collect comprehensive information on surgical interventions followed by patient follow-up, thus guiding subsequent surgical treatment and standards in pediatric cardiac care. By fostering a culture of ongoing education and research, pediatric surgery as a field can continually evolve its management and treatment of congenital heart disease, ultimately leading to improved health outcomes for children. The treatment of congenital heart disease must be managed by a multidisciplinary team involving cardiologists, surgeons, anesthesiologists, and nurses, each of whom plays an important role in optimizing patient care. Aortopexy, for instance, has proven to be successful in treating left mainstem bronchus compression, which is typically associated with congenital heart defects, highlighting the complexity of cases in children. The technique, as well as specific surgical corrections of CHDs, requires strict preoperative evaluation and follow-up for the best results. Secondly, the significance of long-term follow-up cannot be overemphasized since most of these patients will require subsequent evaluations or interventions for comorbid conditions upon reaching adulthood. With an interprofessional approach involving the medical team, surgical correction of congenital heart defects can significantly impact the prognosis and health of children with such defects, much as it supports the role of pediatric surgery in the scenario.

8.2.3. Hernia Repair

Management of pediatric hernias is unique in that it is accompanied by both challenges and opportunities for surgical repair. Hernias, which typically present as inguinal, umbilical, or epigastric masses, require careful evaluation because their occurrence can result in complications unless repaired promptly. Surgical repair is the primary method of treatment for hernias, and in deciding whether or not to do surgery, the decision typically falls on the size and symptoms of the hernia, as well as the child's age and overall health. Techniques of surgery have also been improved, particularly with the addition of laparoscopic minimal invasive procedures, significantly enhancing the results of hernia repair in children. These techniques minimize incision size, thus resulting in less postoperative pain, quicker recovery, and lower complication risk in the form of wound infection, which further adds to higher patient safety and satisfaction (Berloco et al., 2012). Laparoscopic herniorrhaphy has become more popular in pediatric operations due to its numerous advantages over the open technique. Among the significant benefits is reduced postoperative pain, which in children is particularly important as they are more likely to be anxious about surgical interventions. In addition to pain relief, the reduced length of hospital stay associated with laparoscopic repair is credited with optimal use of health resources, allowing for a quicker return to regular life for the child (Adamek et al., 2018). Furthermore, the precision of laparoscopy significantly reduces the risk of injury to nearby structures, a primary concern in the delicate anatomy of children. An amalgamation of these points underscores the necessity of incorporating laparoscopic techniques for herniorraphy to achieve improved operating results. Proper pain management, despite advancements in techniques, remains an essential aspect of pediatric herniorraphy. The European Society of Pediatric Anesthesiology appreciates the need for individualized pain management strategies for every child with respect to the unique physiological and psychological needs of children. Adequate analgesia combined with minimization of opioid use is essential to improve overall recovery results. The ESPA Pain Management Ladder is a guideline to help clinicians manage perioperative pain, ensuring all children receive an optimal level of care with potential individualized adjustments based on the individual surgical context (Adamek et al., 2018). With the development of pediatric surgery, integration of effective pain management with new operative strategies will be essential to optimize patient care in hernia repair operations (Figure 8.7).

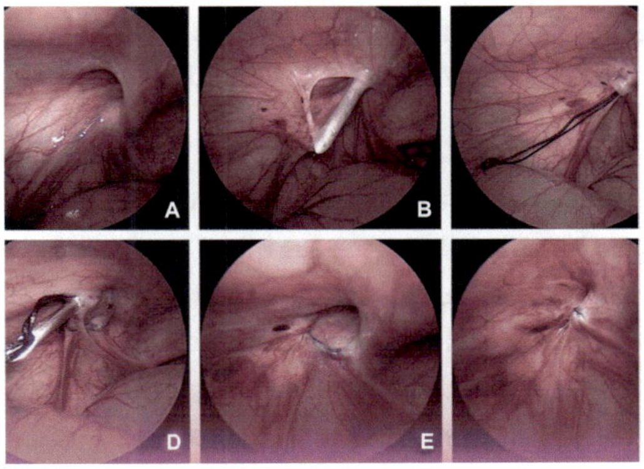

Figure 8.7. Hernia repair.

Source: https://burjeel.com/wp-content/uploads/2025/05/Minimally-Invasive-Surgery-Advances-Laparoscopic-Hernia-Repair-in-Neonates.png.

Test Your Knowledge

1. What is the standard surgical treatment for congenital inguinal hernia in children?
2. Which procedure is commonly performed for pyloric stenosis in infants?

8.3. Surgical Techniques and Innovations

Learning Outcome

1. Explain the minimally invasive surgery for pediatric surgery
2. Define the robotic-assisted pediatric surgery
3. Describe the advances in anesthesia for children

Over the past few years, the advancement that has been achieved in surgical techniques, particularly tailored for pediatric surgery, has revolutionized the pediatric healthcare landscape to a great extent. One of the significant advancements is the evolution of minimally invasive surgical techniques, with an emphasis on smaller incisions and shorter recovery times for children. Techniques such as laparoscopic surgery have become extensively utilized, allowing surgeons to perform complex operations with greater precision and reduced postoperative morbidity. The applicability of these techniques is most relevant in disease operations for conditions such as pediatric stone disease, in which ureteroscopy and shockwave lithotripsy are progressively more common procedures, indicating a trend towards less intrusive treatments that least interfere with a child's developing body. The increasing number of reports on such interventions highlights the rapid pace of research and application within this vital area of pediatric surgery, inevitably leading to improved outcomes and reduced healthcare expenses for families and healthcare facilities alike (Aboumarzouk et al., 2017).

Furthermore, the integration of newer imaging tools has driven the field of pediatric surgery into newer arenas of precision and effectiveness. High-resolution imaging modalities such as intraoperative ultrasound and three-dimensional imaging offer surgeons the ability to visualize anatomical structures in real-time, allowing them to interact with highly complex surgical environments more easily. Not only does this innovation improve the precision of surgery, but it also improves preoperative planning and intraoperative decision-making. Moreover, the integration of imaging with surgical simulation tools offers the promise of practicing highly complex procedures, thereby improving surgeon readiness and potentially reducing intraoperative complications. With the further advancement of these technologies, their implementation into children's surgical processes will lead to improved safety in operating rooms and better outcomes for patients, representing a dedication to excellence in the care of young patients (Loewenstein et al., 2017).

Further advancement and utilization of robotic-assisted surgical systems represent another significant breakthrough in pediatric surgery. These systems offer more dexterity, accuracy, and visualization than traditional methods. Robotic platforms provide pediatric surgeons with greater comfort in performing complex operations, offering improved technical control, reduced tissue trauma, and faster patient recovery. The use of robotic technology is constructive in surgeries on delicate or complex anatomical regions, such as enabling procedures previously deemed too risky. As more evidence emerges about robotic surgery in children, it is evident that such advancements not only enhance the quality of care but also pave the way for future developments in surgical technique. The relentless pursuit of innovation in surgical techniques is at the heart of overcoming the unique challenges of surgical management in children, ultimately leading to enhanced therapeutic outcomes (Aboumarzouk et al., 2017) (Figure 8.8).

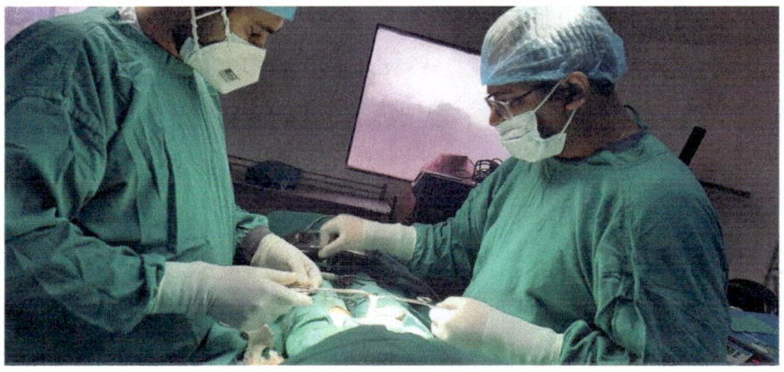

Figure 8.8. Neonatal and pediatric surgery.

Source: https://surgeonforkids.com/wp-content/uploads/2025/06/WhatsApp-Image-2025-06-21-at-12.04.08-PM.jpeg.

8.3.1. Minimally Invasive Surgery

The evolution of minimally invasive surgery (MIS) has significantly transformed pediatric surgery, with numerous advantages over open surgeries. With advancements in technology and surgical improvements, operations that were once deemed complicated can now be performed minimally, resulting in reduced recovery time and fewer complications. For instance, laparoscopic surgery provides the utilization of smaller incisions, which translates to less postoperative pain and shorter hospital stays. With the prevalence of childhood disorders requiring surgical treatment on the rise, MIS procedures are proving to have considerable potential for minimizing the physical and psychological loads on children patients with a view to facilitating faster and more favorable recovery outcomes. The successful application of these techniques is now widespread across various fields of surgery, including nephrolithiasis procedures and other urology procedures, which speaks to the overall trend towards the adoption of MIS in pediatric surgery that is not outside of current paradigms of patient treatment. Recent evidence from systematic reviews has reported trends of rising publication rates of minimally invasive pediatric kidney stone disease (KSD) treatment interventions. A literature systematic review over the past 16 years has recognized a significant increase in published studies on technologies such as ureteroscopy (URS), shockwave lithotripsy (SWL), and percutaneous nephrolithotomy (PCNL), among others. Of notable interest, however, is the advent of newer minimally invasive PCNL methods that have had a striking fivefold surge in publications concerning this intervention, as much a testament to increased awareness and practice of MIS in managing pediatric KSD (Aboumarzouk et al., 2017). The increasing trend in published literature not only signals a shift towards adopting minimally invasive approaches but also an investment into maximizing patient outcomes by enhanced procedural safety and efficiency, ultimately reshaping the management of complex cases in pediatric surgery. Additionally, the benefits of laparoscopic techniques extend beyond nephrolithiasis and encompass all pediatric surgical specialties. The integration of laparoscopic surgery has been said to have the capability to execute delicate intra-abdominal procedures with better precision, minimizing the dangers of traditional open techniques significantly. For example, the application of laparoscopic methods in liver transplantation has been a landmark that has benefited patients with essential advantages such as reduced postoperative morbidity and increased functional recovery (Berloco et al., 2012). These early applications are merely a part of the larger trend towards decreasing invasiveness in surgical interventions, all part of the broader goal of prioritizing patient safety and well-being. As pediatric surgery advances further in the direction of minimally invasive procedures, the need for ongoing research and development remains central to ensuring that surgical interventions are not only effective but also considerate of the unique needs of pediatric patients (Figure 8.9).

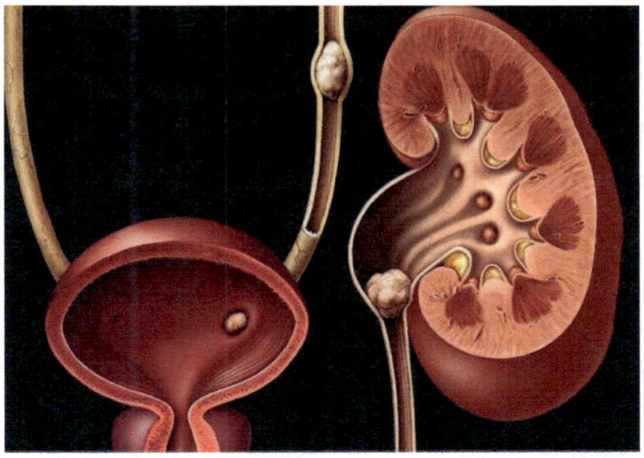

Figure 8.9. Paediatric kidney stone disease (KSD).

Source: https://www.mayoclinic.org/-/media/kcms/gbs/medical-professionals/images/2024/06/17/14/08/kidney-stones-767x535.jpg.

8.3.2. Robotic-Assisted Surgery

The evolution of robotic-assisted surgery (RAS) has transformed pediatric surgery in ways that are fundamental and far-reaching, extending enhancements explicitly designed for the anatomical and physiological specificity of children. Unlike traditional surgery, RAS employs enhanced accuracy and minimally invasive techniques that are particularly advantageous for pediatric patients, given their smaller and more delicate structures. This technology allows surgeons to be more nimble and perform more complex operations, thereby reducing tissue trauma and improving recovery. As a result, several pediatric procedures that once needed bigger incisions can now be performed using smaller ports, very much in keeping with the overall philosophy of pediatric surgery aimed at minimizing discomfort and postoperative complications. Guiding pediatric surgical practice with robotic technology requires not only technical expertise but also careful consideration of patient outcomes and safety. Evidence indicates that robotic surgery can lead to reduced operative time, reduced post-operative pain, and shorter hospital stays, hence enhancing the overall patient experience (Berloco et al., 2012). Moreover, the precision offered by robotic devices enables delicate dissection and suturing, most importantly, pediatric urologic and oncologic surgery.

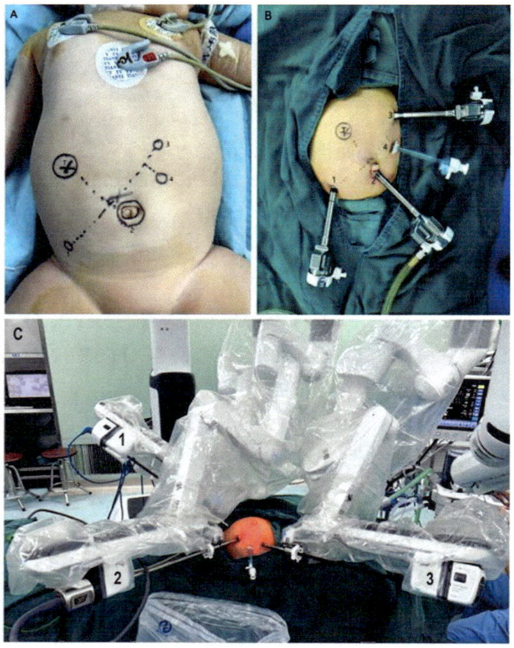

Figure 8.10. Robotic-assisted surgery of pediatric.

Source: https://media.springernature.com/lw685/springer-static/image/art%3A10.1186%2Fs12893-024-02625-7/MediaObjects/12893_2024_2625_Fig1_HTML.png.

Being able to see three-dimensional, high-definition images provides the surgeon with an unrivaled perspective of the operating field, enabling increased cooperation within the operating theater and leading to improved surgical outcomes. As pediatric surgery increasingly adopts robotic technology, research and development remain vital for addressing evolving surgical challenges and enhancing patient care. The prophesied benefits of robotic-assisted surgery are utilized across a host of specialisms, including gastrointestinal and thoracic surgery. Still, a cohesive understanding of its application in the pediatric community remains integral (Chan et al., 2016). Surgical training courses for building robotic system surgical skills are necessary to ensure that practitioners are adequately equipped to handle the complexity of the instruments. There is, hence, a common mandate among the medical community to share best practices, facilitate mentorship, and conduct extensive research that examines the long-term impacts of robotic-assisted surgeries on pediatric patient populations (Figure 8.10).

8.3.3. Advances in Anesthesia for Children

The face of pediatric anesthesia has undergone a massive transformation in recent years to enhance safety and efficiency in children who undergo surgery highly. At the core of such developments are technological advances in innovative airway management devices and techniques. Historically, securing the pediatric airway relied heavily on conventional methods employing tracheal intubation with a laryngoscope. However, in recent decades, specialized equipment has been designed to address the specific anatomical challenges of children, ranging from supraglottic airways to fiberoptic laryngoscopes. These have allowed anesthesiologists to handle challenging airway conditions effectively, enhancing perioperative care and outcome (Hammer et al., 2009). With technological improvements, the increased availability of newer imaging techniques also increases confidence in airway and patient safety management in pediatric surgery. Apart from airway management, the incorporation of regional anesthesia techniques has played a crucial role in creating pediatric anesthesia practice. The use of thoracic epidural analgesia has proven to be a beneficial technique, especially for the patient who has a low-level spina bifida condition. Recent studies have shown that epidural catheters can successfully reduce opioid consumption and improve pain relief following major surgeries, such as lower urinary tract reconstruction (Cain et al., 2018). Such benefits are crucial because pediatric patients are more susceptible to systemic opioid side effects. By facilitating proper pain control with less narcotic use, thoracic epidurals provide a two-fold advantage, allowing pediatric patients to postoperatively recover comfortably with fewer complications. This use of regional anesthesia is part of a broader trend toward multimodal pediatric surgical pain management. Furthermore, more research into emerging anesthetic technologies aims to tailor interventions for the pediatric patient even more precisely. Technologies such as fiber-optic cameras and video displays on a portable base enhance visualization in procedures, allowing for real-time assessment that can be applied for decision-making purposes (Hammer et al., 2009). Additionally, the availability of several more effective anesthetic agents makes tailoring of anesthesia protocols to specific patient needs easier. This patient-centered paradigm is fundamental within pediatric surgery, where developmental age, physiological variations, and customized medical histories each contribute importantly to treatment outcomes. Considered collectively, these advances demonstrate a commitment to improving the quality of care provided to children undergoing surgery, with safety and efficacy always at the forefront of pediatric anesthetic practice.

Test Your Knowledge

1. How has laparoscopic surgery improved recovery in pediatric patients?
2. What are the benefits of using robotic-assisted techniques in complex pediatric procedures?

8.4. Challenges in Pediatric Surgery

Learning Outcome

1. Identify the anatomical differences between children and adults
2. Define the psychological impact on young patients
3. Describe the ethical considerations in surgical decisions

The specialty of pediatric surgery presents a multifaceted set of challenges uniquely affected by the anatomical and physiological distinctions between child and adult physiology. One significant challenge is the minute dimensions and unusual developmental stages of pediatric patients, which render the surgical procedure more complicated. For instance, critical surgery in areas such as the inferior vena cava or the heart needs particular techniques and equipment tailored to the nuances of a child's anatomy. As illustrated by the abdominal tumor and simultaneous thrombus case, technical challenges of surgery are compounded by the need for cardiopulmonary bypass, posing additional risks such as overwhelming bleeding and undue anesthesia time (Li et al., 2025). This subtle interaction between surgical achievement and complication avoidance is characteristic of pediatric surgery. Another frequent pediatric surgical problem is the management of postoperative recovery and care, which has a very different approach in children compared to adults. Because of their ongoing growth and development, children will have a differing response to surgeries, such that individualized management of post-surgical monitoring and rehabilitation is necessary. Complication risks, such as anesthesia reactions or infections, can be heightened as an after-effect of the immaturity of their organ systems. In addition, recovery times can differ widely depending on the individual child's health status and the type of surgery performed.

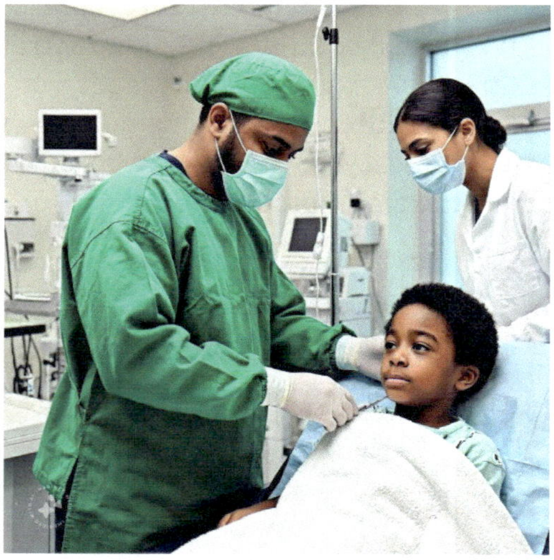

Figure 8.11. Challenges in pediatric surgery.

Source: https://www.hi-techhospital.in/blogs/wp-content/uploads/2024/11/WhatsApp-Image-2024-11-29-at-4.52.52-PM.jpeg.

The outcomes of complex operations emphasize the importance of careful postoperative planning and follow-up management, which are crucial to achieving optimal recovery and preventing long-term complications (Li et al., 2025). In addition to physiological concerns, psychological factors also play a significant role in pediatric surgery, affecting both the patient and their family. The anxiety that children feel when undergoing surgery can be profound, requiring processes of communication and emotional reassurance to calm fears and establish trust. Moreover, the involvement of guardians during the procedure is essential as their knowledge and explanations can significantly help shape a child's experience. The evolution of techniques in pediatric cataract surgery, for example, illustrates a broader trend towards more patient-centered care with family participation in decision-making. Psychological issues are not only made easier with improved surgical treatment for pediatric patients, but also general health outcomes following surgery are prioritized, with a suggestion towards a holistic approach for pediatric surgery (Figure 8.11).

8.4.1. Anatomical Differences Between Children and Adults

The pediatric/adult anatomical differences are profound and have very significant implications in pediatric surgery. A fundamental aspect of these differences is anatomical structure, size, and shape, particularly in the respiratory system. In pediatrics, the airway is relatively small and compliant, and this places them at risk for respiratory complications such as obstructive sleep apnea syndrome (OSAS). The greater prevalence of OSAS in children, particularly between the ages of 2 and 8 years, highlights the peculiarities of their upper airway, such as adenoid size, which typically results in airway obstruction. Although adult OSAS is well understood, the idiosyncratic presentation in children necessitates specialized diagnostic approaches and therapeutic strategies that consider these anatomical aspects to reduce complications and improve operative results (Bellini et al., 2019). In addition to respiratory concerns, the pediatric musculoskeletal system also differs markedly from that of adults. Children possess developing growth plates that produce unique patterns of injury and healing.

Children's fractures, for instance, preferentially occur near growth plates, and the risk for growth disturbance complicates treatment planning. Conventional injury severity scoring systems, primarily used in adults, often fail to account for these differences and can lead to erroneous medical decisions. Injury severity scoring system development for the pediatric patient can more accurately guide surgical intervention, with the guarantee that the delivered intervention is tailored to the specific developmental level of the patient. This need for personalized assessment tools highlights the importance of understanding anatomical variation when planning surgical interventions in children (Aber et al., 2016).

Finally, variations in organ function and size between adults and children need careful attention in surgical approaches. Organs such as the liver and kidneys in children are relatively smaller in relation to body size, which affects drug and anesthetic dosing calculations. Further, the body's response to surgical stress, including inflammatory and healing processes, may differ considerably between these two populations. Consequently, procedures employed during surgery must be adapted to the child's individual anatomical and physiological characteristics to minimize peril. This requires ongoing research and innovation in the field of pediatric surgery to develop procedures that take these differences into consideration, thereby enhancing safety and efficacy in surgical procedures for younger patients. Understanding the relationship between these anatomical differences and surgical methods is an essential in maximizing outcomes in pediatric surgery patients.

8.4.2. Psychological Effect on Adolescent Patients

Patients who are young and being operated upon often experience severe psychological consequences that may impact their health as well as healing. Surgery-induced stress can express itself in various ways, including fear of the unknown, fear of being separated from caregivers, and anxiety due to postoperative pain. This emotional distress is not only confined to the children. Still, it is also seen to affect their families, particularly mothers, who are at risk of high levels of anxiety and depression during such a critical time. Research indicates that mothers of babies with complex medical conditions, such as those with single-ventricle disease, have substantially higher scores on measures of depression and anxiety than normative samples. By addressing these psychological problems with targeted interventions, medical providers can potentially mitigate maternal distress while improving maternal and child outcomes during the course of the surgery (Aiyagari et al., 2018). More recent emphasis has been placed on pediatric intervention for preoperative anxiety relief. Procedures such as clown therapy have been studied, whereby professional clowns interact with children before surgery. One study found that despite the interventions failing to exhibit any discernible decrease in the anxiety of children, they played a significant role in lowering the anxiety of caregivers. Caregivers felt less stressed, which may have a positive impact on their children by offering them a more comforting and stress-free environment during the operation. In addition, caregivers' satisfaction with such interventions suggests that the addition of these strategies will enhance the overall surgical procedure for young patients and thus provide a more holistic care approach in pediatric surgery (Arriaga et al., 2016).

In addition to the preoperative anxiety, the psychological impact of surgery on young patients impacts post-operative recovery as well. The children's psychological status potentially influences their rating of pain and satisfaction with care, and, therefore, prior and post-operative psychological management is necessary. Interventions such as early palliative care introduction in newborn babies with severe medical conditions show that identification of and intervention into parental anxiety may lead to overall improved family functioning and improved communication. By encouraging positive coping mechanisms and enhancing familial relationships, healthcare workers can minimize the psychological effects of surgery, thus improving pathways to recovery for young patients (Aiyagari et al., 2018) (Figure 8.12).

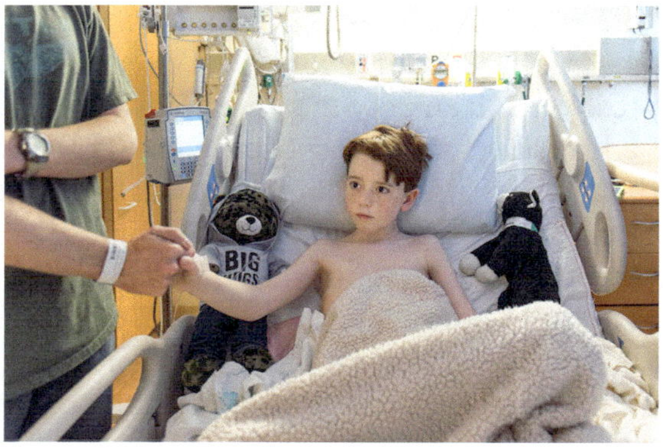

Figure 8.12. Psychological impact on young patients.

Source: https://media.npr.org/assets/img/2016/06/22/distraction-7_edited_custom-8892c2b8d8f4c2049dc810dd5034d7d71de64a3d.jpg?s=1100&c=50&f=jpeg.

8.4.3. Ethical Considerations in Surgical Decisions

In pediatric surgery, ethical implications are paramount in decision-making because the patient population is vulnerable. Surgeons must balance the potential good of surgical procedures with the risks associated with them, particularly when they are operating on children who may not comprehend or may not be able to give proper consent to their procedure. Such ethical subtlety is further compounded by asking parents or guardians to provide informed consent, at times under conditions of stress when the best interest of the child must be the primary consideration. Ethical considerations, such as the principles of beneficence, non-maleficence, autonomy, and justice, must be well-balanced in all instances of surgery. This suggests that pediatric surgeons are not only tasked with medical capability but also with an ethical responsibility to engage in serious conversations with families, ensuring they understand the risks and benefits of the operation that will impact the child's future health experiences. Equally important is the realization that medical decision-making, especially in disorders of sex development (DSD), must be multidisciplinary in scope, affirming ethical values throughout the planning of surgery. Involvement of specialists, ranging from endocrinologists to psychologists, provides a comprehensive understanding of the patient's individual condition. As highlighted in the management of ambiguous genitalia in a multidisciplinary team environment, ethical issues extend beyond the immediate surgical outcome to include long-term implications on the quality of life of the individuals.

This combined effort, taking into consideration both medical and psychosocial factors, underscores the need for an approach to shared decision-making that respects the desires of the child and their family while upholding the highest standards of professionalism. Informed consent must be an accurate representation of the challenges and choices ahead, and thus, the role of the multidisciplinary team becomes critical in providing ethical pediatric care. Additionally, the ethical climate in pediatric surgery is ever-changing with advances in technology and social trends in values towards healthcare. The introduction of new operating methods and the increased emphasis on health-related quality of life raise subtle ethical concerns, particularly in non-life-threatening surgeries. Requiring evaluations of the potential impacts of operations on a child's overall health necessitates that surgeons remain current regarding the latest research and outcomes of various interventions. For instance, the improvements of patient quality of life measures are indicative of the increasing emphasis on valuing patient experience as more than mere clinical results, and hence surgeons consider their operative choices' short-term impact on the child's overall well-being (Stevens, 2025). With such ethical issues in transition, it is essential that participants in pediatric surgery continue to learn and reflect on their practice to ensure that what they do remains consonant with changing expectations for the ethical provision of care and patient advocacy (Achermann et al., 2010).

Test Your Knowledge

1. How does the small size and fragility of pediatric patients affect surgical technique?
2. What ethical issues commonly arise in decision-making for pediatric surgical care?

8.5. Postoperative Care in Pediatric Patients

Learning Outcome

1. Describe the pain management strategies
2. Define the monitoring for pediatric surgery
3. Discuss the importance of family involvement in recovery

Pediatric postoperative care is a crucial component of surgical care with significant implications for recovery. Postoperatively, children are at great risk of complications due to physiological variations from the adult population. Effective postoperative monitoring plays a crucial role in the early detection of complications, such as respiratory distress or infection. The application of formal measurements, including the Vasoactive-Ventilation-Renal score, has been valuable in predicting cardiac surgery complications in neonates. Not only does this provide a valid method of measuring severity, but it also allows for timely interventions that can decrease mechanical ventilation length to a lesser degree, thereby enhancing recovery patterns (Cashen et al., 2018). Optimizing postoperative care with these devices enables healthcare providers to personalize management strategies tailored to the specific needs of pediatric patients, ultimately improving overall clinical outcomes. Pain management in pediatric patients following surgery is essential in facilitating recovery and enhancing the quality of care. The ESPA Pain Committee has built a Pain Management Ladder for facilitating the provision of analgesia across a variety of surgical procedures. This expert-consensus, evidence-based system provides support for administering a baseline level of pain care in children that can be tailored to the nature and complexity of the surgery performed (Adamek et al., 2018). By controlling pain effectively with evidence-based practices, healthcare professionals can minimize distress, facilitating earlier mobilization, improved feeding, and shorter hospital stays. Therefore, the inclusion of systemic pain management algorithms is a critical component of maximizing the postoperative experience for pediatric patients, ultimately leading to patient satisfaction with recovery and physical well-being. Furthermore, the psychological and emotional components of pediatric postoperative care should not be overlooked. Hospitalization and surgery are inherently intimidating and anxiety-evoking for children and, therefore, potential complicators of recovery and lengtheners of hospitalization. Effective communication with the child and their family is consequently critical to avoiding these psychological problems. The use of child-centered approaches, such as maintaining a regular environment, play therapy, and involving families in care plans, greatly enhances children's emotional resilience during recovery. Additionally, the interdisciplinary postoperative care approach, which involves pediatric nurses, child life specialists, and psychologists, ensures comprehensive physical and emotional rehabilitation. Therefore, integrating psychological support into postoperative plans ultimately results in quicker recovery and increased satisfaction with the surgical procedure, illustrating the importance of balanced care protocols in pediatric surgery (Figure 8.13).

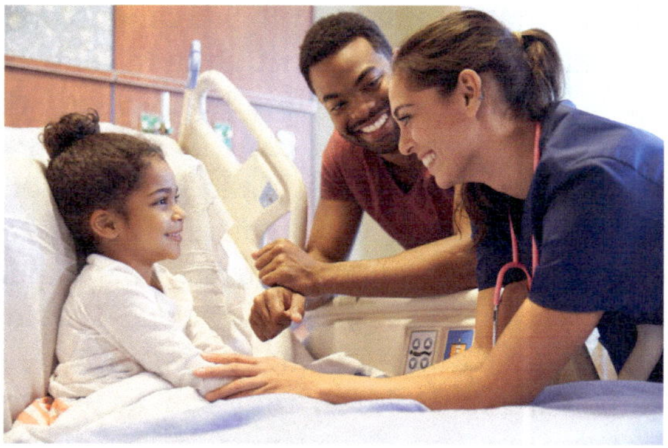

Figure 8.13. Preoperative and postoperative care.

Source: https://www.newarkadvocate.com/gcdn/presto/2021/10/15/PNEW/66047610-9b7b-458e-bda7-f8e401c09fed-Active_Fit_Surgery.jpg.

8.5.1. Pain Management Strategies

Effective pain management strategies are crucial in pediatric surgery to minimize pain and facilitate recovery. Increasing evidence favors the use of enhanced recovery after surgery (ERAS) protocols, with a focus on multimodal pain management, as a method to facilitate improved postoperative recovery in children. The strategies involve the implementation of a combination of analgesics, along with non-pharmacological interventions specifically tailored to the child's special needs. For instance, combining opioids with non-steroidal anti-inflammatory drugs (NSAIDs) will optimize pain control while minimizing opioid-induced side effects. Additionally, the psychological aspect of pain can be explored by management strategies, such as involving the family in care, and constructing a positive environment that optimizes the effectiveness of pain management procedures. However, their current application within pediatric facilities remains limited, underscoring the need for broader research and implementation in this critical area of surgical practice (Kim et al., 2024).

Non-pharmacological interventions are often employed in conjunction with pharmacological interventions in the management of pain for pediatric surgical patients. Among the methods employed are hypnosis, which has gained attention due to the fact that it successfully reduces procedural pain without the adverse impact of pharmacological interventions. Studies have identified hypnosis, particularly administered over the course of multiple sessions before surgery, as an effective means of lowering levels of pain when compared with traditional methods of care. The findings suggest that these psychological interventions can be especially beneficial in simpler surgical interventions where there is a higher risk of anxiety and pain awareness. Although the existing literature identifies the possibility of hypnosis in the control of pain in children, the natural constraints need consideration, including bias in study design and the demands for rigorous controls. Working towards customizing these interventions to their optimal effect on children who are about to have an operation (Elkins et al., 2014). Lastly, proactive application of multimodal pain management with both pharmacological and non-pharmacological methods is necessary to improve the operating room experience in children. The combined method not only tackles the physical aspects of pain but also considers emotional and psychological elements that may influence pain experience and recovery. As research matures, greater attention will have to be placed on tailoring pain management guidelines to the unique demands of pediatric populations. Health care professionals must advocate for early intervention practices that facilitate effective pain management, enhanced communication with families, and the implementation of creative strategies. Such a commitment to maximizing pain control in pediatric surgery will lead to improved patient satisfaction and overall health outcomes, resulting in a more healing-promoting environment (Kim et al., 2024) (Figure 8.14).

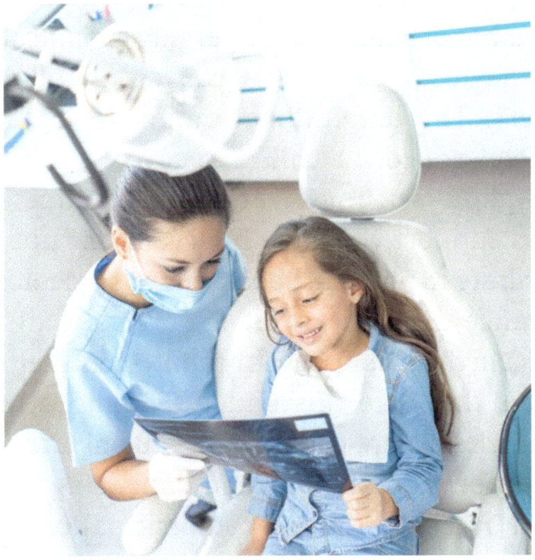

Figure 8.14. Using non-pharmacological behaviour management techniques.

Source: https://media.springernature.com/full/springer-static/image/art%3A10.1038%2Fs41406-021-0268-5/MediaObjects/41406_2021_268_Fig1_HTML.jpg.

8.5.2. Monitoring for Complications

Complication monitoring is crucial in children's surgery to ensure optimal patient outcomes. Due to the unique physiological characteristics of children, as well as the potential for instantaneous changes in their clinical status, close monitoring must be maintained during the perioperative period. Multidisciplinary vigilance, involving contributions from surgeons, anesthesiologists, nurses, and other healthcare personnel, must be employed to recognize warning signs of potential complications. Appropriate monitoring can significantly reduce the risks of surgery, with advancements in technology enabling the detection of complications to occur much faster. This combination of innovative monitoring methods, such as constant pulse oximetry and sophisticated hemodynamic monitoring, has transformed care for pediatric surgery, enabling more precise interventions to meet the specific needs of younger patients. Postoperative complications have been reported to play a significant role in recovery and long-term prognosis in children. These can include respiratory distress, infection, and cardiovascular instability secondary to existing conditions, the complexity of the procedure, or the risk associated with anesthesia. For instance, as pointed out by Li et al. (2025), preoperative assessment can be effective in identifying high-risk patients who may be more susceptible to such complications. Having standardized postoperative monitoring practices provides a blueprint for healthcare practitioners to systematically assess the well-being of the pediatric patient while undergoing the critical recovery phase. Early detection of complications not only enhances patient safety but also helps meet the overall goal of improving surgical outcomes and reducing healthcare burdens. Moreover, research and development of monitoring practice must also be ongoing to optimize results in pediatric operating settings. As targeted in research, patient-centered interventions, such as inspiratory muscle training and targeted postoperative management, enhance patient resilience and outcomes with a decrease in complications (Ahmed et al., 2025). Continuously evaluated are the practices that inform evidence-based monitoring strategies to ensure patient care is maintained in accordance with the latest advancements in medical science. Additionally, establishing guidelines for educating healthcare workers on effective monitoring procedures will foster a culture of safety in pediatric surgery. By doing this, monitoring for complications proves to be more than just a procedural courtesy; it becomes an active and inherent aspect of delivering high-quality pediatric surgical care.

8.5.3. Importance of Family Involvement in Recovery

The role of family involvement in recovery processes, particularly that of children's surgery, cannot be overemphasized. When children undergo surgeries, their emotional and psychological states are very much related to the supportive mechanisms of their families. According to studies, children with supportive families have less anxiety before and after operations, which can actually lead to smoother recovery processes. Effective family participation fosters a healing environment through which parents and caregivers can engage in caregiving rituals and reinforce positive behaviors essential to the recovery process. Further, families can serve as advocates by holding sophisticated healthcare systems accountable, ensuring their child gets the best postoperative care and thus enhancing overall rates of recovery. In addition to providing emotional support, family members often also act as facilitators to bridge the gaps between children and healthcare providers. Open communication regularly reassures children to express their fears and concerns about operations and post-operative life, which can go a long way towards shaping recovery. The integration of family life into care strategies not only helps fulfill the child's immediate needs but also guides interventions that are relevant to the family's beliefs and way of doing things. Pediatric programs have gradually recognized the importance of integrating family training so that they can become effective collaborators in therapeutic interventions. For instance, teletherapy therapies, as noted in the literature, emphasize the importance of long-term family engagement, promoting lasting impacts on a child's recovery process, particularly in feeding and developmental components (Luke et al., 2016).

Family engagement is not only important during the early post-surgical period of healing but also for achieving long-term health outcomes. Continuing support and active participation in postoperative follow-up care enable families to monitor and manage any emerging complications or behavioral issues that can occur following surgery. The longitudinal emphasis of family participation on a child's recovery trajectory is aligned with converging evidence that shows supportive family interventions not only contribute to physical health but to psychological resilience as well. Pediatric surgical units are increasingly advocating for family-centered care models that take this understanding to heart. These models are capable of reducing the work burden of readmissions and enhancing overall health outcomes among pediatric patients, and therefore create a collaborative model that is essential in modern healthcare. Family input is thus needed as they still influence recovery processes long after the physical sites of the surgical environment (King et al., 2017).

Test Your Knowledge

1. How is pain assessed and managed in non-verbal pediatric patients after surgery?
2. What are the key signs of postoperative infection in children?

8.6. Future Directions in Pediatric Surgery

Learning Outcome

1. Describe the research and development in surgical techniques
2. Define the role of technology in pediatric surgery
3. Identify the training and education required for future surgeons

As pediatric surgery continues to progress, future directions are more focused on newer techniques and technologies that yield improved patient outcomes. Tissue engineering, specifically tracheal reconstruction, is one such area of development. Traditional methods, such as tracheal resection, are limited in that the longest resectable segment in children is significantly shorter compared to adults. This has led researchers to investigate the construction of synthetic scaffolds and decellularized organs that would potentially provide a better alternative to children suffering from airway diseases. The ideal tracheal scaffold would require multiple needs such as mechanical stability, biocompatibility, and the ability to accommodate vascular invasion, along with remaining pliable enough to accommodate normal airway function. Subsequently, further research on hybrid scaffolds, which potentially combine the strengths of these two novel techniques, will be at the forefront of pediatric airway surgical interventions (Birchall et al., 2016). Additionally, advancements in extracorporeal membrane oxygenation (ECMO) technology will revolutionize pediatric surgery. As a lifesaving backup system for acute cardiac and respiratory failure, ECMO has already seen high survival rates in infants and children, redefining the prognosis of irreversible lung injury. The future may hold the prospect of self-contained ECMO systems being used beyond intensive care units, allowing for greater patient management flexibility. These developments would not only decrease the load on healthcare facilities but also lay the groundwork for home-care systems, greatly benefiting the quality of life for pediatric patients undergoing surgery. International cooperation, as exemplified by conferences such as the International Conference of ECMO-Life Support for Pakistan in the 21st Century, reflects the world's dedication towards the formulation of ECMO procedures and maintaining healthcare levels in the developing world (Elahi et al., 2017). Furthermore, the integration of minimally invasive surgical techniques is also changing the face of pediatric surgery. The and methods not only reduce recovery periods but also reduce risks of complications associated with open surgeries. Robotic-assisted surgery is also an emerging future trend that can enhance precision, minimize intraoperative blood loss, and reduce pediatric patient hospitalization times. As pediatric patients are defined by a complex set of anatomical and physiological differences, continuous development of these methods, tailored particularly for children, remains an area of critical importance. A dialogue between pediatric surgeons, engineers, and technology developers is required to overcome current limitations and optimize new surgical approaches, making them effective and safe for children. This confluence of advances heralds a brighter future for pediatric surgery, where innovation leads to improved care and outcomes for children (Figure 8.15).

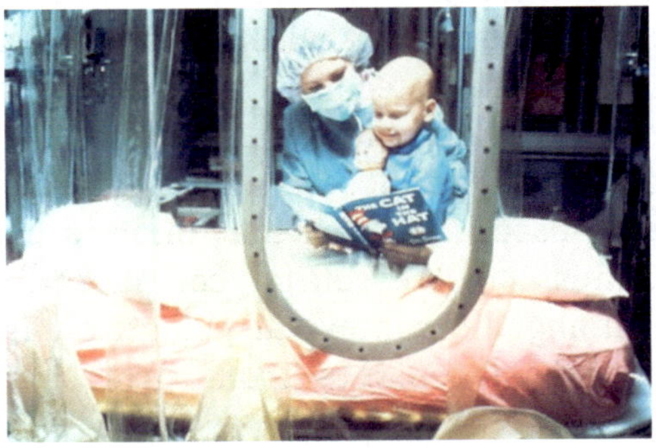

Figure 8.15. The future of pediatric surgery.

Source: https://images.unsplash.com/photo-

1631201036665-35d8815f97e8?crop=entropy&cs=tinysrgb&fit=max&fm=jpg&ixid=M3w3MDgyMDR8MHwxfHNlYXJjaHwxfHxwZWRpYXRyaWMlMjBzdXJnZXJ5JTIwdHJlbmRzJTJDJTIwaW5ub3ZhdGlvbnMlMjBpbiUyMHBlZGlhdHJpYyUyMGNhcmUlMjBmdXR1cmUlMjBvZiUyMHBlZGlhdHJpYyUyMHN1cmdlcnl8ZW58MHwwfHx8MTc0OTkxMzc5NXww&ixlib=rb-4.1.0&q=80&w=500&?utm_source=numberanalytics&utm_medium=referral.

8.6.1. Research and Development in Surgical Techniques

The evolution of surgical techniques within pediatric surgery has been significantly influenced by research and advances in technology. As more surgeons work to maximize patient outcomes, the adoption of minimally invasive techniques has gained momentum. These procedures, including laparoscopic approaches, not only reduce the recovery time but also decrease post-operative complications. Research has shown that these approaches lead to improved visualization and precision in surgery, enabling more delicate dissection and tissue removal in children. Further investigation into robotic-assisted surgery is another ideal example of where technology and patient care intersect. The increased dexterity and three-dimensional vision provided by robots are proving invaluable, particularly in delicate anatomical environments typical of children. As these technologies advance, there are encouraging avenues to improving surgical outcomes and patient satisfaction. Additionally, evidence-based research that informs clinical guidelines is an essential consideration in determining the context of pediatric surgery. Consensus statements from professionals, such as those developed for handling complex conditions like Mucopolysaccharidosis (MPS) VI and MPS IVA, indicate the need for standardized care protocols. These suggestions, developed by multidisciplinary groups of experts and guided by patient representatives, aim to promote uniform and widespread approaches to treatment. The consensus reached through modified-Delphi processes reflects evidence of meeting the challenge of clinical demands while incorporating patients' perspectives. For instance, consensus guidelines for anesthetic management and preoperative surgical planning of such rare disorders illustrate the need for specialist strategies that can have significant impacts on surgical outcomes and children's quality of life. Such consensus guidelines are essential to ensure not only the optimization of clinical effectiveness but also models of caring collaboration. Moreover, the demand for ongoing pediatric surgery research cannot be overstressed. With increasingly sophisticated surgery, the demand for robust evidence to confirm procedural efficacy and safety increases. Observational studies and clinical trials conducted in pediatric populations shed light on best practices and indicate areas for development. Evaluating long-term outcomes of intervention, as with the development of guidelines for MPS disorders, underscores the necessity for continued research. It is these efforts that will bridge knowledge gaps and keep the practice of medicine abreast of emerging science. Lastly, the interplay of research, technological innovation, and standardized guidelines sets the stage for pediatric surgical breakthroughs, paving the way for a future where surgery is safer, more efficient, and patient-centered.

8.6.2. The Role of Technology in Enhancing Outcomes

The use of software technology in pediatric surgery has significantly transformed patient care, leading to improved clinical outcomes. One of the most important innovations is the creation of Pediatric Early Warning systems (PEWs) that enable healthcare providers to identify deteriorating states of children quickly admitted into hospitals. With improved early recognition via structured screening, PEWs have been associated with reduced Pediatric Index of Mortality (PIM2) and the need for invasive intervention like ventilatory support. This modification not only minimizes ICU stays but also reduces total bed occupancy, thereby optimizing the utilization of hospital beds. Better outcomes, such as reduced PICU lengths of stay and other similar improvements, show the significant role technology plays in today's pediatric surgical practices, and ultimately benefit patient and healthcare system demands. Moreover, technology's role extends beyond monitoring systems; it also encompasses rehabilitation processes. In pediatric posterior fossa tumor surgery, several developments have enabled the personalization of the treatment process. A recent e-survey indicated that physiotherapists use a wide range of modern interventions, including balance rehabilitation and gait re-education, to manage ataxia among children. The use of adjuncts, such as mobility aids and orthotics, has also increased these rehabilitation processes. But issues such as a shortage of physiotherapy after discharge highlight the need for sustained technological support and evidence-based treatment. The use of technology to aid physiotherapy not only facilitates the rehabilitation process but sets the stage for continued research into improved outcomes for this at-risk population, demonstrating another way technology creates positive outcomes in pediatric surgery. Besides improving immediate clinical outcomes and rehabilitation, the use of technology enhances communication and data management among healthcare providers. Effective systems of communication, backed by technological advances, enable the open flow of information among the specialists involved in pediatric surgery. An interdisciplinary approach guarantees a smooth flow of information among all members, such as surgeons, anesthetists, and physiotherapists, so that they may design and execute care strategies in sync. EHR implementation enhances document availability and facilitates real-time updates of patient status, which is critical for timely decision-making in ever-changing clinical settings. With pediatric surgical practice ongoing in the face of these advances in technology, the common goal remains the same: to leverage technology not only to streamline processes but also to achieve the highest level of care and improve outcomes for pediatric patients (Figure 8.16).

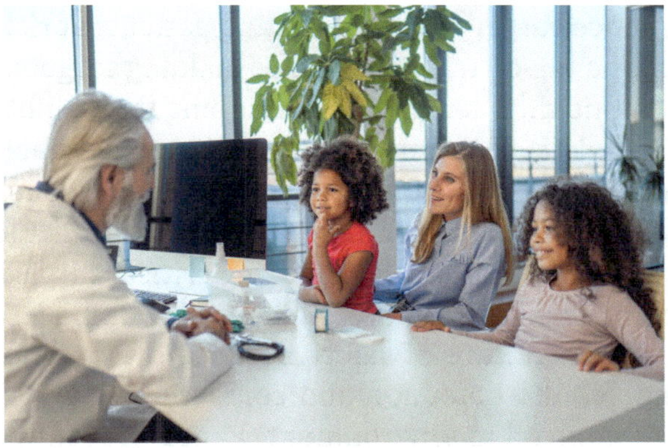

Figure 8.16. Pediatric HER.

Source: https://www.itransition.com/static/744cb15bf717d94466d23050d0c5de37/70a8e/iStock-1356160972.jpg.

8.6.3. Training and Education for Future Surgeons

The dynamic pediatric surgery environment demands an efficient training and education framework for the next generation of surgeons. The complexity of the surgery on children, along with their unique physiological and psychological difficulties, highlights the necessity for comprehensive training programs. In addition to technical skills, surgical education must also involve interdisciplinary approaches to training the next generation of surgeons, not only in the operating room but also in team environments with pediatricians, anesthesiologists, and nurses. Such an overall emphasis on surgical education is consonant with more recent programs that encourage teamwork and communication among various medical specialties integral to the management of complex pediatric cases. Through the enhancement of these models of education, new surgeons can safely navigate the intricacies present in pediatric surgical practice, ultimately leading to improved patient care quality and safety. Simulation-based training has been viewed as one of the significant advances in pediatric surgeon education for the future. Simulators and virtual reality systems provide real-time environments where residents can practice surgery without putting patients at risk. This hands-on training enables budding surgeons to refine their technique, developing their ability through repetition and immediate feedback. More recent studies have found that such novel training can enhance cognitive recall and decision-making abilities during critical surgical moments. Furthermore, simulation training also fosters a culture of safety because the practice enables the detection and correction of errors in a controlled environment, hence preventing future surgeons from facing difficulties in actual operating rooms. With the inclusion of these high-tech teaching tools, prospective pediatric surgeons are adequately skilled with the technical skills and confidence necessary for them to succeed. Moreover, mentorship also plays a significant role in the training of future surgeons. Healthy mentor-mentee relationships can strongly support learning among surgical residents. Experienced surgeons can provide insight, not only in technical skill but also in the management of the nuances of patient interactions and multidisciplinary teamwork. A model of mentorship enables the sharing of tacit knowledge, which cannot be easily taught in a formal classroom setting, allowing for the development of individual attributes such as resilience and flexibility. In ensuring that mentorship is encouraged among surgical residency programs, it is, consequently, crucial, particularly in pediatric surgery, where there are high stakes and emotional intelligence is essential. Establishing effective mentorship networks can enhance the psychosocial well-being of trainees, leading to increased job satisfaction and retention in the high-stress practice of pediatric surgery.

Test Your Knowledge

1. How might tissue engineering impact the treatment of congenital anomalies in the future?
2. What role is artificial intelligence expected to play in improving pediatric surgical outcomes?

SUMMARY

In pediatric surgery, the general finding emphasizes the necessity of making pre-operative education a central part of patient care. Evidence suggests that this form of education is most effective in enhancing patient outcomes, resulting in higher recovery rates and increased patient and family satisfaction. In a Saudi Arabian study, for instance, it was found that children who underwent pre-operative education showed remarkable improvement in achieving their surgical procedure and managing post-surgical pain, as knowledgeable patients typically have smoother recovery courses (Alhajjaj et al., 2024). Thus, the imperative to integrate formal preoperative education programs is clear; these not only explain procedures but also foster a trusting relationship between the patient and healthcare providers. Robotic surgical techniques are also a primary advancement in pediatric surgery, particularly for complex procedures such as those involving Hirschsprung disease or inflammatory bowel disease. New systematic review results indicate that robot-assisted procedures have remarkable benefits, including greater accuracy and a reduced rate of complications compared to conventional techniques (Prato et al., 2024). Despite having positive evidence to support robotic operations, the cost and specific training required remain common barriers to their widespread application. Hence, there has to be a concerted effort to overcome these challenges to expand the field of robot-assisted surgery in the healthcare of children and grant children the safest and best means of treatment. Ultimately, the future of pediatric surgery lies not merely in technological advancement but in comprehensive patient management, including education and psycho-support. By prioritizing preoperative education, clinicians can significantly improve patient satisfaction and postoperative success. Ongoing research into robotic surgery could revolutionize the treatment of complex disease scenarios. As the field continues to evolve, an ongoing investment in clinician and patient education will become imperative. These two strategies together create a path toward improved quality care, ultimately offering the possibility of a brighter future for children placed under the knife. The integration of modern surgical methods with a well-developed educational system will undoubtedly contribute to the continued success and growth of pediatric surgery as a whole.

When considering pediatric surgery, several key issues emerge that underscore its significance within the broader surgical context. A key aspect is the unique physiological and anatomical considerations that distinguish pediatric patients from adults. Children have unique tissue reactions, metabolic rates, and recovery courses that necessitate unique surgical approaches. As emphasized in surgery literature, these aspects need to be understood to deliver optimal results in pediatric surgeries. Also, the daily psychological and emotional development of children complicates surgery; hence, the ability of a pediatric surgeon does not solely lie in the technical field of surgery but also encompasses effective child-oriented preoperative management and good communication (Slade, 2015). By having the ability to engage children and their families in the surgery, anxiety is greatly diminished, and compliance is improved, which can travel far in influencing postoperative recovery. Another critical factor in the area of pediatric surgery is the development of minimally invasive techniques, which are revolutionizing surgical practice for children. Not only do these techniques reduce the recovery time, but they also lower the risk of complications arising from larger incisions, which is particularly useful in a pediatric setting. Other advances, such as robotic and laparoscopic surgery, reflect the shift towards minimally invasive procedures that have proven successful in a variety of surgical interventions, from appendectomies to more complex surgical corrections. Additionally, technological innovations and instrumentation continue to refine precision and reduce intraoperative trauma, reflecting the impetus for ongoing research and education in the field of pediatric surgery (Lung, 2014). Consequently, the convergence of such sophisticated methods is vital in maximizing the outcomes of surgery and minimizing the long-term impact of surgical interventions on children's health. Finally, the multi-professional nature of pediatric surgical management cannot be emphasized enough, as the maximum outcome is usually a product of multidisciplinary teamwork. Surgeons, anesthesiologists, nurses, and allied healthcare professionals must work together to synchronize care pre-operatively, intra-operatively, and post-operatively. A multidisciplinary approach ensures that the individual needs of each child are addressed comprehensively and all components of the care are optimized for successful recovery. Most importantly, the involvement of families as intrinsic partners in the care process fosters a supportive culture, enabling better compliance with postoperative care. As continued development in healthcare systems unfolds, effective communication with staff and families becomes increasingly important, establishing the need for effective strategies to facilitate this cooperation in the practice of pediatric surgery (Slade, 2015).

KEY TERMS FROM THIS CHAPTER

- Choledochal cyst
- Congenital diaphragmatic hernia
- Hirschsprung's disease
- Imperforate anus
- Minimally invasive pediatric surgery
- Neuroblastoma
- Pediatric appendicitis
- Pediatric trauma management
- Congenital anomalies
- Gastroschisis
- Hypospadias
- Intussusception
- Neonatal intestinal obstruction
- Omphalocele
- Pediatric hernia repair
- Posterior urethral valves

CRITICAL THINKING QUESTIONS

1. **Which of the following is the most common type of tracheoesophageal fistula (TEF)?**
   a. Isolated tracheoesophageal fistula
   b. Esophageal atresia with proximal fistula
   c. Esophageal atresia with distal fistula
   d. H-type fistula
2. **The classic "olive-shaped" mass in the right upper quadrant of an infant suggests:**
   a. Intussusception
   b. Hypertrophic pyloric stenosis
   c. Duodenal atresia
   d. Umbilical hernia
3. **Which investigation confirms the diagnosis of Hirschsprung's disease?**
   a. Abdominal ultrasound
   b. Barium enema
   c. Rectal biopsy
   d. Plain abdominal X-ray
4. **In intussusception, which sign is typically seen on ultrasound?**
   a. Double bubble sign
   b. String sign
   c. Target sign (or doughnut sign)
   d. Gasless abdomen
5. **At what age is surgical correction of an undescended testis (orchidopexy) ideally performed?**
   a. At birth
   b. By 6 months
   c. Between 6–12 months
   D. After puberty

Short Answer Questions

1. What is the most common cause of abdominal mass in neonates?
2. At what age is orchidopexy ideally performed for an undescended testis?
3. What is the diagnostic imaging of choice for hypertrophic pyloric stenosis?
4. Name two cardinal symptoms of Hirschsprung's disease.
5. What is the most common type of tracheoesophageal fistula?
6. Which sign on an abdominal X-ray is suggestive of duodenal atresia?
7. What is the typical age group affected by intussusception, and what is its classical presentation?
8. What are the components of the VACTERL association?

Answers to Critical Thinking Questions

1. (c); 2. (b); 3. (c); 4. (c); 5. (c)

REFERENCES

1. Aber, R. (2016). *Improving health literacy: Parental medical decisions regarding lower extremity amputations.* https://core.ac.uk/download/84402968.pdf (accessed on 12th July 2025).
2. Pietropaolo, A., Proietti, S., Jones, P., Rangarajan, K., Aboumarzouk, O., Giusti, G., & Somani, B. K. (2017). Trends of intervention for paediatric stone disease over the last two decades (2000–2015): A systematic review of literature. *Arab Journal of Urology, 15*(4), 306–311. https://doi.org/10.1016/j.aju.2017.10.006Achermann, J. C., Barnicoat, A., Brain, C. E., Carmichael, O., et al. (2010). *Holistic management of DSD.* https://core.ac.uk/download/1854753.pdf (accessed on 12th July 2025).
3. Adamek, D., Al-Zaben, F., Alm, J., Amminnikutty, M., Amoli, M., Anderson, P., et al. (2018). *Postoperative pain management in children: Guidance from the Pain Committee of the European Society for Pediatric Anesthesiology (ESPA Pain Management Ladder Initiative).* https://core.ac.uk/download/157582937.pdf (accessed on 12th July 2025).
4. Ahmed, M. A. K., Bahurmuz, M. A., & Muthanna, F. M. S. (2025). *General anesthesia in cardiac surgery: A narrative review for evolving techniques and patient-centered best practices. Yemeni Journal for Medical Sciences.* https://www.semanticscholar.org/paper/b9f20626e344f524ee83d5ae25eff4809116ebe2 (accessed on 12th July 2025).
5. Aiyagari, R., Bhat, P., Donohue, J., Fifer, C., et al. (2018). *A randomized trial of early palliative care for maternal stress in infants prenatally diagnosed with single-ventricle heart disease.* https://core.ac.uk/download/212864275.pdf (accessed on 12th July 2025).
6. Akyol, M. U., Alden, T. D., Amartino, H., Ashworth, J., et al. (2019). *Recommendations for the management of MPS VI: Systematic evidence- and consensus-based guidance.* https://core.ac.uk/download/323074857.pdf (accessed on 12th July 2025).
7. Alhajjaj, Z., Alshammari, A. S., Alamoudi, S., Alanazi, H. T., Alshahrani, R., Aleid, A. F., Khan, A., et al. (2024). *Pediatric surgical outcomes and pre-operative education in Saudi Arabia: A cross-sectional investigation. Journal of Advanced Trends in Medical Research.* https://www.semanticscholar.org/paper/7c2f8a55c69ca32398ce099f8acf1d84c26d5f6b (accessed on 12th July 2025).
8. Arcieri, L., Assanta, N., Baggi, R., Di Maurizio, M., et al. (2016). *The role of posterior aortopexy in the treatment of left mainstem bronchus compression.* https://core.ac.uk/download/74319435.pdf (accessed on 12th July 2025).
9. Arriaga, P., & Pacheco, C. (2016). *Effects of clown doctors on child and caregiver anxiety at the entrance to the surgery care unit and separation from caregivers.* https://core.ac.uk/download/46603912.pdf (accessed on 12th July 2025).
10. Attenhofer Jost, C., Auf der Maur, C., Bonassin, F., Bouchardy, J., et al. (2017). *Swiss Adult Congenital Heart Disease Registry (SACHER) – Rationale, design and first results.* https://core.ac.uk/download/149207799.pdf (accessed on 12th July 2025).
11. Audor, G. A. A., Caguana, J. P. C., Carrillo, L. A. M., Charris, F., et al. (2024). *Comparative outcomes of early surgical versus conservative management in pediatric congenital cataracts: A systematic review of visual acuity and long-term ocular health.* https://core.ac.uk/download/635338667.pdf (accessed on 12th July 2025).

12. Beez, T., Campbell, E., & Todd, L. (2017). *Prospective review of 30-day morbidity and mortality in a pediatric neurosurgical unit.* https://core.ac.uk/download/80696876.pdf (accessed on 12th July 2025).
13. Bellini, C., Cammaroto, G., Colizza, A., de Vincentiis, M., et al. (2019). *Risk factors for obstructive sleep apnea syndrome in children: State of the art.* https://core.ac.uk/download/231747914.pdf (accessed on 12th July 2025).
14. Berloco, P. B., Di Laudo, M., Frattaroli, F. M., Guglielmo, M., et al. (2012). *Laparoscopy in liver transplantation: The future has arrived.* https://core.ac.uk/download/154948504.pdf (accessed on 12th July 2025).
15. Bhangu, A., Schneider, A., Toki, A., Gasior, A. C., Pierro, A., Malik, A. H., Myers, A. L., et al. (2015). *Outcome reporting in randomized controlled trials and meta-analyses of appendicitis treatments in children: A systematic review.* https://core.ac.uk/download/pdf/81088334.pdf (accessed on 12th July 2025).
16. Bhattasali, O., Geller, D., Gill, J., Gorlick, R., et al. (2015). *Variability in the reported management of pulmonary metastases in osteosarcoma.* https://core.ac.uk/download/323068150.pdf (accessed on 12th July 2025).
17. Birchall, M. A., Bogan, S. L., & Teoh, G. Z. (2016). *Tissue engineered airways: A prospects article.* https://core.ac.uk/download/79506677.pdf (accessed on 12th July 2025).
18. Bonica, M., Students of Health Management 721.01, University of New Hampshire. (2017). *Healthcare management primer.* https://core.ac.uk/download/215509297.pdf (accessed on 12th July 2025).
19. Bunn, L., Carter, B., Cassidy, E., Hartley, L., et al. (2018). *E-survey of current international physiotherapy practice for children with ataxia following surgical resection of posterior fossa tumor.* https://core.ac.uk/download/286357576.pdf (accessed on 12th July 2025).
20. Burgess, A., George, S., Gerard, K., Lathlean, J., et al. (2005). *Integrated out-of-hours care arrangements in England: Observational study of progress towards single call access via NHS Direct and impact on the wider health system.* https://core.ac.uk/download/2709866.pdf (accessed on 12th July 2025).
21. Cain, M. P., Green, M. C., Horn, N. D., Misseri, R., et al. (2018). *Epidural analgesia decreases narcotic requirements in low level spina bifida patients undergoing urologic laparotomy for neurogenic bladder and bowel.* https://core.ac.uk/download/160755276.pdf (accessed on 12th July 2025).
22. Carrol, E. D., Lane, S., Lisboa, P. J. G., McGrath, J., et al. (2014). *What impact did a pediatric early warning system have on emergency admissions to the pediatric intensive care unit? An observational cohort study.* https://core.ac.uk/download/42136646.pdf (accessed on 12th July 2025).
23. Cashen, K., Costello, J. M., Gowda, K. M. N., Grimaldi, L., et al. (2018). *Multicenter validation of the vasoactive-ventilation-renal score as a predictor of prolonged mechanical ventilation after neonatal cardiac surgery.* https://core.ac.uk/download/227054193.pdf (accessed on 12th July 2025).
24. Chan, H. Y. I., Chung, H. Y., Lan, C. L. L., Leung, K., et al. (2016). *Outcomes of re-intervention for laparoscopic transperitoneal pyeloplasty in children.* https://core.ac.uk/download/45606867.pdf (accessed on 12th July 2025).

25. Elahi, M. M., & Matata, B. (2017). *Meeting report on the International Conference of ECMO-Life Support for Pakistan in 21st Century held May 11–12, 2017, Lahore.* https://core.ac.uk/download/131166373.pdf (accessed on 12th July 2025).

26. Elkins, G., Fisher, W., Johnson, A., Kekecs, Z., et al. (2014). *Hypnosis for acute procedural pain: A critical review.* https://core.ac.uk/download/77011633.pdf (accessed on 12th July 2025).

27. Galliers, J. R., Randell, R., Wilson, S., Woodward, B., et al. (2009). *Reconceptualizing clinical handover: Information sharing for situation awareness.* https://core.ac.uk/download/5230495.pdf (accessed on 12th July 2025).

28. Gaskin, J., Singh, R. P., Boyer, D., Elenora, L., Holz, F., Bliss, C., et al. (2022). *Sunday 30 October speakers. Clinical & Experimental Ophthalmology, 50.* https://www.semanticscholar.org/paper/83517ae9841853597e8ac24482ba8c01f32d64b9 (accessed on 12th July 2025).

29. Hammer, G. B., & Morton, N. S. (2009). *Editorial.* https://core.ac.uk/download/6159453.pdf (accessed on 12th July 2025).

30. Isawumi, M., & Ademola-Popoola, D. (2024). *A review of pediatric cataract surgery techniques and practices: Past, present and future. Nigerian Journal of Ophthalmology.* https://www.semanticscholar.org/paper/fba9a786cdc9ee9828c9d23e04ccb65a6f1f6928 (accessed on 12th July 2025).

31. Kim, K. (2024). *Preserving pediatric wellness: Enhanced recovery after surgery protocols and pain management in pediatric surgery.* https://core.ac.uk/download/624274599.pdf (accessed on 12th July 2025).

32. King, J., Lehrnbecher, T., Pana, Z.-D., Steinbach, W. J., et al. (2017). *Recognition and clinical presentation of invasive fungal disease in neonates and children.* https://core.ac.uk/download/131024549.pdf (accessed on 12th July 2025).

33. Kowalska-Bobko, I., Mokrzycka, A., Sagan, A., Włodarczyk, C., et al. (2016). *The 2014 primary health care reform in Poland: Short-term fixes instead of a long-term strategy.* https://core.ac.uk/download/pdf/82388853.pdf (accessed on 12th July 2025).

34. Lee, Y., & Ross, A. (2018). *Projected specialty career choices amongst undergraduate dental students in Scotland.* https://core.ac.uk/download/132211318.pdf (accessed on 12th July 2025).

35. Li, M., Fu, G., Mo, W., & Yan, Y. (2025). *Summary of best evidence for prevention of postoperative pulmonary complications after surgery for patients undergoing gastric cancer operations. Frontiers in Oncology, 15.* https://www.semanticscholar.org/paper/152c2702c1b6d12b7a3bbb0ca0b7ea9858ef26f9 (accessed on 12th July 2025).

36. Li, S., Xu, H., Li, J., Zhang, T., & Cui, J. (2025). *Management of anesthesia and cardiopulmonary bypass in pediatric patients with abdominal tumors invading the inferior vena cava and right atrium: A case series of a tertiary children's medical center in China. Cancer Reports, 8.* https://www.semanticscholar.org/paper/1766a6b28910b52858e36ee8a11c64881542be59 (accessed on 12th July 2025).

37. Loewenstein, A., Moisseiev, E., Moshiri, A., Nemet, A. Y., et al. (2017). *A review of innovations in rhegmatogenous retinal detachment surgical techniques.* https://core.ac.uk/download/323069919.pdf (accessed on 12th July 2025).

38. Luke, T. A. (2016). *The role of telehealth technology in the remediation of pediatric feeding*

disorders. https://core.ac.uk/download/211336814.pdf (accessed on 12th July 2025).

39. Lung, M. (2014). *Physical therapy case files: Orthopedics. Physiotherapy Canada, 66*, 331–332. https://www.semanticscholar.org/paper/fc15a8ee663d25813a5286218cebf517c5d80d42 (accessed on 12th July 2025).
40. Pini Prato, A., & Lacher, M. (2024). *Advancing pediatric robotic colorectal surgery: Trends, outcomes, and future directions—A comprehensive review. European Journal of Pediatric Surgery*. https://www.semanticscholar.org/paper/88373fcb2581b042d7561575a1b12b67039a4de2 (accessed on 12th July 2025).
41. Slade, D. (2015). *Recent advances in surgery 29. Annals of The Royal College of Surgeons of England, 90*, 269. https://www.semanticscholar.org/paper/4d419fcfa0cb9520ed847ba39a7391ec575249e6 (accessed on 12th July 2025).
42. Stevens, K. (2025). *Assessing the performance of a new generic measure of health related quality of life for children and refining it for use in health state valuation*. https://core.ac.uk/download/49644.pdf (accessed on 12th July 2025).
43. Uba, A. F., Christianson, A. L., Measham, A. R., Nandi, B., Warf, B. C., Murray, C. J. L., Adeyemi, D., et al. (2014). *Congenital anomalies in low- and middle-income countries: The unborn child of global surgery*. https://core.ac.uk/download/323070414.pdf (accessed on 12th July 2025).
44. Weissman, J. S., Betancourt, J. R., & Kim, M. K. (2007). *Resident physicians' preparedness to provide cross-cultural care: Implications for clinical care and medical education policy*. https://core.ac.uk/download/71354412.pdf (accessed on 12th July 2025).

MAJOR TRAUMA SURGERY

9

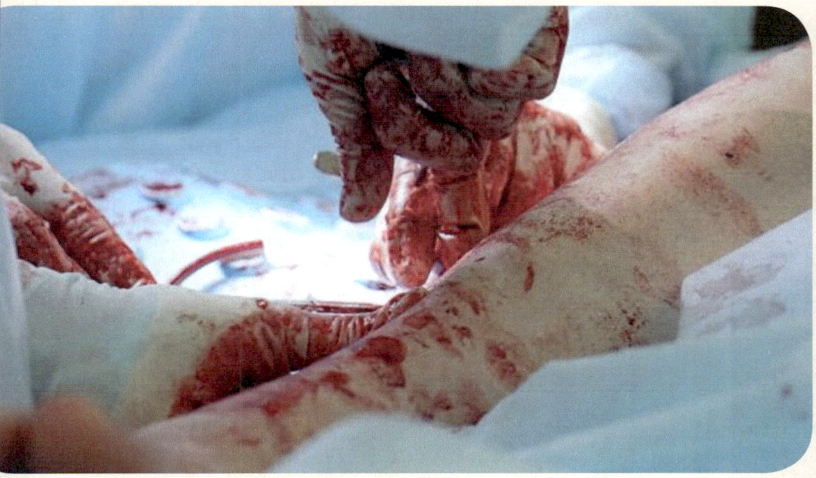

Introduction

The primary trauma surgery specialty has evolved significantly after advances in medical technology and a better understanding of trauma management. By common usage, major trauma means life-threatening injuries, which are frequently surgical and require well-organized action from trauma centers, surgical teams, and training. So much complexity surrounding it, timely diagnosis and treatment are significant to improve patient outcome. The complexity of trauma surgery calls not only for surgical competence but also for multidisciplinary collaboration between various medical disciplines to provide integrated care. Through embracing the principles of recovery from trauma as a complex issue in the context of trauma, medical practitioners can leverage interventions for optimal surgery and optimal recovery outcomes for patients. Due to the complexity of trauma surgery, which often requires advanced technologies, the implementation of computer-assisted surgery systems represents a significant milestone in technology. Using modern technology, such as computer-aided orthopedic surgery (CAOS)

LEARNING OBJECTIVES

After studying this chapter, you will be able to:

1. Understand the types of major trauma
2. Explain the mechanisms of injury of trauma
3. Discuss the assessment and diagnosis of trauma
4. Focus on surgical interventions of trauma
5. Learn about postoperative care of trauma
6. Evaluate the assessment and diagnosis

systems, surgeons can now achieve a level of accuracy previously unattainable when treating musculoskeletal trauma. These systems utilize a variety of imaging modalities, including CT, MRI, and ultrasound, allowing for customized planning and execution of surgery that takes into account the individual patient's anatomy. Such technological advances not only increase accuracy in surgery but also lower the risk for procedure-related complications. Consequently, the advancement and implementation of CAOS systems are a crucial step towards optimizing outcomes in major trauma surgery, potentially improving the quality of care for victims of serious injury. In addition to advanced surgical technology, the role of team research efforts cannot be overstated in major trauma surgery.

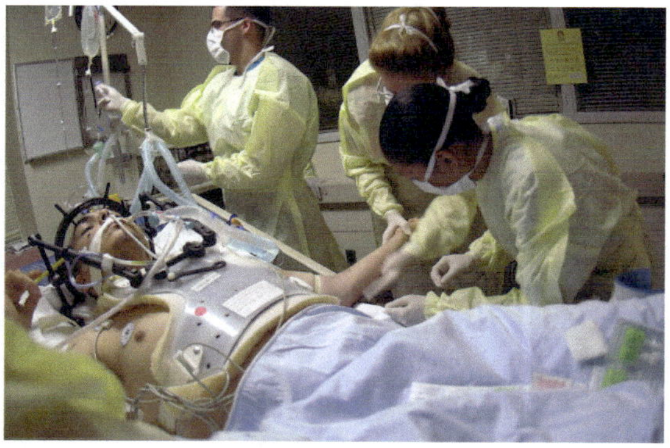

Figure 9.1. Major trauma surgery.

Source: https://upload.wikimedia.org/wikipedia/commons/a/aa/US_Navy_040723-N-8977L-008_Navy_Hospital_Corpsmen_and_Medical_Officers_assess_the_treatment_and_prognosis_of_a_patient_with_a_gunshot_wound.jpg.

Multi-center trials have now become essential in gathering robust data required to improve clinical practices. Initiatives such as the Brain Monitoring with Information Technology group (BrainIT) and the Cooperative Study on Brain Injury Depolarisations (COSBID) demonstrate the importance of inter-institutional coordination in addressing complex trauma cases. These networks focus on maximizing data access and validation processes, thereby facilitating a better understanding of trauma patterns and treatment efficacy. The potential of such collaborative endeavors is enhanced by initiatives like the AVERT-IT project, which aims to address many of the issues with data collection and reliability. By creating such a platform, facilitating such collaborations, major trauma surgery can nonetheless evolve and, ultimately, advance enhanced patient care and outcomes (Figure 9.1).

Definition of Major Trauma Surgery

Major trauma surgery involves the assessment and management of patients with major injuries, particularly blunt and penetrating trauma. The majority of these patients require urgent surgery and more than one discipline. As a result, the definition of major trauma surgery could be established within critical care, emergency medicine, and the surgical specialties. It involves not only the direct surgical care of injury but also the overall facility for the round-the-clock management of trauma patients, resuscitating them, monitoring them, and implementing multi-modal recovery protocols. The American College of Surgeons welcomes the mandate of such treatment of traumatic injuries, which frequently involve acute life-threatening conditions like devastating hemorrhage, ruptured viscera, and complicated fracture patterns needing advanced surgical techniques and instant decision-making. In trauma surgery, the levels of injury are based on grading scales that have been developed and standardized, such as those of the American Association for the Surgery of Trauma (AAST). In the scales, injuries are graded based on anatomical and clinical features, and these grades are used to guide surgical decisions as well as predict the patient's outcomes. For instance, adaptations of the renal injury grading system reflect changes in management, with an increased focus on imaging and non-operative management (NOM) of certain injury grades.

The 2018 revision has led to the reclassification of established patterns of injury, aligning with advancements in radiological techniques and the increasing pressure for conservative management, particularly for high-grade renal trauma (Allen et al., 2020).

This grading revolution outsources the complexity involved in managing injuries and the need for accurate diagnosis to achieve optimal patient care. In addition, the debate regarding significant trauma surgery broadens to cover the clinical benefit of non-operative management as an option, especially in high-grade injury patients. Research indicates that NOM is an option that can be used with reduced mortality and morbidity compared to operative management. Systematic reviews provide evidence indicating that NOM is not only beneficial for lesser grades of renal injuries but also holds validity for greater grades, contrary to the traditional trend favoring surgical intervention (Brachini et al., 2017). The shift highlights the role of trauma surgeons in keeping themselves updated with the evolving paradigms of management so that they can provide an optimal approach to therapy. Lastly, adopting methods like NOM is a reflection of an interest in maintaining organ function and optimizing long-term recovery, representative of the continued evolution in the practice of major trauma surgery.

Importance in Emergency Medicine

Understanding the role of emergency medicine in the context of major trauma surgery is crucial to improving patient outcomes. Intervention in situations corresponds directly to survival in cases of severe injury. Research supports that delays in definitive care will have a quantifiable effect on morbidity and mortality, particularly in pediatric patients with blunt trauma. The implementation of an effective trauma response has been shown to enhance the quality of care provided in emergency departments. For instance, a study indicated that after this response was implemented, the time from emergency department to CT acquisition decreased substantially, making diagnoses and treatments much quicker. This is an indication of the requirement of protocols aimed at rapid assessment and intervention, ultimately resulting in improved management of traumatic injuries and time to definitive care, thereby improving survival rates for all patients experiencing major trauma.

Classification of injuries through the use of standard grading systems, such as the American Association for the Surgery of Trauma (AAST) classification for liver injury, underscores the value of systematic approaches to practice in the field of emergency medicine. In the management of liver trauma, the injury grade provides guidelines to inform decisions regarding care, but the patient's overall physiology and related injuries must also be taken into account. The World Society of Emergency Surgery (WSES) has established guidelines that incorporate anatomical and physiological elements into the treatment of traumatic liver injury. This integrated treatment approach ensures not only that immediate trauma is addressed but also that patients' overall clinical condition is evaluated and treated. In emergency medicine, where rapid decision-making under chaotic circumstances is a standard requirement, such guidelines and categorizations form important tools for medical professionals, enabling timely and accurate treatment that is invaluable in managing serious trauma cases.

In addition, the integration of technology and advanced imaging modalities in emergency medicine further enhances the possibility of rapid and well-considered decision-making. The use of imaging tests, such as focused assessment with sonography for trauma (FAST), has improved the diagnosis of intra-abdominal injury and hemorrhagic events among traumatized patients considerably. As can be seen from the following-quoted study, not only did the use of FAST increase in numbers, but it also shortened the time taken to perform such tests. This directly affects the trajectory of patient care, enabling surgical intervention to be initiated earlier when needed. Both imaging and treatment paradigms in emergency medicine evolve in tandem, playing a significant role in shaping the direction of care for trauma patients and thereby confirming the value of a timely, evidence-based response to severe surgical dilemmas (Figure 9.2).

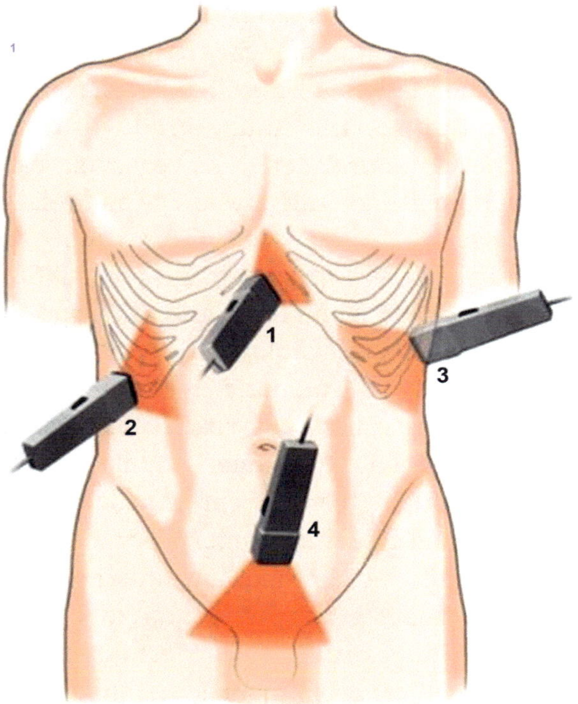

Figure 9.2. Focused assessment for sonography in trauma.

Source: https://www.researchgate.net/publication/305887929/figure/fig1/AS:11431281129852868@1679654568945/Fast-focused-assessment-for-sonography-in-trauma.png.

9.1. Types of Major Trauma

Learning Outcome

1. Describe the blunt trauma
2. Define penetrating trauma
3. Discuss burn injuries

Primary trauma classification is a group of injuries with significant impacts on human health and requires immediate surgical treatment. The most prevalent is blunt trauma, typically due to car crashes or falls. Such trauma tends to affect large body areas and may induce intricate conditions like intracorporeal hemorrhage, organ laceration, or compartment syndrome. The mechanisms of injury in blunt trauma are often related to vast kinetic forces that propagate through body tissues and produce extensive injury. The operative teams must assess the extent of organ involvement and internal hemorrhage rapidly. The subsequent need for a multidisciplinary approach highlights the complexity of being involved in the treatment of cases of blunt trauma, thereby confirming the necessity for timely and coordinated surgical action to enhance survival rates and patient recovery outcomes.

The other significant class of severe trauma is penetrating trauma, caused more frequently by gunshot wounds or stabs. Unlike blunt trauma, penetrating injuries are characterized by their ability to disrupt body structures cleanly and directly, often causing more severe complications. The potential for harm to internal organs, blood vessels, and secondary infections is an indication that immediate surgery is essential. Due to the uncertainty of the trajectory of penetrating objects, surgical assessment must incorporate advanced technology imaging modalities to ascertain the severity of injury and design an adequate surgical plan. Progress in surgical technology, as outlined in Frang et al.

(2011), has also enabled the handling of penetrating trauma more effectively, allowing surgeons to employ minimally invasive techniques that reduce postoperative complications and shorten recovery periods. Last, the creation of trauma in modern warfare presents particular challenges to mass trauma surgery. This includes blast injuries, which are, for the most part, seen in war and result not only in a single injury but a combined presentation of polytrauma. The blast wave creates much secondary trauma, including organ laceration, fractures, and soft tissue damage, at the same time setting the stage for vivid psychological impact through traumatic experiences. Advanced surgical techniques and military medicine have adapted to address these traumas, utilizing computer-aided orthopedic surgery (CAOS) systems, as reported in Kalová et al. (2019). These technologies enable surgeons to handle complex trauma cases more effectively, delivering timely and comprehensive critical surgery interventions that ultimately improve prognosis in an environment where conventional trauma management may not be sufficient (Figure 9.3).

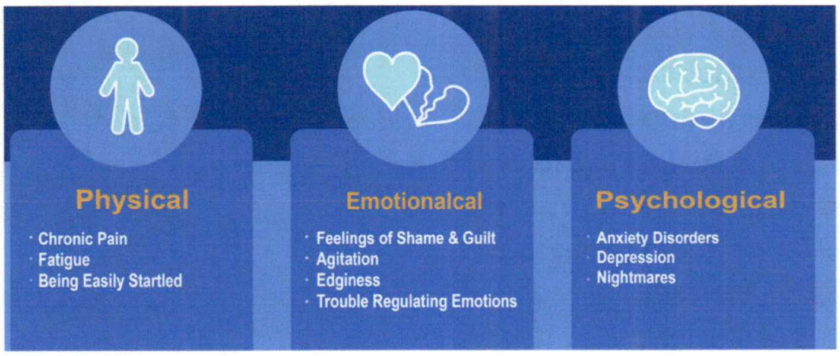

Figure 9.3. Types of major trauma.

Source: https://www.sandstonecare.com/wp-content/uploads/2021/08/Trauma-Symptoms.png.

9.1.1. Blunt Trauma

Blunt trauma is a predominant area of traumatic surgery, which is caused by non-penetrating injuries such as collisions, falls, or impacts. Injuries caused may affect more than one organ system, thereby causing a spectrum of conditions ranging from minor contusions to death-sustaining injury of vital organs. Among the most significant elements in managing blunt trauma is the hemodynamic stability of the patients. The treatment may vary based on this status; stable patients usually are subjects for nonoperative care with observation and management as needed. Clinical evidence indicates that high-grade blunt liver injury may be treated successfully without operation, provided no peritoneal signs and instability are evident, indicating the way of conservative treatment approaches in some instances (Ferrada et al., 2017). This shift is fueled by improvements in imaging and supportive care that enhance patient outcomes. In renal injury, the options for management also reflect the growing acceptance of nonoperative approaches. A systematic review identifies that nonoperative management (NOM) significantly reduces rates of mortality and morbidity in patients with renal trauma as compared to operative management (OM). This is particularly relevant for minor and severe blunt kidney injuries, as NOM has been shown to lead to favorable outcomes in a broad spectrum of injury grades (Brachini et al., 2017). The emphasis on preserving renal function underscores the new paradigms of trauma surgery that prefer approaches minimizing invasiveness and maximizing recovery. With the continued accumulation of data in support of NOM even in more serious-grade injuries, surgeons increasingly stress the importance of personalized approaches that consider the specific conditions of patients and the severity of their injuries.

Despite the success of nonoperative techniques, surgical intervention remains invaluable in cases of hemodynamic instability or severe injury. For those patients who present with extreme blunt trauma, especially those who exhibit evidence of intra-abdominal bleeding or severe organ injury, early operative intervention is indicated to avoid complications and stabilize the patient. For complex trauma surgery, a multidisciplinary treatment approach is generally shown, integrating advanced surgical techniques with modern anesthetic modalities to optimize patient care. While nonoperative care is the preferred option in stable cases, the case requires an exquisite balance between the risks of operation and delay. Trauma surgeons must understand the nuances of the management of blunt trauma to make a distinction between outcomes of treatment and salvaging lives in severely injured patients.

9.1.2. Penetrating Trauma

Penetrating trauma represents a significant area of focus in the practice of major trauma surgery due to its potential for causing catastrophic injury to vital organs and structures. Penetrating external injuries, including gunshot wounds or stabbings, most commonly create these injuries. Diagnosis and management of penetrating trauma both require an intimate knowledge of the mechanism of injury as well as the anatomy of involved pathways. Some effective evaluation measures involve employing diagnostic imaging, physical examination, and clinical judgment to assess injury severity. The complexity of penetrating trauma involves a variety of potential complications, such as hemorrhage, organ perforation, and infection, and hence requires early surgery to avoid systemic consequences. An essential factor in the treatment of penetrating trauma is grading of injuries based on the extent of severity, particularly for those due to the liver, as classified by the American Association for the Surgery of Trauma (AAST). The grading of liver injury ranges from mild to severe, and the hemodynamic stability of patients, as well as their comorbidities, are highly significant in determining the course of treatment. As Abu-Zidan et al. (2016) indicate, the management of liver trauma cannot only be about anatomical characteristics of the trauma but also about the physiological response of the patient.

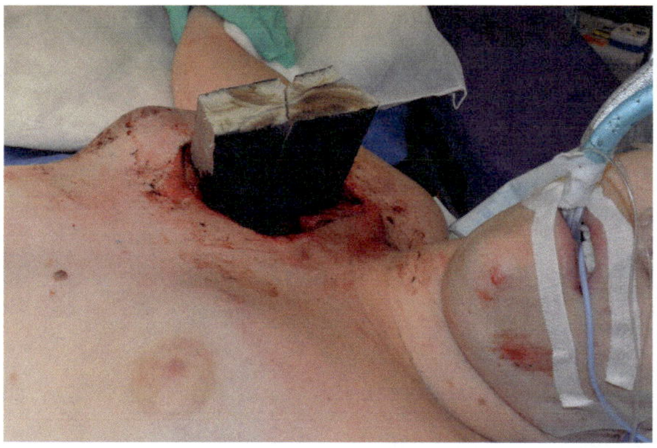

Figure 9.4. Penetrating trauma.

Source: https://www.pedsurglibrary.com/apsa/repview?type=571-438&name=2_829111_Standard.

This double consideration results in a more personalized and effective treatment protocol, greatly influencing the outcome of patients following major trauma surgery. In the last decade, improvements in treatment practices have significantly enhanced trauma care, particularly with the advent of damage control (DC) surgery. Initially instituted through the application of therapeutic liver packing, this has developed into broader-based applications within trauma management. As Ball et al. (2017) indicate, DC applies abbreviated laparotomy and accelerated surgical techniques for stabilizing severely injured patients and restricting the immediate consequences of trauma. This evolution is an indication of a greater understanding of the physiology of trauma, resulting in improved strategies for managing complicated injuries effectively. As trauma care continues to evolve, the integration of DC practices into operating room protocols demonstrates a commitment to achieving higher rates of recovery and optimizing patient safety in penetrating trauma (Figure 9.4).

9.1.3. Burn Injuries

Burn injuries constitute an essential area of concern for major trauma surgery as they are varied and complicated in the extent to which they can be severe. Assessing burn depth and extent is crucial in determining the most suitable management strategy. Burn injuries are categorized into three broad categories: first-degree, second-degree, and third-degree burns, with varying degrees of tissue destruction, such that third-degree burns require more vigorous surgical treatment. Ideal initial management is essential and may include rapid cooling of the burn, cleaning, and stabilization to prevent infection and complications. Particularly in cases with poor outcomes, surgical intervention may include debridement or skin grafting, highlighting the need for multidisciplinary care to optimize results. Early and proper assessment also guarantees the preventability of long-term complications, including scarring, dysfunction, and psychological trauma due to severe burns. The management of burn injuries involves an intimate understanding of trauma's multilateral impacts, specifically concerning concomitant complications. Burn patients, in most cases, also have a set of other issues, including trauma to the lungs from inhalation of smoke, as well as potential hypovolemic shock from fluid loss from the body. Furthermore, the vulnerable nature of managing comorbid conditions complicates surgical procedures and can also extend hospital stay. Studies depict that burn injuries tend to be associated with other trauma incidents, including road traffic accidents, that make injury severity worse and complicate recovery processes. As suggested in research conducted in places such as Tanzania, polytrauma, encompassing burn injuries, is still a common issue, which reflects an urgent need for greater strategies for trauma management, prioritizing global healing for burn patients along with their associated injuries (Khan et al., 2013). An essential component of burn care is psychological support offered to patients throughout the recovery process. Physical consequences of burn injuries tend to cause severe emotional disturbance, making it necessary to have a comprehensive treatment plan that includes psychological support services. Burn injuries can cause drastic changes in the appearance and functioning of a patient, leading to anxiety, depression, and post-traumatic stress disorder. Initiatives to integrate mental health care with trauma surgery have been observed to have prospects of improving the world's patient outcomes, healing, and quality-of-life restoration. In dealing with trauma management, particularly in low-resource settings, initiatives to prevent burn injuries through public education and increased safety become essential. This multi-level approach not only serves to improve surgical performance but also supports the general public health goal of reducing burn incidence and facilitating community education on safety procedures (Claes et al., 2019).

Test Your Knowledge

1. What are the primary categories of major trauma, and how are they typically classified?
2. How do blunt and penetrating traumas differ in mechanism, severity, and clinical management?

9.2. Mechanisms of Injury

Learning Outcome

1. Define the road traffic accidents
2. Describe the falls from heights
3. Understand the gunshot wounds

Understanding the mechanisms of injury is essential in major trauma surgery since it influences not just the treatment plan but also the eventual clinical outcomes for the patients. Various mechanisms of injury, which are mainly divided into blunt, penetrating, and thermal categories, determine the character of trauma and therefore dictate surgical intervention plans accordingly. Blunt trauma, which is common in road traffic accidents and falls, can lead to complex internal injuries that are not readily apparent. For instance, effects from high-impact velocities are likely to cause contusions and lacerations of internal organs. An understanding of these mechanisms enables trauma surgeons to anticipate potential complications and address them proactively during surgery. Furthermore, having specific knowledge of the types of injuries associated with each mechanism is crucial in creating effective management plans that ultimately facilitate patient survival and recovery. IPV injuries also illustrate the traumatic mechanisms trauma surgeons face in terms of diversity and complexity. IPV injuries are very challenging because they are associated with high mortality and patterns of injury. A Malawian study revealed that a significant proportion of trauma patients (34.5%) presented with IPV-related injuries, and most were male (Charles et al., 2018).

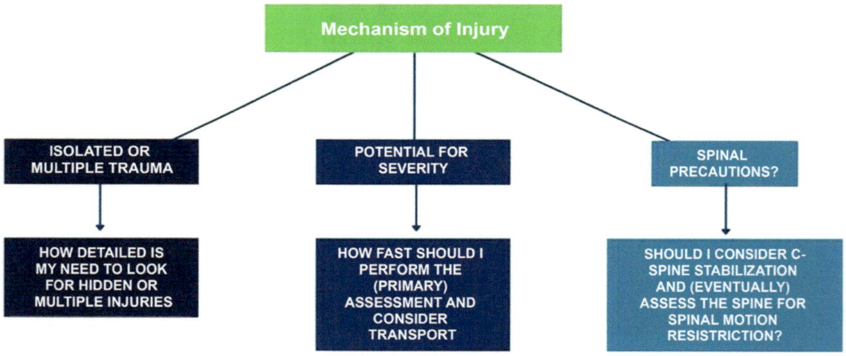

Figure 9.5. Mechanisms of injury.

Source: https://limmereducation.com/storage/media/trauma-assessment_mechanism-of-inury_flowchart.jpg.

Such complicated IPV injuries typically necessitate multidisciplinary management of the patient, not only surgery but also psychosocial intervention and rehabilitation. Surgeons should be skilled in distinguishing between injury patterns resulting from different types of IPV and be aware of the context of the situation, as this will determine the selection of surgical intervention and postoperative management specific to the individual circumstances of each patient. The sequence of injuries inflicted in the event of major trauma also includes significant instances of ear, nose, and throat (ENT) injuries, indicating the urgent need for focused surgery on these areas. Foreign bodies were identified to be the most common etiology for ENT injuries and were followed by road traffic crashes, based on a study at Bugando Medical Centre (Okoye et al., 2013). This trend requires more specificity regarding the precise risk factors and mechanisms of injury that lead to such trauma, toto guide preventive and operative techniques more effectively. The majority of ENT injuries are salvable on an outpatient basis; however, the formation of complications increases the rate of hospitalization. These results underscore the importance of early detection of the mechanism of injury in order to optimize the efficacy of treatment and reduce the morbidity of ENT trauma. Instruct:. An in-depth understanding of how and why injuries occur is thus fundamental to establishing effective treatment strategies in major trauma surgery (Figure 9.5).

9.2.1. Road Traffic Accidents

Road traffic injuries (RTIs) are a public health burden, as they contribute a significant proportion of trauma cases in the world. RTIs have the propensity to produce a variety of injuries ranging from superficial abrasions to life-threatening conditions requiring extensive surgery. The type of injury resulting from RTIs varies with numerous factors, including vehicle speed, seatbelt use, and road type. RTA in the majority of countries is the leading cause of mortality among youth, thus further augmenting the necessity for the implementation of trauma management guidelines. Surgeon preparedness and system response are key determinants in managing the implications of RTAs, with a specific emphasis on trauma surgeons becoming accustomed to the typical forms of injury usually encountered in such accidents, thereby improving patient outcomes and recovery patterns. As such, successful trauma care begins much earlier than a trip to the operating theatre, and that highlights the importance of pre-hospital care and rapid transportation to trauma centers. The extent of the damage done by RTAs usually necessitates a multidisciplinary trauma surgery. Oral and maxillofacial injuries have been found to commonly result from RTAs, constituting over 64.2% of them in studies conducted at medical institutions. These types of injury most typically include fracture and laceration of the jaw, among other facial structures, and often have profound effects upon both function and form. Surgeons are challenged with the challenging task of fixing not only the immediate, but also the long-term effects of these injuries, which may require not only surgical repair, but also reconstructive surgery. The ramifications of RTAs extend beyond physical damage; they also encompass psychological impacts. While survivors labor in recovery, the complex interplay between surgery and mental health cannot be overestimated, with the emphasis laid on the holistic nature of care needed after RTAs. Furthermore, RTAs also leave an impact at a large scale in society and the economy, and interventions are required at the policy level. As in most studies, the prevalence of severe injury from RTAs has elicited controversy on whether there should be more road safety infrastructures, enforcement of traffic laws, and campaigns to the public. Increasing accident rates also underscore the critical need for increased investment in upgrading infrastructure and trauma care centers. By addressing the root causes of RTAs—driver behavior, vehicle safety technologies, and road infrastructure—communities can strive to reduce the number of these collisions. As trauma surgeons continue to grapple with the physical effects of RTAs, they must also speak out for preventive strategies that may reduce the overall trauma burden, ultimately improving the safety of all road users.

9.2.2. Falls from Heights

Height-related falls are a significant area of focus in major trauma surgery due to their prevalence and morbidity. Falls from height tend to result in severe orthopedic and head injuries that need specialized surgical interventions. The mechanism of injury is a predictor of patient outcomes, as findings have indicated that falls from a height rank among the leading causes of head injury in children, leading to higher rates of death and disabilities in patients (Ghazwan et al., 2019). This susceptibility is most pronounced in the pediatric patient population, for whom even low-height falls can be calamitous in their consequences, affecting the overall trajectory of rehabilitation and recovery. For trauma surgery following a fall from a height, familiarity with the demographic and circumstances underlying falls from a height can inform treatment protocols and prevention efforts. Fall injuries among children, especially under 10 years, are usually caused by playground equipment or play activities, hence the significance of heightened vigilance and safety measures (Se et al., 2019). Treatment for such victims usually involves operations for multiple injuries, including fracture of the femur, which presents with associated patterns of presentation and management based on age and severity. The impact of these injuries can be modulated by factors such as the timing of intervention and related injuries, and makes the surgical situation even more challenging. The long-term implications of height falls extend beyond immediate medical needs to impact not only the patient but also the public healthcare system. Surgical teams must adopt an interdisciplinary approach that fosters integrated care and rehabilitation of these trauma patients. An emphasis on preventive methods, such as injury risk prevention and public safety education, is essential in cutting down on the incidence of falls from heights. As the statistics indicate a significant proportion of pediatric injury due to falling, initiating community programs to provide awareness and heighten safety provisions can play a primary role in lessening incidences and intensity of trauma thereafter (Ghazwan et al., 2019; Se et al., 2019). Having clear guidelines for post-surgical rehabilitation and care will be key in efforts to reverse the long-term effects of trauma, ultimately optimizing significant trauma surgery results.

9.2.3. Gunshot Wounds

The treatment of gunshot wounds (GSWs) remains a big issue in major trauma surgery due to their propensity to create complex and potentially life-threatening injuries. Learning the ballistic dynamics and tissue damage caused by such events forms part of the fundamental principle that should guide the treatment of GSWs. GSWs distinguish from other forms of trauma in that they can inflict enormous destruction not only where they enter and exit, but anywhere within the body since kinetic energy is being transferred and cavitation results. This necessitates adequate assessment of the anatomical and physiologic consequences of the injury. The intensity of the injury is often associated with the nature of the weapon, the distance of the shot, and the location of the injury, and thus requires a certain level of complexity in treating each case. Successful and early surgical intervention is crucial in managing GSWs, particularly in assessing the associated injuries. The American Association for the Surgery of Trauma (AAST) has developed classification grading systems for such injuries, specifically those affecting organs like the liver. In the case of liver injury from GSWs, the system helps in deciding on surgery versus non-surgery, depending upon the hemodynamic stability of the patient and the anatomy of the injury. Adding to the difficulty in assessing a patient's status can be the presence of two or more trauma mechanisms. In such situations, multidisciplinary care is necessary, combining multiple specialties to provide the most effective type of care. In this context, awareness of the injury patterns and proper management protocols becomes essential for surgeons to handle such complex cases (Abu-Zidan et al., 2016).

The prognosis for GSW patients can be fatal, especially for injuries involving the central nervous system. The mortality of gunshot head injury highlights the urgency of prompt evaluation and resuscitation maneuvers in trauma care. It has been found through studies that in gunshot wound victims to the brain, the survival rate is extremely low, with one study recording a mere 2.1% survival rate amongst patients who were subjected to cardiopulmonary resuscitation (CPR). This number underscores the time-critical urgency of the interventions required to enhance patient outcomes in these high-risk settings. Complicating management is also the consideration of donor appropriateness for organ donation in non-survivors, raising an ethical consideration of the priorities of treatment. While trauma surgeons make essential decisions in these difficult situations, they need to consider the possible advantages of forceful treatments against the dismal odds of refractory brain injuries (Babcock et al., 2019) (Figure 9.6).

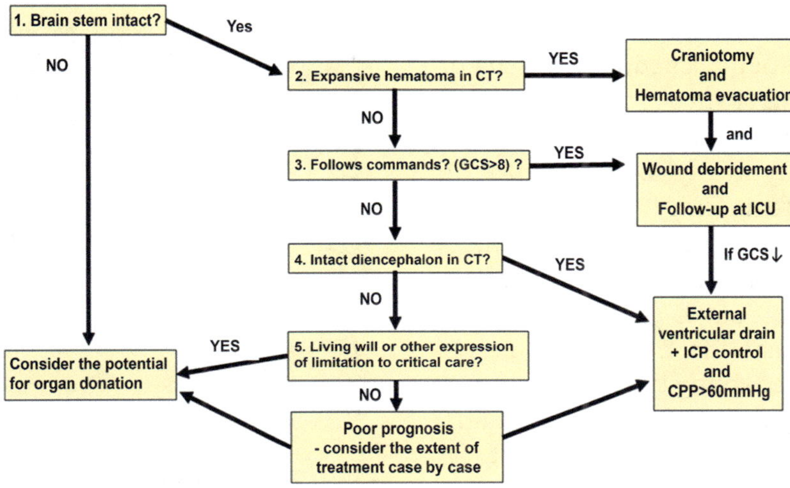

Figure 9.6. Management of gunshot wounds (GSWs) in trauma surgery.

Source: https://www.researchgate.net/publication/333383495/figure/fig2/AS:960313818099712@1605968064298/Proposed-algorithm-for-the-management-of-gunshot-shot-wounds-with-brain-injury-GSWB.png.

Test Your Knowledge

1. How do different forces, such as blunt, penetrating, and rotational, cause specific patterns of injury in trauma patients?
2. Why is understanding the mechanism of injury critical for guiding initial assessment and management in trauma care?

9.3. Assessment and Diagnosis

Learning Outcome

1. Define primary survey protocol for trauma
2. Discuss secondary survey protocol for trauma
3. Understand the imaging techniques used for trauma

Assessment of a patient scheduled for major trauma surgery is imperative since it will make the diagnosis in follow-up and management plans. A general typically begins with an initial assessment to identify potentially life-threatening injuries using the ABCDE method, which addresses Airway, Breathing, Circulation, Disability, and Exposure. The systematic approach ensures that the most basic issues are addressed first, enabling quick life-support measures. Following stabilization, a secondary assessment is performed to document all injuries, assess neurological status, and begin making a differential diagnosis. Higher imaging technologies, such as computed tomography (CT) scan and magnetic resonance imaging (MRI), play a crucial role in revealing occult injuries, especially in the case of complex trauma. Together with extensive clinical data, adequate imaging significantly improves worldwide diagnostic precision, ultimately equating to improved surgical treatment and intervention, especially in patients with significant trauma. In the management of complications from major trauma, like compartment syndrome, early evaluation is the method that prevents irreversible damage. Compartment syndrome is characterized by increased pressure within muscle compartments, leading to compromised blood supply and resulting tissue death. The early detection of high-risk groups, such as young men under the age of 35 with diaphyseal fractures in the tibia, is essential for early intervention. Pain disproportionate to the injury and pain at rest are key symptoms for diagnosis, along with signs such as paresis or paralysis, which would suggest progression. Clinical measurement of compartment pressures, in conjunction with close observation for the above symptoms, remains the best method of diagnosing acute limb compartment syndrome. Hence, a full awareness of risk factors and a high level of suspicion on the part of the treating surgeon enhance the effectiveness of evaluation in major trauma surgery (Ali et al., 2014).

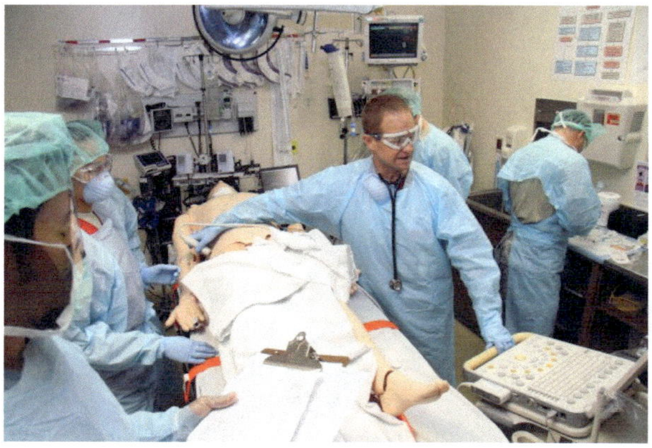

Figure 9.7. Initial trauma assessment.

Source: https://coreem.net/content/uploads/2017/11/US-in-Trauma.jpg.

Moreover, the diagnostic process is tremendously aided by interdisciplinary collaboration in major trauma centers. Trauma surgeons, emergency physicians, and allied health staff must communicate effectively with one another so that there can be a thorough assessment of patients. Teamwork will present more than one opinion regarding the clinical scenario, and less palpable injuries can thereby be detected that may otherwise go undetected. Standardized assessment tools and protocols also facilitate even assessment of patients by various practitioners, which is essential during emergencies. The incorporation of evidence-based guidelines into clinical practice further strengthens the assessment process, allowing for timely and accurate diagnosis. Lastly, a concerted effort to improve collaborative practices and education for assessing trauma can significantly influence outcomes in major trauma surgery, highlighting the role of effective communication and collaboration (Acosta et al., 2020) (Figure 9.7).

9.3.1. Primary Survey Protocol

The Primary Survey Protocol is the primary guideline for handling cases of major trauma, mainly dictating the initial survey and approach for immediate intervention. It is designed to identify life-threatening conditions in a systematic manner that require urgent medical attention. Adopting an organized approach, trauma teams can list injuries based on the severity of the patient's condition. Enactment of this protocol, in addition to facilitating rapid diagnosis, also facilitates early intervention and directly influences the patient's outcomes. For instance, previous research has established that optimized imaging, such as CT scans and limited assessment with sonography in trauma (FAST), significantly reduces time to definitive treatment, which is of vital importance in the setting of trauma where every second matters (Cross et al., 2019). Besides, the integration of a coordinated team response has been proven to enhance the effectiveness of emergency care. Through the implementation of organized training and team protocols, medical professionals can achieve a more coordinated response in cases of trauma. A retrospective analysis of pediatric trauma patients highlighted that protocols resulted in a decrease in the time spent from emergency department presentation to CT scan acquisition, demonstrating a significant correlation between the use of protocols and improved clinical outcomes (Cross et al., 2019). Therefore, having an efficient Primary Survey Protocol is not only a procedural nicety but also a pivotal building block that facilitates the success of trauma care. This model encourages an environment where medical staff can easily adapt to the constantly changing requirements of trauma surgery. In addition, the challenge posed by unforeseen situations, as brought about by the COVID-19 pandemic, calls for a flexible Primary Survey Protocol. The global health emergency emphasized the need for trauma services to change their practice habits in terms of infection control without compromising the provision of timely trauma patient care. The innovations observed across various specialties, such as maxillofacial surgery, reflect this responsive interplay between situational realities and clinical practice. Trauma departments are forced to continue adapting, not simply responding to immediate clinical concerns but also to the effect of larger public health realities. These evolving dynamics underscore the importance of maintaining flexibility in the Primary Survey Protocol to achieve optimal standards of patient care in primary trauma surgical settings.

9.3.2. Secondary Survey Protocol

The secondary survey protocol is a crucial component of the major trauma surgery pathway, serving as a rational way of uncovering occult injuries following the initial assessment. Following the initiation of lifesaving interventions during the primary survey, medical practitioners conduct an in-depth evaluation of the patient's status. This involves a complete assessment of all body systems for potential internal trauma not readily apparent but which could significantly influence patient prognosis. Specifically, clinical personnel must assess neurological status, respiratory status, and abdominal status, correlating clinical findings with imaging studies where necessary. This comprehensive protocol is complemented by evidence from various studies emphasizing the importance of standard procedures, such as postoperative monitoring of lower limb free flap reconstructions, aimed at enhancing patient safety and recovery success (Glynou et al., 2024).

The effectiveness of the secondary survey protocol is enhanced by its integration with a range of diagnostic tools and standard procedures. For instance, the application of advanced imaging modalities provides rapid identification of fractures, hemorrhages, or organ perforations that might otherwise escape detection on a physical examination. Further, adherence to protocols strictly can lead to a decrease in complications of trauma, a topic of particular interest in high-trauma surgery. Current evidence suggests that well-organized guidelines for surveillance, as in the case of infection-related fractures, can enhance decision-making and optimize treatment protocols in trauma centers (Kavi et al., 2023).

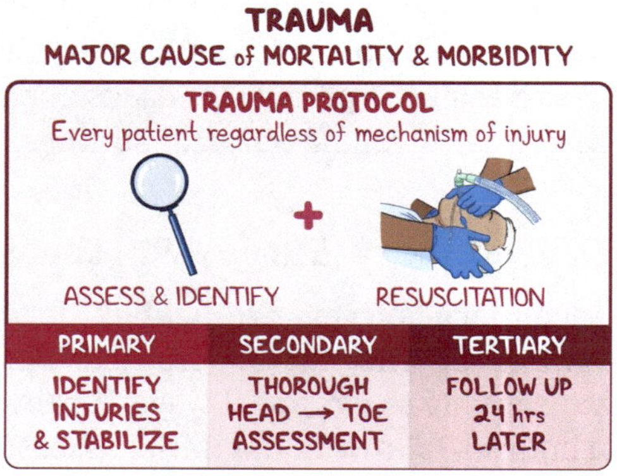

Figure 9.8. The secondary survey protocol is a major component of primary trauma surgery.

Source: https://d16qt3wv6xm098.cloudfront.net/hojsjF-7QTSjnTo_97kp-EQvSimwcQE8/_.jpg.

This ensures that all medical personnel are aware of the protocols and their applications, leading to an optimized trauma care environment. Lastly, the secondary survey procedure is not merely an organized assessment instrument but also a philosophy of trauma care that promotes what is best: completeness and safety for the patient. Because trauma patients can present so clinically heterogeneously, having a standardized method enables surgical teams to provide comprehensive and effective management. In emulating the good practices observed in the discipline, such as the need for proper microbiological profiling of infections associated with fractures, the secondary survey protocol is an essential component towards successful trauma surgery. By constant improvement of these protocols through research and cross-talk between trauma centers, the discipline will be headed towards a future in which trauma care is better in terms of patient outcome, with fewer morbidities and mortalities significantly (Figure 9.8).

9.3.3. Imaging Techniques Used

In trauma surgery, imaging modalities play a crucial role in the assessment and management of trauma. Computed tomography (CT) scans and magnetic resonance imaging (MRI) are the most frequently employed modalities, both with unique strengths in imaging trauma. CT scans are particularly favored for their speed and high-resolution cross-sectional imaging of internal structures, making them indispensable in the acute setting for quickly diagnosing life-threatening conditions such as hemorrhage or organ laceration. The quick acquisition of data enables timely decision-making, which is of utmost importance in trauma surgery, as seconds count. Furthermore, CT imaging has been shown to significantly reduce the number of exploratory surgeries, thereby lowering the risk involved with invasive procedures (Acosta et al., 2020).

Besides CT, MRI has also proven to be a valuable resource, particularly in assessing soft tissue injuries that are less readily identified using other imaging technologies. Improved high contrast resolution of MRI enhances visualization of the brain, spinal cord, and musculoskeletal trauma, thereby guiding surgical and nonsurgical treatment. Less common in acute trauma due to longer scan times, its sensitivity for detecting subtle trauma renders it a component of extended trauma evaluation. Apart from that, advancing techniques such as diffusion-weighted MRI have the potential to make early detection of brain injuries a reality, demonstrating the ongoing progression in imaging technology that renders better surgical results in challenging cases (Ansel et al., 2019). Ultrasound is a significant imaging technique in the trauma environment, particularly in point-of-care settings. Its portability and ability to provide real-time images allow surgeons to assess conditions such as fluid accumulation or organ injury quickly. The FAST (Focused Assessment with Sonography for Trauma) protocol is a routine application of ultrasound in trauma surgery, as it provides a quick assessment of patients for internal bleeding. This non-invasive technique not only aids in the diagnosis of injury but can even impact later management, whether surgery or observation. With the ongoing development of trauma protocols, consolidating various imaging modalities ensures that operating teams are as well-prepared as possible, generally improving patient management and outcomes in major trauma.

Test Your Knowledge

1. What are the key components of a primary and secondary survey in the assessment of a trauma patient?
2. How do imaging and laboratory investigations complement clinical evaluation in diagnosing traumatic injuries?

9.4. Surgical Interventions

Learning Outcome

1. Discuss emergency resuscitation of trauma
2. Understand the damage control surgery of trauma
3. Define the definitive surgical procedures of trauma

Surgical procedures in the management of severe trauma are critical, involving effective and timely decision-making to provide the best possible patient outcome. Among all the surgical procedures available, thoracic procedures like pneumonectomy and limited lung resections (LLR) are critical while managing traumatic lung injuries. Pneumonectomy has long been linked with considerable mortality, much greater than 50%, due to complications like shock and right ventricular failure. In a recent study, scientists established that the mortality rate was much higher in patients who were undergoing pneumonectomy when compared to those who were undergoing LLR, with rates posted at 64.9% compared to 27.2%, respectively (Doben et al., 2020). This observation highlights the need for assessing the viability of surgical procedures in trauma patients, promoting an individualized approach that prioritizes survival over minimizing morbidity. One key trauma surgical innovation is damage control (DC), which upends conventional practice by prioritizing the expeditious stabilizing process over the complete repair. Having originated in such initial practices as therapeutic liver packing, DC has evolved to encompass abbreviated laparotomy techniques. This method permits surgeons to stabilize complex injuries without subjecting patients to undue operative times that may augment coagulopathy and other complications of severe trauma (Ball et al., 2017). By applying early control of bleeding and avoidance of further physiological derangement, damage control surgery promotes necessary resuscitation maneuvers to combat shock and improve patient survival. These innovative alterations track shifting dynamics of operative intervention as trauma care responds to advances in understanding patterns of injury and patient physiology. The adoption of damage control techniques signals a paradigm shift within trauma surgery, one placing a premium on the necessity for continuous review and innovation in procedural technique. With the increasing application of DC, long-term implications within patient care are significant. The creation of this surgical model also raises legitimate questions regarding the timing of interventions like these, and how they might be used to augment resuscitation protocols. Furthermore, heightened awareness of potential issues, such as abdominal compartment syndrome, demands vigilant monitoring during the post-surgical period (Ball et al., 2017). Surgeons, then, need not only skill in performing these procedures initially but also skill in managing complications that can arise as part of post-trauma recovery. This deep understanding of surgery is fundamental to improving results in major trauma, with the patient maintained at the forefront of surgical management (Figure 9.9).

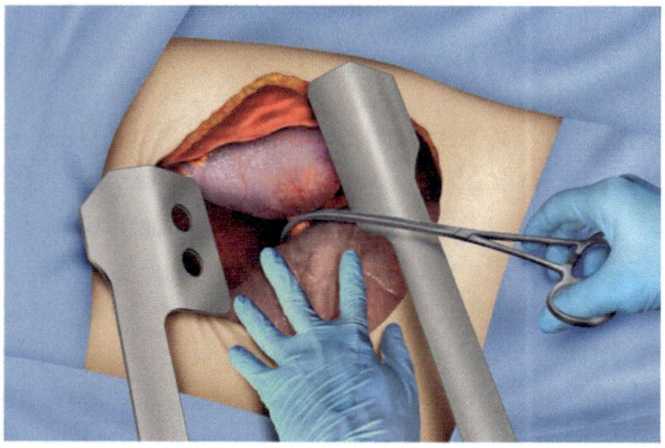

Figure 9.9. Damage control surgery in lung trauma.

Source: https://www.redalyc.org/journal/283/28366681010/1657-9534-cm-52-02-e4044683-gf4.jpg.

9.4.1. Emergency Resuscitation

Resuscitation in emergency is crucial in major trauma surgery, significantly affecting patient outcomes in acute care. Once trauma patients arrive in medical facilities, there is a need to perform resuscitation procedures promptly to prevent compromised physiological stability and management of life-threatening conditions. These include the management of hypovolemia, monitoring of vital signs, and securing the airway. Systematic management, involving the prompt assessment of the patient's hemodynamic status, is necessary to guide further care. Furthermore, understanding of the injury mechanisms allows surgical teams to apportion treatment modalities appropriately, tailoring resuscitation practices to meet the individual needs of each patient. Increasingly, damage control resuscitation is aimed at adopting a balanced approach, restoring hemostatic function without excessive crystalloid infusion, and utilizing early transfusion protocols where necessary (Ball et al., 2017).

Treatment of the major trauma surgery for injury to organs such as the liver requires taking into account emergency resuscitation protocols. The AST grading system is employed to classify the grade of liver injury, and it provides a platform for individualized treatment interventions according to the anatomy of injury and concomitant physiological status of the patient (Abu-Zidan et al., 2016). Of importance, trauma surgeons must assess not only the liver but also the patients' global hemodynamic stability and associated injuries. This combined evaluation directs the choice between conservative management and more invasive surgical treatments. Thus, emergency resuscitation extends beyond the immediate stabilization, influencing surgical choice and post-operative management. Successful resuscitation has been correlated with improved survival, emphasizing the importance of education and adherence to established protocols in the pressure-cooker environment of trauma management. The evolution of resuscitation methods, and in particular the emergence of damage control, highlights the adaptive quality of emergency treatment in severe trauma surgery. Damage control resuscitation tries to reverse the physiological derangements with massive blood loss and trauma using judicious fluid administration and early transfusion practice to get the patient into a state for surgery. Historical accounts indicate that damage control innovation emerged as a result of a growing understanding of trauma physiology, leading to updated strategies for surgical management (Ball et al., 2017). As progressive emergency protocol follows, the addition of process improvements and evidence-based practices continues to dominate. Lastly, the success of emergency resuscitation in trauma surgery depends on impeccably coordinated multidisciplinary teams, trauma care education in an advanced manner, and continuous refinement of protocols to enhance patient outcomes in this area.

9.4.2. Damage Control Surgery

Damage Control Surgery (DCS) represents a paradigm shift in the management of severely wounded patients, particularly in severe trauma surgery. Traditionally, trauma surgery has worked towards having complete anatomical restoration. With the accompanying high mortality and morbidity following big procedures during the initial resuscitation, the approach has been questioned. DCS tries to balance urgency for expeditious operation with patients' severely ill conditions, and instead of definitive repair, attempts to stabilize them.

This novel technique is adopted from the age-old method of therapeutic liver packing. It has gained popularity due to an improved understanding of the physiology of trauma and the dynamics of hemorrhagic shock. Thus, DCS enables clinicians to focus on appropriate resuscitation and temporary closure techniques, ultimately improving patient outcomes in a measured, stepwise surgical strategy (Ball et al., 2017). DCS has progressively been adapted to be applied in various complex injuries, beyond the initial usage trend in abdominal trauma, to thoracic, vascular, and orthopedic injuries. This massive application of DCS proves the versatility and effectiveness of DCS in treating trauma patients with different and complex injuries. Studies show that using abbreviated laparotomy and the following therapies, such as packing or temporary closure of the abdomen, has been effective in controlling hemorrhage and achieving critical time for physiological recovery. By early management of life-threatening hemorrhage, DCS not only decreases the risk of immediate death but also decreases the risk of complications like abdominal compartment syndrome, which may be caused by aggressive resuscitation (Ball et al., 2017).

Thus, DCS is a valuable principle in major trauma surgery programs, enabling the optimization of patient care in emergency conditions. Research on the specific consequences of surgical techniques, such as DCS, reveals glaring differences in patient outcomes based on the type of surgical procedure performed. For instance, comparison of trauma pneumonectomy (TP) and limited lung resections (LLR) in traumatic lung injury demonstrates much higher mortality with TP. The findings indicate that patients treated with TP had a mortality rate of 64.9% as opposed to only 27.2% of the LLR patients. Additionally, the independent risk of TP underscores the challenge faced in the management of severe thoracic injuries. This supports the need for application of strategies like DCS, which are aimed at stabilization and risk reduction, and which could lead to worse outcomes in patients under aggressive surgical techniques. Thus, DCS not only reshapes the landscape of trauma surgery but also calls for ongoing research to expand care practice and surgical decision-making in the critically injured cohort (Figure 9.10).

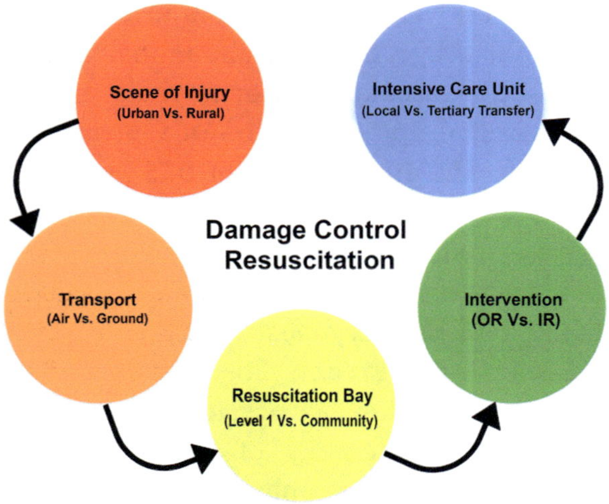

Figure 9.10. Damage control resuscitation across the phases of major injury care.

Source: https://media.springernature.com/lw685/springer-static/image/art%3A10.1007%2Fs40719-017-0096-9/MediaObjects/40719_2017_96_Fig2_HTML.gif.

9.4.3. Definitive Surgical Procedures

As far as major trauma surgery is concerned, definitive surgical management is the basis for the best possible management of complex injuries. They are not only designed to stabilize a patient's condition but also to reestablish anatomical function and improve overall outcomes. Among the definitive techniques employed, some surgeries, such as Open Reduction and Internal Fixation (ORIF) and Minimally Invasive Plate Osteosynthesis (MIPO), have gained popularity for fracture treatment. The latest studies confirm the efficacy of these interventions, with findings showing them to yield favorable radiographic outcomes, particularly in articular tibial pilon fractures, where fracture comminution heavily determines recuperation. In fact, the choice of surgical technique should be guided by the type of injury, the status of adjacent soft tissues, and the anticipated long-term functional outcomes, as illustrated by the results of aggregate studies comparing these surgical methods (Angelini et al., 2018).

The historical progression of surgical methods underscores the necessity of innovation in trauma surgery, especially in the case of definitive operations. Damage control surgery is a valuable innovation that has emerged in response to the challenge of controlling traumatic, life-threatening injuries. It has developed from therapeutic liver packing but thereafter expanded to include abbreviated laparotomies and other conservative rapid surgical methods. Systematic application of damage control principles has now been extended not only to abdominal trauma but also to orthopedic trauma, highlighting the need for a paradigm shift in managing challenging injuries. With improved understanding of trauma resuscitation and patient physiology, the role of damage control surgery has been better understood, illustrating the relationship between surgical innovation and clinical practice (Ball et al., 2017). Finally, definitive surgical intervention in major trauma surgery is possible only with a multi-modal approach combining expert surgical skills with innovative techniques tailored to the individual patient presentation. In addition to optimizing emergent care for trauma patients, these interventions minimize complications and maximize the potential for rehabilitation. A comparison between various methods has demonstrated that no single method is superior to any other; however, outcomes can be significantly impacted by fracture type and patient-related factors, such as the integrity of soft tissues. In the future, continued research will be pivotal to further advancing these surgical techniques, yielding the best possible outcomes for myriad traumatic injuries and evolving with the new face of trauma care through strategic planning and execution of surgical interventions (Angelini et al., 2018).

Test Your Knowledge

1. What factors determine whether a trauma patient requires emergency surgical intervention versus conservative management?
2. How do damage control surgery and definitive surgical repair differ in the management of major traumatic injuries?

9.5. Postoperative Care

Learning Outcome

1. Define monitoring for complications for post-major trauma
2. Discuss on pain management strategies
3. Explain the rehabilitation and recovery

Optimal postoperative care is essential to optimizing patient outcomes following definitive trauma surgery. Optimized postoperative care is designed to minimize complications, reduce pain, and expedite recovery, ultimately enhancing satisfaction with surgical intervention. Of particular interest, of course, is the increasing emphasis on opioid stewardship, particularly in the context of today's opioid epidemic. Surgeons must work to optimize pain relief without the risk of opioid abuse. Studies have found that trauma surgeons write more opioids more often, depending on the history of opioid use among the patients and other considerations, which highlights the urgency for tailored pain management practices. Such findings regarding trends in prescribing highlight the surgeon's role in optimizing discharge practices to minimize postoperative opioid addiction among patients (Anderson et al., 2019). Early postoperative observation and assessments also play a crucial role in the early detection of complications such as infections, hemorrhage, and thromboembolic events. Patients recovering from major trauma surgery will have complicated medical histories that require close observation. There are numerous diagnostic modalities available to healthcare teams to monitor a patient's postoperative course, allowing for early intervention when necessary. This observation is essential for patients who are to undergo bariatric surgery, where complications may arise long after hospital discharge. A study referred to the importance of emergency surgeons being aware of the frequent complications following such procedures, believing that a strict follow-up protocol would significantly influence patient outcomes (Abu-Zidan et al., 2020). Having a definite postoperative care plan that emphasizes close follow-up can enable early identification and management of complications, thus ensuring better recovery patterns. Open communication between patients and healthcare professionals is a crucial aspect of postoperative care. This involves educating patients on their recovery process, complications risks, and when to come in for further medical attention. Open channels of communication can help minimize anxiety among patients significantly, promote compliance with postoperative instructions, and facilitate active patient involvement in the recovery process. As part of interprofessional healthcare, involving patient feedback in postoperative care plans can help address individual needs and expectations, enhance patient satisfaction, and lead to improved outcomes. By emphasizing appropriate education and establishing a sound communication system, medical professionals can create an environment that enables patients throughout the recovery process, thereby laying the foundation for effective postoperative care in major trauma surgery (Figure 9.11).

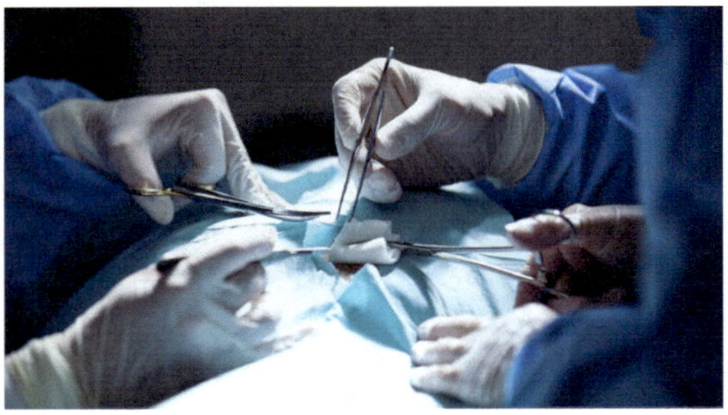

Figure 9.11. The critical role of a trauma surgeon in emergency care.

Source: https://centersurgentcare.net/wp-content/uploads/2025/03/What-Can-X-Rays-Detect-8-3.jpg.

9.5.1. Monitoring for Complications

Impeccable monitoring for post-major trauma surgery complications is paramount to patient security and optimizing the result of recovery. This is particularly true in the case of penetrating cardiac injuries (PCIs), where there is a risk of significant hemodynamic instability and therefore the need for more attentive monitoring. There have been emerging studies highlighting the intervention of procedures like the pericardial window (PCW) that can potentially be a less invasive approach for specific cardiac injuries. Specifically, hemopericardium patients are typically closely monitored post-procedure in an intensive care unit (ICU) environment for their cardiovascular status and any residual bleeding. This strict postoperative observation has proven to be significant; results show that patients who were initially treated with PCW had good outcomes, and no in-hospital mortality was reported in either the PCW or sternotomy groups (Chestovich et al., 2018). Thus, awareness of the monitoring guidelines following PCI procedures is crucial in preventing complications after surgery. Apart from cardiac complications, patients who undergo major trauma surgery are also at risk for a range of postoperative complications, particularly if there exist conditions like obstructive sleep apnea syndrome (OSAS). These patients are usually predisposed to heightened sensitivity to anesthesia and sedative drugs, deteriorating their respiratory condition, and leading to adverse postoperative outcomes. A significant prevalence of OSAS in elective surgical patients calls for perioperative care, demanding meticulous preoperative assessment to identify such patients. Effective monitoring strategies should involve the identification of at-risk patients and the implementation of measures to regulate sedation levels, thereby avoiding risks in recovery. Heightened alertness and awareness in the ICU can significantly help in the prevention of complications due to untreated sleep apnea in recovery from major trauma surgery (Doghramji et al., 2012).

Eventually, the integration of multiple aspects of monitoring strategies can significantly impact patient outcomes following major trauma surgery. Near-real-time monitoring tools such as telemetry and high-fidelity imaging also assist clinical staff in identifying deviations from expected recovery patterns early. Nursing staff also play an essential role in checking vital signs and symptomatology that will indicate impending complications. Regular bedside evaluation, coupled with interprofessional collaboration among surgical teams, intensivists, and nurses, fosters a culture that promotes the early detection and treatment of suspected complications. With protocols dedicated to all-inclusive monitoring—varied from hemodynamic stability to respiratory function—this also enhances the surgical teams' ability to and adequately cater to patients' evolving needs during that all-important postoperative period. A symphony, therefore, of coordinated, interprofessional management with an emphasis on diligent monitoring can lead to improved postoperative outcomes and ultimately, patient survival (Chestovich et al., 2018) (Figure 9.12).

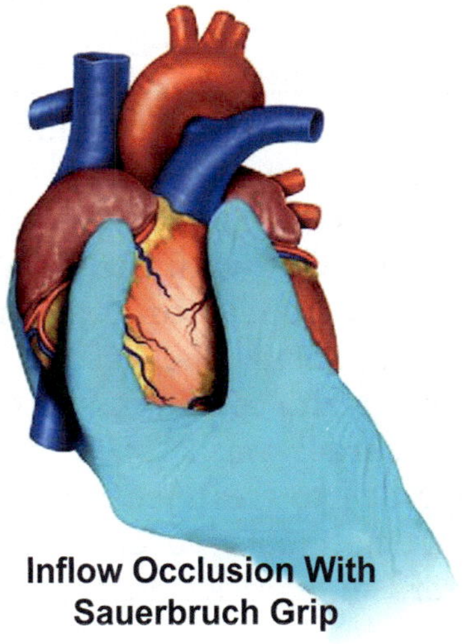

Figure 9.12. Damage control in penetrating cardiac trauma.

Source: https://www.redalyc.org/journal/283/28366681002/1657-9534-cm-52-02-e4034519-gf3.jpg.

9.5.2. Pain Management Strategies

Optimal management of pain is an essential component of significant trauma surgery, particularly about patient satisfaction and recovery. Previously, much reliance has been placed on opioid medications; however, this has contributed to the ongoing opioid crisis in the United States. Physicians are encouraged to adopt a more multifaceted method of pain management that involves a multitude of methods beyond narcotics. With the development of their repertoire, clinicians can employ physical interventions such as physiotherapy, cognitive-behavioral techniques for coping, and multimodal analgesic regimens involving non-opioid analgesics in combination with regional anesthesia. The practices not only enhance pain mitigation but are essential in averting risks of opioid addiction and dependence, ultimately resulting in higher recovery rates for trauma patients (Hsu et al., 2019). There was a strong push in recent years to advance the issue of nonoperative management of certain blunt liver injuries, illustrating how treatment paradigms keep changing in the field of trauma care. It is aimed at stability among stable hemodynamic patients in whom the operation should not be done urgently. Utilization of this policy enables the most appropriate use of advanced imaging techniques and interventional methods, such as embolization and percutaneous drainage, to reduce the need for more invasive surgery. Pain management in such patients can thus be made possible with the vision of restricting narcotic therapy by means of conservative monitoring and supportive treatment. This paradigm not only reflects the development of critical care medicine but also addresses practices at the time, favoring patient-focused treatment and personalized care systems (Ferrada et al., 2017).

Moreover, the ongoing development of clinical practice guidelines by national medical societies seeks to make pain management practices uniform in the context of major trauma surgery. These guidelines encourage the implementation of a multimodal approach, utilizing multiple diverse modalities, to enhance safety and efficacy in pain management. The key to the success of these interventions is education for clinicians, which is vital for understanding addiction and pain pathophysiology. Preventing opioid misuse but safeguarding patients is also accomplished by expanding access to such resources as naloxone. Clinicians and policymakers must collaborate to redefine pain management practices in accordance with modern medical standards, ensuring these approaches are effective and responsible in addressing the complexities of pain management in trauma surgery (Hsu et al., 2019).

9.5.3. Rehabilitation and Recovery

Rehabilitation and recovery are fundamental components of the rehabilitation process following major trauma surgery. Rehabilitation from surgery to recovery is a multidisciplinary process involving physical therapy, psychological counseling, and patient education. Rehabilitation is not just restoring one's physical function but also addressing the emotional and psychological scars left by trauma. Patients exhibit depression, anxiety, and post-traumatic stress symptoms, which inhibit their recovery process. Thus, an integrated system of trauma-informed care and traditional rehabilitation methods is most important. Adhering to such a system will enhance patients' resilience and quality of life, paving the way for an integrated process of whole-person recovery involving body and mind. Physical rehabilitation strategies, particularly after severe trauma requiring surgical stabilization, focus on regaining mobility and functional autonomy. Early mobilization within the process of rehabilitation has been proven to reduce complications arising from prolonged immobilization, such as muscular atrophy and thromboembolic events. Where more than one trauma has occurred, individually tailored physical therapy measures will accelerate the recovery rate, with targeted exercises designed to optimize strength and range of motion simultaneously while minimizing pain. Tailored rehabilitation protocols cannot be overestimated, since these need to adapt to the specificity of the trauma and to the needs of the individual patient. Secondly, a patient-centered approach ensures that individuals are continuously encouraged and motivated to participate in their rehabilitation process, which is equally crucial for achieving long-term recovery results. Psychosocial factors play a vital role during recovery and rehabilitation following major trauma surgery. Survivors are likely to go through challenging emotions related to their trauma, including feelings of isolation and powerlessness, which can hinder their participation in rehabilitation interventions. Coupling cognitive-behavioral therapies and supportive counseling with the rehabilitation will enable individuals to overcome such psychological barriers. The possibility of co-morbid mental health conditions, such as Major Depressive Disorder and PTSD, necessitates a holistic approach to treatment involving both physical and emotional recovery. In addressing these matters, integrative interventions can enable not only the recovery of function but also improved emotional resilience, allowing one to re-engage in life with a newfound purpose and agency (Tr, 2025; Maaroufi, 2024) (Figure 9.13).

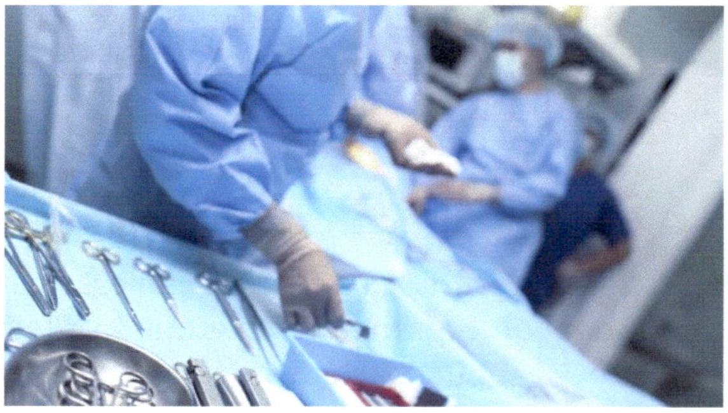

Figure 9.13. The current and future role of nurses within enhanced recovery after surgery pathways.

Source: https://www.britishjournalofnursing.com/content/professional/the-current-and-future-role-of-nurses-within-enhanced-recovery-after-surgery-pathways/.

Test Your Knowledge

1. What strategies are essential to prevent complications such as infection, hemorrhage, or organ dysfunction after trauma surgery?
2. How does early mobilization and rehabilitation influence recovery outcomes in postoperative trauma patients?

9.6. Ethical Considerations

Learning Outcome

1. Understand the informed consent for trauma surgery
2. Describe the resource allocation in trauma cases
3. Define end-of-life decisions

Ethical problems in major trauma surgery are multifaceted, reflecting the complexity of surgical practice and patient care. Beneficence requires surgeons to act in the best interests of their patients, underscoring the need for precision and effectiveness in trauma interventions. This raises a myriad of ethical issues with the introduction of new technologies, like robotic surgery. For instance, while robotic systems represent the pinnacle of progress insofar as they enhance precision and surgical efficacy, concerns are voiced regarding potential depersonalization of care and substitution of human clinicians. Surgeons must weigh the benefits of improved performance through automation against ethical losses of reduced human oversight of vital procedures (Das et al., 2017). Finally, patient autonomy and informed consent remain the paramount considerations, as patients will require these technological subtleties and potential dangers to be explained to them. The ethical dilemma is also made more complex by demographic shifts in trauma patients, particularly elderly patients. Increased numbers of elderly trauma patients emphasize the necessity for age-specific consideration during operative planning. Incidence suggests that older patients develop injuries more frequently from falls and assault, which tend to result in more extended hospitalization periods and greater complications (Chalya et al., 2012). Surgeons are then confronted with ethical issues in allocating limited resources when patients present with comorbidities or severe injuries that may pose a higher risk of mortality. Satisfying these requirements requires a balance between the demands for total care and the need to consider each situation with measured restraint, weighing patients' quality of life following intervention. Furthermore, the ethical implications of pre-hospital and surgical trauma intervention help define a critical area of ethical concern. Trauma victims usually experience delays in treatment that exacerbate their injuries and have worse outcomes. In developing nations, where medical care might not always be timely, the problem is even more pronounced (Chalya et al., 2012). This test evaluates the ethical values of justice and fairness in the provision of medical care. Policymakers in the medical field and trauma surgeons must collaborate to demand improved emergency response systems that ensure everyone, regardless of socioeconomic status or origin, receives effective and timely surgery. These disparities need to be resolved to uphold the ethical standard of equal care while being capable of delivering the best results to all trauma patients.

9.6.1. Informed Consent for Trauma Surgery

Trauma surgery-informed consent is complicated due to the urgency and dynamic nature of the situations upon which both patients and health teams must operate. Trauma patients generally present with incapacitating injuries that prevent them from being completely capable of grasping the extent or nature of their ailment or the treatment options suggested. Despite the pressing need for speedy surgery, medical professionals must do their best to uphold the ethical hallmark of informed consent. Consent is not just an element of legal safeguarding, but also a step for upholding the patient's autonomy and ensuring they are being involved in decisions regarding their care. This challenge is particularly amplified in cases where patients are unable to express their preferences or where family members must be involved, complicating decision-making in ways that can have profound impacts on patient outcomes. Legal and ethical frameworks involving informed consent are exceptionally complicated in the setting of traumatic injuries that require emergency surgical intervention. For surgeries such as open reduction and internal fixation (ORIF) of fractures, benefits and risks must be fully explained to the patient or surrogates when the patient is incapacitated. Physicians must balance the urgency of surgery and the requirement for informed consent, and balance the sensitive tension between ethical and legal requirements. For instance, Belluzzi et al. (2019) indicate the relevance of understanding the effects of the timing of surgery on outcomes in a clinical context, for example, risk of complications like avascular necrosis.

This broaches a highly relevant point: one concerning the balancing act between when timely surgery must be performed and how to guarantee that patients or consents are maximally informed about risks. In exceptional circumstances where obtaining informed consent is impracticable or time-consuming, such as in some cases of acetabular fractures requiring prophylaxis, medical professionals must adhere to established protocols following set ethical and legal standards. For instance, Bosshard et al. (2018) prescribe protocols for the use of prophylactic irradiation against heterotopic ossification among trauma patients, arguing that consent can only be postponed when it is unavoidable. It is this proactive planning that makes sure patients are instructed as early as possible and families are included in decision-making. Through these habits, trauma surgeons can effectively manage the complexities of informed consent while ensuring patient safety, rights, and dignity. Therefore, having an ethical system in place for informed consent not only complies with the law but also induces trust and openness between the patient and surgeon, key elements of successful trauma care (Figure 9.14).

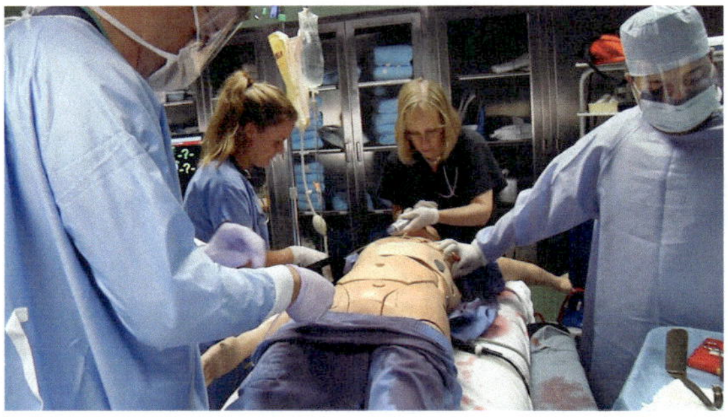

Figure 9.14. Informed consent in trauma surgery.

Source: https://static01.nyt.com/images/2014/06/10/science/10SURG/10SURG-superJumbo.jpg.

9.6.2. R-esource Allocation in Trauma Cases

Trauma case resource management is a critical component of major trauma surgery, requiring the effective allocation of limited resources to meet varying levels of patient need. In high-stress environments such as in trauma units, healthcare practitioners need to allocate treatment when prioritizing based on injury severity, likelihood of survival, and likely prognosis for a favorable outcome. This decision-making process is further complicated by the need to consider not only the individual case of each patient but also systemic factors such as operating room suite availability, surgical staff, and post-operative capacity. Practical evaluation and timely mobilization of resources will maintain morbidity and mortality rates at an optimum, thereby emphasizing the importance of organized protocols in trauma centers. These frameworks ensure the timely and ethical provision of life-saving interventions that achieve the best patient outcomes under limited conditions. Furthermore, evidence-based guidelines incorporated into the resource allocation process will enhance decision-making in trauma surgery. These guidelines, derived from continuing research and funded work such as that addressed by the NIHR Health Technology Assessment program, provide clinicians with up-to-date information on optimal practice and emerging technologies to support surgical efficacy (Mendelow et al., 2015). While clinician-level judgment cannot be replaced, reliance on a standardized protocol can help to reduce variability between units in treatment approaches and outcomes. Empirical research findings can elucidate effective strategies for allocating resources, allowing trauma centers to cater to patients' needs while maximizing the use of available resources. Thus, a keen emphasis on evidence-based practice not only improves the quality of patient care but also ensures accountability in the allocation of healthcare resources. Beyond short-term interventions for surgeries, resource allocation has long-term implications for patient recovery and the sustainability of healthcare. The right and timely allocation of resources can lead to reduced hospital stays, fewer complications, and better rehabilitative outcomes, ultimately relieving healthcare systems (Boto et al., 2015). Alternatively, inappropriate resource management can result in delayed interventions and increased morbidity, highlighting the importance of active measures in trauma care. The application of evidence-based measures in assessing patient flow and resource utilization enables healthcare managers to forecast requirements and prepare for potential eventualities accurately. In general, an understanding of ethical issues and empirical data in the distribution of resources is crucial in major trauma surgery, significantly contributing to improved healthcare delivery and overall public health improvement.

9.6.3. End-of-Life Decisions

In trauma surgery, end-of-life decisions are often a major ethical dilemma for both patients and medical professionals. The trauma care scenario can evoke perplexing situations where injury severity, patient prognosis, and the viability of life-sustaining procedures must be balanced accordingly. As surgical teams act with urgency to stabilize and treat life-threatening injuries, the danger of unfavorable outcomes can provoke debate about potential limitations of care. Such debates should involve not just clinical realities but also the patient's values and prior expressed wishes for preferences in care. Having such a framework early in the process of treatment ensures patient autonomy because individuals can communicate their preferences regarding life-sustaining interventions, which can lead to a more patient-centered approach within the high-risk environment of primary trauma care. In addition, end-of-life decisions in major trauma surgery have implications that extend beyond the short-term clinical outcomes, affecting the emotional and psychological well-being of patients and medical staff. When patients sustain life-threatening injuries, their families are most often placed in the impossible position of begging for care decisions on a mixture of hope and despair. Clear communication among the medical staff and families is essential to steer through these turbulent waters. This communication can be used to provide information on treatment options and help families understand the chances of recovery or deterioration. Moreover, involving the families in decision-making may decrease feelings of helplessness, fostering an environment of care in which emotional trauma burden is acknowledged. Thus, integrating family participation and emotional support becomes an integral part of the model of care for trauma surgery.

Lastly, ethics in decision-making for end-of-life care is imperative in the context of major trauma surgery. Medical professionals often need to operate within ethical models that encourage the use of principles such as beneficence, non-maleficence, and respect for autonomy to guide their clinical interventions. As trauma patients typically present with severe conditions, the urgency of intervention creates particular ethical dilemmas; professionals must reconcile the need to save lives with an understanding of the quality of a patient's life and individual preferences. Moreover, research funded by institutions such as the National Institute for Health Research has provided significant evidence on patient decision-making in life-threatening conditions, specifically regarding long-term consequences (Boto et al., 2015). A critical analysis of such research reveals that end-of-life care must prioritize integrating patient-centered approaches into discussions, fostering compassionate and ethically driven settings in traumatic scenarios (Figure 9.15).

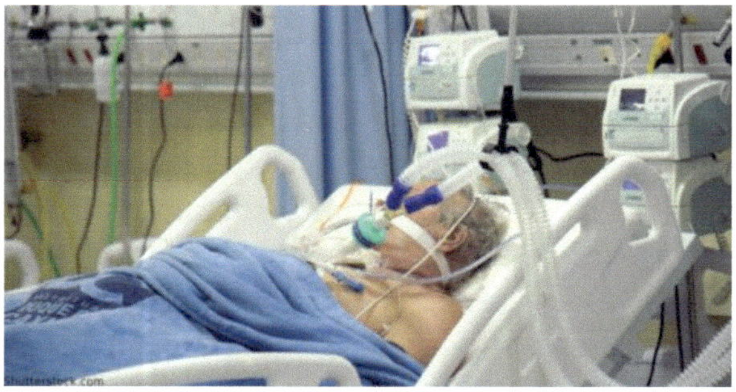

Figure 9.15. Difficult decisions in the intensive care unit.

Source: https://www.acepnow.com/wp-content/uploads/2023/03/diff-decisions-art-mar-2023-500x261.jpg.

Test Your Knowledge

1. What ethical dilemmas arise when prioritizing treatment for multiple trauma patients in mass casualty situations?
2. How does informed consent and patient autonomy influence decision-making in emergency trauma interventions?

SUMMARY

Major trauma surgery entails a complex interaction of surgical interventions required to correct potentially lethal injuries. This complex discipline takes precedence in stabilizing and restoring patients in recuperation, often utilizing evidence-based care for optimal outcomes. The integration of nonoperative management (NOM) in the treatment of certain types of trauma, such as renal trauma, has gained more widespread recognition, which accounts for the shift in treatment paradigms. In particular, NOM has been shown to be advantageous for lower-grade injuries and may even be applicable to high-grade renal trauma, suggesting a possible reconsideration of conventional operative strategies in some instances (Kawish et al., 2020). These developments point to an increasing recognition of trauma care, where selective regimens can result in less morbidity and improved function preservation. Additionally, the role of follow-up after operation cannot be overemphasized in major trauma surgery. Monitoring on a real-time basis enables medical professionals to assess the course of recovery and take appropriate action accordingly. A clinical study comparing scleral buckling surgery for retinal detachment found that patients may experience more ocular motility restrictions post-surgery, emphasizing the need for optimal post-surgical care (Kawish et al., 2020). This emphasis on inclusive follow-up not only serves to identify complications, but also empowers patients through education and informing them during the process of recovery, emphasizing the integral role of trauma surgery. Ultimately, the evolution of major trauma surgery will depend on ongoing research and adoption of new, patient-centered practices. As the specialty evolves, providers must remain vigilant to new evidence that undermines traditional management paradigms. Through both surgical and non-surgical approaches, clinicians can tailor interventions to meet the specific needs of each patient, ensuring increased outcomes and quality of life. Outcomes of studies in favor of NOM show a paradigm-changing approach that maximizes effectiveness and safety for patients, supporting further extended use in the context of major trauma surgery (Brachini et al., 2017).

In examining the complexity of major trauma surgery, there are salient points that highlight the importance of surgery in the treatment of specific conditions, including patellar dislocation. The evidence suggests that operative management may result in lower recurrent dislocation rates compared to non-operative rehabilitation strategies. That said, the quality of this evidence is not high, and most of this can be attributed to the presence of biases in studies and varying levels of methodological quality across trials. For example, a systematic review illustrated that patients who had undergone surgical treatment for primary patellar dislocation had a recurrence rate of 21/162 compared with 32/136 in the non-surgical group, with the benefit of a risk ratio in favor of surgery to be addressed in further research. The pressing need for well-executed, multicenter trials is evident, as the available studies have drawbacks and fail to adequately address recurrent dislocations, a serious deficiency in the trauma surgery literature (Apostolovic et al., 2015).

Furthermore, improved techniques in clinical research play a crucial role in shaping the course of trauma surgery. Multi-center trials, through collaboration, are now essential, especially in the field of complicated injuries, such as those to the brain. These group efforts can consolidate data collection and validation mechanisms, addressing the multi-dimensional nature of trauma. The Cooperative Study on Brain Injury Depolarizations and the Brain Monitoring with Information Technology team are good illustrations of how data infrastructure is being improved. They raise concerns about data protection and access issues, which are crucial in facilitating and adequate multi-center studies. The ongoing focus on developing IT solutions, such as the AVERT-IT project, is an indication of a commitment to overcoming technological barriers in trauma research, ultimately leading to changes in clinical practices in major trauma surgery (Piper et al., 2009).

Ultimately, the successful deployment of data-driven methods in trauma surgery can lead to clinical innovations that enhance patient outcomes. As the horizon of trauma care shifts toward an interdisciplinary approach, the ability to share wisdom and data between institutions will be a valuable boost for surgical algorithms and patient management strategies. Enhanced technical infrastructures will place researchers in a better position to perform well-informed studies addressing multiple treatment modalities, surgical considerations, and nonsurgical. Such a collaborative approach not only facilitates comprehensive evaluations of therapeutic success but also offers the potential for new and innovative practice according to patient-specific needs. Thus, the incorporation of evidence from multi-center trials will play a crucial role in defining best practices, minimizing complications, and enhancing the overall effectiveness of major trauma surgery (Piper et al., 2009; Apostolovic et al., 2015).

KEY TERMS FROM THIS CHAPTER

- Airway management
- Blunt abdominal trauma
- Compartment syndrome
- Head injury
- Massive transfusion protocol
- Pelvic fracture
- Polytrauma
- Spinal cord injury
- ATLS (Advanced Trauma Life Support)
- Chest trauma
- Damage control surgery
- Hemorrhagic shock
- Open fractures
- Penetrating trauma
- Resuscitative thoracotomy
- Thoracotomy

CRITICAL THINKING QUESTIONS

1. **What is the first step in the primary survey of a trauma patient according to ATLS protocol?**
    a. Circulation with hemorrhage control
    b. Airway with cervical spine protection
    c. Breathing and ventilation
    d. Disability assessment
2. **Which of the following findings is most consistent with a tension pneumothorax?**
    a. Bilateral breath sounds
    b. Tracheal deviation toward the affected side
    c. Hyperresonance on percussion and distended neck veins
    d. Bradycardia and hypotension
3. **The "lethal triad" in trauma includes all of the following EXCEPT:**
    a. Hypothermia
    b. Acidosis
    c. Coagulopathy
    d. Hyperkalemia
4. **Which of the following is the most appropriate imaging modality for a hemodynamically unstable patient with suspected intra-abdominal bleeding?**
    a. CT abdomen with contrast
    b. Diagnostic peritoneal lavage
    c. FAST (Focused Assessment with Sonography for Trauma)
    d. MRI abdomen
5. **Damage control surgery primarily aims to:**
    a. Perform definitive repair of all injuries immediately
    b. Reduce the need for blood transfusion
    c. Limit operative time to correct life-threatening issues and stabilize physiology
    d. Minimize surgical incision size

Short Answer Questions

1. What are the components of the primary survey in trauma according to the ATLS protocol?
2. What is the role of the physical examination in abdominal trauma?
3. What are the clinical signs of tension pneumothorax, and how is it managed?
4. Define the "lethal triad" in trauma and explain its significance.
5. When is an emergency thoracotomy indicated in a trauma patient?
6. What are the indications for surgical intervention in blunt abdominal trauma?
7. How is hemorrhagic shock classified, and what guides fluid resuscitation?
8. What is the purpose of damage control surgery, and when is it performed?

Answers to Critical Thinking Questions

1. (b); 2. (c); 3. (d); 4. (c); 5. (c)

REFERENCES

1. De Simone, B., Ansaloni, L., Sartelli, M., Kluger, Y., Abu-Zidan, F. M., Biffl, W. L., Heyer, A., Coccolini, F., Baiocchi, G. L., & Catena, F. (2020). The Operative management in Bariatric Acute abdomen (OBA) Survey: long-term complications of bariatric surgery and the emergency surgeon's point of view. *World Journal of Emergency Surgery, 15*(1). https://doi.org/10.1186/s13017-019-0281-yAcosta, S., Azuma, N., Bastos Gonçalves, F., Björck, M., et al. (2020). *Editor's choice: European Society for Vascular Surgery (ESVS) 2020 clinical practice guidelines on the management of acute limb ischaemia.* https://core.ac.uk/download/286570102.pdf (accessed on 12th July 2025).
2. Adin, D., Bostwick, D., Breznock, E., Bright, R., Bussadori, R., Greenhalgh, S., et al. (2017). *Treatment of intrahepatic congenital portosystemic shunts in dogs: A systematic review.* https://core.ac.uk/download/146489756.pdf (accessed on 12th July 2025).
3. Ali, P., Santy-Tomlinson, J., & Watson, R. (2014). *Assessment and diagnosis of acute limb compartment syndrome: A literature review.* https://core.ac.uk/download/151161255.pdf (accessed on 12th July 2025).
4. Allen, L., Anderson, R. E., Askari, R., Baradaran, N., et al. (2020). *The American Association for the Surgery of Trauma renal injury grading scale: Implications of the 2018 revisions for injury reclassification and predicting bleeding interventions.* https://core.ac.uk/download/287623169.pdf (accessed on 12th July 2025).
5. Anderson, J. E., Cocanour, C. S., & Galante, J. M. (2019). *Trauma and acute care surgeons report prescribing less opioids over time.* https://core.ac.uk/download/323070594.pdf (accessed on 12th July 2025).
6. Angelini, A., Biz, C., Carniel, D., Iacobellis, C., et al. (2018). *Medium-long-term radiographic and clinical outcomes after surgical treatment of intra-articular tibial pilon fractures by three different techniques.* https://core.ac.uk/download/154330599.pdf (accessed on 12th July 2025).
7. Ansel, G. M., Dake, M. D., Johnson, M. S., Mendes, R., et al. (2019). *The clinical rationale for the Sentry bioconvertible inferior vena cava filter for the prevention of pulmonary embolism.* https://core.ac.uk/download/228066254.pdf (accessed on 12th July 2025).
8. Apostolovic, D., Arnbjörnsson, E., Atkin, J., Baier, C., Beasley, T., Bennell, K., Bitar, K., et al. (2015). *Surgical versus non-surgical interventions for treating patellar dislocation.* https://core.ac.uk/download/41990248.pdf (accessed on 12th July 2025).
9. Babcock, J. M., Berne, J., Bosarge, P., Bruns, B., et al. (2019). *Outcomes in patients with gunshot wounds to the brain.* https://core.ac.uk/download/287624186.pdf (accessed on 12th July 2025).
10. Ball, C. G., Fabian, T. C., Feliciano, D. V., Ivatury, R., et al. (2017). *History of the innovation of damage control for management of trauma patients: 1902–2016.* https://core.ac.uk/download/84402892.pdf (accessed on 12th July 2025).
11. Belluzzi, E., Biz, C., De Cicco, M., Fantoni, I., et al. (2019). *Long-term radiographic and clinical-functional outcomes of isolated, displaced, closed talar neck and body fractures treated by ORIF: The timing of surgical management.* https://core.ac.uk/download/224995443.pdf (accessed on 12th July 2025).

12. Bosshard, G., Keel, M., Lütolf, U., Oertel, M., et al. (2018). *Prophylaxis of heterotopic ossification in patients sedated after polytrauma: Medical and ethical considerations.* https://core.ac.uk/download/159149081.pdf (accessed on 12th July 2025).

13. Boto, G. W., Brain Trauma Foundation, American Association of Neurological Surgeons (AANS), Briggs, M., Broderick, J., Bullock, R., et al. (2015). *Surgical trial in traumatic intracerebral hemorrhage (STITCH): A randomized controlled trial of early surgery compared with initial conservative treatment.* https://core.ac.uk/download/42130685.pdf (accessed on 12th July 2025).

14. Brachini, G., Cirillo, B., La Torre, M., Migliori, M., et al. (2017). *Operative and nonoperative management for renal trauma: Comparison of outcomes. A systematic review and meta-analysis.* https://core.ac.uk/download/98349100.pdf (accessed on 12th July 2025).

15. Cascone, P., Fontanari, M., Maffia, F., Mercuri, L., et al. (2020). *Impact of COVID-19 on maxillofacial surgery practice: A worldwide survey.* https://core.ac.uk/download/323192162.pdf (accessed on 12th July 2025).

16. Chalya, P. L., Dass, R. M., Gilyoma, J. M., Mabula, J. B., et al. (2012). *Geriatric injuries among patients attending a regional hospital in Shinyanga, Tanzania.* https://core.ac.uk/download/pdf/18410878.pdf (accessed on 12th July 2025).

17. Charles, A. G., Gallaher, J. R., Kincaid, J. A., Maine, R., et al. (2018). *Interpersonal violence in peacetime Malawi.* https://core.ac.uk/download/213444928.pdf (accessed on 12th July 2025).

18. Chestovich, P. J., Clark, E., Fildes, J. J., et al. (2018). *Selective use of pericardial window and drainage as sole treatment for hemopericardium from penetrating chest trauma.* https://core.ac.uk/download/215451049.pdf (accessed on 12th July 2025).

19. Claes, K., De Wolf, E., Opsomer, D., Roche, N., et al. (2019). *Free flaps for lower limb soft tissue reconstruction in children: Systematic review.* https://core.ac.uk/download/286548693.pdf (accessed on 12th July 2025).

20. Cross, K., Fallat, M. E., Laniewicz, M., Nti, A., et al. (2019). *A novel streamlined trauma response team training improves imaging efficiency for pediatric blunt abdominal trauma patients.* https://core.ac.uk/download/187423820.pdf (accessed on 12th July 2025).

21. Das, N., & Yip, M. (2017). *Robot autonomy for surgery.* http://arxiv.org/abs/1707.03080 (accessed on 12th July 2025).

22. Doben, A. R., Dolich, M., Grigorian, A., Gross, C., et al. (2020). *Outcomes after pneumonectomy versus limited lung resection in adults with traumatic lung injury.* https://core.ac.uk/download/323308579.pdf (accessed on 12th July 2025).

23. Doghramji, K., Grewal, R. G., Vasu, T. S., et al. (2012). *Obstructive sleep apnea syndrome and perioperative complications: A systematic review of the literature.* https://core.ac.uk/download/83049558.pdf (accessed on 12th July 2025).

24. Ferrada, P., & Peysha, J. (2017). *Operative and nonoperative management of blunt liver injuries.* https://core.ac.uk/download/84404215.pdf (accessed on 12th July 2025).

25. Frang, D., Jako, G. J., & Repassy, D. L. (2011). *Minimal and direct access surgery in urology.* https://core.ac.uk/download/142040468.pdf (accessed on 12th July 2025).

26. Glynou, S., Georgiannakis, A., Ackling, E., Bystrzonowski, N., Pafitanis, G., & Diver, A. (2024). Postoperative protocols for lower extremity free flap reconstructions: Literature review and

a national survey of the United Kingdom's major trauma centers. *Journal of Reconstructive Microsurgery Open, 9*, e121–e128. https://www.semanticscholar.org/paper/2ed4ae92e314c16de76f36b5bf4a7b309b81d5cf (accessed on 12th July 2025).

27. Goldberg, A., Macgregor, A. J., Pfeil, M., Zaidi, R., et al. (2013). *How do patients with end-stage ankle arthritis decide between two surgical treatments? A qualitative study.* https://core.ac.uk/download/19595159.pdf (accessed on 12th July 2025).
28. Hsu, J. R., Jahangir, A. A., Miller, A. N., Mir, H., et al. (2019). *Confronting the opioid crisis: Practical pain management and strategies: AOA 2018 critical issues symposium.* https://core.ac.uk/download/286537307.pdf (accessed on 12th July 2025).
29. Ibeanusi, S. J. C. (2019). *Femoral fractures in children treated in a regional trauma center in Nigeria. International Journal of Critical Care and Emergency Medicine.* https://www.semanticscholar.org/paper/07503bfaeec7735799c61e5f8a271e4be7b46e33 (accessed on 12th July 2025).
30. Kalová, M., Kubíček, J., Oczka, D., Tomanec, F., et al. (2019). *Recent trends, technical concepts and components of computer-assisted orthopedic surgery systems: A comprehensive review.* https://core.ac.uk/download/287649034.pdf (accessed on 12th July 2025).
31. Kawish, A. B., Nawaz, S., & Tahir, Q. (2020). *Extraocular muscle imbalance and outcomes of scleral buckling surgery for primary rhegmatogenous retinal detachment.* https://media.neliti.com/media/publications/301074-extraocular-muscle-imbalance-and-outcome-2a99bee0.pdf (accessed on 12th July 2025).
32. Khan, A., Kuzuku, A., Chandika, A. B., Solagberu, B. A., Mutasingwa, D. R., Norberg, E., Twagirayezu, E., et al. (2013). *Citywide trauma experience in Mwanza, Tanzania: A need for urgent intervention.* https://core.ac.uk/download/pdf/19726063.pdf (accessed on 12th July 2025).
33. Kileo, B. F. (2012). *The pattern of oral and maxillofacial injuries among patients attending Muhimbili National Hospital, Dar es Salaam, Tanzania.* https://core.ac.uk/download/pdf/11307821.pdf (accessed on 12th July 2025).
34. Lafta, G. A., Dolachee, A. A., Al-Zubaidi, A., & Hoz, S. S. (2019). A death calls from unsafe heights: A study of factors influencing the outcome of surgically treated pediatric head trauma patients in Baghdad. *International Journal of Research in Pharmaceutical Sciences.* https://www.semanticscholar.org/paper/08da6ff8bf75999feb1fcc2d26f1742714b541f0 (accessed on 12th July 2025).
35. Maaroufi, A. (2024). *Anesthetic management of multiple traumas for trauma surgery in the Moroccan 5thMSC in Errachidia. ARC Journal of Anesthesiology.* https://www.semanticscholar.org/paper/7510d979e31a7266d7c8ff374dfb56ca72674cb6 (accessed on 12th July 2025).
36. Mendelow, A. D., Unterberg, A., Gregson, B. A., Boyers, D., McColl, E., Rowan, E. N., Chambers, I. R., et al. (2015). *Early surgery versus initial conservative treatment in patients with traumatic intracerebral hemorrhage [STITCH(Trauma)]: The first randomized trial.* https://core.ac.uk/download/30435926.pdf (accessed on 12th July 2025).
37. Okoye, B. C., Bugando Medical Centre (BMC), Trunkey, D., Kang, E. G., Orji, F. T., Matilda, I., et al. (2013). *Ear, nose and throat injuries at Bugando Medical Centre in northwestern Tanzania: A five-year prospective review of 456 cases.* https://core.ac.uk/download/pdf/11307767.pdf (accessed on 12th July 2025).

38. Patel, K. H., Gill, L. I., Tissingh, E. K., Galanis, A. S., Hadjihannas, I., Iliadis, A. D., Heidari, N., et al. (2023). Microbiological profile of fracture-related infection at a UK major trauma center. *Antibiotics, 12.* https://www.semanticscholar.org/paper/312f781981807deca390ac982eb227923949d1e3 (accessed on 12th July 2025).

39. Piper, I., & Sinnott, R. O. (2009). *E-infrastructures fostering multi-center collaborative research into the intensive care management of patients with brain injury.* https://core.ac.uk/download/1396979.pdf (accessed on 12th July 2025).

40. Reji, T. R. (2025). *Healing from trauma: A comprehensive psychosocial approach to recovery from sexual abuse, depression, and suicidal ideation. International Journal of Social Science Exceptional Research.* https://www.semanticscholar.org/paper/57ad4e759de956b4ed55a32f4df530b3ab67356e (accessed on 12th July 2025).

ORTHOPEDIC SURGERY

10

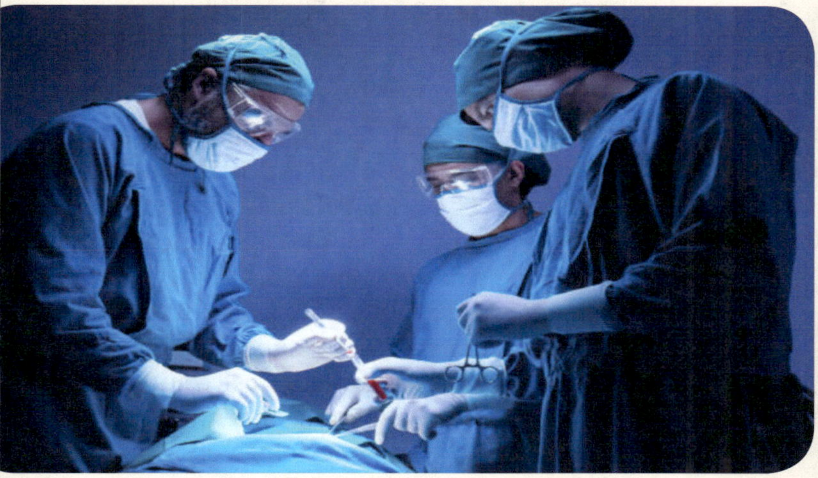

LEARNING OBJECTIVES

After studying this chapter, you will be able to:

1. Understand the history of orthopedic surgery
2. Explain the common orthopedic conditions
3. Discuss the diagnostic techniques of orthopedic surgery
4. Focus on surgical procedures of orthopedic surgery
5. Learn about postoperative care of orthopedic surgery
6. Evaluate the advances in orthopedic surgery

Introduction

Orthopedic surgery then becomes a vital field of medicine that is fundamentally concerned with the diagnosis, treatment, and rehabilitation of disorders of the musculoskeletal system. As a highly complex discipline, it entails many techniques and technologies, treating conditions and injuries involving bones, joints, ligaments, tendons, and muscles. With the rising prevalence of musculoskeletal disorders precipitated by aging and increasing activity in high-load sports, the importance of orthopedic surgery cannot be overstated. Moreover, advancements in surgical techniques and minimally invasive procedures have revolutionized patient care, offering the benefits of quicker recovery and improved outcomes. An understanding of the extent of orthopedic surgery is necessary because, besides playing an enormous role in restoring mobility and functionality, patients' quality of life and well-being are significantly influenced by it. The trend of orthopedic literature points toward key challenges that bring to the fore the necessity of solid research methods. Concerns persist over the quality of such literature due to reliance on low levels of evidence to inform clinical practice. Practitioners believe there needs to be stronger research, with only around 3% of orthopedic literature being reported through randomized trials—a figure that reflects severe deficiencies in high-quality work. Such a shortage primarily results from the lack of unique difficulties in conducting randomized trials in surgical settings, including difficulty in patient populations and heterogeneity in surgical technique. It is crucial to tackle such challenges to foster knowledge enhancement and improve patient safety in orthopedic surgery because improved studies can guide clinical decisions and propel innovations in procedural techniques (Bhandari et al., 2008). No less significant is research into complications following orthopedic surgery, such as postoperative infection.

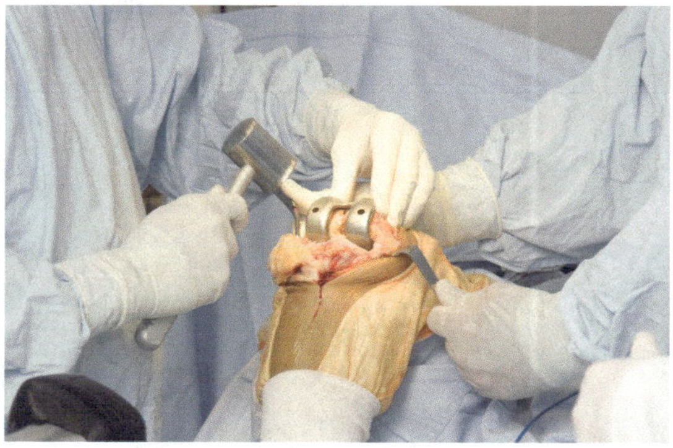

Figure 10.1. Orthopedic surgeon.

Source: https://maggohospital.com/wp-content/uploads/2019/11/130218_1518507771.jpg.

These can lead to disastrous outcomes, with neurological impairment and prolonged morbidity of patients. Research into the causative mechanisms behind such diseases is a widening field of interest, with existing animal models being valuable for studying postoperative outcomes. While highly efficacious in replicating surgery, current models are deficient in their ability to assess infection over time and across various techniques. Improvements to these models through the incorporation of high-resolution imaging modalities and bioluminescent bacterial strains could enhance the productivity of future research studies. These technologies have the potential to make significant advancements in creating preventive measures and treatment protocols for controlling postoperative infections in orthopedic procedures, ultimately resulting in improved patient care and fewer complications (Bernthal et al., 2015) (Figure 10.1).

Definition of Orthopedic Surgery

Orthopedic surgery is a specialized branch of medicine committed to the diagnosis, cure, and treatment of musculoskeletal injuries and diseases. The branch of medicine encompasses a wide range of conditions, including fractures, degenerative diseases, soft tissue trauma, and congenital deformities. Orthopedic surgeons use surgical as well as non-surgical treatments in order to restore function and alleviate pain, thereby making their specialty a critical one for enhancing the quality of life of patients with various musculoskeletal problems. The specialty not only addresses acute physical trauma but also plays an integral part in chronic conditions that affect mobility and overall well-being, thereby ensuring patient resilience in returning to normal activities. Orthopedic surgery has been dramatically affected by ongoing research and advancements in healthcare technology. Techniques such as minimally invasive surgery and the design of sophisticated prosthetics have revolutionized treatment procedures, enabling faster recovery periods and improved patient outcomes. The significance of provider diversity in quality and innovation enhancement in healthcare services has also been pointed out in recent research. For instance, studies on orthopedic surgery have found that varying kinds of providers can equally meet the quality standards established by traditional hospital networks, with patient experience mainly being influenced by case mix and hospital-specific factors (Allen et al., 2011). This necessitates context and specificity even within known models for the adoption of surgery. The role of orthopedic surgery extends beyond single-treatment intervention to encompass health outcomes at a more general level, in a sense, treating issues observed in populations afflicted by such conditions as cerebral palsy. Adding orthotic interventions, such as prescription splits and braces, demonstrates potential for cross-link among medical and rehabilitative interventions (Bowers et al., 2009). Interdisciplinary treatments, in this manner, not only foster physical rehabilitation but also facilitate greater functional independence among patients. The integration of surgical therapy with rehabilitative treatment highlights the need for a high-order understanding of orthopedic surgery, involving continued evolution in surgical technique and in patient-centered models of care dedicated to long-term outcomes (Figure 10.2).

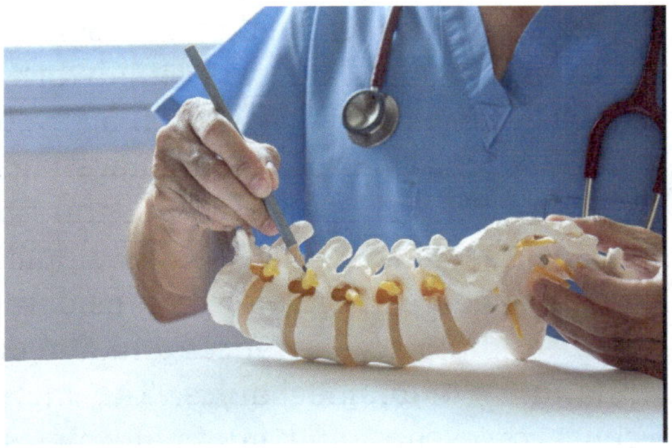

Figure 10.2. Orthopaedic surgery represents a specialized branch of medicine focused on the diagnosis, treatment.

Source: https://cdn.prod.website-files.com/6419c6455bd31b5d09bbe049/641c81bff32a256d5fc1119a_orthopedic-surgeon-in-dallas-explain-spine-surgery.jpeg.

Importance in the Medical Field

In the orthopedic surgery field, mentorship becomes an essential element that highly affects the dynamics of medical training and professional growth. Mentors are vital in facilitating the trajectories of young surgeons, influencing not only technical skills but also decisions that affect their careers. Having access to diverse role models is valuable in its own right; with women occupying only 15% of orthopedic surgery residents and racial/ethnic minorities representing only 3% to 10% of US orthopedic surgeons, the profession is in desperate need of increased representation. Studies have shown that successful mentorship programs can narrow this gap and foster an environment in which individuals from the underrepresented group feel safe and empowered. By effectively bridging these differences, the profession can not only enhance the professional competencies of future surgeons but also improve overall workplace satisfaction and retention through inclusive mechanisms (Domalaon et al., 2021). Research contributions in orthopedic surgery have broad implications for patient care, particularly in surgical outcomes as well as innovation. The identification of post-operative care practices, such as antibiotic therapies, has emerged as the need of the hour in the prevention of complications such as surgical site infections. A pilot international multi-center randomized controlled trial (RCT) was able to establish the feasibility of the same, having enrolled a heterogeneous group of patients from different countries. With a completion rate of 93% in administering post-operative doses, the study shed light on how collaboration can yield more accurate and generalizable findings across various health settings. This research not only illustrates the potential for enhancing patient outcomes using evidence-based procedures but also highlights the need for systematized multi-center trials to solve intricate medical questions (Investigators P, 2015). Lastly, research incorporation and mentorship in orthopedic surgery demonstrate the discipline's concern for enhancing medical practice and knowledge. A robust mentorship framework fosters a culture of inquiry, encouraging surgeons to engage with ongoing research and partake in clinical advances. As patient demographics continue to evolve, being able to treat a diverse population becomes increasingly important. This entails not only providing clinical care but also understanding the socio-economic and cultural factors that influence patient outcomes and decision-making. By building a new generation of capable orthopedic surgeons who have the knowledge and ability to provide holistic care, the specialty is capable of significantly affecting its overall effectiveness and sustainability within the health industry (Domalaon et al., 2021). So, the place of mentorship and research cannot be overworked, given that they are at the heart of ensuring the continued evolution of orthopedic surgery as a vital medical specialty.

10.1. History of Orthopedic Surgery

Learning Outcome

1. Describe early practices and techniques of orthopedic surgery
2. Define evolution of surgical procedures of orthopedic
3. Discuss key figures in orthopedic history

The history of orthopedic surgery is characterized by dramatic advances consistent with the evolving concept of musculoskeletal disease. Early treatment was often rudimentary and based on tradition. The Egyptians and Greeks employed splints and rudimentary surgical techniques, with stabilization being the primary objective and healing often an afterthought. It was in the Middle Ages that these principal works began to appear, detailing surgical methods and anatomy; however, within a restricted empirical context. The Renaissance marked the resumption of anatomical studies, spearheaded by Andreas Vesalius's work, which laid the groundwork for modern knowledge of the human body. This shift was a turning point, and it allowed subsequent generations to practice orthopedic surgery in a more scientific way, leading to better treatment techniques and more integration of surgery into the management of musculoskeletal trauma. With the arrival of the 19th century, the landscape of orthopedic surgery fundamentally altered with improvements in surgical techniques and anesthesia. Notably, the advent of ether and chloroform revolutionized surgery, enabling more complex procedures to be performed with minimal pain for patients. Pioneers like Sir Robert Jones during the early half of the 20th century contributed a great deal towards the evolution of orthopedic surgery as an independent branch of medicine. His work in specialized training made it a respectable profession and added to its standing in the larger medical professional community. Notably, this was also a time when specialized musculoskeletal clinics and hospitals began to emerge, offering facilities that were favorable for research and teaching. These advancements not only established orthopedics as a legitimate field of study but also laid the groundwork for the establishment of a formal teaching system that would set the precedent for generations of surgeons to come. The latter 20th century and early 21st century saw unparalleled development in orthopedic surgery, driven to a considerable extent by technological advances and a deeper understanding of biomechanics. The merger between arthroscopy and minimally invasive surgery represented a significant paradigm shift, revolutionizing the management of joint disorders and injuries. For instance, current studies have compared traditional open surgical interventions, such as open gluteal tendon repair (OGR), with emerging endoscopic techniques (EGR), where there has been a shift towards less invasive procedures with shorter recovery periods and less postoperative pain (Bini et al., 2020). This is part of a broader movement in medicine towards precision and personalized treatment options. The collaborative effort of surgeons, researchers, and engineers continues to extend the boundaries of what is possible in orthopedic surgery, paving the way for approaches that promise to improve patient results and health. The rich history of the specialty is at once a foundation and stimulus for ongoing progress and innovation in the practice of orthopedic surgery (Figure 10.3).

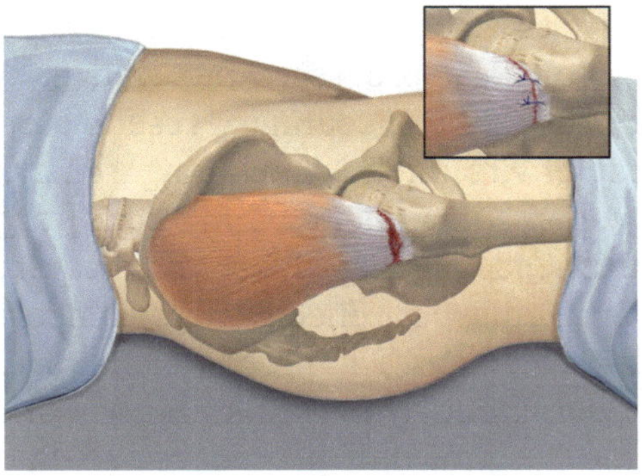

Figure 10.3. Open gluteal tendon repair (OGR).

Source: https://www.ochsnerjournal.org/content/ochjnl/19/4/405/F4.large.jpg.

10.1.1. Early Practices and Techniques

The early practice and method in orthopedic surgery opened the way for the modern approaches towards treating musculoskeletal disorders. At first, these practices were controlled by primitive procedures, but they came a long way after the post-19th century and early 20th century with the improvement of surgical methods and an enhanced knowledge about human anatomy. Among these early advancements, employing skeletal traction and immobilization methods was one, and it assisted in stabilizing fractures and promoting healing. Early practitioners of the field began to recognize that precise surgical methods, followed by protracted immobilization, were essential for successful recovery. As these initial practices evolved, practitioners attempted to merge them with advancing practices in anesthesia, creating ways for increasingly advanced procedures and improved patient safety and comfort in the process, entirely reshaping the parameters of orthopedic intervention. In the mid-20th century, epic breakthroughs in orthopedic surgery transformed treatment methods, particularly through the use of new materials and prosthetic technologies. Surgeons began utilizing advanced alloys and surgical instruments that enabled greater precision and efficiency during operations. Key breakthroughs included the development of total hip replacements, which were found to successfully reduce serious degeneration of joints and improve mobility in patients. The interaction between surgeons, the engineering community, and manufacturing firms fueled an environment of innovation that led to the evolution of improved surgical practices and the application of aseptic procedures in operating rooms. These procedures were designed to minimize infection rates while maintaining the extended lifespan of implants, thus dramatically improving patient outcomes. The constant search for better material and procedure showed how dynamic orthopedic surgery was during this revolutionary period. With the advancement of the field, the development of national hip registers in the 1970s provided robust data on implant survival rates, such that it was now feasible to compare prostheses systematically. Loosening and infection failures early on prompted researchers and surgeons to conduct detailed studies on the causes, which in turn led to the development of successful materials and fixation techniques. These registries not only gave essential tools for monitoring the performance of implants but also functioned as knowledge stores that shaped future innovation in orthopedic care. Contributions to the history of joint replacement from key individuals and organizations informed the knowledge base, and this dedication to ongoing critique and reform reflected the profession's concern with patient safety and quality treatment. Ultimately, these initial methods and procedures are significant pages in the evolution of orthopedic surgery, opening the door for further innovation in the field.

10.1.2. Evolution of Surgical Procedures

The evolution of surgical techniques in orthopedics is a significant milestone in the history of medical intervention for treating musculoskeletal diseases. Early surgical practice was primitive, with an utmost focus on open procedures and immediate resolution of problems, irrespective of the outcome. However, with greater knowledge of anatomy and physiology came improvements in surgery techniques. New technologies created towards the latter half of the 20th century began concentrating on less invasive surgery, culminating in a revolution within orthopedic surgery. This advance reflects growing concern for patient-focused care with an aim towards shorter recovery times and improved overall surgery success, which has become a key measure for orthopedic practice.

The integration of the latest technology into surgical procedures is a revolutionary shift in orthopedic surgery. Such technologies, such as 3D printing and robot-assisted equipment, enable surgeons to perform surgery with increased accuracy and personalization. These technology-based procedures not only improve the accuracy of joint replacements but also guarantee proper implant alignment and longevity, addressing previous complications that arose from traditional methods. Additionally, computer-assisted navigation has become an integral component of the surgical process, guiding surgeons in real-time and complementing their expertise during intricate procedures. These technologies support the commitment to minimization of postoperative complications and optimization of recovery, in accordance with today's philosophy of orthopedic surgery emphasizing patient satisfaction and enhanced functional outcomes (Gaonkar et al., 2023). ecent clinical reports illustrate the promising applications of new operations, further validating their places in current-day orthopedic practice. For instance, osteochondral scaffold culture has been of interest owing to its potential to treat chondral and osteochondral defects, reflecting the trend towards regenerative medicine (Brittberg et al., 2017). These developments not only reflect the role of engineered materials in surgery but also signal a growing understanding of the biological processes involved in tissue repair. Despite the encouraging results observed in most environments, including remarkable improvement in patient populations targeted for treatment, ongoing research is required to confirm unequivocal effectiveness compared to traditional methods. This process of improvement and assessment will undoubtedly continue to refine surgical and procedures so that the evolution of orthopedic techniques not only meets immediate patient needs but also encourages optimal long-term health results (Figure 10.4).

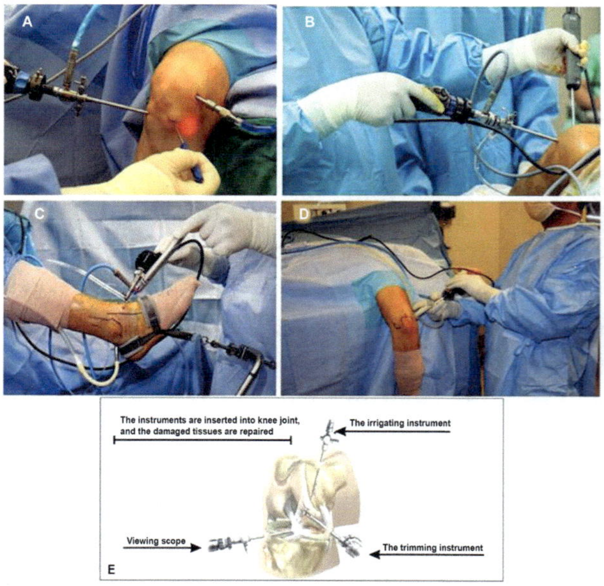

Figure 10.4. Current advancements in therapeutic approaches in orthopedic surgery.

Source: https://images-provider.frontiersin.org/api/ipx/w=1200&f=png/https://www.frontiersin.org/files/Articles/1328997/fbioe-12-1328997-HTML/image_m/fbioe-12-1328997-g001.jpg.

10.1.3. Key Figures in Orthopedic History

The enhancement of orthopedic surgery is furthered by the contributions of the key players who have shaped its principles and practice. One of these key players is the highly renowned Sir Robert Jones, who is often described as the father of orthopedics. His pioneering work in surgical technique, particularly in the handling of fractures, paved the way for contemporary practice in the specialty. Jones emphasized the need for fresh and creative ways of attending to patients and advocated bringing educational and clinical innovation together in orthopedic education. His establishment of specialty training programs and clinics not only improved patient results but also assisted in cultivating a new generation of orthopedic surgeons who would carry on his legacy. Thus, Jones's gigantic contributions were most significant in changing orthopedics from a rudimentary division of medicine to a sophisticated medical specialty handling complicated musculoskeletal abnormalities. Hugh Owen Thomas is another prominent figure in the history of orthopedic surgery who introduced some groundbreaking approaches that have remained relevant to this day. Thomas's approach was centered on the utilization of concepts related to mechanics to drive surgical techniques. His input towards the development of the Thomas splint, a device applied to immobilize fractured limbs, revolutionized trauma care in the late 19th and early 20th centuries, an entirely different process. Notably, his emphasis on the role of biomechanical science in orthopedic treatments paved the way for the kinds of developments that aim not only at healing but also at rehabilitation and mobility as well. Thomas's commitment to integrating engineering concepts with medical practices illustrated a profound understanding of the body's mechanics, making his contributions invaluable to the orthopedic field as a whole. His legacy remains evident in the continued use of splinting techniques in modern surgery. Along with this, the contributions of medical voluntarism at key moments in history have also shaped orthopedic practices to a significant degree, as evident from the efforts witnessed in Lancashire during World War I. The region became a center for providing rehabilitation orthopedic treatment to disabled ex-servicemen, revealing the intersection of social duty and medical creativity. As research indicates, institutions like Grangethorpe Hospital played a crucial role in rehabilitating soldiers, demonstrating a collaborative effort between medical professionals and local volunteers in the face of epidemic health crises. This era of advanced medical voluntarism not only motivated the excellence of rehabilitative treatment available but also spurred the emergence of charities dedicated to adapting to the shifting needs of individuals with disabilities. Thus, the commitment of leaders and community efforts contributed towards the overall understanding and development of orthopedic surgery during a record social need (Smith et al., 2024).

Test Your Knowledge

1. Who were the pioneers in the development of modern orthopedic surgical techniques?
2. How have major historical milestones, such as the introduction of internal fixation devices, shaped orthopedic surgery practices?

10.2. Common Orthopaedic Conditions

Learning Outcome

1. Define fractures and trauma
2. Describe arthritis and joint disorders
3. Explain the sports injuries

Routine orthopedic complaints cover a wide variety of musculoskeletal diseases that heavily affect people's daily lives. Among them, osteoarthritis is particularly significant, resulting from the degeneration of cartilage and bone in the joints, which leads to pain, stiffness, and decreased mobility. The disease not only affects patients' physical functioning but also their psychological state. As a degenerative condition, osteoarthritis usually leads to surgeries, particularly joint replacement, if conservative therapy fails. The multidisciplinary treatment of such diseases necessitates an interdisciplinary care model, comprising various forms of treatment, including physical therapy, pharmacotherapy, and, as needed, surgery. Optimization of the result in osteoarthritis patients is a classic example of the significant role of orthopedic surgery in quality-of-life improvement and return of function. Recurrent lateral epicondylitis (LE), or more commonly called tennis elbow, is another common condition that is encountered in orthopedic surgery. The disease is characterized by pain and tenderness over the lateral aspect of the elbow, resulting from chronic overuse of the forearm tendons and muscles. The challenge in treating LE is the variability of treatment modalities available, from more conservative to more invasive techniques. Recent studies have proposed that platelet-rich plasma (PRP) injections can significantly enhance symptoms of refractory LE. Specifically, it was found that a combination of PRP and one of several percutaneous needling therapies can lead to substantial improvements in pain and function. However, the utility of the specific needling technique is problematic (Culp et al., 2017). This complexity points to the necessity of evidence-based practice in orthopedic surgery to provide optimal care to patients with this disabling disorder. Second, fractures are generally considered a critical situation in the scenario of common orthopedic disorders. Fractures are classified into types, including complete, incomplete, and compound fractures, each requiring different treatment modalities depending on their severity and location. Orthopedic surgeons commonly employ both surgical and non-surgical techniques for the management of fractures. Surgery may involve internal fixation, employing plates or screws to stabilize fractured bones, particularly in complex conditions. Despite enhanced surgical techniques, methodological flaws in studies investigating these conditions remain an issue. Research highlighted glaring deficits in statistical design and reporting of orthopedic articles, with the observation that in most instances the conclusions reached were not appropriately supported by the results reported (Achten et al., 2012). This highlights the importance of greater rigor in orthopedic research to fuel higher patient outcomes by evidence-based practice (Figure 10.5).

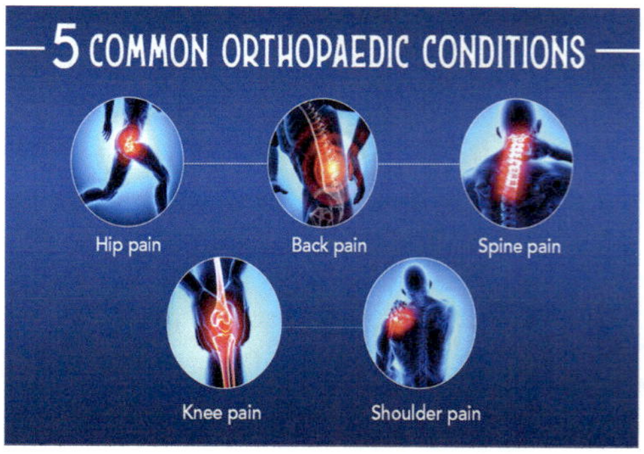

Figure 10.5. Common orthopedic conditions.

Source: https://kdahweb-static.kokilabenhospital.com/kdah-2019/tips/1714655085.jpg.

10.2.1. Fractures and Trauma

Fractures and trauma are significant issues in orthopedic surgery, primarily due to the complexity of treating various types of bone trauma. Trauma can result from varied mechanisms, including falls, motor vehicle accidents, and interpersonal violence, and thus urgent treatment is required. Principles of damage control orthopedics are most effective in such cases, with an emphasis on rapid and effective treatment to minimize morbidity and optimize patient outcomes during recovery. The treatment guidelines are designed to integrate early surgical fixation with subsequent definitive procedures, which dictate the overall management of fractures. Knowledge of these guidelines is essential in depth, especially in combat areas, where the injuries sustained may be complicated by limited resources and urgent medical needs, as noted in the experiences reported in trauma care during the Libyan civil war crisis (Borg et al., 2015). The character of the fracture has a significant influence on the treatment strategy and the patient's outcome. Fractures are classified in accordance with different criteria, such as the Gustilo-Anderson system, which classifies open fractures according to the extent of the soft tissue damage. Class III and IIIB or IIIC fractures are critical fractures needing a complex treatment plan employing a multi-disciplinary approach to achieve rapid healing and minimize the chances of complications. Furthermore, the unique challenge of war injuries underscores the imperative for specially crafted management strategies that account for the increased level of injury typical of modern warfare, requiring innovative surgical procedures and rehabilitative interventions beyond routine civilian trauma treatment protocols (Borg et al., 2015). In the context of certain types of fractures, studies have demonstrated that talar neck fractures, for instance, require meticulous treatment to achieve an optimal outcome. Evidence indicates that open reduction and internal fixation (ORIF) can yield satisfactory clinical results despite related long-term complications, such as avascular necrosis (AVN) or post-traumatic arthritis. The influence of timeliness has been under intense scrutiny; on-time surgical treatment is positively linked with patient satisfaction and recovery trends. Of special interest, the Hawkins sign was recognized as a useful prognostic indicator, helping clinicians formulate treatment strategies that take into consideration underlying complexities while facilitating optimal healing. These findings illustrate the intricate interplay between fracture mechanics, surgical timing, and outcomes in patients, all indicating the need for strong clinical assessment paradigms in the treatment of orthopedic trauma (Figure 10.6).

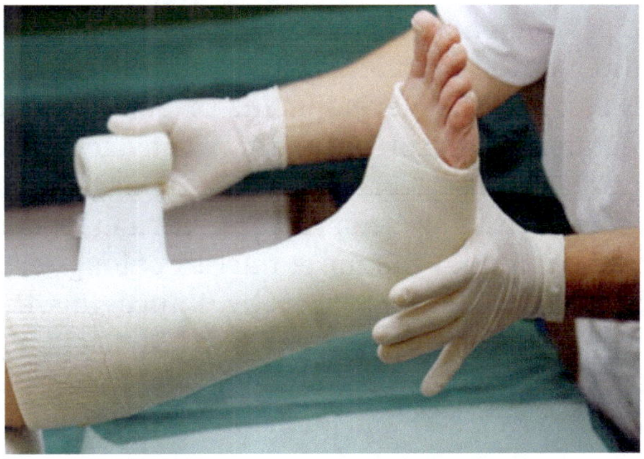

Figure 10.6. Trauma and fracture treatment.

Source: https://www.myorthoclinic.in/assets/images/services/traumaandfracture.jpg.

10.2.2. Arthritis and Joint Disorders

The intricate relationship between joint disorders and arthritis is crucial in orthopedic surgery since they directly affect patients' quality of life and function. Arthritis, which is joint inflammation, exists in two forms: rheumatoid and osteoarthritis. Both have their own specific pathologies on which subsists their mode of treatment, with the most common of it leading to unbelievable agony, swelling, and limited mobility. Over time, these inflammatory processes have the potential to lead to joint damage and deformities, and, therefore, early intervention is vital. Surgical intervention is typically considered when conservative measures cannot provide relief and restore function. As an illustration, surgical interventions such as arthroscopy or joint replacement can provide excellent relief and improved joint function, and, thus, a personalized approach to management of patients in orthopedic clinics is further critical. In managing the complexity of joint disorders, early detection and effective treatment methods are crucial for preventing long-term consequences. Hemophilic arthropathy is a condition that illustrates the multifaceted nature of joint disorders, characterized by recurrent intra-articular bleeding that leads to prolonged inflammation and progressive joint deterioration. Such complications necessitate the development of an extended treatment protocol with both prophylactic and interventionist treatments. Early, aggressive therapy, including factor replacement and regular monitoring, may minimize the risk of long-term joint complications, thereby improving the overall outcome for patients. Multidisciplinary care with the involvement of hematologists, physiotherapists, and orthopedic surgeons is very important for successful management, particularly in patients with systemic conditions like hemophilia that exacerbate disorders of joints. Long-term outcomes in patients with arthritis and joint disease are generally determined by numerous factors, including the timing of surgery and the pathologic type of the joint. Evidence indicates that patients with displacement fractures due to diseases such as arthritis may develop severe complications, including avascular necrosis (AVN) and post-traumatic arthritis (PTA). Studies have shown that prompt surgical intervention can lead to favorable outcomes, with a substantial number of patients expressing satisfaction following the procedure. Late complications, however, demand long-term follow-up and accommodative management. Therefore, orthopedic surgeons ought to be cautious to monitor their patients closely for PTA and AVN symptoms, particularly for complex or high-risk cases, rendering interventions proactive and reactive depending on the needs of individual patients, as maintained in the literature (Berntorp et al., 2011; Belluzzi et al., 2019) (Figure 10.7).

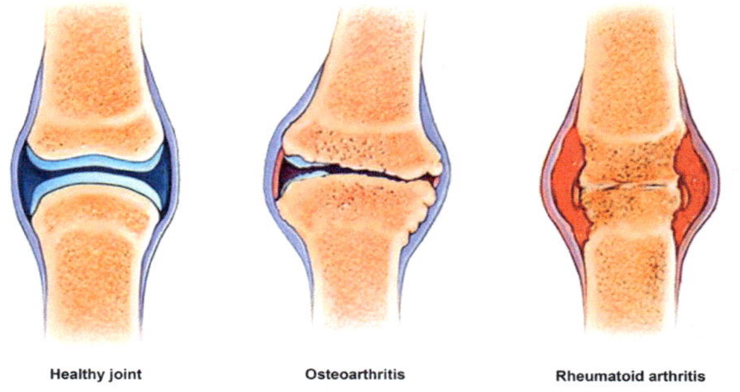

Figure 10.7. Arthritis – symptoms and causes.

Source: https://www.mayoclinic.org/-/media/kcms/gbs/patient-consumer/images/2013/11/15/17/44/ds01122_ds00020_im03689_mcdc7_arthritis_typesthu_jpg.jpg.

10.2.3. Sports Injuries

Sports injuries are a prevalent problem in orthopedic surgery, often needing surgery to return athletes to playing status. Among numerous injury types, sprains of the ankle are particularly prevalent and affect athletes in numerous sports. In one study of talocrural joint chondral injuries, high numbers of athletes suffer from recurrent exertion ankle pain that can be caused by inadequate treatment after injury. The study reveals that 93% of the studied athletes experienced this complaint, underscoring the importance of early and effective management in sports medicine. In addition, the study elucidates that conventional MRI is not highly sensitive in the diagnosis of cartilage lesions, with a note of emphasis on the observation that suggestive clinical features, such as swelling and pain, should prompt earlier surgical investigation to maximize opportunities of successful recovery and subsequent return to sport (Hintermann et al., 2006). Elbow dislocation is one example of how sports injuries affect athletes, particularly those in contact sports like football. In a review of the clinical course of the professional football player, it was discovered that elbow dislocations most often occurred in defenders who had attempted tackles. The National Football League (NFL) statistics indicate that although these injuries represent a tiny proportion of all injuries, they can cause significant loss of time out from playing. To our surprise, 75.8% of the injured athletes returned to their field within the same season, with those treated conservatively being off for a mean of 25.1 days compared with 46.5 for those treated surgically. This recovery diversity underscores the need for customized treatment regimens that consider both the nature of the injury and the athlete's position, ultimately allowing for a better return to competitive functioning (Bishop et al., 2018).

Sports injury management requires an interdisciplinary approach that incorporates surgical skill coupled with rehabilitative principles. Surgeons need to collaborate with athletic trainers and physiotherapists to develop a proven protocol for healing that incorporates both post-operative rehabilitation and surgical repair. Based on outcomes from comparative recovery pathways in athletes who suffer recurring injuries, such as those related to ankle and elbow conditions, these protocols can be enhanced. For example, in ankle injuries, the identification of clinical signs and the timing of surgeries can allow for optimal results to a greater degree. Similarly, drawing a complete picture of average recovery times for each injury enables teams and doctors to create realistic expectations for athletes. This coordinated plan ultimately achieves the highest possible chances for the athletes at an efficient and sustained return to competition, indicative of the role of orthopedic surgery in sports medicine today.

Test Your Knowledge

1. What are the most prevalent musculoskeletal conditions that require orthopedic intervention?
2. How do degenerative and traumatic orthopedic conditions differ in their presentation and management?

10.3. Diagnostic Techniques

Learning Outcome

1. Define the imaging technologies (X-rays, MRIs)
2. Discuss the physical examination methods
3. Describe laboratory tests and assessments

In orthopedic surgery, accurate diagnosis of musculoskeletal diseases is paramount in achieving successful treatment and management of the patient. Radiography, or commonly referred to as X-rays, is one of the first diagnostic procedures utilized. These radiological examinations allow orthopedic surgeons to visualize bone anatomy and test for fractures, dislocations, or other bone dysmorphias. Additionally, advancements in imaging technology, such as computed tomography (CT) and magnetic resonance imaging (MRI), offer enhanced detail and three-dimensional visualization of bone and soft tissue anatomy. These modalities aid in the detailed assessment of multifaceted joint conditions and degenerative diseases. Utilizing these diagnostic techniques, clinicians are able to formulate well-rounded treatment plans, thus enabling patient-specific care decisions to optimize outcomes. One key feature of diagnostic approaches in orthopedic surgery is the application of functional assessments and patient self-report outcomes. These assessments are extremely valuable in providing information regarding a patient's orthopedic function, which can include strength, range of motion, and pain. These tools not only provide clinicians with information regarding the severity of a condition but also enable tracking of progress during and after treatment. For instance, applying scales such as the Western Ontario and McMaster Universities Osteoarthritis Index (WOMAC) enables the quantification of a patient's subjective disability and quality of life. When combined with objective imaging outcomes, practitioners will be able to have an integrated perception of every patient's condition, which eventually translates to enhanced intervention effectiveness. Moreover, in some conditions, such as Morquio A syndrome, the significance of early and accurate diagnosis during multidisciplinary approaches becomes the focal point of treatment. The syndrome features an extensive list of complications, predominantly orthopedic, particularly involving extremities, necessitating meticulous examination by a group of orthopedic specialists, pediatricians, and geneticists.

The synergy ensures a comprehensive study, identifying not only skeletal deformity but also associated concurrent soft tissue issues. Clinical research guidelines emphasize the importance of early intervention and treatment planning tailored to each patient, underscoring the complexity of diagnosing unique complications of Morquio A syndrome. To maximize patient outcomes, it is essential to incorporate high-tech imaging and multidisciplinary expertise into the diagnostic process (Bache et al., 2014). The comprehensive framework improves the quality of care offered to patients with complex orthopedic disorders (N/A, 2004) (Figure 10.8).

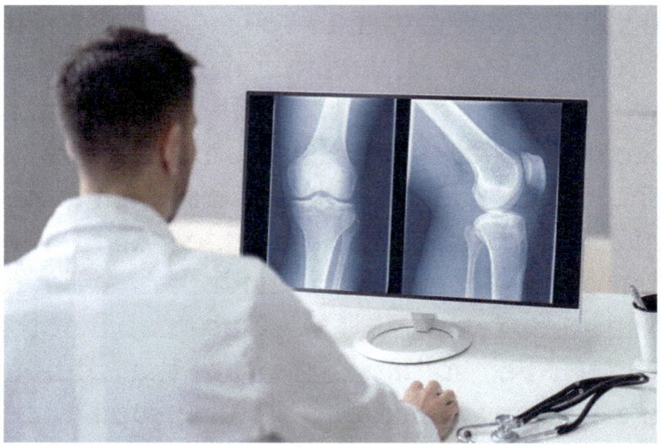

Figure 10.8. Orthopedic diagnostics.

Source: https://dearbornassoc.com/wp-content/uploads/sites/274/2023/12/shutterstock_1619489473.jpg.optimal.jpg.

10.3.1. Imaging Technologies (X-rays, MRIs)

Imaging equipment is of utmost significance in orthopedic surgery, as it enables better diagnosis and results in the treatment of patients. Of these imaging modalities, X-rays and magnetic resonance imaging (MRI) hold a special significance. X-rays are generally the first imaging utilized in orthopedics because they are fast and well-suited for visualizing bone fractures and joint malalignment issues. They are effective in demonstrating the presence of abnormalities in bone structure, allowing surgeons to promptly ascertain the severity of the injury. Despite their widespread use, X-rays have certain limitations, particularly in assessing soft tissues. The advent of MRI technology redresses some of these deficiencies by enabling greater contrast in soft tissues and satisfactory visualization of ligaments, cartilage, and surrounding muscles. Hence, the combination of both imaging technologies aids in developing an overall treatment plan, particular to the specific needs of the patient. New technology advances in imaging equipment have also revolutionized orthopedic practice through the integration of new techniques that aid in diagnosing multifactorial conditions such as osteoarthritis. A consensus study highlighted the potential of new imaging methods, such as MRI and proteomics, to improve diagnosis and treatment options by effectively subcategorizing osteoarthritic patients. The study cites agreement among specialists that novel approaches would optimize patient management through the segregation of separate treatment lines based on unique conditions. This becomes important because traditional X-rays may not accurately represent the heterogeneity of osteoarthritic changes, thereby leading to false negatives. Methods like MRI not only overcome such gaps but also enable surgeons to obtain vital information regarding soft tissue integrity, thereby making more informed surgical decisions and interventions, as demonstrated by the agreement reached by experts. The ongoing development of imaging technologies necessitates keeping pace with evolving modalities that enhance diagnostic precision. Physics takes the lead in these technologies, enabling the creation of imaging techniques that can replace or reduce the need for invasive procedures. Recent reports indicate that imaging technologies, such as MRI and X-rays, have opened new avenues for non-invasive assessment, promoting patient safety and recovery. The priority given to the integration of these imaging modalities in orthopedics not only provides a more articulate comprehension of trauma but also justifies treatment protocols. This way, the outcomes of surgery can be significantly improved, substantiating that precise use of imaging technologies is now an integral part of the modern orthopedic practice and thereby justifying the reasons why advancements in this field need to be addressed and invested in by the medical world (Anderson et al., 2020; Nagessar et al., 2023).

10.3.2. Physical Examination Methods

The initial phase of the orthopedic surgical physical examination involves a thorough review of the patient's history and symptoms, and directs the remainder of the physical examination procedures. A methodical approach involves searching for any gross deformity, edema, or change in color before palpating the involved area. The thorough evaluation goes deeply into the patients' functional impairments, range of motion, and pain level. Specifically, the examination must be done on common orthopedic trauma, such as ligament injuries or fractures. Importantly, the utilization of techniques such as diagnostic imaging alongside clinical assessment allows for a comparative analysis of observations, thereby enhancing diagnosis and treatment planning. A combination of subjective patient complaints with objective observation has the capacity to create useful information regarding the state of the patient, which is crucial in coming up with effective surgery plans in dealing with musculoskeletal disorders. Aside from visual inspection and palpation, specialized orthopedic tests play a vital role in narrowing down the diagnosis. These tests, which include maneuvers like the Lachman test for assessment of the anterior cruciate ligament (ACL) integrity or the Thompson test for Achilles tendon rupture, are designed to produce unequivocal responses that indicate injury or dysfunction. The relevance of such special tests lies in their capacity to differentiate between the nature of injuries, thereby guiding treatment options. Furthermore, the integration of these tests with advanced imaging techniques, such as quantitative magnetic resonance imaging (QMRI), yields more profound insights into the biomechanical alterations associated with injuries. For example, long-term changes in tibial positioning and internal rotation, as assessed by MRI evaluations after injury, are closely associated with cartilage degradation, as emphasized by new research findings (Amano et al., 2016). This integration of physical exam and special testing with imaging enhances the practitioner's accuracy in making an informed treatment plan. Finally, compartment syndrome demonstrates the importance of precise physical examination methods in orthopedic practice. Compartment syndrome, an intra-compartmental pressure elevation that leads to complications if not promptly detected, has symptoms typically comprising grossly disproportionate pain, and diagnosis of such symptomatology is imperative for an early diagnosis. Both clinical presentation and measurement of compartmental pressure in high-risk patients—for example, those with tibial or forearm fractures—provide a valuable tool for early identification of this potentially injurious condition (Ali et al., 2014). Since clinical presentations, such as pain with passive stretching, can present late in the course of the disease, vigilant observation is necessary. Using a complete physical examination to identify symptoms and risk factors, the potential to intervene early is enhanced, hence enhancing patient outcomes in orthopedic surgery (Figure 10.9).

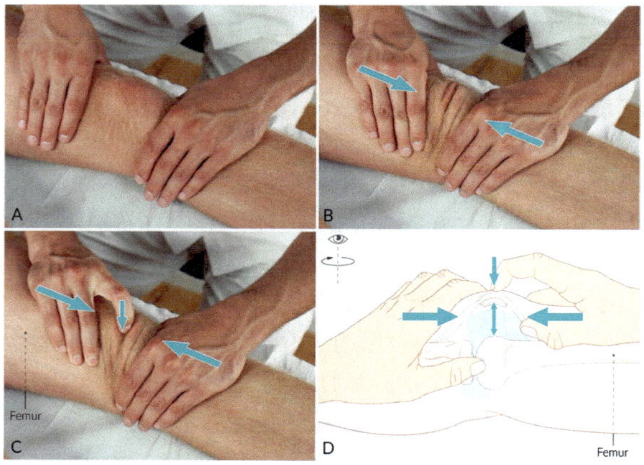

Figure 10.9. Orthopedic examination.

Source: https://media-us.amboss.com/media/thumbs/big_5e787f74c79ab.jpg.

10.3.3. Laboratory Tests and Assessments

In orthopedic surgery, laboratory evaluation and testing are the most critical factors in preoperative and postoperative monitoring. These evaluations not only affect surgical planning but also are integral to patient recovery monitoring. For example, knee ligamentous compliance testing may provide decisive information about the integrity of joint structures following procedures such as anterior cruciate ligament reconstruction. These measurements provide quantitative data that reflects the functional capacity of the knee, and it is critical in the management of the rehabilitation process (Bailey et al., 2008). By using diagnostic equipment, practitioners can identify compensatory strategies and areas that require specific rehabilitation, thereby enhancing patient outcomes. Furthermore, emotional and psychological factors have a significant influence on the success of rehabilitation following orthopedic interventions. Studies have shown a link between musculoskeletal fitness and psychological well-being, indicating that psychological assessments should be integrated into postoperative management (Bailey et al., 2008).

With this ability to differentiate the emotional pictures of patients, health practitioners can optimize rehabilitation programs with a more personalized approach, incorporating both physical and psychological recovery. Identifying the value of these multidimensional tests enhances an improved model of patient care, creating an environment that maximizes recovery and rehabilitation. Within broader healthcare systems, laboratory tests also play a crucial role in demand management programs. The application of reforms such as Payment by Results has emphasized the importance of having proper monitoring approaches in measuring patient outcomes and utilization of resources in orthopedic surgery. By documenting patient progress using proper assessment, doctors can record the performance of various interventions, minimize adverse outcomes, and enhance the delivery of services. This data, based on experience, not only provides individual benefits to patients but also assists in informing changes at the system level in how healthcare systems manage differential demands for surgical services. Consequently, drawing from laboratory tests and assessments is imperative in enhancing patient outcomes and healthcare efficiency as a whole within orthopedic settings.

Test Your Knowledge

1. What imaging modalities are commonly used to diagnose fractures, joint disorders, and other orthopedic conditions?
2. How do clinical examination and patient history complement imaging in accurately diagnosing orthopedic problems?

10.4. Surgical Procedures

Learning Outcome

1. Describe the arthroscopy
2. Define the joint replacement surgery
3. Describe the spinal surgery

Operative intervention is paramount in orthopedic surgery, revolutionizing the quality of life in patients with musculoskeletal disorders. Among the many interventions, hip and knee replacements are among the most frequently performed operations worldwide. These operations aim to alleviate pain, restore function, and enhance mobility, particularly among patients with osteoarthritis or advanced joint failure. Nevertheless, despite their prevalence, debate continues regarding the assessment and quantification of their success. The advent of newer surgeries, such as hip resurfacing and unicondylar knee arthroplasty, serves to highlight the necessity for rigorous clinical trials to identify their performance measures and results in various populations, with a need for ongoing research in this field. Randomized controlled trials (RCTs) are the gold standard for quantifying surgical interventions, but their use in orthopedic surgery has been complicated. Surgical procedures have inherent methodologic challenges that can complicate trial design. Unlike pharmacologic intervention, surgical intervention is often complex to standardize because techniques and the surgeon's ability may differ. Additionally, patient demographics and the mix of cases for operations can further complicate the evaluation process. These are issues that need to be resolved for surgical innovations to receive adequate scrutiny. Collaboration between researchers and surgical clinicians is required to develop well-planned trials that not only compare the results of existing procedures but also provide avenues for discoveries, promoting a culture of evidence-based practice in orthopaedic surgery (Cook et al., 2009). Revision rates following such procedures are part of assessing long-term efficacy and safety. An extensive review of the England and Wales National Joint Registry data sheds light on the performance of hip and knee replacements. The study found that revision rates during the first three years varied substantially based on the type of prosthesis implanted. For instance, in the case of hip replacements, the revision rate was found to be higher in resurfacing compared to cemented and hybrid procedures, particularly in women, indicating the requirement for gender considerations during planning for surgery. Similarly, knee replacements exhibited varying rates of success that were patient-age- and prosthesis-nature-dependent, highlighting the requirement for tailored approaches in orthopedic surgery (Alex et al., 2008). These findings highlight the imperative for ongoing research and development of surgical techniques to achieve optimal patient outcomes (Figure 10.10).

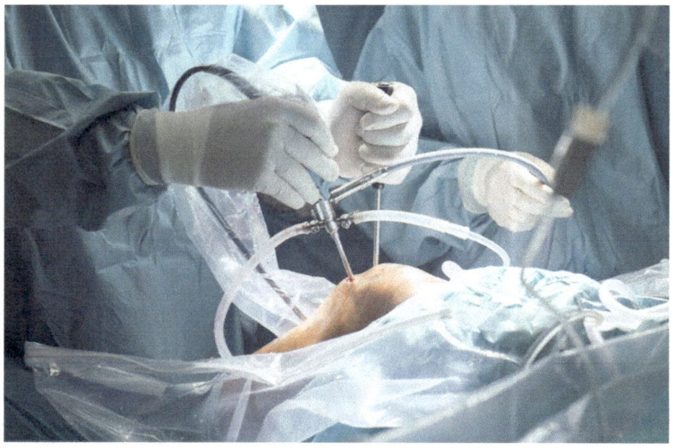

Figure 10.10. Surgical procedures in orthopedic surgery.

Source: https://www.chaudharyhospital.in/wp-content/uploads/2021/03/orthopedic-surgery-in-udaipur.jpg.

10.4.1. Arthroscopy

Arthroscopy is now an indispensable technique in the domain of orthopedic surgery, offering a less invasive alternative to the traditional open surgery method for joint pathology diagnosis and treatment, through the use of a compact camera device known as an arthroscope, orthopedic surgeons can view inside joints, such as the knee and shoulder joints, without inflicting severe damage on surrounding tissue. This visualization enables precise interventions, such as the repair of torn ligaments or the removal of loose cartilage fragments. Compared to open surgery, arthroscopy is associated with smaller incisions, reduced postoperative pain, and faster recovery for patients.

Thus, the procedure not only enhances surgical outcomes but also meets the increasing demands of patients for minimally invasive interventions in orthopedics. Evidence supports the effectiveness of arthroscopic procedures in reducing postoperative pain and narcotic needs. Evidence in one study assessing the use of positive-pressure air arthrography and venting in hip arthroscopic surgery showed a significant reduction in patient-reported levels of pain and opioid intake following surgery. The patients undergoing these procedures had lower ratings for pain and required less pain medication upon recovery compared to those who were not. Such reduction is significant, as maximized pain control can lead to shorter hospital stays as well as greater surgical satisfaction, testifying to the success of integrating new techniques into outpatient orthopedic surgery (Cheung et al., 2019).

Most importantly, it highlights arthroscopy's potential to enhance the safety of patients through minimized complications due to opioid abuse. Perhaps most importantly, arthroscopy enables quick rehabilitation protocols that are specifically designed to meet the needs of elite athletes recovering from joint injuries, in a research study involving athletes who underwent osteochondral autograft plug transfer for chondral injury, application of an accelerated return-to-sport program delivered encouraging results.

Athletes claimed to have returned to activity levels before injury within approximately 82.9 days, proving that intervention with arthroscopy at the onset can yield favorable clinical outcomes without long-term negative consequences. The long-term satisfaction of players with their performance following arthroscopic procedures underscores the potential of arthroscopy not only in the treatment of injuries but also in achieving optimal recovery, thus its position as a fundamental technique of contemporary orthopedic surgery (Brockmeier et al., 2017) (Figure 10.11).

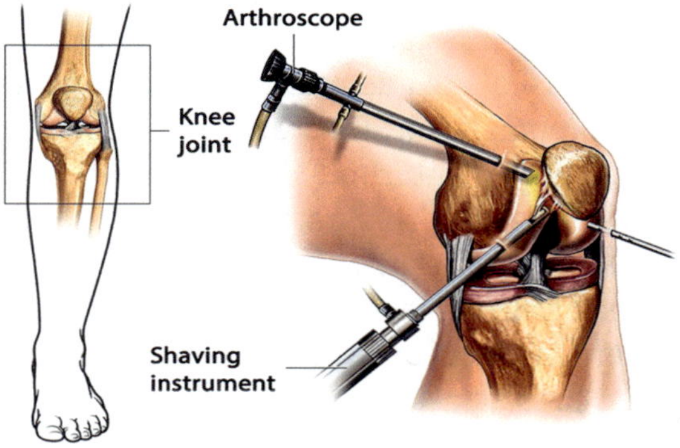

Figure 10.11. Arthroscopy.

Source: https://media.healthdirect.org.au/images/inline/original/arthroscopy-illustration-8ee5e5.gif.

10.4.2. Joint Replacement Surgery

Joint replacement is a revolutionary innovation in orthopedic surgery that provides relief from debilitating pain to patients and restores joint function seriously compromised by injury or degenerative illness. It is one of the most prevalent elective surgeries, with hundreds of thousands of patients undergoing total hip replacement and total knee replacement annually. Specifically, nearly 700,000 patients undergo total knee replacements and roughly 330,000 have total hip replacements annually in the United States. The success of the procedures can be attributed to the excellent success rates of modern implants, with over 90% having chances of remaining effective for over 10 years following surgery, and thus consolidating the position of joint replacement surgery in enhancing the quality of life of patients (Allen et al., 2016). Routine as it may be, the surgery still poses many risks and necessitates considerable contemplation by both patients and surgeons. The technological innovations in joint replacement surgery have revolutionized the specialty, enabling enhanced patient outcomes and satisfaction. Advanced materials and techniques are among the innovations that have resulted in improved longevity and performance of implants. Individually designed prostheses and highly cross-linked polyethylene are among such advancements, offering patient-specified alternatives that fulfill individual anatomical and lifestyle needs. Additionally, computer-assisted navigation technology and robot-assisted surgery have enhanced the accuracy of surgery, reducing tissue trauma and shortening recovery times. The advances underscore a paradigm shift toward less invasive treatments, leading to fewer postoperative complications and enabling quicker patient rehabilitation (Gaonkar et al., 2023). Therefore, innovations like these are crucial to the success of joint replacements, in that patient satisfaction remains the foremost priority of orthopedic care. Furthermore, patient choice and preoperative assessment are some other critical determinants of joint replacement surgery success.

The meticulous evaluation of patients, including their clinical background, psychological readiness, and physical condition, ensures that only those who could benefit from the surgery are considered as candidates. This customized approach has become top priority on the agenda, as it optimizes surgical operations in relation to a patient's goals and lifestyle. Alongside advancements in surgical techniques, postoperative care protocols have also been revised to incorporate effective rehabilitation protocols that further enhance recovery outcomes. Such multifaceted processes, including collaboration between surgeons, physiotherapists, and psychological support systems, aim to maximize long-term outcomes and address secondary complications that may arise during the recovery process (Gaonkar et al., 2023). Thus, the convergence of technology, patient-specific care, and informed patient selection positions joint replacement arthroplasty as an archetype of orthopedic practice today (Figure 10.12).

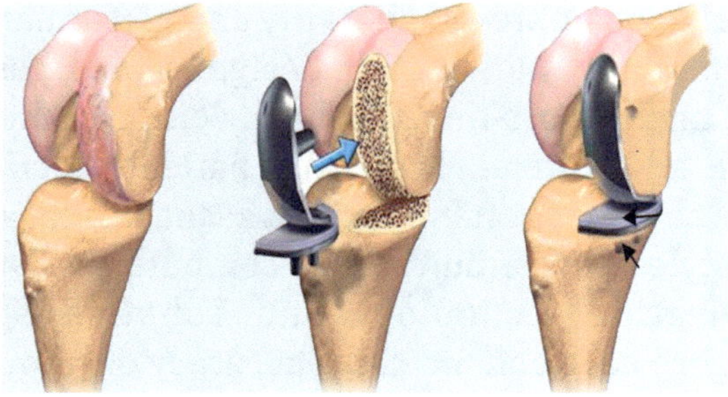

Figure 10.12. Joint replacement surgery.

Source: https://productimages.withfloats.com/serviceimages/actual/62c6466f9f5d31b7f2cdf291JOINT%20REPLACEMENT%20SURGERY.

10.4.3. Spinal Surgery

Spinal surgery plays a crucial role as part of the broader orthopedic surgery, fixing all kinds of spinal conditions. It exists primarily to alleviate pain, restore functionality, and improve patients' quality of life for spinal disorders such as herniated discs, degenerative disc disease, and stenosis. The increasing prevalence of such diseases among the geriatric population underscores the significance of spinal surgery in contemporary times. Effective surgical operations involve decompressive laminectomies, spinal fusions, and anterior cervical discectomies, which aim to stabilize the spine, alleviate compression of the nerves, and maintain alignment. With advancements in surgical techniques and technology still ongoing, spinal surgery has undergone considerable evolution, resulting in improved outcomes and reduced rehabilitation time for patients. Recently, the incorporation of electrical stimulators has been on the debate list when it comes to spinal fusion surgery. A study indicated that the use of bone growth stimulators can have the potential to increase the likelihood of successful fusion, especially in complex cases such as multi-level fusions. In a study comparing patient outcomes following anterior lumbar interbody fusion (ALIF), it was observed that approximately 19% of patients received post-operative external stimulators. The research indicated a potential correlation between the use of stimulators and surgery revision rates, particularly in patients exposed to multi-level surgery. This finding emphasizes the importance of individualized treatment protocols, as the selection of grafting material and the application of stimulators can play a critical role in determining success in surgery and recovery patterns, thereby enhancing overall patient outcomes (Brodke et al., 2018). The complexity of spinal surgery is also compounded by the inherent risks and complications associated with the various procedures. For instance, extrusions are among the complications that can occur following anterior cervical fusion, though comparatively rare. In a multi-institutional analysis of thousands of patients, implant extrusion rates ranged from 0.0% to 0.8%, with the highest rates occurring most frequently in more complex, multi-level cases. Although the vast majority of patients have good function after reoperation, the necessity for avoidable revision procedures is a challenge to spinal surgeons. This emphasizes the critical significance of accurate preoperative planning and patient-specific consideration of variables in an attempt to minimize risk, ensuring that spinal surgical interventions are safe and effective (Arnold et al., 2017).

Test Your Knowledge

1. What factors determine whether a patient requires conservative management or surgical intervention for an orthopedic condition?
2. How do joint replacement and fracture fixation procedures differ in technique and expected outcomes?

10.5. Postoperative Care

Learning Outcome

1. Understand the rehabilitation and physical therapy
2. Describe the pain management strategies
3. Identify the monitoring for complications

Postoperative care is a critical link in the orthopedic surgery chain since it directly influences patient outcomes and patterns of recovery. After surgery, particularly in orthopedics, where postoperative complications such as surgical site infections (SSIs) are prevalent, close surveillance and intervention are crucial. Effective postoperative care programs aim to address several key issues, including pain management, infection prevention, and rehabilitation. Studies emphasize that prevention of SSIs is of utmost value because such complications can lead to more extended hospital stays, morbidity, and even mortality, prompting the importance of strict prevention strategies during the postoperative period. Prevention is the best approach, achieved through meticulous wound management, patient education, and control of comorbid health states, and is paramount to prevent the dangers of SSIs, which may otherwise impede worldwide recovery and long-term results (Atesok et al., 2020).

The Enhanced Recovery after Surgery (ERAS) protocol has gained traction in orthopedic postoperative care, providing evidence-driven recommendations to maximize patient recovery after major spinal surgery. This approach prioritizes optimization of perioperative care by coordinating evidence-based practice in all facets of patient care. Key features of the ERAS protocol include extensive preoperative counseling, nutrition support, multimodal analgesia, and early mobilization. The evidence suggests that implementing an ERAS pathway for major spine surgery results in lower complication rates, a decreased length of hospital stay, and higher patient satisfaction. These advancements have been attributed to an integrated approach to treatment that emphasizes early intervention and minimizes the physiological stress associated with surgical interventions, resulting in a rapid recovery process and reducing overall healthcare expenditure for healthcare systems (Aasvang et al., 2016).

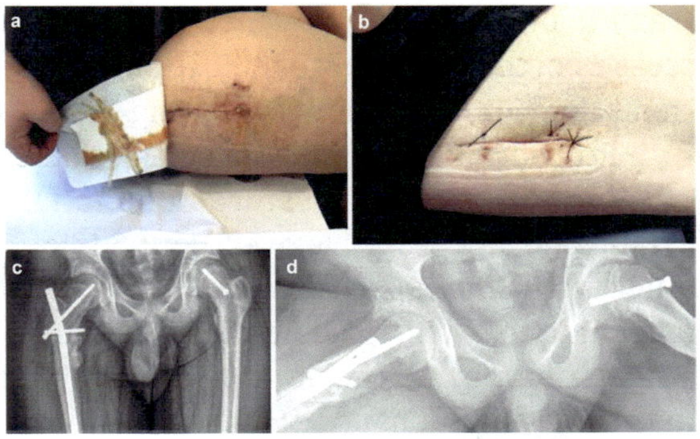

Figure 10.13. Surgical site infections (SSIs).

Source: https://media.springernature.com/lw685/springer-static/image/chp%3A10.1007%2F978-3-030-95794-0_16/MediaObjects/492685_1_En_16_Fig3_HTML.png.

Besides, successful postoperative management of orthopedic surgery also demands a multidisciplinary process, where surgical teams, nurses, and rehabilitation practitioners cooperate to improve patient outcomes. Such coordination is necessary for monitoring recovery and treating complications early, before they aggravate. Effective communication among all parties involved, including patients, is essential in developing an integrated recovery plan tailored to each patient's specific needs. Such an atmosphere offers reassurance to patients during their postoperative period through continuous support, ensuring effective compliance with rehabilitation protocols and lifestyle changes necessary for recovery. With the ongoing evolution of the practice of orthopedic surgery, the integration of advanced postoperative care protocols, including the ERAS approach and strict infection control policies, will remain vital in maximizing surgical outcomes and patient satisfaction within the specialty (Aasvang et al., 2016) (Figure 10.13).

10.5.1. Rehabilitation and Physical Therapy

The function of rehabilitation and physical therapy is of utmost significance to the overall success of orthopedic surgery. Post-surgery, the patient tends to experience varying levels of pain, reduced mobility, and muscle weakness. Rehabilitation aims to restore functionality, alleviate pain, and improve overall quality of life through the use of specific treatment exercises and techniques. This is essential not only for physical healing but also for mental well-being, as it helps ensure that patients regain independence and self-assurance. Effective rehabilitation programs are individually tailored, considering the type of surgery performed and the patient's existing medical conditions. With compliance to an established rehabilitation program, patients are most likely to experience improved outcomes, validating the importance of physical therapy in the continuum of care for orthopaedic surgery. Rehabilitation is also achieved by incorporating assistive devices and education to ensure safe post-operative practice. The provision of such devices assumes a leading role in patients who undergo procedures like hip arthroplasty. As mentioned earlier in the literature, whole-person rehabilitation programs are supplemented with activities of daily living (ADL) and extended activities of daily living (EADL) training that is specific to patients' mobility needs. Hip precautions and environmental modifications are integral to such programs, as they help prevent complications and ensure safety during recovery. A review was conducted to assess the impact of these varied strategies on patient outcomes, with the goal of understanding the effects of device usage and education on the overall effectiveness of rehabilitation (Ackerman et al., 2013). Multidisciplinary interventions ensure that physical therapy is not only exercises but includes accommodations that facilitate the patient through their rehabilitation. Furthermore, advances in physical therapy have been built upon extensive research and systematic reviews that consider outcomes across diverse patient groups. Specialized studies, such as those involving cerebral palsy, have provided critical knowledge about best practices for orthotic intervention to complement rehabilitation approaches. By considering literature available over defined time intervals, scholars can establish effective treatment interventions and the role of orthoses in rehabilitation. These systematic reviews have informed the current practice procedures in physical therapy, leading to improved rehabilitation outcomes for patients who undergo orthopedic surgery. Emphasis on evidence-based interventions allows for continuous improvement in treatment strategies, ensuring that patients receive the highest quality care adapted to their individualized rehabilitation needs (Bowers et al., 2009). This cyclical perspective highlights the significance of research in shaping the future of physical therapy and rehabilitation, pointing to their core role in the provision of orthopedic surgical care.

10.5.2. Pain Management Strategies

Management of post-orthopedic surgical pain is a key aspect of patient management with considerable ramifications for recovery and satisfaction with the surgical procedure. Effective pain management alleviates suffering but also facilitates functional recovery. The multimodal approach, which involves the use of more than one analgesic modality to achieve optimal analgesia, is increasingly emphasized in contemporary practice through the implementation of a range of analgesic techniques tailored to individual patients. This includes the utilization of non-opioid medication, such as acetaminophen and nonsteroidal anti-inflammatory drugs (NSAIDs), that can work synergistically to minimize pain and limit narcotic requirements. It is welcomed that clinicians adopt this multimodal strategy, one that has shown decreased opioid use and thus lowered risks of addiction and abuse, a growing problem in the context of the opioid crisis (Hsu et al., 2019). In addition, the integration of physical and cognitive assessments further extends pain management guidelines. Physical therapy interventions, in the form of rehabilitative exercises, can play a vital role in relieving pain and improving post-surgery mobility. Utilizing cognitive-behavioral techniques, in the form of relaxation and mindfulness, has also been found to extend coping strategies against pain in patients. These integrative techniques not only address the physiological aspect of pain but also the psychological characteristics that can amplify the sensation of pain. Thus, attention by educational programs toward pain management is paramount, as learning about the various modalities is empowering for both patients and clinicians to manage postoperative pain more effectively. By integrating holistic, patient-specific methods of pain management, healthcare providers can optimize patient outcomes for orthopedic surgery. Specifically, postoperative sleep quality significantly impacts healing and patient satisfaction, making the control of pain essential. Research indicates that pain is an important variable explaining postoperative sleep disorders, where night-time awakening due to pain following surgery is common in most patients (Camilleri-Brennan et al., 2016). This is a determinant of why pain management is not only critical during the daytime but also at night during recovery. To improve postoperative recovery, steps should include changes in analgesia regimens and nocturnal pain relief. Enhancing the sleeping environment, such as introducing single-bed bays in hospitals, can help minimize noise disturbance and create a more comfortable environment for healing. In general, incorporating these factors into pain management planning is key to facilitating holistic recovery and allowing patients to experience a more uneventful postoperative process in orthopedic surgery (Figure 10.14).

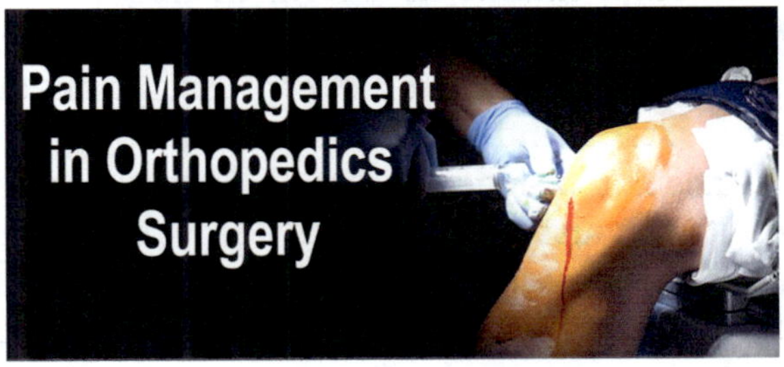

Figure 10.14. Pain management in orthopedic surgery.

Source: https://conferencepanel.com/dashboard/public/blogs/Pain-Management_1744884699.jpg.

10.5.3. Monitoring for Complications

In orthopedic surgery, vigilant monitoring for complications is crucial to allow optimal patient outcomes. This is particularly necessary in surgical cases involving high-risk patient groups, such as pregnant women, who may present unique challenges. For instance, when a pregnant woman requires surgery for an ankle fracture dislocation, the operating team must take care of not only the usual risks of the operation but also fetal well-being. Effective monitoring using devices such as heart tone monitors is crucial in these scenarios. A chilling case report was of a pregnant woman who had intraoperative fetal distress necessitating an urgent cesarean section. It stresses the need for there to be a coordinating team effort from obstetricians to anesthesiologists where both fetal and maternal welfare receive priority during the perioperative period (Coopersmith et al., 2013). These illustrations underscore the need for robust monitoring regimens to avoid inherent complications in the context of orthopedic surgery. In addition, complication monitoring is not merely an isolated intraoperative procedure but demands vigilant postoperative observation. Pain control after orthopedic procedures is one of the most critical areas where adequate monitoring becomes indispensable to avoid such complications as opioid addiction. The United States opioid epidemic has placed the adverse effects of overprescription on center stage and has necessitated a review of analgesic practice in orthopedic medicine. Providers must be more knowledgeable about addiction science and other strategies for pain management that reduce narcotic use. Employing multimodal treatment modalities—integrating physical therapies, cognitive strategies, and alternative pharmacology—has been shown to improve not only pain management but also minimize the risk of opioid abuse. With advancement in the specialty, it is essential for orthopedic surgeons to stay updated on clinical practice guidelines aimed at optimizing pain management while safeguarding patients against potential complications relating to narcotics (Hsu et al., 2019). Finally, regular patient assessment throughout the postoperative process is a requirement for early recognition of complications so that interventions can be undertaken in a timely fashion able to alter prognosis significantly. Infection, thromboembolic events, and delayed wound healing are the complications that must be prevented and monitored closely by the surgical team. Frequent follow-up visits, careful observation of surgical wound locations, and education for patients regarding signs and symptoms of potential complications are critical components of this monitoring regimen. In addition, the incorporation of patient-reported outcomes into the monitoring regime will enhance understanding of recovery progress and enable the detection of developing issues. This holistic policy fosters cooperation between the patient and the healthcare team, again emphasizing teamwork in orthopedic surgery. Ultimately, adequate monitoring not only enhances patient safety but also provides a superior outcome for the surgery, reflecting dedication to orthopedic excellence.

Test Your Knowledge

1. What are the key measures to prevent complications such as infection or deep vein thrombosis after orthopedic surgery?
2. How does physiotherapy and early mobilization influence recovery and functional outcomes in postoperative orthopedic patients?

10.6. Developments in Orthopedic Surgery

Learning Outcome

1. Define the minimally invasive techniques
2. Discuss use of robotics and technology
3. Identify the regenerative medicine and stem cell therapy

Evolution of orthopedic surgery has significantly improved the outcome of the patient, particularly through the advent of advanced imaging modalities and minimally invasive operative procedures. Technologies such as arthroscopy and computer-aided surgery allow for more precise diagnosis and treatment of musculoskeletal trauma. These technologies allow surgeons to visualize the structures of a joint better, enabling them to treat complex cases more precisely with reduced recovery times. The rising trend in outpatient surgical interventions further explains these advancements, as patients can often be sent home on the day of surgery. The inclusion of advanced imaging equipment, therefore, not only optimizes the efficiency of surgery but also aligns with the general aim of promoting patient quality of life, which translates to a revolutionary influence on the practice of orthopedics. Another crucial innovation in orthopedic surgery is the application of regenerative medicine, particularly in tissue engineering and stem cell therapy. These techniques can revolutionize the management of diseases such as osteoarthritis and tendon injuries, in which conventional surgical methods can only give minimal relief. By applying biologically active scaffolds or leveraging stem cell regeneration capabilities, surgeons can enhance the body's own healing mechanisms and restore tissue function more effectively. Furthermore, with the integration of 3D printing technology, there is the capability to create personalized implants and prosthetics tailored to patient anatomy. This customized plan not only enhances surgical outcomes but also facilitates faster patient rehabilitation, thereby shifting the paradigm from reactive surgery to proactive, customized treatment pathways that prioritize long-term health. The role of technology in shaping orthopedic surgery cannot be overstated, as evidenced by the incorporation of telemedicine and artificial intelligence (AI) into clinical practice. Telemedicine, particularly in the context of the COVID-19 pandemic, has enabled clinicians to maintain continuity of care while reducing the risk of infection. Patients can receive consultations and follow-up evaluations remotely, thereby improving access to specialized care regardless of geographic limitations. Likewise, AI's capacity to process vast amounts of surgical information is transforming preoperative planning and postoperative evaluation. Through pattern recognition and prediction of surgical outcomes, AI helps orthopedic surgeons make better-informed decisions that are unique to each patient's needs. As these technologies advance, the combined impact on improving the effectiveness and efficiency of orthopedic surgical practice holds a lot in store for the future of healthcare globally, with the emphasis of advocating for the right of all to equal access to quality health care as brought out by Farooq et al. (2017) (Figure 10.15).

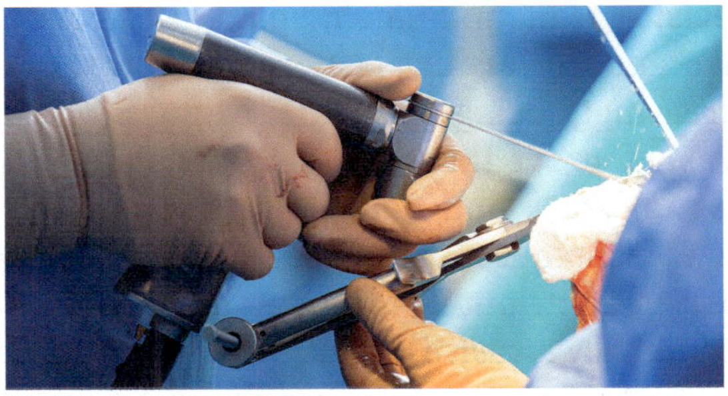

Figure 10.15. Advances in orthopaedic surgery.

Source: https://www1.racgp.org.au/getattachment/df422065-d5de-4516-b634-2c2da1bb04b9/Advances-in-orthopaedic-surgery.aspx.

10.6.1. Minimally Invasive Techniques

Minimally invasive techniques have made orthopedic surgery a new world, and patients today benefit from reduced recovery time and minimal surgical trauma. One such technique that departs from the traditional open reduction internal fixation (ORIF) is minimally invasive plate osteosynthesis (MIPO). The MIPO technique has been shown to yield acceptable clinical outcomes, particularly in terms of radiographic quality and functional recovery, as demonstrated in studies of articular pilon fractures. The reduced soft tissue damage associated with MIPO facilitates easier preservation of the surrounding anatomy, which is critical in ensuring joint health and functionality. Therefore, these advancements serve only to underscore the necessity of accepting minimally invasive methods of maximizing patient outcomes for orthopedic surgery, as the ability to benefit from their lower rate of complications continues to encourage increasing application in clinical practice (Angelini et al., 2018). The application of minimally invasive techniques is not limited to fracture surgery, but also extends to joint replacement and reconstruction surgeries. Minimally invasive surgery and more advanced imaging modalities have enabled surgeons to perform complex procedures with improved precision while minimizing patient discomfort. Knee and hip arthroplasties, for instance, are increasingly being performed using minimally invasive procedures, leading to shorter in-hospital stays and quicker recoveries. These newer techniques reduce postoperative pain and scarring, contributing to patient satisfaction. Use of minimally invasive techniques also contributes to the strides we see in orthopedic surgery's progress over the last 50 years, from crude fracture management to sophisticated joint reconstructive capability (Grixti et al., 2005). While the benefits of minimally invasive surgery are meaningful, it is crucial to consider the learning curve associated with its use. Surgeons will need to undergo rigorous training to master the finesse of these procedures, as the small working space and limited visualization area present unique challenges. Beyond that, selecting appropriate patients for minimally invasive procedures is paramount; not every patient or condition is suitable for such approaches, and due consideration of the likely risks versus benefits is necessary. As technology and science progress further, however, it can be predicted that both safety and efficacy will improve, and so usage will become more widespread across a broad spectrum of orthopedic applications. Lastly, persistent work on enhancing minimally invasive methods will be responsible for the future of orthopedic surgery (Angelini et al., 2018) (Figure 10.16).

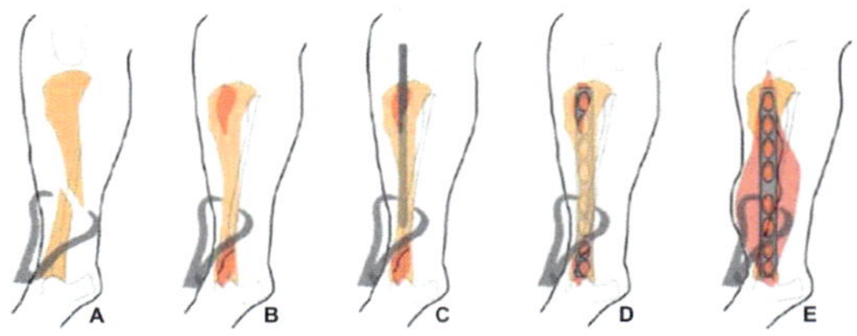

Figure 10.16. Minimally invasive plate osteosynthesis.

Source: https://www.researchgate.net/profile/Suyoung-Heo/publication/273260204/figure/fig2/AS:669073935437845@1536531065666/Schematic-illustrations-of-the-minimally-invasive-plate-osteosynthesis-MIPO-and-the.png.

10.6.2. Use of Robotics and Technology

The combination of state-of-the-art technologies and robotics in orthopedic surgery is a significant shift in the way surgical procedures are conducted and patient results. Robotics, with the help of state-of-the-art tools such as artificial intelligence and augmented reality, enhances accuracy in surgeries, potentially reducing complications and recovery periods. The technologies allow for intricate procedures to be carried out with a precision that human hands may not have. Thus, the reliance on robotics not only paved the way for minimally invasive surgery but has also improved the ability to perform complex surgeries that were once considered impractical. Thus, the advances necessitate a reevaluation of training protocols and surgical norms, as well as an awareness of the need to pursue continuous professional development to adapt to the evolving technological landscape in orthopedics. In addition, the application of technologies like 5G connectivity is about to revolutionize healthcare systems, including orthopedic surgery. The integration of Internet of Things (IoT) devices and machine learning algorithms enables real-time data analysis and patient monitoring during surgery. This will enhance decision-making processes and intraoperative communication among surgical teams. By optimizing workflows and streamlining the exchange of information, these technologies have the potential to address some of the long-standing challenges in healthcare, such as inefficiencies in resource allocation and patient management. As identified in recent studies, 5G technology and orthopedic practice at the intersection clearly demonstrate how essential systematic reforms are in the creation of a more efficient healthcare system that prioritizes the well-being of patients while maintaining high standards of surgery (Farooq et al., 2017). Nevertheless, the transition to the widespread use of robotics and new technologies in orthopedic surgery is not without its share of problems. Key among them are the cost aspects of investing in new technologies and the need for specialist training to utilize these innovations fully. Patients' acceptance and learning curves of new technologies are equally key factors that are responsible for their uptake within clinical practice. Research indicates that such challenges necessitate a structured framework that seeks cost-effectiveness, training, and an innovation culture in operating rooms (Buser et al., 2025). By considering such elements, the orthopedic surgical community can harness the benefits of technological innovations while ensuring that surgical procedures adapt to mitigate the challenges of innovations.

10.6.3. Regenerative Medicine and Stem Cell Therapy

The intersection of orthopedic surgery and regenerative medicine is key in further advancing the use of musculoskeletal disease management. Ongoing research suggests the potential of stem cell therapy in regeneration, utilizing the patient's own cells to initiate repair and restoration. Unlike traditional treatments characterized by extensive surgery, stem cell treatments can activate endogenous repair, resulting in reduced recovery time and fewer associated complications. The establishment of such techniques based on these cellular activities follows the increasing demand for less invasive procedures in orthopedic surgery. Advances in regenerative medicine, thus, not only enhance healing but also challenge previous paradigms in disease management and recuperation in musculoskeletal treatment, which demand more patient-focused approaches. One significant hindrance in the expanded application of stem cell therapy in orthopedic surgery is the logistical intricacies associated with the cultivation of autologous cells. The ex vivo culture undertaken to maximize such cells prior to their implantation is not only time-consuming but also costly and manpower-intensive. Moreover, questions related to the usage of exogenous cells, including their safety and availability, are further making the clinical acceptability of such treatments more challenging. Against these challenges, researchers are directing attention towards endogenous tissue engineering methods that utilize cells within the body to harness their regenerative capacity. These processes can prove to have the advantage of an efficient therapeutic regimen, which makes sophisticated regenerative techniques more feasible while remaining within the paradigms of orthopedic surgery (Adam et al., 2012). Such a focus on the use of the patient's own biological factors is evidence of a paradigm shift in orthopedic treatment of musculoskeletal trauma and degenerative disease. Current progress in regenerative medicine, including the use of stem cell therapy, portends the potential for new paradigms in orthopedic disease treatment. Most crucially, perhaps, the integration of biologic medicines, for example, the use of autologous stem cells, into routine surgical procedures holds the potential to expedite functional outcomes. Not only do these interventions aim to repair damaged tissues, but they also control the inflammatory reaction that typically occurs after musculoskeletal injury. With the advancement of science, continued trials are illuminating the safety and efficacy of these emerging treatments. Promising results from stage-stage studies generate optimism for their eventual role as standard of care in orthopedics (Baron et al., 2016). These developments not only underscore the importance of continued research in this area but also underscore the need for strict regulatory frameworks for ensuring the responsible application of regenerative technologies to clinical practice.

Test Your Knowledge

1. How have minimally invasive and robotic-assisted techniques advanced the field of orthopedic surgery?
2. What recent innovations in implants and biomaterials have improved patient outcomes and recovery in orthopedic procedures?

SUMMARY

The orthopedic surgery practice is witnessing unprecedented advances that enhance operating room outcomes and recovery processes of patients. When we compare the open gluteal tendon repair (OGR) and endoscopic gluteal tendon repair (EGR), we find that both procedures exhibit remarkable enhancements in clinical results, but their efficacy is considerably similar. Current studies have shown that the nature of surgical technique is not immediate in diminishing pain or promoting functional recovery, as indicated by patient outcomes. This remains vital since clinicians base decisions on approaching the surgery with individual patient conditions and not necessarily on the absolute superiority of one procedure over another (Bini et al., 2020). The versatility of these methods enables surgeons to treat complex gluteal tendon ruptures more effectively, aligning with the diverse needs of their patient populations. Furthermore, the evolving landscape of digital health technologies is a tipping point for the approach of orthopedic surgery to heal patients. The COVID-19 pandemic has accelerated the adoption of telehealth services in clinical care, introducing a novel paradigm for care delivery that extends beyond traditional face-to-face encounters. These technologies, which gained prominence during the health crisis, have not only contributed to patient management but also increased access to specialist musculoskeletal care (Ast et al., 2020). Looking back on these developments, we can now appreciate how the long-term implications of digital health for orthopedics will redefine patient expectations and lay the groundwork for continuous interaction throughout the entire continuum of care.

In the end, as orthopedic surgery matures, there must be emphasis on the convergence of both revolutionary surgical practices and digital health technologies. By drawing upon evidence-based findings from comparative analyses of EGR and OGR, and through commitment to ongoing development of digital health approaches, orthopaedic surgeons are well positioned to enhance patient care outcomes significantly. Trust in diverse methods of surgery and prudent deployment of technology is testimony to the responsiveness of the profession in addressing patient needs in a changing healthcare environment. With these developments continuing to evolve, orthopedic surgery's future is one that promises a new frontier where more sophisticated models of care delivery will optimize recovery alongside improved quality of life for patients (Bini et al., 2020; Ast et al., 2020).

Orthopedic surgery practice entails a number of forms of operative procedures that are performed to manage musculoskeletal disorders, with varying objectives and mechanisms. One is patient care that undergoes hip arthroplasty, and preoperative education coupled with the provision of assistive devices can significantly enhance recovery outcomes. A systematic review of these interventions defines education on hip precautions and environmental adaptations as a significant intervention in making postoperative rehabilitation feasible for patients. This method not only prevents complications but also allows patients to become more independent in activities of daily living (ADL) and instrumental activities of daily living (EADL). By assessing the effects of such strategies, clinicians can optimize preoperative planning to the point where patients not only learn about their care but also become empowered to maximize their recovery (Ackerman et al., 2013).

Another region of focus in orthopedic surgery is the management of end-stage arthritis of the ankle and, more specifically, the decision between ankle fusion and replacement. Understanding factors influencing the patient's decision in these cases is vital in the development of patient-specific treatment planning. Research indicates that the patient's expectation of function, lifestyle concerns, and potential outcomes of each surgical option can greatly influence their choice. Ankle fusion is commonly associated with increased stability, but at the expense of mobility. In contrast, ankle replacement offers improved range of motion, albeit at the expense of attachment loss. By examining critically how decisions are made by patients, surgeons can engage in shared decision-making, where patients are given information on the outcomes of each option and can make their decisions based on personal values and goals (Goldberg et al., 2013). Briefly, the breadth of orthopedic surgery necessitates a broad understanding of both patient-oriented care and procedural intervention. The intersection of educational pathways and assistive technology in hip arthroplasty represents a paradigm shift in which patient engagement leads to improved functional outcomes. Concurrently, examination of decision-making strategies in the selection between ankle fusion and ankle replacement also emphasizes the importance of patient-individualized treatment pathways in orthopedics. As the field continues to advance, research and evidence-based practice must continue to be paramount in maximizing surgical efficiency as well as patient satisfaction, ultimately towards the ultimate goal of orthopedic surgery: restoration of optimal function and quality of life for the patient.

KEY TERMS FROM THIS CHAPTER

- Arthroscopy
- Closed reduction
- Compartment syndrome
- Fracture fixation
- Joint dislocation
- Orthopaedic implants
- Osteomyelitis
- Rotator cuff repair
- Bone grafting
- Clubfoot
- Degenerative joint disease
- Intramedullary nailing
- Open reduction internal fixation (ORIF)
- Orthopaedic trauma
- Pathological fracture
- Scoliosis correction

CRITICAL THINKING QUESTIONS

1. **Which of the following is the most common site for avascular necrosis (AVN)?**
   a. Tibial plateau
   b. Scaphoid bone
   c. Femoral head
   d. Patella
2. **Which nerve is most commonly injured in a mid-shaft fracture of the humerus?**
   a. Ulnar nerve
   b. Radial nerve
   c. Median nerve
   d. Axillary nerve
3. **Which of the following findings is characteristic of compartment syndrome?**
   a. Joint instability
   b. Swelling relieved by elevation
   c. Pain out of proportion to injury and pain on passive stretch
   d. Hyperesthesia and brisk reflexes
4. **The most common location of osteosarcoma in adolescents is:**
   a. Proximal tibia
   b. Distal femur
   c. Pelvis
   d. Humeral shaft
5. **Which of the following is considered a complication of long bone fractures?**
   a. Deep vein thrombosis
   b. Pneumonia
   c. Hypertension
   d. Diabetes mellitus

Short Answer Questions

1. What is the difference between an open and a closed fracture?
2. Name the components of the neurovascular examination for a limb injury.
3. What are the clinical features of compartment syndrome?
4. How is a supracondylar fracture of the humerus classified in children?
5. What are the indications for internal fixation of fractures?
6. Define avascular necrosis and mention one common site where it occurs.
7. What is the mechanism of injury in anterior cruciate ligament (ACL) tears?
8. What are the common complications of long bone fractures?
9. What are the differences between osteoarthritis and rheumatoid arthritis in terms of joint involvement?
10. List the common sites for metastatic bone disease.

Answers to Critical Thinking Questions

1. (c); 2. (b); 3. (c); 4. (b); 5. (a)

REFERENCES

1. Wainwright, T. W., Immins, T., & Middleton, R. G. (2015). Enhanced recovery after surgery (ERAS) and its applicability for major spine surgery. Best Practice & Research Clinical Anaesthesiology, 30(1), 91–102. https://doi.org/10.1016/j.bpa.2015.11.001Achten, J., Costa, M. L., Hiskens, R., Parsons, N., et al. (2012). An evaluation of the quality of statistical design and analysis of published medical research: Results from a systematic survey of general orthopedic journals. https://core.ac.uk/download/9846544.pdf (accessed on 12th July 2025).
2. Ackerman, I. N., Altman, R. D., Bellamy, N., Birrell, F., Boutron, I., Canadian Joint Replacement Registry, Collin, C., et al. (2013). Assistive devices, hip precautions, environmental modifications and training to prevent dislocation and improve function after hip arthroplasty. https://core.ac.uk/download/19595821.pdf (accessed on 12th July 2025).
3. Adam, C. (2012). Endogenous musculoskeletal tissue engineering – a focused perspective. https://core.ac.uk/download/10908942.pdf (accessed on 12th July 2025).
4. Ali, P., Santy-Tomlinson, J., & Watson, R. (2014). Assessment and diagnosis of acute limb compartment syndrome: A literature review. https://core.ac.uk/download/151161255.pdf (accessed on 12th July 2025).
5. Allen, M. (2016). Cerebral fat microembolism and its potential role in postoperative cognitive dysfunction after major orthopedic surgery: Commentary on an article by Anna N. Miller, MD, et al.: "Use of the Reamer/Irrigator/Aspirator decreases carotid and cranial embolic events in a canine model." https://core.ac.uk/download/35280153.pdf (accessed on 12th July 2025).
6. Amano, K., Li, X., Ma, C. B., Pedoia, V., et al. (2016). Persistent biomechanical alterations after ACL reconstruction are associated with early cartilage matrix changes detected by quantitative MR. https://core.ac.uk/download/323079514.pdf (accessed on 12th July 2025).
7. Anderson, A., Bailey, C., Barter, L., Braun, H. J., Cox, L. G., Dell'Isola, A., Deveza, L., et al. (2020). The use of technology in the subcategorization of osteoarthritis: A Delphi study approach. https://core.ac.uk/download/326325068.pdf (accessed on 12th July 2025).
8. Angelini, A., Biz, C., Carniel, D., Iacobellis, C., et al. (2018). Medium-long-term radiographic and clinical outcomes after surgical treatment of intra-articular tibial pilon fractures by three different techniques. https://core.ac.uk/download/154330599.pdf (accessed on 12th July 2025).
9. Arnold, P. M., Bumpass, D. B., Bydon, M., Corriveau, M. R., et al. (2017). Incidence and outcomes of acute implant extrusion following anterior cervical spine surgery. https://core.ac.uk/download/129191221.pdf (accessed on 12th July 2025).
10. Ast, M. P., Bini, S. A., Chung, C. C., Kalore, N. V., et al. (2020). Digital orthopedics: A glimpse into the future in the midst of a pandemic. https://core.ac.uk/download/323308683.pdf (accessed on 12th July 2025).
11. Atesok, K., Gokaslan, Z. L., Heffernan, M. J., Papavassiliou, E., et al. (2020). Current strategies in prevention of postoperative infections in spine surgery. https://core.ac.uk/download/299811520.pdf (accessed on 12th July 2025).
12. Bache, C. E., Harmatz, P. R., Jester, A., Mackenzie, W. G., et al. (2014). Orthopedic management of the extremities in patients with Morquio A syndrome. https://core.ac.uk/download/323062594.pdf (accessed on 12th July 2025).

13. Bailey, A., Gleeson, N., Minshull, C., Parfitt, G., et al. (2008). Influence of surgery and rehabilitation conditioning on psychophysiological fitness. https://core.ac.uk/download/30640181.pdf (accessed on 12th July 2025).
14. Baron, D. A., Bergman, P. J., Bryan, J. N., Calvet, J., et al. (2016). A One Health overview, facilitating advances in comparative medicine and translational research. https://core.ac.uk/download/323068355.pdf (accessed on 12th July 2025).
15. Belluzzi, E., Biz, C., De Cicco, M., Fantoni, F., et al. (2019). Long-term radiographic and clinical-functional outcomes of isolated, displaced, closed talar neck and body fractures treated by ORIF: The timing of surgical management. https://core.ac.uk/download/224995443.pdf (accessed on 12th July 2025).
16. Bernthal, N. M., Dworsky, E. M., Hu, Y., Loftin, C., et al. (2015). Current animal models of postoperative spine infection and potential future advances. https://core.ac.uk/download/323066862.pdf (accessed on 12th July 2025).
17. Berntorp, E., & Knobe, K. (2011). Hemophilia and joint disease: Pathophysiology, evaluation and management. https://core.ac.uk/download/pdf/29572290.pdf (accessed on 12th July 2025).
18. Bhandari, M., Chaudhry, H., Einhorn, T. A., Mundi, R., et al. (2008). How good is the orthopedic literature? https://core.ac.uk/download/142041949.pdf (accessed on 12th July 2025).
19. Bini, S. A., Jäger, M., Maslaris, A., Patel, V., et al. (2020). Equivalent mid-term results of open vs endoscopic gluteal tendon tear repair using suture anchors in forty-five patients. https://core.ac.uk/download/323073887.pdf (accessed on 12th July 2025).
20. Bishop, M., Chang, E. S., Ciccotti, M. G., Cohen, S. B., et al. (2018). Management of elbow dislocations in the National Football League. https://core.ac.uk/download/155271710.pdf (accessed on 12th July 2025).
21. Borg, J. N., Mifsud, M., Mizzi, C., Ng, K., et al. (2015). The Libyan civil conflict: Selected case series of orthopedic trauma managed in Malta in 2014. https://core.ac.uk/download/323186351.pdf (accessed on 12th July 2025).
22. Bowers, R., ISPO (Funder), & Ross, K. (2009). A review of the effectiveness of lower limb orthoses used in cerebral palsy. https://core.ac.uk/download/9024488.pdf (accessed on 12th July 2025).
23. Brittberg, M., Busacca, M., Condello, V., Engebretsen, L., et al. (2017). A multilayer biomaterial for osteochondral regeneration shows superiority vs microfractures for the treatment of osteochondral lesions in a multicenter randomized trial at 2 years. https://core.ac.uk/download/91120498.pdf (accessed on 12th July 2025).
24. Brockmeier, S. F., Cosgrove, C. T., Diduch, D. R., Gilmore, A., et al. (2017). Accelerated return to sport after osteochondral autograft plug transfer. https://core.ac.uk/download/83101110.pdf (accessed on 12th July 2025).
25. Brodke, D. S., Buser, Z., D'Oro, A., Hsieh, P. C., et al. (2018). Trends and costs of external electrical bone stimulators and grafting materials in anterior lumbar interbody fusion. https://core.ac.uk/download/213444606.pdf (accessed on 12th July 2025).
26. Buser, Z., Chen, X., Cho, S., Demetriades, D., et al. (2025). Framework for adoption of enabling technologies for improved outcomes in spine surgery. https://core.ac.uk/download/644524688.pdf (accessed on 12th July 2025).

27. Camilleri-Brennan, J., Dolan, R., Huh, J., Sproat, I., et al. (2016). A prospective analysis of sleep deprivation and disturbance in surgical patients. https://core.ac.uk/download/84591804.pdf (accessed on 12th July 2025).
28. Cheung, E. C., Flores, S. E., Hodax, J. D., Zhang, A. L., et al. (2019). Use of air arthrograms to aid in joint distraction during hip arthroscopic surgery decreases postoperative pain and opioid requirements. https://core.ac.uk/download/323062560.pdf (accessed on 12th July 2025).
29. Cook, J. A. (2009). The challenges faced in the design, conduct and analysis of surgical randomized trials. https://core.ac.uk/download/177136.pdf (accessed on 12th July 2025).
30. Coopersmith, A., Gidumal, R., Gross, S. C., Schwarzkopf, R., et al. (2013). Ankle fracture surgery on a pregnant patient complicated by intraoperative emergency caesarian section. https://core.ac.uk/download/323075671.pdf (accessed on 12th July 2025).
31. Culp, R. W., Gaspar, M. P., Jacoby, S. M., Kane, P. M., et al. (2017). Platelet-rich plasma injection with percutaneous needling for recalcitrant lateral epicondylitis: Comparison of tenotomy and fenestration techniques. https://core.ac.uk/download/155271598.pdf (accessed on 12th July 2025).
32. Domalaon, K., Henderson, L., Kim, J., Kroin, R., et al. (2021). The perceived value of same-sex or race mentors and role models in academic medicine. https://core.ac.uk/download/621696193.pdf (accessed on 12th July 2025).
33. Farooq, S., Imran, M. A., Latif, S., Qadir, J., et al. (2017). How 5G wireless (and concomitant technologies) will revolutionize healthcare? https://core.ac.uk/download/143476480.pdf (accessed on 12th July 2025).
34. Gaonkar, K. L., et al. (2023). Advancements in joint replacement surgery: Improving long-term outcomes and patient satisfaction. https://core.ac.uk/download/596247506.pdf (accessed on 12th July 2025).
35. Goldberg, A., Macgregor, A. J., Pfeil, M., Zaidi, R. K., et al. (2013). How do patients with end-stage ankle arthritis decide between two surgical treatments? A qualitative study. https://core.ac.uk/download/19595159.pdf (accessed on 12th July 2025).
36. Grixti, C. J. (2005). Orthopedic surgery. https://core.ac.uk/download/46602006.pdf (accessed on 12th July 2025).
37. Hintermann, B. A., Friemert, B. Y., Rolf, C., Barclay, C., Rolf, C. G., et al. (2006). The importance of early arthroscopy in athletes with painful cartilage lesions of the ankle: A prospective study of 61 consecutive cases. https://core.ac.uk/download/55432.pdf (accessed on 12th July 2025).
38. Hsu, J. R., Jahangir, A. A., Miller, A. N., Mir, H. R., et al. (2019). Confronting the opioid crisis: Practical pain management and strategies: AOA 2018 critical issues symposium. https://core.ac.uk/download/286537307.pdf (accessed on 12th July 2025).
39. MacGregor, A. J., Archibeck, M., Baker, P., Berger, R., Charnley, J., Coventry, M. B., Daniel, D., et al. (2008). Revision rates after primary hip and knee replacement in England between 2003 and 2006. https://core.ac.uk/download/1394863.pdf (accessed on 12th July 2025).
40. Mannion, A. F., Coll, A. M., Ransford, A. O., Provenzano, D. A., Ohnmeiss, D. D., Felix, E. R., Felix, E. R., et al. (2011). 2D vs. 3D pain visualization: User preferences in a spinal cord injury cohort. https://core.ac.uk/download/9633514.pdf (accessed on 12th July 2025).

41. Nagessar, K. (2023). Applications and topics of physics in surgery. https://core.ac.uk/download/639335195.pdf (accessed on 12th July 2025).

42. PARITY Investigators. (2015). Prophylactic antibiotic regimens in tumor surgery (PARITY): A pilot multicenter randomized controlled trial. https://core.ac.uk/download/323068137.pdf (accessed on 12th July 2025).

43. Reynolds, L. A., & Tansey, E. M. (2007). Early development of total hip replacement. https://core.ac.uk/download/30696185.pdf (accessed on 12th July 2025).

44. Smith, N. (2024). Medical voluntarism and orthopedic advancements: Lancashire and the disabled ex-servicemen of the First World War. https://core.ac.uk/download/624083462.pdf (accessed on 12th July 2025).

45. Street, A., & Mannion, R. (2025). Payment by results and demand management: Learning from the South Yorkshire laboratory. https://core.ac.uk/download/pdf/6833648.pdf (accessed on 12th July 2025).

46. Zellweger, C. (2009). Keynote address: Foreign bodies / jewellery as prosthesis. https://core.ac.uk/download/99988.pdf (accessed on 12th July 2025).

PLASTIC SURGERY

11

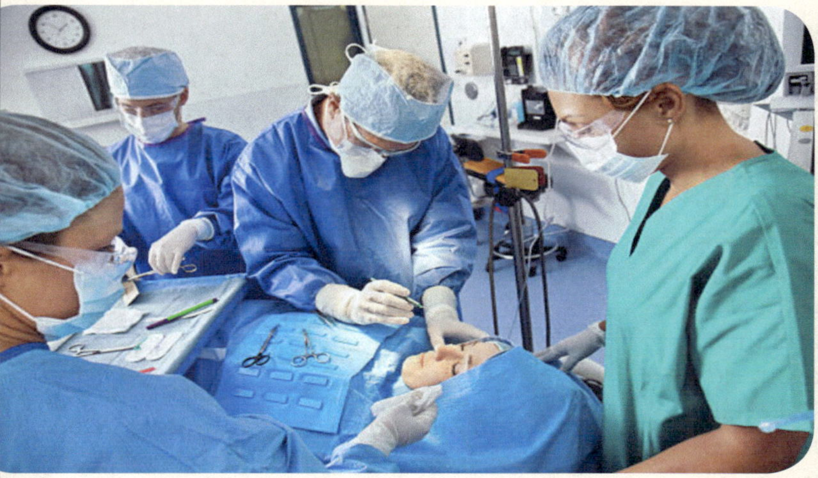

LEARNING OBJECTIVES

After studying this chapter, you will be able to:

1. Understand the types of plastic surgery
2. Explain the reasons for undergoing plastic surgery
3. Discuss the risks and complications of plastic surgery
4. Focus on the role of technology in plastic surgery
5. Learn about ethical considerations in plastic surgery
6. Evaluate the cultural perspectives on plastic surgery

Introduction

The history of plastic surgery has been marked by profound shifts in cultural attitudes, significant advances in medicine, and complex ethical questions. Initially focused on reconstructive surgery for repairing physical malformations from accident or birth, plastic surgery broadened its scope significantly to encompass cosmetic procedures. This reflects the growing significance of physical beauty in modern society, where outward appearances increasingly determine personal and social success. Notably, cosmetic surgery enhances body image and self-esteem, which are important factors in the psychological well-being of individuals. However, the cosmetic procedure issues, particularly in vulnerable populations such as adolescents, unveil complex ethical issues that require careful consideration. The increase in demand for these treatments complicates patient motivation issues and the roles of healthcare providers in ensuring informed consent and emotional readiness (Luca et al., 2018). With plastic surgery as a wider field, clinicians must tread carefully between enhancing appearance and upholding ethical procedures, particularly when dealing with adolescent patients. The decision to undergo cosmetic surgery at an early age involves psychological, social, and familial issues that must be extensively deliberated. Adolescents may be subject to specific pressures to conform to current views of beauty and attractiveness, leading to decisions based on appearance over mental and emotional health. Furthermore, through inadequate psychological evaluations, clinicians may unwittingly endorse harmful motivations linked to body image disorders or hidden psychiatric illnesses. The requirement of detailed counseling sessions for both patients and their families prior to undergoing surgical procedures is key to facilitating an understanding of the risks and benefits that cosmetic procedures pose (Luca et al., 2018). The multipronged strategy ensures that choices are made on behalf of the minor patient in their best interest, considering not only aesthetic preferences but also their psychological well-being. Given these considerations, it is most essential to have definite regulations governing plastic surgery, particularly that done on children. There must be limitations on what can be performed to avoid unnecessary or overly invasive procedures, ensuring that operations are based on the body's objective needs and not on subjective beauty standards. Studies indicate that following post-operative evaluations, practitioners need to measure breast position, for instance, to consider how body positioning may change depending on factors such as clothing. Such findings emphasize the need for ongoing research and a commitment towards improving normalized breast procedures that prioritize patient care over trends in beauty. Lastly, plastic surgery ethics rely on practitioners' professionalism to act in the patient's best interest, ensuring a setting where healthy-minded, balanced, and well-informed decisions can be made (Figure 11.1).

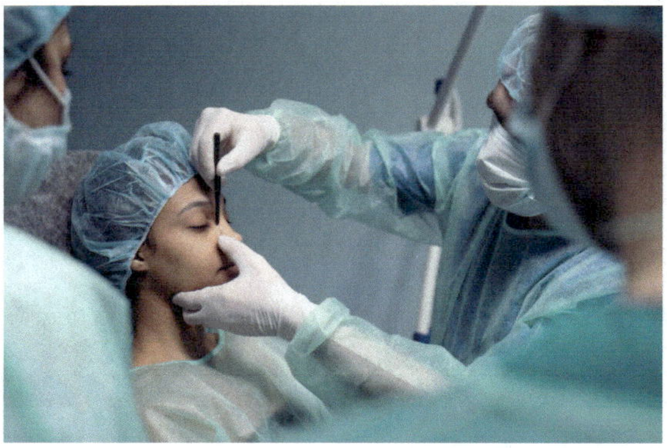

Figure 11.1. Plastic surgery.

Source: https://sukhmanihospital.in/wp-content/uploads/2024/03/jpeg-optimizer_side-view-doctor-checking-patient-before-rhinoplasty.jpg.

Definition of Plastic Surgery

Plastic surgery is a subspecialty of medicine with the correction, reconstruction, or alteration of the human form. Plastic surgery is predominantly classified into two broad categories: reconstructive plastic surgery and aesthetic (or cosmetic) plastic surgery. Reconstructive plastic surgery is designed to restore form and function in body structure with congenital deformity, trauma, or disease. They are breast reconstruction after mastectomy or surgery in a burn patient, where the aim is not only cosmetic but also resumption of normal functioning. Aesthetic plastic surgery, however, seeks to enhance one's appearance through procedures such as facelifts, liposuction, or breast augmentation. This contrast highlights the accommodation of plastic surgery to cope with both health and cosmetic medical interventions. Social expectations have significantly impacted the field of plastic surgery, along with concerns regarding the psychological impact and ethics. Cultural perspectives often dictate beauty ideals, prompting individuals to undergo surgical alterations for enhancement or social advantage. Specifically, studies have shown that patients may approach plastic surgery with preconceptions about beauty, such as those associated with social measures, including the golden proportion, which posits that certain facial measurements are considered beautiful (Rossetti et al., 2018). A growing body of evidence contradicts the applicability of those standards to all people, particularly those from diverse backgrounds. For instance, studies indicate that the facial measurements of professional African American models fall short of the golden proportion, suggesting an even more individualized response to beauty standards is required (Rossetti et al., 2018).

In addition, plastic surgery motivations are frequently inextricable from broader sociocultural circumstances, specifically those of immigration. Immigrants do practice body modification, for example, plastic surgery, as a means of negotiating their identity in the consumer culture they find themselves in. The practice demonstrates the complex relationship between social pressure and personal wants, with the explanation of how plastic surgery is employed as a conduit for self-adjustment and adaptation to the new cultural landscape. Even as the perilous situations that plague most immigrants persist, body modification remains in strong demand, and this suggests that looking good is an integral aspect of identity in the modern world. It emphasizes the urgency to view plastic surgery not just as a medical procedure but also as a cultural trend that reflects and responds to shifting forces of identity and beauty standards in an age of globalization.

History Background of Plastic Surgery

The evolution of plastic surgery can be traced back to ancient times, where primitive techniques were primarily used for repair. The oldest examples of surgical operations for the correction of physical defects are recorded in ancient Indian texts, such as the Sushruta Samhita around 600 BCE. This text outlines methods for restoring the nose, which is frequently destroyed as a consequence of cultural retribution. Advances in India quickly influenced nearby cultures, especially in the Mediterranean world, where Greek and Roman physicians started to fashion analogous practices. These early practices laid the groundwork for modern plastic surgery through the display of a deep early understanding of anatomy and the application of surgical technique, and they emphasized the significance of physical appearance in social and cultural life. During the Renaissance, a renewed interest in the human body emerged, with a significant impact on the history of plastic surgery. Painters and anatomists, such as Leonardo da Vinci and Andreas Vesalius, observed the human body with great care, which in turn promoted surgical knowledge. Surgical practice became more acceptable and advanced during this period, and newer reconstruction techniques were developed. However, it wasn't until the 19th century that the topic gained momentum. Surgeons began employing more systematic approaches to healing injuries and defects, particularly as advances in antiseptic treatments and anesthesia made surgery more secure. The introduction of these medical methods into the field of plastic surgery revealed a growing social awareness of the importance of both form and function, laying the groundwork for the specialized surgical fields of the 20th century. World War I marked a milestone that brought the practice of plastic surgery into the 20th century. The war produced horrific facial injuries on soldiers that necessitated the intervention of surgeons like Sir Harold Gillies, who developed novel reconstructive techniques to restore not only the appearance but also the identity of injured servicemen. This period of medical advancement was characterized by an interdisciplinary collaboration between surgeons, engineers, and the military to fix complex injuries. Furthermore, advances in surgery and materials have set the stage for further innovation in cosmetic surgery, enabling greater societal tolerance for procedures that enhance one's appearance. As technology and science grew, questions regarding body modification ethics arose, shaping the modern plastic surgery scene as one that reconstructs and aesthetically alters, reflecting the complex dyad between identity and body image in the contemporary world (Reynolds et al., 2007; Shilling et al., 2016).

Importance of the Topic in Contemporary Society

The problem of plastic surgery is very significant in contemporary society, reflecting higher cultural norms and values concerning beauty, aging, and identity. While individuals become more enthusiastic about surgical treatments in an attempt to live up to the expectations of the world, plastic surgery becomes a gesture of personal empowerment as well as a reflection of social status. This is particularly evident in societies where appearance is closely tied to self-worth and success. A recent study emphasizes how individuals utilize plastic surgery to manage the look of aging, which results in better mental health and sexual satisfaction, implying surgery is being contemplated as a normal aspect of personal grooming in an emerging world (Edmonds et al., 2014). This transformation reveals the growing acceptability of body modification as a means of coping with the relentless stress of contemporary life, and raises important questions regarding authenticity and the influence of consumer culture on individual self-knowledge. Moreover, the landscape of plastic surgery is inextricably intertwined with shifting narratives of feminism and femininity in agency in the 21st century. Post-feminist discourse encourages women to take charge of their bodies and realize their freedom in terms of decisions, like surgical enhancement. This reconceptualization of empowerment aligns with contemporary values that uphold agency, consumer choice, and sexual emancipation, as evident in various cultural texts that celebrate self-transformation and autonomy (Adriaens et al., 2014). These accounts show that the need to undergo plastic surgery is not necessarily a reflection of social pressure, but rather an acknowledgment of people's right to alter their appearance according to individual needs and aspirations. With these ideas gaining prominence in popular culture, they redefine the notion with which society perceives beauty standards, misleadingly interchanging self-improvement with social expectation.

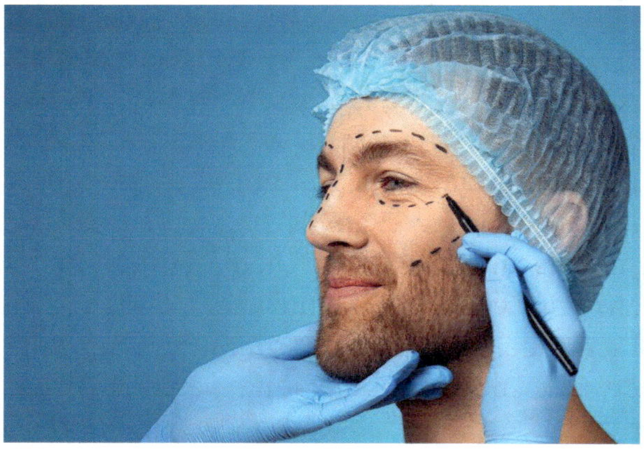

Figure 11.2. Cosmetic plastic surgery.

Source: https://max-website20-images.s3.ap-south-1.amazonaws.com/Plastic_Surgery_b9690e9803.jpg.

In addition, the interfusion of technology, media, and plastic surgery has created an active culture that promotes and legitimates such beauty choices. Social media platforms, for example, amplify the visibility of cosmetic procedures through the use of before-and-after photographs, generating desirable discourses that can potentially influence public perceptions of beauty and attractiveness. These websites are more likely to have individuals who embrace plastic surgery as a lifestyle, which influences others to do the same. The rise of the influencer and celebrity culture, who are extremely forthcoming about their procedures, further assists in altering public perception—moving from being stigmatized to a routine procedure. The normalization process that this creates leads to significant discussions around authenticity, the consumerism of beauty, and the psychological effects of attempting to achieve idealized appearances, making the topic integral to understanding the body image and self-esteem trends of our current society (Figure 11.2).

11.1. Types of Plastic Surgery

Learning Outcome

1. Define cosmetic surgery
2. Discuss on reconstructive surgery
3. Describe the non-surgical procedures

The field of plastic surgery encompasses a wide range of procedures designed to address various physical enhancements and reconstructive needs. The best-known categories are aesthetic and reconstructive procedures. Aesthetic surgery, also referred to as cosmetic surgery, is directed towards improving appearance and is in demand from individuals seeking to enhance a specific aspect of their appearance, such as breast enhancement or nose reconstruction. These procedures tend to reflect the greater cultural ideals of beauty and self. In contrast, reconstructive surgery has a more functional purpose to rebuild shape and function following trauma, birth defect, or disease. Breast reconstruction following mastectomy or facial reconstructive surgery following an accident are examples. The difference between these categories highlights the dual aspect of plastic surgery, demonstrating its ability to both enhance beauty and promote healing. One of the most major subcategories of aesthetic surgery is minimally invasive procedures, which have gained widespread popularity due to their brief recovery time and minimal risks. Techniques such as Botox injections and dermal fillers have revolutionized the way people approach cosmetic modification since they allow people to make drastic changes without much surgery required. This becomes part of the trend for a pliable body in today's time, where identity can be actively constructed through aesthetic choices. There is typically a media influence on people, and as such, there is more treatment involving the promise of fitting in with society's expectations, as discussed in Ricciardelli et al. (2011). Therefore, these developments in cosmetic surgery provide a space in which to investigate identity and resilience, as well as a new narrative around body autonomy and augmentation. Reconstructive surgery, while utilitarian in its intention to repair function and form, also has an overlap with emotional well-being. Patients who receive these surgeries often deal with the emotional impacts of physical trauma, as well as with congenital defects.

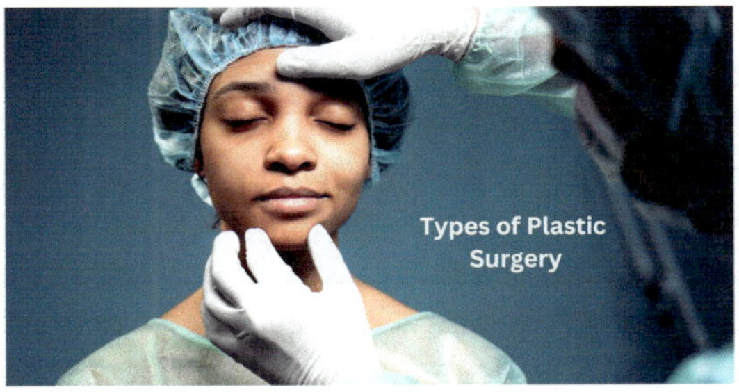

Figure 11.3. Types of plastic-surgery.

Source: https://www.bmcosmetic.com/wp-content/uploads/2023/08/Types-of-Plastic-Surgery-2.png.

For example, successful reconstructive surgery can significantly help progress the self-esteem of patients in addition to re-integrating them into society in which they might have struggled before the surgery. Further, the aftermath of reconstructive surgery proceeds to encompass gender identity, body image, language, and social norms. The reports of individuals who undergo surgery place greater emphasis on how such surgeries influence their constructions of femininity and masculinity, suggesting an underlying dynamic between body, self, and social membership, as quoted by Ricciardelli et al. (2011). Overall, these results put the complexity of plastic surgery and its relevance to individual and shared experiences at the forefront (Figure 11.3).

11.1.1. Cosmetic Surgery

The face of cosmetic surgery has undergone drastic changes over the years, reflecting the shifts in society and advancements in technology. Formerly stigmatized, they are now more widely accepted as methods to enhance body aesthetics or correct perceived imperfections. Notably, breast reconstruction procedures, which have been on the rise in recent years, capture this change. Statistics also demonstrate a growth in autologous flap procedures, as implant-only reconstructions have declined, illustrating an increased acceptance of diverse surgical treatments. Notably, during the period from 1996 to 2012, the relative decline in latissimus dorsi flap procedures, in comparison to the growth in autologous and implant procedures, illustrates the dynamic nature of patient demand and medical capability. This evolving perspective not only influences surgical practice but also reflects the integration of cosmetic surgery within overall healthcare systems, resulting in controversies over its ethical implications in the broader field of plastic surgery (Athanasiou et al., 2015).

While the developments in cosmetic surgery have numerous benefits, ethical concerns become particularly evident when addressing the teenage group. Adolescents, being immensely susceptible to social pressures as far as appearance goes, must be dealt with carefully before they are subjected to surgery. Cosmetic surgeons have the responsibility of conducting adequate psychological tests to examine the reasons that bring adolescents to surgery. Implementing such tools as the Derriford Appearance Scale (DAS-59) can prove to be highly effective in assessing the emotional and psychological condition of adolescent patients. Before surgery, there is a crucial need to go through adequate counseling sessions involving not just the adolescents but also their families, where the setting is made to facilitate any existing body image and self-esteem issues. Such practice establishes the ethical principles concerning informed consent, as well as the need to protect vulnerable subjects from potentially risky decisions (Luca et al., 2018). The moral argument of cosmetic surgery extends far beyond that of adolescent patients and extends to societal implications. The very nature of beauty is often controversial when individuals seek surgery in the hopes of achieving an ideal appearance. These activities may unwittingly perpetuate unrealistic expectations that impact self-esteem and societal values. Surgeons must be proactive in making a definitive evaluation of the reasons for a patient's request for surgery, distinguishing between requests based on objective physical flaws and those driven by social pressures or insecurity. This entails not recording requests as consumerist demands, but prioritizing the patient's well-being and ensuring that any degree of surgery truly improves their quality of life. From this ethical perspective, cosmetic surgery is not only for enhancing appearance but also for maintaining bodily and mental well-being, emphasizing the importance of a responsible approach in the practice of plastic surgery (Luca et al., 2018).

11.1.2. Reconstructive Surgery

Reconstructive surgery is a critical part of restoring both the shape and the function in patients who have undergone radical changes to their body form via trauma, disease, or birth. This branch of plastic surgery encompasses a broad range of procedures designed to restore deformity, rehabilitate body segments, and regain quality of life. Of its myriad applications, reconstructive surgery is specifically employed in the treatment of breast cancer, wherein it forms a standard procedure following mastectomy. Due to the variety of reconstructive techniques available, ranging from autologous tissue reconstruction to implant-based techniques, patients can be treated on an individual basis, tailored to their unique needs. Thus, reconstructive surgery not only considers the physical aspects of the treatment consequences of breast cancer but also has a profound psychological impact on the emotional well-being of the individual having an identity and selfhood crisis following cancer. The changing landscape of reconstructive surgery reflects the advancement in surgical treatment as well as patient-centered care. Increasing numbers of breast cancer patients are being informed of their reconstruction options, and this enables them to take an active role in their treatment plans. Recent research has underscored the significance of such consultations in affecting the decision of the patient; importantly, most individuals change their initial surgical decisions after consulting plastic surgeons. For instance, studies have shown that many patients opt for more aggressive interventions, such as opting for mastectomy instead of lumpectomy, based on the comprehensive education given on reconstructive methods and cosmetic outcomes. This change represents the evolving role of reconstructive surgery in multidisciplinary breast cancer treatment, with plastic surgeons positioned at the forefront of the oncological management model (Blair et al., 2019). In addition, changing reconstructive surgical trends are important for both patients and clinicians to be aware of. Trends over the past year indicate a significant increase in autologous free flap surgery, accompanied by a decrease in implant-based reconstructions in certain contexts. The trend reflects more educated patients and the need to choose more complex but conceivably more fulfilling operations with natural form and long-term outlook. For instance, monitoring trends in reconstructive techniques over the years confirms shifting tendencies from latissimus dorsi flap procedures towards more diverse techniques, likely meeting personal desires for body autonomy and beauty (Athanasiou et al., 2015). As reconstructive techniques improve, healthcare practitioners need to stay updated on the latest changes to offer integrated care that meets modern patient needs (Figure 11.4).

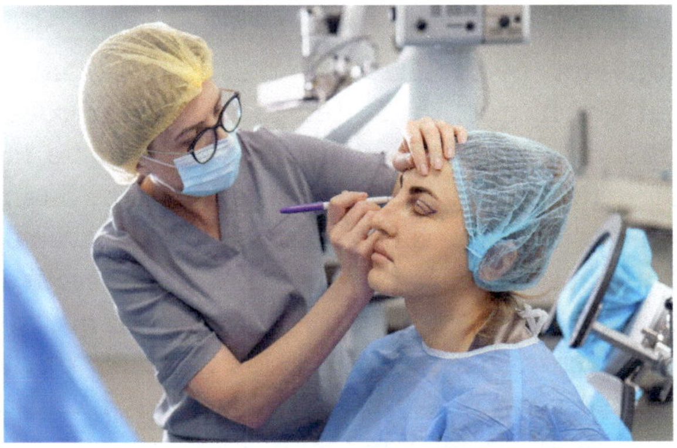

Figure 11.4. Reconstructive-surgery.

Source: https://cachevalleyent.com/storage/2023/10/Reconstructive-Surgery-by-Cache-Valley-ENT-in-Logan-UT-scaled.jpeg.

11.1.3. Non-Surgical Procedures

The area of non-surgical interventions in plastic surgery has experienced tremendous growth over the last few years, primarily due to advances in technology and technique. Such interventions offer alternatives that reduce the need for the extensive healing times typically associated with traditional surgical interventions. Non-surgical interventions such as dermal fillers, Botox, and laser therapy have been increasingly sought by individuals in pursuit of aesthetic enhancements without the risk factors associated with surgery. The appeal of these minimally invasive procedures is in their ability to produce instantaneous results with minimal downtime, allowing patients to plan treatments within their busy lifestyles. Moreover, as cultural beauty ideals continue to change, non-surgical treatments are increasingly viewed as active, autonomous choices for self-improvement, aligning with contemporary desires for individualization and instant gratification of one's appearance. Besides the aesthetic grounds, non-surgical growth may also be explained by more general socio-cultural dynamics. Higher social media usage has had an impact on how the public perceives beauty and themselves, leading to increased demand for aesthetic augmentation. Individuals are often motivated by idealized representations online that are frequently edited to reflect improved appearances, creating the aspiration to be the same. Research indicates that patients pursuing non-surgical interventions are not only driven by self-beauty but also by sociocultural imperatives in order to achieve certain beauty standards. Such factors need the greatest vigilance of the medical community as they are most likely to be behind rising trends in some operations, such as female genital cosmetic surgery, where one feels obligated to meet the pace of the moment (Malone, 2025). The range of non-surgical procedures available has also created controversy regarding the long-term impact and effectiveness of these processes. Although cosmetic outcomes are instant and aesthetic, the question of long-term outcomes has to be examined thoroughly. Most non-surgical procedures require repeat sessions to sustain their effects, which pose challenges to patient satisfaction and cost. Furthermore, emerging trends in breast reconstruction, such as the trend away from traditional implant-only methods in favor of autologous free flaps, are indicative of ongoing change under non-surgical and surgical approaches for treatment of patients (Athanasiou et al., 2015). As practice evolves, it is essential that medical professionals continue to address, through ongoing communication, the efficacy, safety, and psychosocial implications of non-surgical interventions in helping patients manage their experiences within plastic surgery.

Test Your Knowledge

1. What are the main differences between reconstructive and cosmetic plastic surgery procedures?
2. How do burn reconstruction and craniofacial surgery fit within the spectrum of plastic surgery types?

11.2. Reasons for Pursuing Plastic Surgery

Learning Outcome

1. Define the aesthetic enhancement
2. Discuss on medical necessity
3. Explain the psychological factors of plastic surgery

A complex combination often makes the decision to undergo plastic surgery of personal, social, and cultural factors. The majority of individuals seek cosmetic reconstruction to improve their own self-image and self-esteem. It appears that higher self-esteem is linked with lower levels of acceptance of cosmetic therapy, and thus, individuals who are confident with their appearance do not see the necessity for surgical alteration. On the other hand, in collectivistic societies where social acceptance is crucial, people may be more likely to seek plastic surgery to conform to societal notions of beauty. Here, it is clear that the reasons why people undergo plastic surgery are not just individual decisions, but also indicators of prevailing cultural values that influence judgments of beauty and value (Han et al., 2017). Moreover, the psychological aspects are the significant determinants of surgery demand. Patients experiencing body shame or non-acceptance of their body appearance tend to consider surgery as a solution for their problems. A qualitative study of patients' experience of plastic surgery presented themes of Shame of the hidden body and Lack of acceptance; the future-focused body. The subjects regularly expressed dissatisfaction with their bodies, blaming this on societal pressures that idealize the way one should look. The pursuit of bodily change through surgery is strongly rooted in these psychological struggles, highlighting a significant connection between an individual's sense of self and the reasons why people feel the need to alter their bodies (Smith et al., 2012).

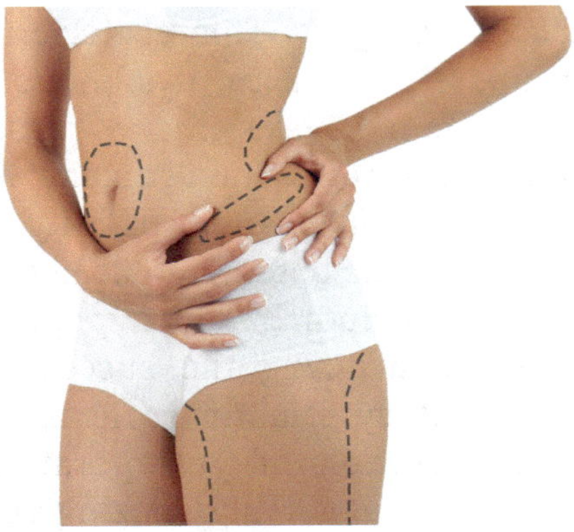

Figure 11.5. Reasons to undergo cosmetic plastic surgery.

Source: https://d3b3by4navws1f.cloudfront.net/226718791.jpg.

In addition to psychological and cultural considerations, external society influences quite significantly contribute towards deciding whether one should have plastic surgery. Portrayal of beauty and attractiveness by the media has an overwhelming effect on the ideals and perceptions held by people. People are mostly born with a malfunctioning sense of normal after they see perfect bodies, and they feel unsatisfied with their appearance afterward. Thereby, individuals will turn towards plastic surgery as a means of achieving the standards outlined in television advertisements, films, and social media. The situation is prevalent among most groups of people, illustrating the extensive nature of media influence across various demographic groups and societal segments. Finally, the urge for plastic surgery goes beyond simple aesthetic improvements; it is a complex interplay between self-image and social pressure that may drive individuals to seek out surgical methods in the hope of achieving an idealized expression of beauty (Figure 11.5).

11.2.1. Aesthetic Enhancement

The concept of beauty enhancement has gained considerable momentum in our contemporary world, particularly in the realm of plastic surgery. The phenomenon is driven most of the time by cultural narratives that cling to the ideal of beauty according to societal standards. Aesthetic enhancements can be a tool of empowerment, allowing individuals to change their body shape according to their preferences and orientations. However, such procedural choices are not without complications. As noted in discussions regarding aesthetic surgery, individuals are often bound by societal and personal expectations. The mechanics of subjective and objectified concepts of the body necessitate critical examination of the normalization of surgeries, revealing the complexities of motivation behind perceived beauty and self-worth (Alsop et al., 2017). Moreover, the desire for aesthetic improvement is particularly pronounced in societies such as South Korea, where cultural forces are particularly influential in shaping perceptions of beauty and desirability. The dialectic between modernity and body image is key to understanding the experience of aesthetic improvement. Aesthetic treatments are not merely individual choices within a cultural context, but also societal expectations that aim to achieve idealized beauty standards. This obsession can be interpreted to represent a male-dominated culture of competition and mutual understanding of femininity and beauty.

The expansion of luxury products and surgery interest demonstrates complicated dynamics of creating personal body story and social expectation (Gelézeau et al., 2015).

Lastly, aesthetic improvements represent an extension of social arguments in general about identity and self-expression. In their interaction with the potential for body modification, individuals confront the tension between personal freedom and social pressures. The desire for beauty often aligns with the concept of achieving the ideal self, which is facilitated through the modification of physical features. This tension requires a reevaluation of bodily norms that presently govern aesthetic practices. By encouraging more tolerance for various physical expressions, society can work towards a broader definition of beauty that will enhance all bodies' expressive possibilities while working to supplant the prevailing narratives that result in stigmatizing differences (Alsop et al., 2017) (Figure 11.6).

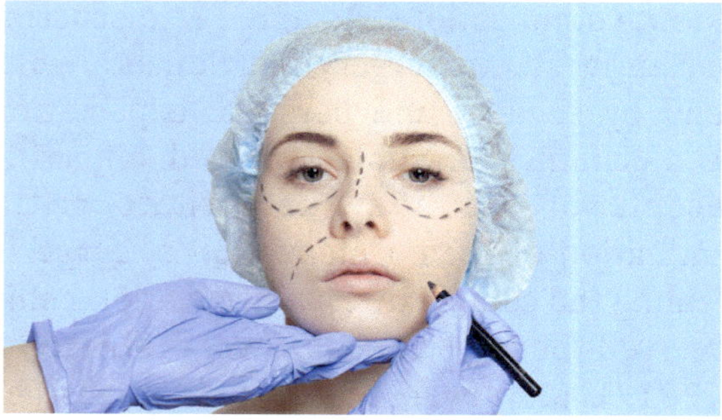

Figure 11.6. Reconstructive and aesthetic plastic surgery.

Source: https://www.polyclinique-djerba.com/uploads/0000/7/2024/08/12/chirurgie-plastique-reconstructrice-et-esthetiqu.jpg.

11.2.2. Medical Necessity

In plastic surgery, the concept of medical necessity is paramount in determining the appropriateness and justification for treatment. Medical necessity refers to treatments or interventions that are deemed essential for the diagnosis or treatment of a medical condition. Plastic surgery is not cosmetic in most cases; it is a necessary intervention to restore function and improve the quality of life in patients. For example, reconstructive operations performed after trauma, disease, or congenital defects are excellent examples of surgery due to medical need. As patients weigh their treatment options, what constitutes medical necessity can often make the difference between insurance coverage and access to proper surgery overall. Additionally, medical necessity considerations apply to complex procedures, such as microvascular reconstructive surgery. This esoteric field of research addresses critical dysfunctions that may ensue from severe injury or surgical resections. Anesthetic management of such procedures is of the highest priority, as any default may have the potential to lead to severe complications, including flap hypoperfusion, potentially jeopardizing the success of the surgery. Recent systematic reviews suggest that standardization of perioperative care pathways is crucial for maximizing recovery and minimizing the risks associated with these complex procedures. Having a well-defined understanding of medical necessity not only assists in optimizing surgical treatment but also results in better outcomes for patients and a higher quality of care (GM et al., 2018). New technologies are also an indication of how crucial medical necessity is in plastic surgery. For instance, the development of desk-based systems to generate quick prototypes of medical replicas shows how new techniques can be applied to enhance preoperative planning. These replicas help surgeons visualize anatomical complexities and enhance their appreciation for the interrelations between organs and pathologies. Practitioners can provide greater accuracy in surgery by utilizing such medical replicas, thereby maintaining the argument for medical necessity. In the end, as plastic surgery continues to advance through the incorporation of technological innovation, patient care and the efficiency of surgery will continue to support the necessity of encapsulating sharp medical necessities in practice (Bici et al., 2018).

11.2.3. Psychological Factors

Psychological determinants in an individual's choice to undergo plastic surgery are multifaceted and entrenched in one's as well as society's beliefs. The desire for physical change most often stems from an individual's perception of self and social expectations of beauty. The majority of patients report that the motivation for surgery is linked to enhanced self-esteem and self-worth, which can be largely influenced by societal narratives and social comparison. As described in the existing literature, patient satisfaction following surgery is greatly influenced by the manner of clinician-patient communication, which can also serve as an intermediary between expectations and outcomes. This highlights the importance of addressing psychological needs during the surgical experience to enhance patient satisfaction and overall experience (Fortier et al., 2019). In addition, the interplay of collectivism, self-esteem, and religion becomes a pertinent consideration in conceptualizing acceptance of cosmetic surgery. In a recent research, higher collectivism is found to be associated with greater acceptance of cosmetic surgery, implying that shared values influence people's attitudes toward cosmetic surgery. In contrast, self-esteem was found to correlate with acceptance of such procedures negatively, indicating that people who have lower self-worth are more inclined towards pursuing surgical enhancement as a way of eliminating insecurities. Notably, religiousness was also found to be negatively correlated with acceptance of cosmetic surgery, indicating moral and ethical beliefs are capable of deeply influencing one's attitude towards modifying physical appearance (Han et al., 2017). Overall, the psychology of plastic surgery emphasizes the complexity of personal identity, social pressures, and cultural impact. The motivations that drive individuals to undergo aesthetic changes are not merely due to physical dissatisfaction; rather, they are an expression of a larger set of psychological forces. It is therefore extremely critical that medical practitioners engaged in plastic surgery conduct thorough psychological assessments and provide comprehensive care. By addressing the inner psychological determinants, surgeons not only improve patient outcomes but also develop a more nuanced understanding of the implications of plastic surgery in relation to individual self-esteem and social expectations. This integrated model ensures that benefits of surgical therapy are in harmony with the psychological well-being of patients, enabling healthier definitions of beauty and self-concept.

Test Your Knowledge

1. What medical conditions commonly necessitate reconstructive plastic surgery?
2. How do psychological and aesthetic considerations influence a patient's decision to undergo cosmetic plastic surgery?

11.3. Risks and Complications

Learning Outcome

1. Define the surgical risks in plastic surgery
2. Describe the long-term health implications in plastic surgery
3. Understand the psychological impact of complications in plastic surgery

The increase in plastic surgery has been accompanied by a growing need for information regarding the risks and complications associated with the procedure. While a majority of patients go in for plastic surgery anticipating an enhancement of their physical appearance, it is essential to mention that the surgery itself has embedded risks. Infection, scarring, and complications from anesthesia are some of the common surgical risks that can result either before or after the operation. Also, patients may become unhappy with the result, leading to emotional distress, and, in some instances, necessitating further surgical correction. These complications serve to highlight the importance of extensive preoperative consultations, during which potential risks are discussed. Patients can make informed decisions about their surgical options. Beyond the physical risks, the psychological consequences of plastic surgery cannot be overlooked. Emotional and psychological well-being play a significant role in a patient's recovery and overall happiness with the outcome. Luca et al. (2018) also point out that there is a requirement for assessing the patient's psychological condition, particularly among adolescents, who are often overlooked when discussing consent and decision-making. The susceptibility of youths may lead them to pursue transformations in response to peer pressure rather than genuine self-improvement. Thus, psychological evaluation and adequate counseling sessions are required in prepping patients for the physical and psychological alterations that accompany surgery. Neglect of these factors can lead to serious outcomes, such as increased vulnerability to body dysmorphic disorders or other psychiatric diseases. Furthermore, some procedures, such as gluteoplasty, carry unique complications that prospective patients should be aware of. Despite procedures like (Blugerman et al., 2011), which provide personalized solutions to enhance body shape, such procedures also yield inherent side effects like asymmetry, overcorrection, or undercorrection of desired body features. The three-dimensional gluteoplasty (3-DGP) procedure, for example, aims to address aesthetic problems simultaneously as it reshapes nearby areas. Regardless of this, like any other surgery, it poses risks like tissue necrosis, chronic pain, or seroma formation. Patients must weigh the cosmetic benefits against these risks, with a sensible attitude and an explicit understanding of potential complications before deciding to proceed (Figure 11.7).

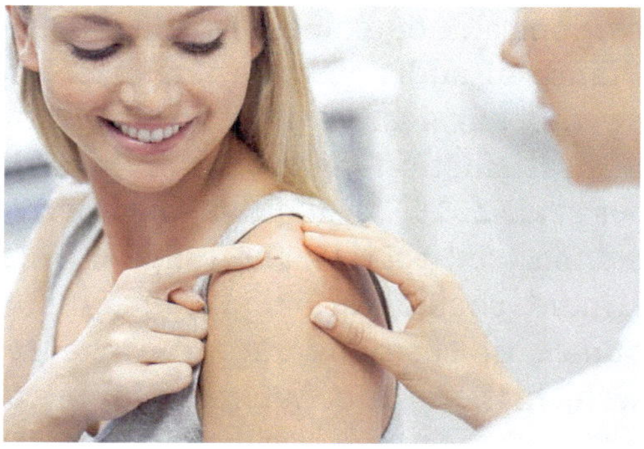

Figure 11.7. Risks-and-complications-of-plastic-surgery.

Source: https://cheshirecosmeticsurgery.com/wp-content/uploads/2024/10/Risks-and-Complications-of-Plastic-Surgery-Featured-Image.jpg.

11.3.1. Surgical Risks

Plastic surgery is typically followed by a number of considerations, and one of the most important ones that the patient must evaluate is the surgical risks. Surgical risks encompass all types of complications that may occur during or after surgery, including infections, complications related to anesthesia, and excessive bleeding. They can significantly impact patient outcomes and satisfaction with the operation process, ultimately influencing their quality of life. For example, a study found that patient-reported outcomes strongly indicate satisfaction with the surgical procedure, highlighting the importance of understanding inherent risks in forming realistic expectations about the outcomes of breast surgery. Overcoming surgery risks is not just about evaluating physical health but also includes psychological preparedness, which plays a crucial role in ensuring the informed decision-making process of the patient for plastic surgery, especially when reconstructive procedures are involved and the results can differ significantly based on personal factors. Additionally, in the case of young patients who are eager to make use of plastic surgery, the risk evaluation turns all the more ethically demanding. The emotional and mental condition of younger patients is the key to understanding why they wish to have surgery done. A concerted psychological evaluation, like the application of the Derriford Appearance Scale (DAS-59), is a good method to establish the actual reasons for having a child opt for surgery. Inadequate assessment can result in patients who are ill-equipped to understand the risks and benefits of undergoing surgery. Hence, plastic surgeons are also obligated to conduct thorough evaluations with teenagers and, if necessary, with their relatives as well, taking into account the results of surgery and the establishment of a realistic body image. Care should be taken to ensure that the procedure is undertaken for the maximum welfare and benefit of the patient based on ethical requirements that prioritize their overall well-being and health. Lastly, the implications of operating risks also extend beyond short-term medical complications into long-term psychological consequences. The majority of patients will endure distress concerning body image, coupled with societal pressure that celebrates specific beauty ideals. Such pressures create unattainable expectations for surgical outcomes, and patients become dissatisfied when there are no physical complications. These dynamics must then be addressed with a conceptual framework emanating from empirical research on patient satisfaction and quality of life post-surgery to inform clinical practice. Plastic surgery should not only focus on cosmetic purposes but also aim for psychological recovery and enhanced quality of interpersonal interaction. Surgeons must therefore balance cosmetic desires with rational evaluations of risks and gains, to ensure that operations benefit the patient's overall health and improve their lives (Cano et al., 2009; Luca et al., 2018).

11.3.2. Long-Term Health Implications

The long-term health consequences of plastic surgery go well beyond the physical changes often spotlighted in popular culture. Most patients undergo these surgeries as a tool to cope with aging and to improve their perceived self-esteem, especially among women. This motive is part of broader cultural trends that prize youthfulness, creating a story of the "de-chronologized life course." This phrase emphasizes how conventional life course paths are becoming more fluid, allowing an individual to assemble their identity through lifestyle choices at various life stages. However, plastic surgery as an anti-aging solution is ambivalently presented because guaranteed optimized aging may be at the cost of enduring sociocultural conceptions of femininity and beauty. The long-term effects then are psychological, as people find it to deal with intrapsychic and extrapsychic pressures regarding their identity and societally defined constructs of health and age, as shown in research that replicates patient narratives and medical discourse (Edmonds et al., 2014). In the field of breast cancer treatment, the results of plastic surgery take on a special hue. The evolution of reconstructive surgical techniques has allowed more favorable results for patients as well as autonomy in decision-making regarding treatment. Studies show that patient consultations with plastic surgeons significantly affect patients' management plan decisions, which can enhance quality of life and mental well-being. In particular, the patients changed their surgical procedures after consulting under these circumstances, which indicates the significant impact that cosmetic concerns have on oncological treatment. This conflict between enhancing the body's appearance and curing potentially fatal diseases highlights the importance of informed choices within the healthcare setting.

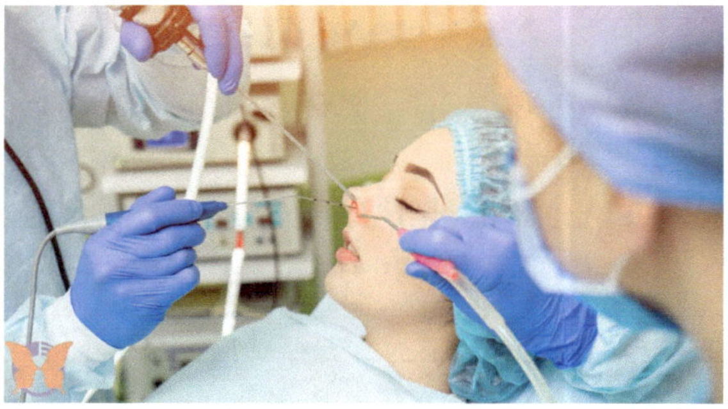

Figure 11.8. Cosmetic surgery side effects.

Source: https://dranmolchugh.com/wp-content/uploads/2025/01/Cosmetic-Surgery-Side-Effects-What-to-Expect-Preparation-Tips.png.

Thus, the long-term health outcomes in this specialty are not solely clinical but also encompass psychological coping capacity and quality of life, demonstrating that, when approached with care, plastic surgery can be a central part of comprehensive cancer care (Blair et al., 2019). The long-term health effects of plastic surgery are not always positive; however, potential complications may be realized afterward. Complications such as scarring, infection, or discontent with outcomes can lead to a vicious cycle of additional procedures or revision operations that prolong physical and psychological stress on patients. Research also suggests that the psychological effects, like anxiety or body-image depression, can last long after the first procedure. Since patients are subjected to multiple surgeries to achieve their desired look, they indirectly become self-bonded to the physical appearance, thus forming a cycle of harmful dependency on surgeries. The complexity of coping with expectations must be recognized in the context of long-term health impact, which only underscores the need for comprehensive pre-surgical counseling and ongoing psychological therapy (Edmonds et al., 2014; Blair et al., 2019) (Figure 11.8).

11.3.3. Psychological Impact of Complications

The psychological impact of complications from plastic surgery is a powerful concern that extends beyond the actual physical outcomes of treatments. Patients approach cosmetic treatments with high expectations, envisioning greater self-esteem and body satisfaction. When complications arise, however, those anticipated benefits can easily dissipate, causing patients to become frustrated, disappointed, and even depressed. There is evidence to indicate that almost 50% of breast cancer patients become psychologically disturbed due to their surgical experience, especially when confronted with complications that negatively impact their quality of life (Bălălău et al., 2018). Such distress is not uncommon to be limited to the postoperative period; it is also likely to be expressed as long-term emotional struggles, such as anxiety and low self-esteem. Hence, the psychological effects of surgical complications warrant serious investigation by the medical fraternity, who play a significant role in shaping the experiences and outcomes of patients. The Breast Implant Illness process is a stark reminder of how complications can significantly alter a patient's psychological setting. There have been reports of increased numbers of dissatisfied patients with their breast implants, reporting a symptomatology from fatigue to autoimmune responses (Ardeleanu et al., 2019). This latest tale about breast implants is also fueled by social media, where patients share their experiences, either positive or negative. The psychological distress caused by perceived complications or unmet expectations may create a vicious cycle of anxiety and despair as the patients grapple with their dissatisfaction and health concerns. Moreover, the possibility of explanation also creates another dimension of emotional complexity, which typically includes feelings of failure and regret. Therefore, the understanding of these psychological consequences is critical to providing holistic care to plastic surgery recipients. Furthermore, the relationship between psychological outcomes and surgical complications justifies preoperative psychological evaluations. As noted, such patients who have already had psychological disturbances, such as depression, typically require more intensive aftercare following surgery, with prolonged hospital admissions and more follow-up visits (Bălălău et al., 2018). These findings reveal a critical element of patient care: predicting those who are at higher risk for undesirable psychological outcomes. Attending to patients' emotional needs in advance will better equip them for potential complications and enhance therapeutic outcomes. Furthermore, surgeons must take responsibility for informing patients about realistic expectations and complications, thus fostering a supportive environment in which patients feel nurtured. By addressing the psychological as opposed to the physical dimensions of plastic surgery, the medical community can act to neutralize the adverse psychological consequences of surgical mishaps, effectively improving patient satisfaction and quality of life.

Test Your Knowledge

1. What are the common surgical and postoperative complications associated with plastic surgery?
2. How do patient factors, such as age and comorbidities, influence the risk of adverse outcomes in plastic surgery?

11.4. The Role of Technology in Plastic Surgery

Learning Outcome

1. Describe the advancements in surgical techniques
2. Discuss on usage of 3D simulation and imaging
3. Define the innovations in recovery and aftercare in plastic surgery

Its impact on plastic surgery is enormous, to the point of transforming many aspects of surgical practice, patient safety, and the final aesthetic outcomes. Advances in imaging technologies, such as 3D imaging and augmented reality, have enabled surgeons to visualize anatomical structures more clearly and in greater detail than before. Such advanced technologies enable better preoperative planning, with surgical methods optimized to address the unique needs of individual patients. For instance, 3D modeling can provide different aesthetic outcomes based on the particular variations of a patient's anatomy, enabling patients to make very informed choices about their procedures. Thus, such technologies encourage greater patient satisfaction and trust in the surgical procedure, which, in turn, improves the overall quality of care delivered in plastic surgery. Besides, the addition of robotic-assisted surgery has ushered in a new era of minimally invasive plastic surgical procedures. The precision and agility offered by robotics allow plastic surgeons to accomplish intricate maneuvers with fewer traumas to surrounding tissues, significantly reducing recovery times and postoperative discomfort for patients. These benefits illustrate the transformative impact of technology on improving surgical outcomes and minimizing complications. In addition, robotic systems offer a more comfortable working condition for surgeons, thus minimizing fatigue during lengthy procedures and maximizing concentration. As accuracy and good outcomes remain an ever-increasing demand in aesthetic medicine, the application of robot-assisted procedures will become increasingly prevalent, becoming a standard procedure in plastic surgery practice. Apart from surgical innovation, technology also plays a critical role in enhancing patient management and safety through data-driven methodology.

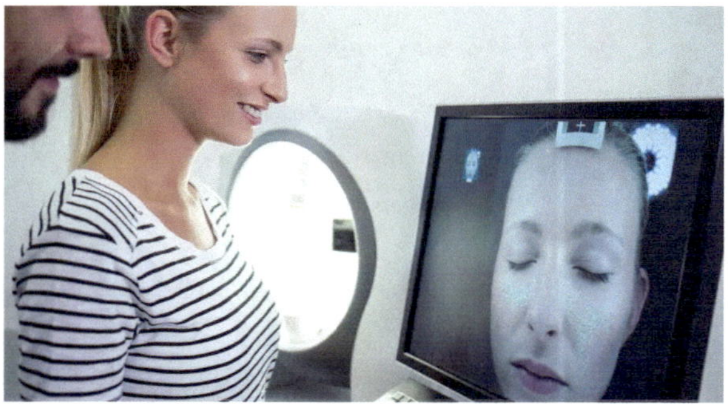

Figure 11.9. Role of technology in modern plastic-surgery.

Source: https://www.trustmedclinic.com/upload/the-role-of-technology-in-modern-plastic-surgery-800x453.webp.

The latest healthcare is more reliant on cutting-edge technologies such as Radio Frequency Identification (RFID) for tracking surgical instruments, inventory management, and workflow automation. These systems not only increase efficiency but also reduce the risk of retained surgical items and other errors in procedures considerably, with an emphasis on safety for the patient. The integration of such technology-based approaches among the plastic surgery group creates a culture of openness and accountability that drives up the level of care delivered to patients. As businesses adopt these innovations, they can utilize lean principles in conjunction with technological advancements to achieve optimal operating room productivity and enhance overall patient experiences, ultimately shaping the future of plastic surgery (Correa et al., 2005) (Figure 11.9).

11.4.1. Advancements in Surgical Techniques

Advances in surgical technology in plastic surgery have significantly altered patient outcomes, reflecting the intersection of medical science and technology. The most significant innovation is the development of minimally invasive surgery, which often utilizes endoscopic techniques. The surgical methods allow surgeons to perform complex operations through small incisions, minimizing scarring, reducing post-operative pain, and shortening recovery periods. The availability of robot-assisted surgery has also improved accuracy in lesser procedures, particularly reconstructive surgery, where precise delicacy is paramount for successful aesthetic outcomes. Not only do they enhance the cosmetic impact of surgery, but they also result in reduced rates of complications and shorter rehabilitation times for patients, demonstrating the vital role technology plays in modern surgery. Moreover, the development in anesthetic modalities has played a critical role in the evolution of plastic surgery procedures. The introduction of regional anesthesia and sedation has enabled surgeons to perform a range of procedures with enhanced patient comfort and security. Compared to the traditional general anesthesia, which is riskier, the modern anesthetic modalities offer quick recovery rates and fewer side effects. This change is particularly observed in outpatient surgeries, which are on the rise due to their ability to lower hospital stays and expenses. Thus, elective cosmetic surgeries are increasingly being opted for by patients, facilitated by an improved patient-friendly strategy that emphasizes convenience and comfort. The continuous evolution of anesthetic techniques is evidence of the continually evolving aspect of the field with focus on both safety and patient satisfaction. Paralleling anesthetic and surgical advancements, the incorporation of 3D printing technology has revolutionized preoperative planning and outcome prediction in plastic surgery. Preoperative simulation with complex designs is now possible through surgeons' ability to create customized models of patients' anatomical structures. Preparation here reduces the margin for error in actual procedures and plays a significant role in reconstructive surgery, where replication of complex facial structures is crucial. In addition, 3D printing offers opportunities for the production of bespoke implants and prosthetics that meet individual patient needs, resulting in even superior aesthetic and functional outcomes. Through these technological integration developments, plastic surgeons can achieve unprecedented precision in their work, ultimately redefining patient care standards in an ever-evolving medical landscape (N/A, 1985).

11.4.2. Usage of 3D Simulation and Imaging

The marriage of 3D imaging and simulation technology is a breakthrough in the field of plastic surgery, transforming preoperative planning and enhancing surgical outcomes. The new technology enables surgeons to create precise three-dimensional models of the patient's anatomy, thereby offering more accurate visualization of the surgical site. The models are employed by surgeons to simulate various methods of surgery and predict potential complications or aesthetic outcome before the procedure is undertaken. The ability to visualize projected results fosters enhanced communication between the surgeon and patient, setting realistic expectations and facilitating informed decision-making. The significance of 3D imaging thus entered the fundamentals of modern practice, bridging the gap between theory and practice in the dynamic field of plastic surgery. One of the applications of 3D imaging in plastic surgery is the reconstructive process, particularly among patients with congenital anomalies or trauma. Three-dimensional models based on imaging data may be utilized by surgeons to plan complex reconstructions accurately. In congenital heart disease, for instance, the applicability of 3D printing has been demonstrated in the reconstruction of anatomical structures, thereby improving the precision of surgery. These developments not only make more complex procedures viable but also reduce operating time, which can lower the risk of long-term complications. As indicated in recent studies, technological advances in 3D visualizations continue to expand the possibilities of surgical interventions that were previously deemed extremely complex or high-risk, ultimately resulting in improved patient survival rates and quality of life (Anwar et al., 2018). Also, the advent of 3D printing technologies brought a revolution in residency training in plastic surgery and medical education for prospective plastic surgeons. Ethical controversies surrounding the application of new technologies, such as 3D imaging and simulation, underscore both their impact and the effect on residency training and patient participation. Physical models developed from 3D imaging are invaluable educational tools, refining the educational process of residents by providing the opportunity to rehearse surgical techniques on accurate anatomical replicas. Furthermore, the careful utilization of such technologies creates fertile ground for healthy discussions among multidisciplinary groups, making patients more aware of available care options. With the evolving landscape of education, embracing such technologies ensures that future plastic surgeons are well equipped to leverage existing methods in their own practices (Białas et al., 2018) (Figure 11.10).

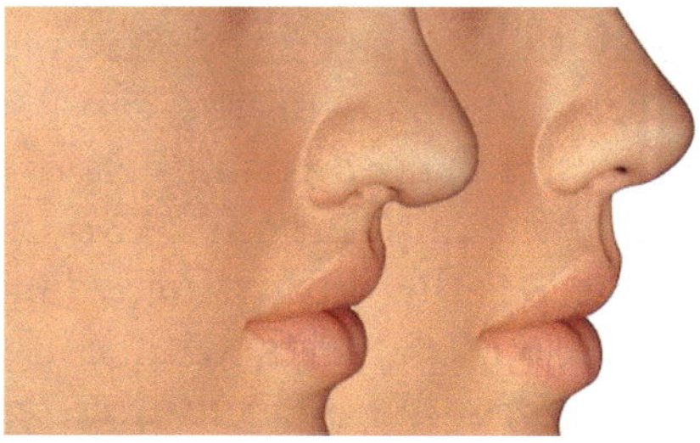

Figure 11.10. The role of 3D simulation in plastic surgery.

Source: https://media.licdn.com/dms/image/v2/D4E12AQHuvNSnJ-GboA/article-cover_image-shrink_600_2000/B4EZbnE_VLHAAU-/0/1747633567409?e=2147483647&v=beta&t=Gf6snaEZL-7qn_tzZQC8pOMsspLFFYxnNufGxQgLiTY.

11.4.3. Innovations in Recovery and Aftercare

The plastic surgery landscape has, to a significant degree, been transformed by recovery and aftercare technologies, which address evolving patient needs of patients undergoing surgery. The application of technology in post-surgical care has enabled enhanced monitoring practices, allowing surgeons to remotely track patients' recovery. Real-time data streamline interventions, reducing the possibility of complications and enabling better rates of patient satisfaction. Moreover, mobile application deployment enables patients to access their recovery plans and learning resources, allowing them to engage in their own recovery actively. In addition to this, these advancements not only improve outcomes but also facilitate patient-centered care philosophy, which emphasizes the individual needs and preferences of patients along their recovery process (Groen et al., 2025). Additionally, new aftercare models are also essential components of the plastic surgery process. Multidisciplinary teams of surgeons, nurses, physical therapists, and mental health professionals form the new normal in aftercare. The interdisciplinary team ensures that a patient's overall recovery—physical, psychological, and emotional—is comprehensively provided. For instance, psychological counseling can manage the emotional aspects of altered body image post-surgery. Evidence shows that this combined strategy yields lower rates of dissatisfaction and higher well-being in patients, hence the overall effectiveness of the procedure. Thus, the evolution of aftercare models indicates a fundamental shift toward integral care in plastic surgery (Galle et al., 2019). In addition, artificial intelligence (AI) and machine learning integration into recovery protocols is an innovation in aftercare practices. AI and machine learning enable personalized recovery plans tailored to the unique needs of each patient, taking into account variables such as medical history, procedure complexity, and individual recovery rates. Machine learning algorithms can search through vast quantities of data to predict potential complications and recommend preventive measures, thereby lowering post-operative complications. These advances represent a revolutionary shift towards evidence-based decision-making in plastic surgery recovery procedures, raising not only the bar for safety but also promoting more efficient use of health facility resources. In summary, these innovations in recovery and aftercare represent a commitment to improving patient experiences and outcomes in plastic surgery practice (Groen et al., 2025).

Test Your Knowledge

1. How have innovations such as 3D imaging and surgical planning improved precision in plastic surgery?
2. What role do minimally invasive techniques and laser technologies play in enhancing patient outcomes and recovery?

11.5. Ethical Issues

Learning Outcome

1. Describe the informed consent of plastic surgery
2. Discuss on social pressures and body image
3. Define the regulation and standards in the industry

The plastic surgery setting is increasingly characterized by ethical issues that reflect the larger cultural attitudes toward beauty and health. A primary problem stems from the marketing practices employed by doctors, and particularly dermatologists, who have a tendency to sell cosmetic surgery along with necessary medical interventions. This dyad can result in a culture where patients are covertly pushed to improve aesthetic value at the cost of their health, infusing a culture that identifies worth with beauty. The ethical implications of this trend are profound, as it promotes unattainable ideals of beauty, thereby placing undue pressure on individuals. By advertising cosmetic products and services, such practitioners not only perpetuate a disfiguring cultural obsession with perfection but also risk infringing on basic bioethical principles, such as autonomy and beneficence, by prioritizing profit over patient interest (Lowe et al., 2017). Another field open to ethical analysis in plastic surgery is the practice of medical tourism, where patients travel to other countries to undergo cosmetic procedures often in pursuit of lower prices or more options. While this practice may appear to be beneficial at first glance, it raises numerous ethical concerns. Patients jeopardize their safety and care after the operation by getting procedures in countries with less stringent medical regulations. In addition, the absence of follow-up visits and the risk of side effects expand the moral obligation of providers, who can inadvertently fuel this trend through their own promotions. General practitioners will also play a key role in this process, as they will need to provide appropriate advice on the risks of treatment overseas and ensure that patients are aware and well cared for upon return (Leggat, 2015). Ultimately, then, ethical issues related to plastic surgery include not only problems of regulation and control but also questions of inequality and accessibility. Most of the discourse regarding beauty treatments is focused on affluent populations that possess the economic means to undergo elective therapies. This a tendency to relegate concerns about the psychological and social pressures faced by various socio-economically positioned individuals regarding beauty norms. The hegemonized focus on cosmetic treatments tends to subtly expand inequalities because people without access to similar means can feel marginalized or devalued. Therefore, an ethical position in responding to plastic surgery must be one of critical examination of such injustices and the demand for greater access to quality treatment, so that everyone can make informed choices and not be victimized by social definitions of beauty and self (Figure 11.11).

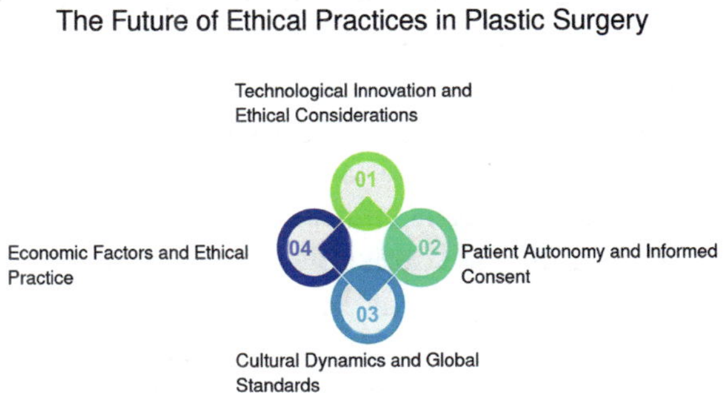

Figure 11.11. Plastic surgery ethics.

Source: https://fastercapital.co/i/Plastic-Surgery-Ethics--Beyond-Aesthetics--The-Business-Side-of-Ethical-Plastic-Surgery--The-Future-of-Ethical-Practices-in-Plastic-Surgery.webp.

11.5.1. Informed Consent

Informed consent is a cornerstone of good ethical medical practice, especially in plastic surgery, where the distinctions between reconstructive and cosmetic surgery are often blurred. Patients have the right to be fully informed of all the risks, benefits, alternatives, and potential outcomes of any surgical procedure. This requirement is also heightened in cases where psychological aspects are involved, such as in cosmetic surgery intended to alter a person's appearance for social approval or self-esteem reasons. The complexity of such motivations may complicate the informed consent process, and therefore a serious consideration of the patient's psychological state and aims is warranted. Thus, professionals must utilize careful assessment tools and have the patient acknowledge the consequences of decisions they are about to make to gain a sense of autonomy without regret or future negative consequences. The process of informed consent also involves more than merely signing on the line; it stems from obtaining an understanding that the patient truly knows what is being provided. Particularly in the adolescent patient cases, as in the case of cosmetic surgery, the ethical duty of considering the psychological and emotional state of such minors takes precedence. Teenagers are more susceptible to societal pressures regarding beauty, which can lead to rash decisions about undergoing surgery. The ethical concerns mandate surgeons to be certain of multiple counseling sessions, not only with the young patient but also with his/her family members. The inclusive process serves to explain the motivation behind requesting the surgery, thereby ensuring the patient's best interest and ensuring that their decision-making capacity is evaluated accordingly.

Secondly, plastic surgeons must tread carefully to fulfill patient expectations while maintaining ethical standards. The temptation of complying with procedures employed to achieve culturally accepted ideals of beauty can place practitioners in compromising positions. These treatments not only reinforce destructive concepts about beauty but also divert attention from treating the specific needs of patients. It is necessary to study the physical and psychological impact of surgical modification so that whatever interventions are being performed are done with warranted intent. Since the moral argument regarding such procedures has been explained, informed consent can be provided solely on the occurrence of a clear-cut, objective physical deficiency or deformity that adversely affects an individual's social life. Hence, the ethical issue is not patient satisfaction, but rather a responsibility to improve health and well-being in accordance with Lowe et al. (2017) and Luca et al. (2018).

11.5.2. Social Pressures and Body Image

The body image concept is well rooted in cultural and social pressures, the result of which, most of the time, prompts people to go to great extremes, including plastic surgery. Beauty trends in the contemporary world are usually dictated by the media, where pictures are doctored to arrive at unattainable expectations. This pervasive influence fosters a culture that associates self-esteem with physical appearance. The chasing of these hyper-idealized bodily ideals can make people feel deficient, prompting them to seek out surgery as a means of rectifying their discontent with their bodies. Such a dynamic is most apparent in situations where there are intense cultural norms about beauty, which beefs up the desire for enhancement and makes body modification a must for social acceptability. The outcomes of these social pressures set the stage for the complex dynamic between plastic surgery's popularity, body image, and mental health. Within some cultural environments, for instance, in South Korea, the historical and social environment adds to the complexity of the dynamic between plastic surgery and body image. With the emergence of advanced technological capabilities and an economic landscape shaped by crises such as the 1997 Asian Financial Crisis, social pressures have intensified, leading to radical transformations in individual identity and self-concept. The emphasis on high-quality appearance has triggered new demand for cosmetic surgery, particularly among teenagers and young adults. As individuals navigate the expectations of their societies, the pressure to conform to ideal body images is overwhelming.

This is not merely a personal but also a deeply interrelated general societal issue, like extreme levels of mental distress and suicide among adolescents in South Korea, illustrating the overarching necessity to resolve underlying cultural forces influencing body image (Porter et al., 2016). Similarly, in Utah, a clash of traditional values and growing numbers of cosmetic alterations is evidence of the body's ambivalence and social expectation. Even though it is famous for being a religious and conservative state, the state has been infamous for its high plastic surgery per capita rates. It has been accorded names like the "Vainest City in America." Interestingly, two-thirds of Mormon women from Utah claim they know somebody who has had aesthetic treatments, indicating a cultural contradiction. This contradictory trend highlights the means by which cultural influencers coexist alongside firmly rooted cultural axioms, instituting a norm into practice for elective surgery that is normalized and even advertised. Plastic surgery billboards along the state's highways alter perspectives regarding beauty and body modification. These trends bear the intricate dynamic of personal agency and social pressure, and they underscore the need for more understanding of cultural contexts impacting body image and plastic surgery decisions (Dillon et al., 2017) (Figure 11.12).

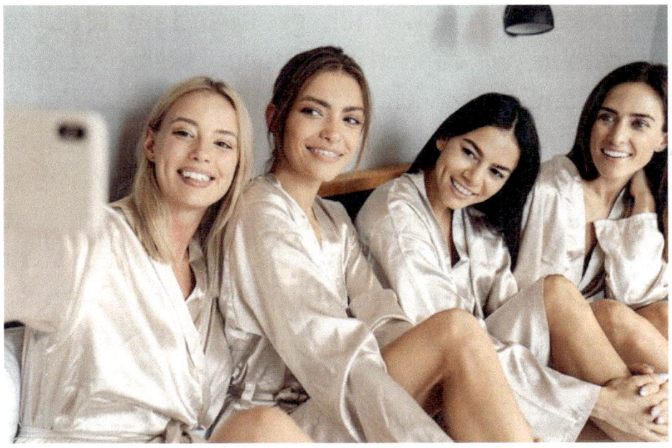

Figure 11.12. Body image for plastic surgery.

Source: https://www.plasticsurgery.org/images/blog/plastic-surgery-body-positivity.jpg?width=700&format=jpg.

11.5.3. Regulation and Standards in the Industry

The plastic surgery environment is highly regulated and standards-based, with both of these conditions being necessary to ensure patients remain safe and the practice maintains its integrity. Regulatory bodies develop procedures plastic surgeons must adhere to, ranging from surgical techniques employed to patient care procedures. The evolving nature of surgical technology and technique generates ongoing controversy regarding the sufficiency of existing regulation. For instance, new procedures can offer greater efficacy but also ethical challenges and dangers that have to be addressed by regulatory devices. Doctor autonomy, while fundamental for innovation, sometimes leads to practices that may not be entirely consistent with set norms and, therefore, present potential risks to patients. This conflict between regulatory oversight and innovative practice is central to the legitimacy of the plastic surgery profession, as argued in recent critiques of new techniques within the discipline (Clinch et al., 2011). The interplay between professional societies and regulatory authorities also raises the complexities of maintaining standards in plastic surgery. Such groups then tend to operate in two capacities: offering best practices advice and then withdrawing to allow individual physicians the space to adopt new practices. This means that there can exist very divergent surgical standards and practices across different regions, making it more difficult to develop a one-size-fits-all regulatory framework. Cosmetic procedures, such as female cosmetic genital surgery (FCGS), further illustrate the challenge of differentiating between acceptable practices in the field. Discussion of such procedures will naturally centre upon ethical concerns and patient outcomes, which require scrutiny of proper industry practice. Ultimately, collaboration among stakeholders—doctors, regulators, and professional organizations—will be necessary to establish a framework that drives innovation while maintaining patient safety in plastic surgery (Reynolds et al., 2007).

Moreover, compliance with stringent regulatory requirements can be viewed as a double-edged sword for the profession of cosmetic surgery. While regulation plays a critical role in maintaining patient safety and quality, very prescriptive rules may stifle innovation and ultimately limit access to beneficial treatments. The development of new materials and techniques, for example, is often bogged down by bureaucratic obstacles that can delay the advancement of patient care. There must be a balance between calls for regulations and calls for surgical innovation to ensure patients achieve the best possible outcomes. Additionally, the establishment of national registries for surgical outcomes can significantly enhance accountability, evidenced by initiatives in other fields of medicine. Based on a review of effective models of regulatory action, the plastic surgery profession can strive to adopt standards that effectively protect patients and foster a culture of continuous improvement and ethical practice (Clinch et al., 2011).

Test Your Knowledge

1. What ethical challenges arise when balancing patient autonomy with realistic surgical outcomes in plastic surgery?
2. How do issues like informed consent and elective cosmetic procedures impact ethical decision-making in plastic surgery?

11.6. Cultural Perspectives on Plastic Surgery

Learning Outcome

1. Define the variations in acceptance across cultures
2. Discuss on influence of media and celebrity culture
3. Describe the trends in plastic surgery

Cultural perceptions of plastic surgery have long-standing effects on people's decisions to undergo procedures, shaping the cultural definition of beauty globally. Collectivism, self-esteem, and religion intersect to form unique attitudes towards cosmetic enhancements. For instance, findings indicate that collectivist culture participants tend to report a greater degree of plastic surgery acceptability based on an inclination to conform to social standards and ideals. But self-esteem and religious values may complicate this acceptance.

Increased religiousness is implied through the findings to have negative attitudes toward cosmetic surgery, suggesting cultural contexts significantly influence individual acceptance. These processes mean that an individual's culture and surroundings need to be considered when examining motivations for plastic surgery, which points to the intricacies of identity and social expectations embedded in this field (Han et al., 2017).

Furthermore, the universalization of beauty concepts has brought about the pervasive effect of Western ideas, which tend to dominate indigenous perceptions and practices of plastic surgery. In Vietnam, for example, global integration of the economy since 1986 modified indigenous beauty norms to facilitate an in-mixing of Western norms and traditional values. This reflects how economic reform has facilitated the mainstreaming of global beauty practices, prompting many to seek cosmetic treatments to fit new standards. The evolving Vietnamese beauty culture serves as a case study that encapsulates the general impact of global dynamics on local practices. In light of this, it can be concluded that cultural attitudes towards plastic surgery are fluid, continually changing in response to shifting economic, political, and social realities, which in turn influence the concept of beauty and its pursuit across cultures (Nguyen et al., 2020). As cultural perceptions of plastic surgery continue to evolve, its implications extend beyond individual choice and reflect broader societal values and expectations. Critical examination shows plastic surgery to be consistently invested with empowerment and self-actualization while simultaneously raising ethical concerns regarding authenticity and self-worth. In most cultures, the quest for cosmetic surgery can stem from internalization of idealized images fueled by media and advertisement, leading to a complex relationship between social acceptance and self-image. Second, the commodification of beauty has implications for the commercialization of identity and the ethics of conformity to externalized norms. By gaining insight into the cultural discourses of plastic surgery, an individual can better understand the motivations of the choices made by others while questioning the ethical ramifications that come with seeking beauty in our globally connected world (Figure 11.13).

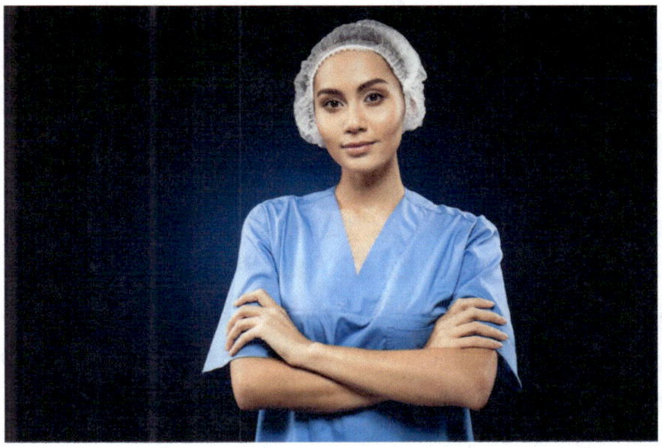

Figure 11.13. Beauty & cultural perceptions of plastic surgery.

Source: https://transform.goalsplasticsurgery.com/wp-content/uploads/2023/12/serious-confident-doctor-looking-holding-hands-folded.webp.

11.6.1. Variations in Acceptance Across Cultures

The acceptance of plastic surgery is strongly influenced by culture, which is shaped by deeply rooted sociocultural values and norms. Cosmetic surgery in Western cultures is generally viewed from a self-enhancement frame of reference, strongly supporting ideals of beauty and personal preference. Media presentations and celebrity promotions contribute to this image, fostering the desire for physical enhancement. Conversely, though, in most Asian cultures, plastic surgery is not necessarily considered a change process but instead as a social necessity to meet the standards of attractiveness in society. Sociocultural perspectives mandate not just individual choice but broader societal acceptance of surgery, and once again, this demonstrates how beauty ideals can drive individuals down the surgical path for social acceptance and self-actualization. Various attitudes towards plastic surgery usually are exhibited through the levels of accessibility and stigma associated with the procedures. In North America, for instance, the growing popularity of cosmetic surgeries facilitates their easier normalization, and social narratives about them persuade individuals to take action to improve their appearance. However, in other societies, plastic surgery remains greatly stigmatized as a rejection of one's original appearance. It is based on notions of authenticity, where people should embrace their natural appearances, thereby creating an imbalance between cultural expectations and individual desires. These cultural beliefs influence not only individuals seeking surgery but also shape the international context of the aesthetic surgery industry, shifting marketing techniques and practitioner strategies. Globalization and increased travel have also facilitated the global exchange of beauty standards, resulting in ever-rising levels of acceptability. Above all, trends in plastic surgery have extended past the traditional borders, as economically diverse countries' citizens increasingly seek procedures generally referred to as part of Western standards. This is a fascinating issue involving cultural appropriation and globalized beauty standards, with individuals weighing the connotations of adopting practices rooted in other cultural contexts. Although certain cultures have adopted these changes by reconciling conflicting beauty ideals, others resist them and instead emphasize the ongoing struggle between tradition and modernity. A thorough understanding of these differences is essential for plastic surgery practitioners and policymakers as they develop culture-sensitive care models that account for and respect the varying views on aesthetic enhancement in society.

11.6.2. Influence of Media and Celebrity Culture

The modern preoccupation with plastic surgery is inextricably tied to media representation and the ubiquitous power of celebrity culture. Celebrities are inspirational icons, setting standards of beauty that are often beyond the reach of the average citizen. The secularization of cosmetic interventions, facilitated by numerous media sources, helps construct surgical augmentation as a norm. As audiences consume images and accounts of celebrities voluntarily disclosing their surgeries, such as on television talk shows and social media platforms, they may perceive these alterations as accessible and worthwhile. This can be viewed as a type of atonement ritual, in which celebrities seek to reclaim their narratives, thereby fostering a culture in which beauty is equated with success. Through this process, cosmetic surgery becomes increasingly trivialized, as identified in research verifying heightened support for the procedures among celebrity culture-oriented audiences, particularly young women (Chae et al., 2012).

Also, the media's homogenization of beauty ideals significantly shapes individual self-perceptions and shared expectations regarding femininity. The image of plastic surgery presented by celebrities is not merely cosmetic but symbolic in kind as a gatekeeper to social acceptance and approval. These images show a frame through which people, especially women, are encouraged to pursue bodily modifications as a means of expression and, at the same time, as a means of gaining social mobility. The rhetoric of enlarging femininity via body work echoes persistently in media accounts, presenting a cultural burden on women to achieve their authentic selves through surgery. The dependence on body modification is a method by which media accounts reinforce the extent to which media representations shape understandings of beauty and self, thereby maintaining an unhealthy equation between self-worth and corporeality (Anon et al., 2017). Furthermore, the incessant reaffirmation of such values and norms by celebrity culture has significant repercussions for psychological health and self-esteem, especially for vulnerable populations. Representing cosmetic surgery as a life-altering wonder cure can generate unrealistic expectations, stimulating belief in surgical reform as equaling fulfillment. This media-bred paradigm also often neglects the psychological subtleties that accompany self-image and the potential consequences of pursuing surgery to alter one's body as a solution to more entrenched emotional issues. When media narratives increasingly celebrate and espouse bodily alteration, they become key determinants of notions of normalcy and beauty. Thus, the effect of celebrity and media culture extends far beyond shallow taste for appearance, and inevitably transforms the way people navigate their own identities and the cultural framework that determines beauty standards in contemporary society (Chae et al., 2012) (Figure 11.14).

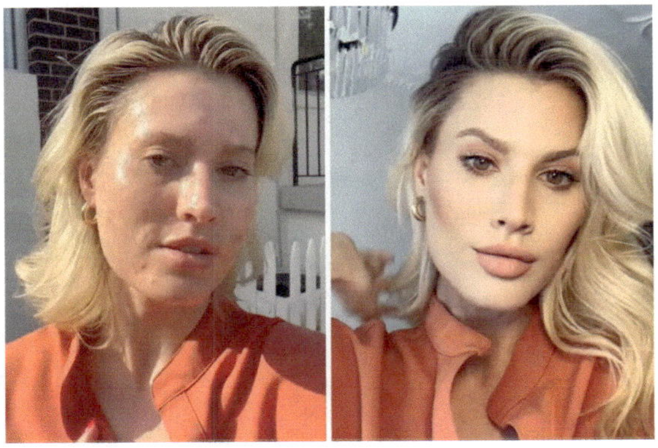

Figure 11.14. Media and celebrity culture of plastic surgery.

Source: https://newlifecosmetic.com/wp-content/uploads/2025/05/8-woman-before-and-after-using-filter-1024x683.webp.

11.6.3. Trends in Plastic Surgery Around the World

With changes in the aesthetic landscape of beauty and self-presentation, plastic surgery trends have immediate social and cultural consequences internationally. In particular, the rise of social media has accelerated the time in which some aesthetic ideals become popular, perpetuating some body shapes and facial features that are consistent with contemporary beauty standards. This phenomenon has led to an increase in procedures aimed at achieving what is now popularly known as the "Instagram body," characterized by a narrow waist, curvy hips, and enhanced facial features. The global dissemination of these beauty ideals highlights the manner in which modern societies are integrated, with individuals becoming increasingly concerned with finding a place within expectations that are transnational in character. The stress that is placed upon such ideals affects self-esteem and identity considerably in the vast majority of cases, prompting individuals to pursue surgical interventions in a quest for the unattainable perfection that is presented on the web (Ginwala et al., 2014).

Furthermore, one should not forget the role of cultural heritage in the perception and practice of plastic surgery. In many areas, people tend to deal with the confluence of ethnic identity and social conception of beauty through surgery. For example, the experiences of women from diverse backgrounds illustrate how outward beauty concepts are intertwined with personal stories and cultural histories. These nuances emphasize that whereas some individuals use plastic surgery as a vehicle of empowerment and self-expression, others may be compelled by social forces to conform to some notion of beauty that verifies stereotypes and shuts out others. This dynamic highlights the complex motivations behind desiring surgical enhancements, showing that plastic surgery trends are not merely surface-level but deeply rooted in individual and group identity (Ginwala et al., 2014). Furthermore, the economic implications of these global trends are substantial. Plastic surgery is now a lucrative industry, driven by widespread consumer interest in procedures aimed at enhancing an individual's appearance. Countries with a reputation for cutting-edge medical centers, such as South Korea and Brazil, are now prime destinations for surgical tourism, offering affordable yet excellent services. This trend not only reflects the desire for bodily change but also the cultural investment in beauty as capital. As funding for cosmetic procedures increases, issues of access to healthcare, ethical marketing of these procedures, and potential long-term psychological impact on individuals struggling with their identity come to the fore. Lastly, trends in plastic surgery globally are a continuous, multidisciplinary discourse on beauty, identity, and the implications of seeking conformity with societal expectations (Uti et al., 2022).

Test Your Knowledge

1. How do cultural attitudes and societal norms influence the demand for cosmetic and reconstructive plastic surgery?
2. In what ways can cultural beliefs affect patient expectations and satisfaction with plastic surgery outcomes?

SUMMARY

Plastic surgery is both aesthetic and reconstructive in nature, evolving into a highly advanced branch of medicine with a profound impact on patients' lives. According to various studies, the life-altering impact of surgical intervention extends beyond the physiological; psychological and social impacts are also observed. For instance, patients undergoing body contouring following weight loss report enhanced satisfaction with body image and overall mental well-being. The outcomes of experiences from participants who have undergone qualitative research demonstrate a rediscovery of self and an enhancement of quality of life following primary surgical intervention. These benefits, however, must be balanced with the necessity for regular research to verify such claims and ensure care is equally available across heterogeneous groups, as argued by proponents of the study and reinforced in recent literature (Gilmartin et al., 2012). Moreover, reasons to seek cosmetic procedures such as dermal fillers are also likely to be multifaceted in nature, influenced by societal expectations, peer perception, and media profile. Recognizing that this motivation is more than just superficial, psychological motivations often require pre- and post-procedure counseling. By engaging patients more comprehensively, practitioners can establish an environment that facilitates informed decision-making and reduces the potential for dissatisfaction after the procedure. As has been revealed through research aimed at the reasons behind dermal fillers, people cited desiring extensive counseling to gain more knowledge and be able to manage expectations better (Hirschfeld et al., 2022). These findings demonstrate that enhancing the patient experience with plastic surgery cannot occur by chance; it must be an integral part of the process. The future of plastic surgery clearly hinges on integrating research-based practices, namely improving safety and quality of life outcomes. Interdisciplinary collaboration among investigators, healthcare practitioners, and policymakers can lead to evidence-based recommendations that are more responsive to patient needs. As noted in the reconstructive intervention studies, it is critical to investigate further how demographic factors such as gender, ethnicity, and socio-economic status affect patients' perceptions and outcomes in plastic surgery (Gilmartin et al., 2012). Emphasis on an interdisciplinary research paradigm can introduce tremendous enhancements to the understanding of the fragile interplay between plastic surgeries and their psychosocial ramifications, permitting a stronger patient care model in the ever-evolving world of plastic surgery.

Over the past decade, techniques used in plastic surgery have undergone significant improvements in patient outcomes and procedure efficacy. Tissue liquefaction liposuction (TLL) is one such advancement that uses the application of a warm, low-pressure saline flow to excise the fat tissue. A comparative study highlights that TLL not only enables surgeons to perform fat excision at a faster rate—42% faster than traditional suction-assisted liposuction (SAL)—but also reduces the level of movement involved, thereby improving accuracy in procedures. Implications for patients' recovery are that smaller levels of bruising and swelling were documented following TLL compared to SAL. These findings highlight the impact of technological advancements on plastic surgery practices, with immediate effects on patient satisfaction and experience. Beyond technological advances in the methods of plastic surgery, the increased phenomenon of medical tourism has emerged as a focal point within discussions of plastic surgery. Increasingly, patients are traveling abroad, particularly to Southeast Asia, for procedures such as cosmetic surgery and dental work, due to the availability of services not accessible locally and lower costs. The trend is of great concern due to a lack of certainty in the quality of care provided, risk of side effects, and complications resulting from follow-up and aftercare. The implications for health professionals are profound, necessitating that general practitioners possess the capacity to inform patients regarding risks of receiving treatment abroad. The context serves to underscore the duality of plastic surgery as both a medical profession and a globalizing enterprise, with a depth of oversight required to ensure patient well-being and outcomes. In summarizing key points in the practice of plastic surgery, the intersection of patient decision and technological capability is all that matters. With advancements such as TLL improving procedural outcomes and the lure of medical tourism luring patients into complex decision-making, the practice itself is evolving at a rapid pace. Of equal importance, it is also imperative to respect the socio-economic determinants of such choices for both practitioners and patients. With the constantly evolving field of plastic surgery, there is always a need for research and training to ensure that medical practitioners are equipped to effectively counsel patients on their options, thereby providing an environment that caters to both aesthetic demands and patient safety. Such issues collectively contribute to the revolutionary nature and challenges inherent in the multidisciplinary field of plastic surgery.

KEY TERMS FROM THIS CHAPTER

- Abdominoplasty (Tummy tuck)
- Aesthetic contouring
- Blepharoplasty
- Breast augmentation
- Burn management
- Cleft lip and palate repair
- Cosmetic surgery
- Facelift (Rhytidectomy)
- Flap surgery
- Hand surgery
- Keloid management
- Liposuction
- Maxillofacial reconstruction
- Microsurgery
- Reconstructive surgery
- Replantation

CRITICAL THINKING QUESTIONS

1. **Which of the following best describes a full-thickness skin graft?**
   a. Includes epidermis only
   b. Includes epidermis and part of the dermis
   c. Includes epidermis and entire dermis
   d. Includes skin, muscle, and bone
2. **What is the correct order of the reconstructive ladder in increasing complexity?**
   a. Flap > Skin graft > Primary closure > Secondary intention
   b. Secondary intention > Primary closure > Skin graft > Flap
   c. Skin graft > Flap > Secondary intention > Primary closure
   d. Primary closure > Flap > Skin graft > Secondary intention
3. **Which of the following is a common early complication of split-thickness skin grafting?**
   a. Graft contracture
   b. Graft necrosis due to poor vascularization
   c. Malignancy in the grafted skin
   d. Hypertrophic scarring at the donor site
4. **What is the most important factor in successful flap survival?**
   a. Antibiotic coverage
   b. Length of the flap
   c. Vascular supply to the flap
   d. Patient's age
5. **In cleft lip repair, the ideal age for primary surgical correction is typically:**
   a. At birth
   b. 1–2 months
   c. 3–6 months
   d. After 2 years of age

Short Answer Questions

1. What are the basic principles of wound healing relevant to plastic surgery?
2. Define the reconstructive ladder and its significance in plastic surgery planning.
3. What is the difference between a skin graft and a skin flap?
4. Name two common complications associated with skin grafting.
5. What is the role of negative pressure wound therapy (VAC) in plastic surgery?
6. Which classification system is commonly used to assess burn depth and extent?
7. What are the indications for microsurgical free tissue transfer?
8. How is a cleft lip and palate typically managed surgically over time?
9. What are the key aesthetic subunits of the face considered in facial reconstruction?
10. Describe the importance of tension-free closure in plastic surgical wound repair.

Answers to Critical Thinking Questions

1. (c); 2. (b); 3. (b); 4. (c); 5. (c)

REFERENCES

1. Adriaens, F., & Van Bauwel, S. (2011). Sex and the City: A Postfeminist Point of View? Or How Popular Culture Functions as a Channel for Feminist Discourse. *The Journal of Popular Culture, 47*(1), 174–195. https://doi.org/10.1111/j.1540-5931.2011.00869.xAguado Correa, F., Barcos, L., & Álvarez Gil, M. J. (2005). *Benefits of connecting RFID and lean principles in health care.* https://core.ac.uk/download/29427288.pdf (accessed on 12th July 2025).
2. Alsop, R., & Lennon, K. (2017). *Aesthetic surgery and the expressive body.* https://core.ac.uk/download/151161362.pdf (accessed on 12th July 2025).
3. Andrew, M. S., Bharti, G., Crantford, J. C., Daniels, K. M., et al. (2018). *A multicenter, prospective, randomized, contralateral study of tissue liquefaction liposuction vs suction-assisted liposuction.* https://core.ac.uk/download/299809007.pdf (accessed on 12th July 2025).
4. Anon, N., Anon, N., Bissinger, B., Bornstein, K., Butler, J., Cave, L., Cave, L., et al. (2017). *Call me Caitlyn: Making and making over the 'authentic' transgender body in Anglo-American popular culture.* https://core.ac.uk/download/41993108.pdf (accessed on 12th July 2025).
5. Anwar, A., Barach, B., Bhatla, N., Biglino, J., Biglino, J., et al. (2018). *3D printing is a transformative technology in congenital heart disease.* https://core.ac.uk/download/212858839.pdf (accessed on 12th July 2025).
6. Ardeleanu, V., Danciu, R., Marin, R., Marina, D., et al. (2019). *Breast implant illness: A step forward in understanding this complex entity and the impact of social media.* https://core.ac.uk/download/232440357.pdf (accessed on 12th July 2025).
7. Athanasiou, T., Aylin, P., Bottle, A., Darzi, A., et al. (2015). *Trends in immediate postmastectomy breast reconstruction in the United Kingdom.* https://core.ac.uk/download/77002746.pdf (accessed on 12th July 2025).
8. Bălălău, D., Cozma, C. N., Jecan, C. R., Popa, F., et al. (2018). *Depression and breast cancer; postoperative short-term implications.* https://core.ac.uk/download/216808123.pdf (accessed on 12th July 2025).
9. Białas, P., Curceanu, C., Czerwiński, E., Dulski, R., et al. (2018). *Evaluation of single-chip, real-time tomographic data processing on FPGA – SoC devices.* https://core.ac.uk/download/161798676.pdf (accessed on 12th July 2025).
10. Bici, M., Bini, F., Campana, F., Cardini, L., et al. (2018). *Digital design of medical replicas via desktop systems: Shape evaluation of colon parts.* https://core.ac.uk/download/188828207.pdf (accessed on 12th July 2025).
11. Blair, S. L., Dobke, M. K., Mackert, G. A., Yee, D. F., et al. (2019). *The influence of patient exposure to breast reconstruction approaches and education on patient choices in breast cancer treatment.* https://core.ac.uk/download/323066881.pdf (accessed on 12th July 2025).
12. Blugerman, G., D'Angelo, J. A., Habbema, L., Lisborg, M., et al. (2011). *Application of the liposuction techniques and principles in specific body areas and pathologies.* https://core.ac.uk/download/17179833.pdf (accessed on 12th July 2025).
13. Brown, N., Loveridge, A., Mills, C., Scurr, J., et al. (2015). *Acute changes in clinical breast measurements following bra removal: Implications for surgical practice.* https://core.ac.uk/download/29588823.pdf (accessed on 12th July 2025).

14. Cano, S. J., Klassen, A. F., Klok, J., Pusic, A. L., et al. (2009). *Satisfaction and quality of life in women who undergo breast surgery: A qualitative study to develop conceptual model.* https://core.ac.uk/download/1715813.pdf (accessed on 12th July 2025).
15. Chae, J. (2012). *"Yes! I had cosmetic surgery": Celebrities' cosmetic surgery confessions in the media and their impact on Korean female college students' perceptions.* https://core.ac.uk/download/56703672.pdf (accessed on 12th July 2025).
16. Clarkin, C. E., Emery, R. J., Gburcik, V., Pitsillides, A. A., et al. (2015). *Local origins impart conserved bone type-related differences in human osteoblast behavior.* https://core.ac.uk/download/36778258.pdf (accessed on 12th July 2025).
17. Clinch, N. C., Osland, A., & Wang, C. (2011). *Legitimizing radical new medical services.* https://core.ac.uk/download/70426040.pdf (accessed on 12th July 2025).
18. Demetris, A. J., Lu, L., Murase, N., Rao, A. S., et al. (1995). *Microchimerism, dendritic cell progenitors and transplantation tolerance.* https://core.ac.uk/download/12205240.pdf (accessed on 12th July 2025).
19. Di Luca, N. M., Marinelli, E., Napoletano, S., Vergallo, G. M., et al. (2018). *Ethics and/or aesthetics? Reflections on cosmetic surgery for adolescents.* https://core.ac.uk/download/188823836.pdf (accessed on 12th July 2025).
20. Dillon, J., Madsen, S. R., & Scribner, R. T. (2017). *Cosmetic surgery and body image among Utah women.* https://core.ac.uk/download/533933917.pdf (accessed on 12th July 2025).
21. Edmonds, A. (2014). *Surgery-for-life: Aging, sexual fitness and self-management in Brazil.* https://core.ac.uk/download/28979727.pdf (accessed on 12th July 2025).
22. Ennes, M., & Ramos, N. (2018). *Immigrants and body modifications in the consumer society.* https://core.ac.uk/download/196575527.pdf (accessed on 12th July 2025).
23. Fortier, M. A., Kain, Z. N., & Trinh, L. N. (2019). *Primer on adult patient satisfaction in perioperative settings.* https://core.ac.uk/download/287622490.pdf (accessed on 12th July 2025).
24. Galle, T. (2019). *Die globale Bewirtschaftung des Körpers. Eine qualitative Fallstudie zum amerikanischen Markt der Ethnochirurgie.* https://core.ac.uk/download/288478944.pdf (accessed on 12th July 2025).
25. Gelézeau, V. (2015). *The body, cosmetics and aesthetics in South Korea: The emergence of a field of research.* https://core.ac.uk/download/47088133.pdf (accessed on 12th July 2025).
26. Gilmartin, J., Long, A. F., & Soldin, M. (2012). *Quality of life following massive weight loss and body contouring surgery: An exploratory study.* https://core.ac.uk/download/13504967.pdf (accessed on 12th July 2025).
27. Ginwala, A. (2014). *Breaking the mold: Four Asian American women define beauty, detail identity, and deconstruct stereotypes.* https://core.ac.uk/download/72048098.pdf (accessed on 12th July 2025).
28. Groen, M., Hertog, F. den, & Weehuizen, R. (2025). *Mapping health care innovation: Tracing walls & ceilings.* https://core.ac.uk/download/pdf/6937006.pdf (accessed on 12th July 2025).
29. Han, E. J. (2017). *Potential predictors that influence women to undergo cosmetic surgery.* https://core.ac.uk/download/158970005.pdf (accessed on 12th July 2025).

30. Hasken, J. (2007). *Coercion in bioethics.* https://core.ac.uk/download/46722270.pdf (accessed on 12th July 2025).

31. Hirschfeld, E. R. (2022). *Motivational factors and post procedure impact of facial dermal fillers: A qualitative descriptive study.* https://core.ac.uk/download/541360040.pdf (accessed on 12th July 2025).

32. Leggat, P. (2015). *Medical tourism.* https://core.ac.uk/download/pdf/30672773.pdf (accessed on 12th July 2025).

33. Lowe, B. (2017). *Slathered, zapped, nipped, and tucked: An ethical analysis of cosmetic dermatology.* https://core.ac.uk/download/129153456.pdf (accessed on 12th July 2025).

34. Malone, J. (2025). *Women and genital cosmetic surgery.* https://core.ac.uk/download/pdf/30677491.pdf (accessed on 12th July 2025).

35. Nguyen, H.-K. (2020). *Beauty culture in post-reform Vietnam: Glocalization or homogenization?* https://core.ac.uk/download/305120711.pdf (accessed on 12th July 2025).

36. Porter, C. (2016). *Youth in crisis: Understanding the surge of adolescent suicide in South Korea.* https://core.ac.uk/download/70984094.pdf (accessed on 12th July 2025).

37. Prucher, G. M., Caporali, L., Lauretta, M. P., & RM, R. M., et al. (2018). *Anesthetic challenging in microsurgical flap reconstruction: A systematic review.* https://core.ac.uk/download/188826841.pdf (accessed on 12th July 2025).

38. Reynolds, L. A., & Tansey, E. M. (2007). *Early development of total hip replacement.* https://core.ac.uk/download/30696185.pdf (accessed on 12th July 2025).

39. Ricciardelli, R., & White, P. (2011). *Modifying the body: Canadian men's perspectives on appearance and cosmetic surgery.* https://core.ac.uk/download/51087617.pdf (accessed on 12th July 2025).

40. Rossetti, A., Peron, A. P. L. M., Kolb, B., Baker, B. W., Borelli, C., Sforza, C., Samuels, C. A., et al. (2018). *Proportions of the aesthetic African-Caribbean face: Idealized ratios, comparison with the golden proportion and perceptions of attractiveness.* https://core.ac.uk/download/161525252.pdf (accessed on 12th July 2025).

41. Shilling, C. (2016). *The rise of body studies and the embodiment of society: A review of the field.* https://core.ac.uk/download/46663852.pdf (accessed on 12th July 2025).

42. Smith, F., & Farrants, J. R. (2012). *Shame and self-acceptance in continued flux: Qualitative study of the embodied experience of significant weight loss and removal of resultant excess skin by plastic surgery.* https://core.ac.uk/download/29017740.pdf (accessed on 12th July 2025).

43. Uti, T. O. (2022). *The lifecycle of a social media beauty trend: A case study of the Instagram body.* https://core.ac.uk/download/586144778.pdf (accessed on 12th July 2025).

44. Zellweger, C. (2009). *Keynote address: Foreign bodies / jewellery as prosthesis.* https://core.ac.uk/download/99988.pdf (accessed on 12th July 2025).

CARDIOTHORACIC SURGERY

12

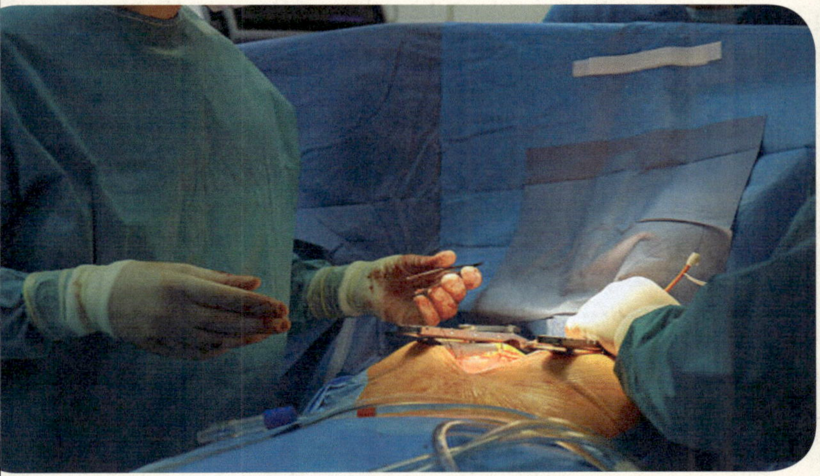

LEARNING OBJECTIVES

After studying this chapter, you will be able to:

1. Understand the history of cardiothoracic surgery
2. Explain the types of cardiothoracic procedures
3. Discuss the preoperative considerations of cardiothoracic procedures
4. Focus on surgical techniques and innovations of cardiothoracic procedures
5. Learn about postoperative care and recovery of cardiothoracic procedures
6. Evaluate the ethical considerations in cardiothoracic surgery

Introduction

Cardiothoracic surgery is a significant branch of the medical field, encompassing the intermixed complexities of cardiac and thoracic conditions. It is considered a surgical subspecialty that primarily concerns operations on the lungs and heart and managing a range of diseases from congenital cardiac disease to neoplastic chest diseases. The rapid advancement of surgical techniques and technologies has not only enhanced the lives of patients but also expanded the range of procedures that can be performed. To this end, cardiothoracic surgery plays a vital role in contemporary medicine, operating at the intersection of innovation and patient needs. This opening aims to establish the significance of this specialty as a foundation for a comprehensive exploration of its history, techniques, and broader impact on global healthcare delivery systems. Furthermore, the evolution of cardiothoracic surgery has been driven by a commitment to achieving greater surgical success through relentless study and innovation. Innovative techniques, such as minimally invasive surgery and robotic-assisted procedures, have transformed traditional practices, enabling surgeons to perform cutting-edge operations with shorter recovery periods and fewer complications. The application of advanced imaging technologies and better anesthetic practices has also increased precision during surgery. These developments not only aid in patient recovery but also contribute to an ever-growing body of literature focused on evidence-based best practices in this area. As we delve deeper into the advancements of cardiothoracic surgery, we should observe how these have aided the advancement of present-day surgical techniques and the ongoing quest for the best possible care for patients, as mentioned in N/A (1981) and N/A (2020).

It is more essential than ever that, as this area of cardiothoracic surgery progresses, we address the issues that are multidimensional in nature to follow this practice. Issues such as ethical application of new technologies, growing costs of advanced surgical procedures, and equitable access to lifesaving interventions are the most critical.

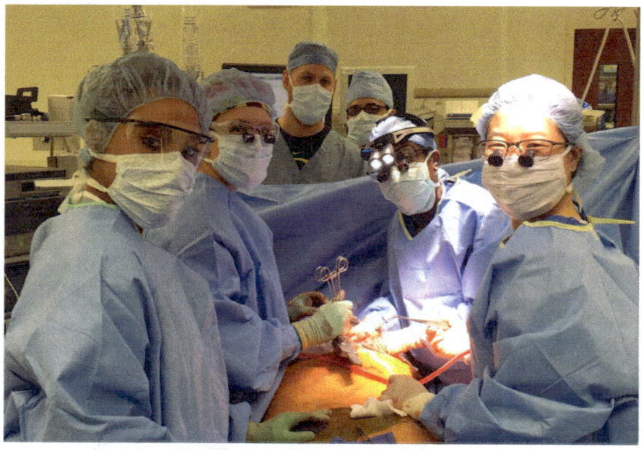

Figure 12.1. Cardiothoracic surgery.

Source: https://glenfieldmallareddybrainhearthospital.com/images/inner_imagese/Cardiothoracic%20Surgery1.jpg.

Additionally, the interprofessional provision of care by cardiologists, pulmonologists, and general surgeons highlights the team-oriented care of patients in this specialty. Analysis of these dimensions not only reveals the complexity inherent to cardiothoracic surgery but also speaks to ongoing debate among medical practitioners regarding patient-centered approaches. This introduction thus serves as a gateway to contemplating both the spectacular innovations and the problematic issues that define the practice of cardiothoracic surgery within modern healthcare (Figure 12.1).

Definition of Cardiothoracic Surgery

The cardiothoracic surgery is a subspecialty of surgery that entails the diagnosis and treatment of disease affecting the thoracic cavity, such as the heart and lungs. This tremendously intricate branch of medicine requires extensive knowledge of patient physiology, alongside surgical techniques. Cardiothoracic surgeons perform a range of procedures from coronary artery bypass grafting to congenital heart defect correction and lung resection. The methods are planned to assist in alleviating symptoms, correcting anatomical distortions, and improving overall patient outcomes. The surgical specialty is extremely challenging and requires extensive training, typically spanning several years of postgraduate education and residency in general and thoracic surgery. With ongoing developments in technology and procedural methods, cardiothoracic surgery is at the forefront of medical technology, improving patient care through enhanced surgery outcomes. One of the essential elements of cardiothoracic surgery is understanding influences on surgical therapy and patient outcomes. Studies have shown that the location of the first diagnosis significantly influences the likelihood of undergoing surgery. For instance, patients first seen in surgical hospitals have a higher probability of surgery for non-small cell lung cancer compared to those first diagnosed in non-surgical centers, with an odds ratio indicating a highly significant advantage in specialist centers (Khakwani et al.,

2014). This dynamic underscores the necessity of developing lung cancer services that ensure equality of access to surgery, the argument being that not all patients are given equal access to treatment when they first present to a healthcare encounter. These dynamics must be understood to optimize patient pathways for cardiothoracic surgery and improve the delivery of care. As well, the specialty of cardiothoracic surgery is not entirely risk-free, as there are numerous potential complications related to both the procedures themselves and the patient population treated. Post-cardiothoracic surgery complications may be slight issues or serious medical events that impact recovery and long-term prognosis. The MultiSocietal Database Committee has established comprehensive categories to define operative complications, including intraoperative and postoperative events in various systems, such as cardiovascular and infectious complications (Bronicki et al., 2017). These categories are essential for creating a greater understanding of surgical morbidity, guiding quality improvement, and enhancing reporting accuracy. As the clinicians forge ahead with the cardiothoracic intricacies, a firm model for the detection and handling of complications will remain at the forefront of ensuring maximum patient safety and surgical outcomes.

Significance in Contemporary Medicine

The significance of cardiothoracic surgery in modern medicine extends beyond its reputation as a single procedure; it is the hope for millions suffering from life-threatening cardiac and thoracic illnesses. The advent of cutting-edge surgical techniques, such as minimally invasive and robotic-assisted surgery, has transformed the treatment options presented to patients. These technologies not only decrease recovery periods but also lower the risks associated with traditional open-heart surgery, thereby improving overall patient outcomes. The importance of precise surgical intervention is even greater because of the rising prevalence of cardiovascular diseases globally, which in turn, contribute immensely to morbidity as well as mortality rates. With its emphasis on treating complex pathological conditions, cardiothoracic surgery highlights the importance of symbiotic relationships between advanced technology and surgical skills in improving patients' quality of life. For this reason, this branch of surgery has become an integral part of comprehensive healthcare in the modern world. Coupled with advancements achieved in surgery techniques, cardiothoracic surgery in contemporary medicine relies primarily on interprofessional collaboration. Surgeons, cardiologists, pulmonologists, and anesthesiologists typically work together to formulate personalized treatment plans, taking into account the complexity of cardiothoracic disease. The interdisciplinary approach ensures that the patient receives integrated care that is both effective and tailored, which is critical in addressing complex conditions such as congenital heart disease and lung cancer. Education and Research are equally instrumental in facilitating this integrated way of thinking, as caregivers constantly upgrade their knowledge about new surgery techniques as well as patient care practices. This reciprocal interaction and sharing of expertise indicates a commitment not only to cure patients but to enhance the practice of cardiothoracic surgery as well. It is on efforts such as these that modern medicine can pursue excellence and innovation for this critical area of medicine. Further, the public influence of cardiothoracic surgery extends beyond individual patient outcomes to encompass public health ramifications. The ability to perform life-saving interventions at an optimal level of effectiveness can significantly reduce the demands that cardiovascular diseases place on healthcare systems, a growing concern as populations age. Successful surgery results in shorter hospitalization, lower healthcare spending, and ultimately a healthier population.

Furthermore, outreach programs aimed at promoting awareness of heart health and preventive measures underscore the need for education in minimizing disease occurrence. With combined treatment and prevention, cardiothoracic surgery not just saves lives but supports sustainable healthcare practices. The synergy between surgical mastery and public health initiatives underscores the pivotal role of cardiothoracic surgery in modern medicine, solidifying its commitment to achieving better global health outcomes in the future (Figure 12.2).

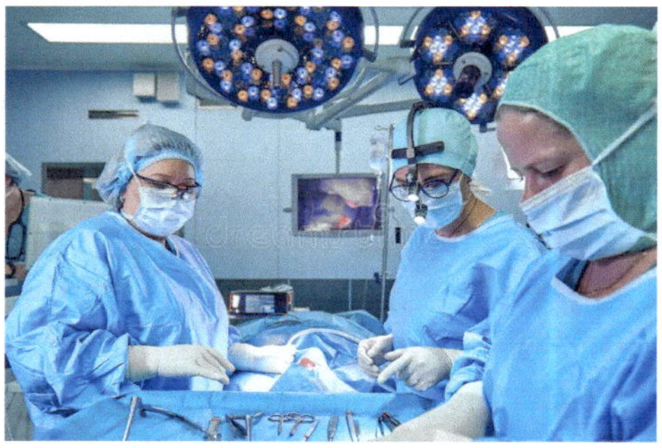

Figure 12.2. Cardiac operation on patient by professional surgeons*Source*: https://thumbs.dreamstime.com/b/surgeon-s-team-uniform-performs-operation-patient-cardiac-surgery-clinic-modern-medicine-professional-surgeons-151975092.jpg.

12.1. History of Cardiothoracic Surgery

Learning Outcome

1. Understand the early developments and pioneers of cardiothoracic surgery
2. Define the milestones in surgical techniques of cardiothoracic surgery
3. Describe the evolution of technology in the field of cardiothoracic surgery

The history of cardiothoracic surgery has been marked by significant milestones that highlight the collaborative process between medical need and innovation. Early experimental attempts at heart surgery date back to the late 19th century, with cases including the first successful repair of a congenital heart defect by Dr. Ludwig Rehn in 1896. These early efforts paved the way for future development, although the discipline remained risky and largely experimental for years. The advent of anesthesia and subsequently antibiotics was instrumental in these developments. During this period, thoracic surgeons faced unparalleled challenges and mortality rates that seemed nearly impossible to overcome, requiring a humble yet hopeful outlook on the surgical potential of thoracic medicine. These initial attempts set a foundation that cleared the way for the more formal and scientific approaches that would develop in mid-20th century, opening the field of cardiothoracic surgery significantly. The mid-20th century witnessed an unparalleled revolution in cardiothoracic surgery, marked by innovative advancements in surgical techniques and technologies. The creation of the heart-lung machine in the 1950s by Dr. John G. D. Ochsner revolutionized the branch of surgery by enabling surgeons to perform complex procedures on the heart without diverting the flow of blood. This technology enabled the first successful open-heart procedures, such as coronary artery bypass grafting (CABG) and valve replacement, and significantly transformed patient outcomes and survival rates. Surgeons who adopted these innovations, such as Dr. Michael DeBakey and Dr. Denton Cooley, emerged as leading pioneers in advancing the field, performing high-risk procedures with increasing confidence and reliability. This period not only solidified the role of surgery in treating most cardiac illnesses but also initiated a shift toward a more multidisciplinary approach to treating patients with complicated cardiovascular diseases. In the past few years, the field of cardiothoracic surgery has continued to thrive, with the addition of minimally invasive and robotic-assisted surgery. Technological advancements in imaging, such as MRI and CT scans, have facilitated preoperative evaluation, enabling surgery to be planned and conducted with increased accuracy. Concurrently, advancements in material and device technology, such as bioprosthetic heart valves and stents, have enhanced surgical outcomes and reduced recovery time. These technologies reflect a movement toward personalized medicine, with therapies selected increasingly according to individual patient needs. Moreover, the introduction of telemedicine has also facilitated follow-up care and teleconsultations, thereby increasing patient access to specialty care. With this field of medicine still evolving, the previous history of cardiothoracic surgery is testament to the resolve and ingenuity of medical professionals who have dedicated their professional lives to advancing this vital area of healthcare (Figure 12.3).

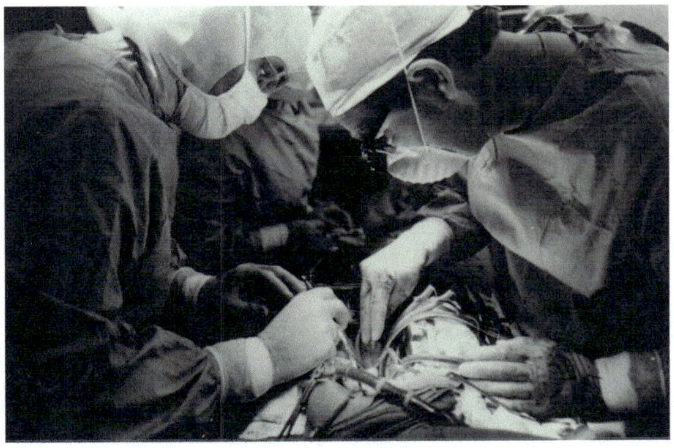

Figure 12.3. History of cardiothoracic surgery.

Source: https://wacohistory.org/files/original/e9b93fbb1b6505e39a3099e134457f6a.jpg.

12.1.1. Early Developments and Pioneers

The initial progress in cardiothoracic surgery can be traced back to the significant medical achievements of the mid-20th century, primarily driven by the demands of complex diseases affecting the lungs and the heart. The founders of this specialty recognized the need for new surgical techniques that could address then-inoperable conditions. This created the integration of improved anesthetics and surgery, including the use of heart-lung machines, which allowed more complex operations. Success with operations such as mitral valve replacement and coronary artery bypass grafting stemmed from a synergy of surgical skill and technology so that the surgeon was able to correct structural abnormalities of the heart successfully. With their relentless passion for achieving better patient outcomes, these initial pioneers laid a solid foundation for modern cardiothoracic surgery, which would dramatically evolve over the decades. The polio epidemic in the early 1950s served as a catalyst for advances in critical care, with immediate ramifications for cardiothoracic surgery procedures. Particularly in Copenhagen, the efficacy of tracheostomy and intermittent positive pressure ventilation demonstrated a revolutionary approach to respiratory failure that significantly improved survival. Such breakthroughs were not isolated incidents, but part of a continuum of medical advancements powered by wartime imperatives, including triage and collaboration among multidisciplinary groups of specialists. With the advent of these challenges, hospitals also began to create specialty intensive care units, resulting in the development of formalized care protocols. Metropolitan cities like Cambridge, London, and Liverpool had also developed specialist units by the early 1960s, which addressed the rising needs of post-operative patients and consequently enhanced the overall quality of care and outcomes in cardiothoracic surgical settings (Reynolds et al., 2011). With the growth of the specialty, the need for rigorous training and education for surgeons as well as nursing staff was realized. The emergence of nursing education, particularly intensive care, made the need for specialized knowledge more evident, which would be capable of handling the challenges of new surgical practices and levels of patient care. Nurse consultants were officially included in the National Health Service (NHS) by 1999, serving as a testament to the multidisciplinary nature of patient care in this field. Additionally, the establishment of national audits and scoring systems created a culture of continuous improvement and responsibility in clinical practice.

This paradigm shift towards evidence-based medicine was crucial in ensuring patient safety and optimizing the efficacy of treatments in cardiothoracic surgery. Thus, the initial pioneers' foundation created not only precedent for high-tech intervention but also laid the groundwork for necessary supportive care mechanisms that provide the foundation for cardiothoracic surgery today (N/A, 1989).

12.1.2. Milestones in Surgical Techniques

The development of surgical practice in cardiothoracic surgery has revolutionized the specialty, with milestones having changed the direction of patient outcomes in fundamental respects. One of the most significant is the development of minimally invasive surgical methods, which began to gain prominence in the later years of the 20th century. Reduced incisions and increased accuracy characterize them and offer several advantages over open-heart surgery, most notably lower recovery times and lower rates of postoperative morbidity.

The introduction of video-assisted thoracoscopic surgery (VATS) and robot-assisted surgical systems embodies this step, enabling surgeons to perform delicate operations with greater finesse than earlier methods. As these technologies advance, they not only expand the scope of surgery but also highlight the importance of integrating advanced methods into clinical practice, improving the quality of care offered to patients in need of cardiothoracic intervention (N/A, 1985). Another milestone in surgical techniques is the advancement in cardiac valve repair and replacement procedures. Patients have undergone risky operations in cardiac valve surgery in the past, and these also had prolonged recovery times with major thoracotomies. Advances in transcatheter aortic valve replacement (TAVR) have revolutionized this field, offering a less invasive option that can be performed without open-heart surgery in some patients. This has been particularly beneficial for elderly patients or those at high risk for surgery, allowing them to receive therapy previously out of reach. The integration of imaging modalities, such as echocardiography and fluoroscopy, has also significantly improved procedural outcomes, allowing surgeons to visualize and manipulate cardiac structures with unprecedented accuracy. The convergence of these various innovations is a testament to the advancement of surgical practice and patient-centered care in cardiothoracic surgery (Bedford et al., 2024).

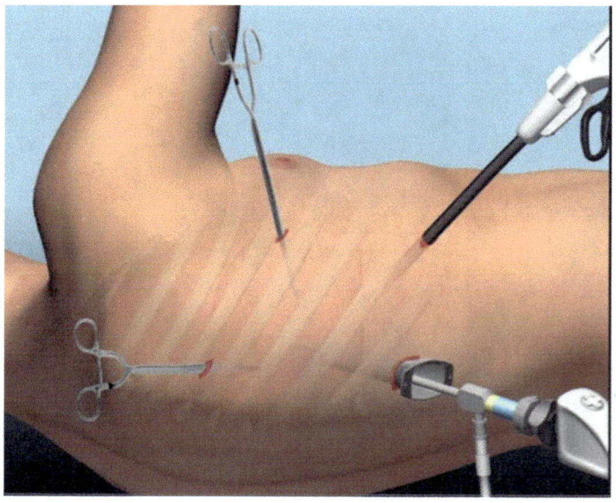

Figure 12.4. Video assisted thoracic-surgery.

Source: https://www.drshilpagandhi.com/wp-content/uploads/2024/12/Video-Assisted-Thoracic-Surgery-VATS.jpg.

Finally, adoption of enhanced recovery after surgery (ERAS) protocols in cardiothoracic management has been a revolutionary shift in surgical practice, getting clinical practice up to date with a contemporary evidence-based approach. ERAS use involves the incorporation of holistic, evidence-based strategies aimed at minimizing the surgical stress response, optimizing pain management, and maximizing patient mobilization during the recovery period. ERAS protocols are not only crucial in addressing physiological recovery but also aim to promote the active involvement of patients in their care process, thereby improving their experience. With the creation of an organizational culture that fosters cooperation and learning, patients recovering from cardiac surgery in intensive care units can have their prognosis significantly enhanced by healthcare teams. These advances highlight the importance of surgical proficiency and holistic patient care, underscoring the necessity of ongoing innovation in cardiothoracic surgery (N/A, 1985) (Figure 12.4).

12.1.3. Evolution of Technology in the Field

The evolution of technology in cardiothoracic surgical intervention has completely transformed the landscape of patient care and surgical outcomes. With ongoing medical advancement, the incorporation of new methods is inevitable in the evolution of surgical methods. Traditional surgical methods are being supplemented, if not replaced, by emerging technologies that are intended to be more accurate and less invasive. For instance, the classical model of training and skill acquisition in cardiothoracic surgery is being modified, with more emphasis placed on the capacity to attain competencies that combine technical proficiency with effective communication and teamwork skills. formulate tried, competency-based curricula in response to these evolving technological advances to promote a high standard of patient safety, which is the ultimate aim of surgical practice (Ahmed et al., 2017). The evolution of minimally invasive techniques has also been closely tied to significant technological advancements, notably the introduction of robotic surgery systems. Robotics has proved to be a revolution in cardiothoracic surgery, and robotic coronary heart surgery alone accounts for a large percentage of the number of robotic cardiac procedures performed today. This is one trend within a broader trend of less invasive techniques, offering patients shorter recovery times and fewer complications. Robotic platforms haveproven both safety and efficacy in the previous two decades, in spite of the revelation that fewer than 1% of coronary artery bypass grafting cases are conducted on these advanced setups. The development of robotics for cardiothoracic surgery holds promise for broadening the scope of new surgical approaches beyond conventional limits, providing alternative pathways for practice even as adoption rates are gradual (D'Auria et al., 2024). The future of cardiothoracic surgery, then, depends on the incorporation of novel technologies, such as robotic assistance, hybrid surgical techniques, and augmented reality systems, into clinical practice. The enhanced optimism regarding these technologies suggests a shift toward more efficient, accurate, and effective surgical methods. With the ongoing development of the field, it is crucial that cardiac surgeons fully leverage these technological developments to the fullest extent of their skill and optimize patient outcomes. Investing in training programs dedicated to these new techniques will better equip surgery professionals for the challenges of today's times. Lastly, the convergence of education and innovation in cardiothoracic surgery will redefine care standards, enabling surgical teams to meet the growing expectations of the specialty and deliver the best possible level of patient care (D'Auria et al., 2024).

Test Your Knowledge

1. Who were the pioneers in the development of modern cardiothoracic surgical techniques?
2. How have major milestones, such as the introduction of heart-lung machines, shaped the evolution of cardiothoracic surgery?

12.2. Types of Cardiothoracic Procedures

Learning Outcome

1. Define coronary artery bypass grafting (CABG)
2. State the heart valve repair and replacement
3. Describe the lung surgeries, including lobectomy and pneumonectomy

Cardiothoracic surgery encompasses a range of operations focused on treating disorders of the heart and thorax. The most common operation is coronary artery bypass grafting (CABG), which is performed to treat clogged coronary arteries leading to heart disease. The surgical procedure can entail two major approaches: mini-thoracotomy and full sternotomy. Mini-thoracotomy is a less invasive operation that has emerged to prominence due to its benefit in reducing postoperative morbidity, including infection and pneumonia. To compare, full sternotomy is an open incision operation and will most probably be followed by longer postoperative recovery times. Research indicates that, although there is limited comparative data on these two techniques, particularly in terms of the length of hospital stay and ventilator utilization in CABG patients, an argument can be explored further (Badrkhani et al., 2019).

Apart from coronary interventions, some of the other cardiothoracic surgical procedures are valve replacement and repair operations, which are critical in the treatment of valvular heart diseases. These operations can restore good blood circulation to the heart and can revolutionize the survival and quality of life for affected patients. The choice between valve repair and replacement depends normally on the individual characteristics of the valve disease, and also on patient factors. Repair techniques can be minimally invasive and may even retain the patient's own valve, whereas replacement may require the use of mechanical or biological prosthetics. New developments in surgical techniques, such as minimally invasive surgery and robotic-assisted surgery, are transforming the way these procedures are performed, leading to shorter recovery periods and improved surgical outcomes (Tilney et al., 2003). Another main class of cardiothoracic interventions is thoracic surgery, which addresses conditions affecting the lungs, esophagus, and mediastinum. Thoracic operations, such as lung resections like pneumonectomy and lobectomy, are performed to treat lung cancer and other respiratory diseases. Thoracoscopic surgery, which employs minor cuts and a telescope, has also gained wide use in thoracic operations because it is helpful in reducing postoperative pain and accelerating patient recovery. Also included are esophageal disease procedures, such as esophagectomy for cancer or achalasia, which demonstrate the range of conditions treated in the specialty. The flexibility to incorporate these newer operations demonstrates the continued evolution and improvement of cardiothoracic surgery, requiring ongoing education and interprofessional collaboration among caregivers to achieve optimal patient outcomes (Badrkhani et al., 2019) (Figure 12.5).

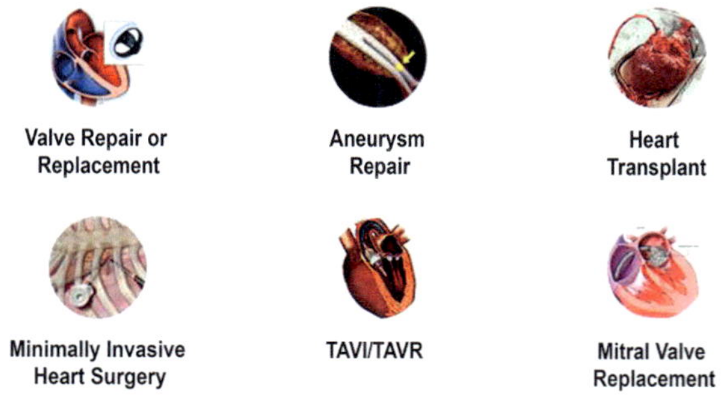

Figure 12.5. Types of cardiothoracic procedures.

Source: https://psrihospital.com/wp-content/uploads/2021/12/heart-surgery.jpg.

12.2.1. Coronary Artery Bypass Grafting (CABG)

Coronary artery bypass grafting (CABG) is a significant cardiothoracic surgery procedure aimed at restoring adequate blood flow to the myocardium of patients with severe coronary artery disease. CABG technique involves creating a passageway beyond blocked or narrowed arteries, typically utilizing a segment of a patient's own vein or artery. The rising prevalence of coronary artery disease calls for effective surgery, as it is among the leading determinants of morbidity and mortality in the world. CABG's technological advances, including minimally invasive surgery and the use of arterial grafts, have made it possible to achieve improved patient outcomes by reducing postoperative complications and enhancing long-term survival. Postoperative care following CABG is of the greatest significance, most importantly concerning the issue that patients will have a longer hospital stay due to many reasons. Recent studies reveal various predictors that have been linked with a stay in the cardiac intensive care unit (CICU), such as non-elective procedures and underlying diseases like congestive heart failure and renal failure. In addition, the intricacy of surgery—whether with combined CABG and valve—increases the difficulty of recovery. .

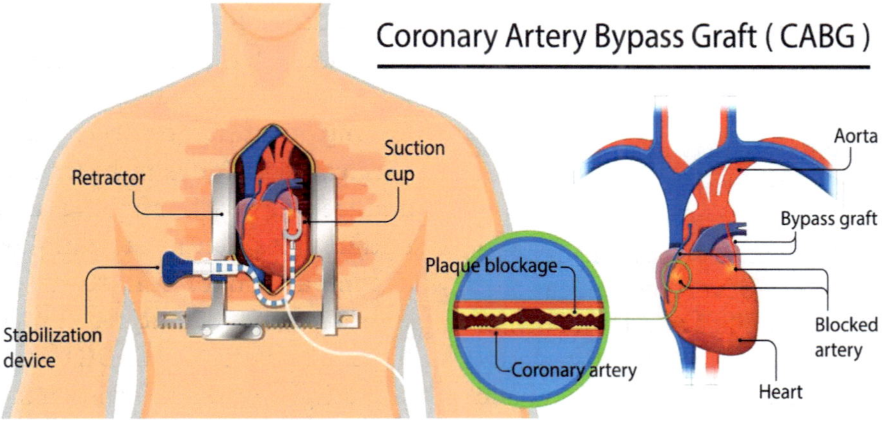

Figure 12.6. Coronary artery bypass grafting.

Source: https://cdn-assets-eu.frontify.com/s3/frontify-enterprise-files-eu/eyJvYXV0aCI6eyJjbGllbnRfaWQiOiJmcm9udGlmeS1leHBsb3JlciJ9LCJwYXRoIjoia WhoLWhlYWx0a GNhcmUtYmVyaGFkXC9hY2NvdW50c1wvYzNcLzQwMDA2MjRcL3B yb2plY3RzXC8yMDlcL2Fzc2V0c1wvMzFcLzMzOTU3XC8yNDA0NDUzYzFlYzEyM2Q3ZGY3Mzc4ZT NiYjE5Y2UyNy0xNjQ3MjY0MDA1LmpwZyJ9:ihh -healthcare-berhad:MMSAakHslcZN81Q3hViCRO7 VApeziSUsQjzaGot7yzA?format=webp.

The direct relationship between complications and total postoperative hospital stay emphasizes the need for individualized patient management pathways. Through predictive models based on preoperative criteria, healthcare teams can proactively intervene against imminent risks, thereby maximizing resource utilization and enhancing patient recovery outcomes (Almashrafi et al., 2016). Furthermore, new management approaches to patients, such as the implementation of fast-track recovery programs, have been common in cardiac surgery, symbolizing efforts aimed at promoting efficiency in postoperative care. The programs are designed to facilitate quick recovery by transferring the patient early to the intermediate care units if they are discovered to have stable circulatory patterns. Despite this, however, a high percentage of patients are likely to experience undesirable readmissions in the intensive care unit, a sign of deteriorating outcomes. The identification of independent predictors, such as greater ASA classes and longer operation times, plays a critical role in optimizing fast-track regimens and overall patient safety. These empirical results underscore the interconnectedness of surgical practice, patient factors, and postoperative care, necessitating an integrated approach to managing the nuances of CABG in modern cardiothoracic surgery (Bingold et al., 2013) (Figure 12.6)

12.2.2. Heart Valve Repair and Replacement

The field of cardiothoracic surgery has made significant advancements in valve repair and replacement techniques, which are crucial in the management of valvular heart disease. This form of surgery corrects malformations of heart valves that may lead to severe complications, including arrhythmias and heart failure. Former methods typically required a full sternotomy, which involves a significant healing period and has added risks. Current practices, however, aim for the least invasive interventions, such as thoracoscopic surgery, that advance patient outcomes. By reducing trauma on the chest cavity and shortening recovery periods, such interventions are better aligned with the new practice of patient-centered care in today's healthcare.

These developments are complemented by the evolution of effective preoperative regimens aimed at optimizing patient selection and outcome prediction, thereby ensuring that surgical interventions are tailored to the patient's unique condition and need. The success of heart valve replacement and repair is as much a function of the technical method utilized as it is of total patient assessment and prudent surgical judgment. With the arrival of minimally invasive mitral valve repair and replacement, healthcare providers have placed greater emphasis on standardizing optimal practice that is patient assessment criterion-based. This not only enhances surgical outcome but also allows risk stratification, thus high-risk patients receive the most appropriate interventions. To this end, the preoperative planning stage establishes vital myocardial protection protocols and cannulation techniques, both of which are crucial to ensuring patient safety and enhancing postoperative recovery. Such meticulous care to detail highlights the interface of surgical acumen and systemic patient care as key factors of successful cardiothoracic surgery, particularly in terms of heart valve processes, thereby profoundly influencing general health outcomes. Early findings continue to drive the development of surgical techniques in heart valve replacement and repair, with ongoing controversy over optimal intervention techniques. For instance, a comparison of full sternotomy and mini-thoracotomy techniques for coronary artery bypass grafting (CABG) outcomes sheds some light on significant debates concerning procedural efficiency and patient recovery. Although the two methods have yielded comparable results regarding postoperative ventilation and hospitalization, further studies are ongoing to determine their respective advantages and disadvantages. Information on these is crucial for guiding protocols aimed at ensuring optimal patient safety by minimizing invasive interventions. Lastly, the development of heart valve surgery reflects broader trends in cardiothoracic surgery, where practice evolution through empirical data and clinical consensus results in more effective and less invasive interventions for patients receiving these life-saving treatments (Figure 12.7).

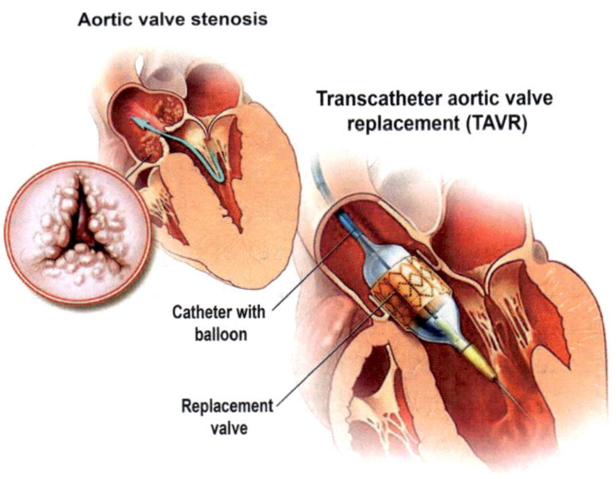

Figure 12.7. Heart valve repair and replacement.

Source: https://www.heartvascularcentre.com/wp-content/uploads/2018/10/tavr-post.jpg.

12.2.3. Lung Surgeries, Including Lobectomy and Pneumonectomy

Lung resections, lobectomy, and pneumonectomy are great significant operations in cardiothoracic surgery employed primarily for malignancy and other severe pulmonary pathologies. Lobectomy is the surgical removal of a lobe of lung. It is most commonly indicated for localized lung carcinoma or a life-threatening infection that cannot be managed with other means. Surgical technique can be performed by way of traditional open surgery or less invasive procedures such as video-assisted thoracoscopic surgery (VATS), which has gained broader popularity due to its associated benefits of less postoperative pain and earlier recovery times. The surgical technique utilized can significantly impact the short-term and long-term outcomes for patients, underscoring the importance of the surgical technique employed in these procedures. Pneumonectomy, however, involves the removal of one lung and is usually reserved for cases of large tumors that occlude the airway or enter adjacent structures such that lobar resection is not possible. The complexity of pneumonectomy necessitates extensive preoperative assessment and planning as the patients inevitably have significant comorbidities. The procedure also carries a higher risk of complications like pneumonia, respiratory failure, and postoperative complications due to low lung function. These factors determine the outcomes, with the volume and experience of the operating team being the most important. A documented positive correlation has been established, where greater surgical volume by a thoracic surgeon leads to improved patient outcomes, particularly in VATS lobectomies compared to traditional open procedures (David et al., 2012). With the evolving landscape of thoracic surgery, structural variations in training and infrastructure can significantly impact the quality of care delivered. The European Society of Thoracic Surgeons' existing guidelines provide the primary structural elements that comprise a successful general thoracic surgery unit, emphasizing the standardization of training and procedural guidelines across Europe (Brunelli et al., 2017). Having surgeons qualified in both the traditional open and the new minimally invasive techniques is the solution to optimizing patient results in lung surgery. As sustained by differences in training programs, coordination of surgery practice can act to close gaps between institutions and toward cultivating an excellence culture in cardiothoracic surgery, ultimately benefiting the patient population at large.

Test Your Knowledge

1. What are the main differences between open-heart surgery and minimally invasive cardiothoracic procedures?
2. How do procedures like coronary artery bypass grafting (CABG) differ from valve repair or replacement surgeries in indications and outcomes?

12.3. Preoperative Considerations

Learning Outcome

1. Describe the patient assessment and evaluation
2. Discuss on contraindications and risk factors
3. Define preoperative education and preparation

A comprehensive assessment of preoperative considerations is critical in cardiothoracic surgery as it lays a basis for successful surgery and optimum patient outcomes. The patient history, physical examination, and preoperative testing all contribute immensely to the understanding of the patient's overall state of health. Cardiovascular risk stratification is crucial, particularly in patients with pre-existing comorbid conditions such as hypertension, diabetes, and obesity, as they can influence intra- and postoperative recovery. Psychological assessment may also be warranted as anxiety and depression can have an impact on surgical outcomes. Having a clear understanding of these variables allows healthcare professionals to tailor surgical procedures to individuals, ensuring complications-related outcomes are sidestepped and ensuring each patient receives individually tailored care. More recent approaches to cardiothoracic surgery, such as minimally invasive and robot-assisted surgery, may have varying preoperative procedures from traditional methods. Preoperative planning of such advanced techniques requires special training and proficiency, as outlined in various expert reviews of robotic-assisted techniques (Agnihotri et al., 2016). Second, patient selection is a crucial element; not all can be candidates for minimally invasive procedures. Excessive care must be exercised when considering anatomical factors, previous surgery, and cardiopulmonary status to determine the appropriateness of these therapies. Measurement of these parameters enables more individualized surgical planning, which may potentially reduce recovery periods and the risk of complications. Thus, assessing appropriateness of advanced techniques forms a pivotal role in preoperative management. Additionally, identifying factors that control postoperative recovery is essential for enhancing patient care in cardiothoracic surgery. Recent research has identified several preoperative factors that correlate with prolonged CICU LOS and the entire postoperative recovery period. A non-elective surgery, renal impairment, and the relative complexity of the surgery all significantly influence these durations (Almashrafi et al., 2016). Creating predictive models that identify at-risk patients for prolonged hospitalization can enable healthcare professionals to distribute resources optimally and conduct targeted presurgical interventions. By addressing these presurgical issues, medical teams can enhance patient outcomes, minimize complications during postoperative recovery, and ultimately elevate the standard of care in cardiothoracic surgery (Figure 12.8).

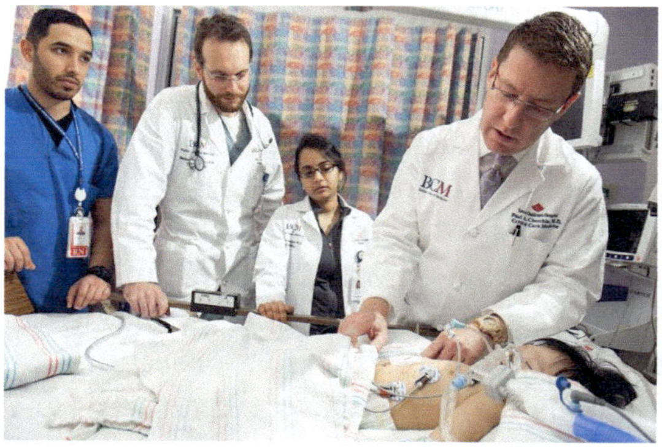

Figure 12.8. Cardiac intensive care unit (CICU).

Source: https://www.texaschildrens.org/sites/tc/files/styles/coh_medium/public/2023-11/2K13-0187-DSC_0952%20Dr.%20Paul%20Checchia%20conducts%20patient%20rounds%20in%20CVICU.jpg?itok=bdljE0WX.

12.3.1. Patient Assessment and Evaluation

The key building block of patient assessment and evaluation in cardiothoracic surgery is a proper understanding of cardiovascular and thoracic underlying conditions. This begins with a comprehensive medical history examination, including the patient's symptoms, previous medical treatments, and comorbidities that may impact surgical treatment. Comprehensive physical examinations also delineate the overall state of health and unique cardiac function of the patient. With advancing minimally invasive technology, such as mitral valve repair and replacement, the proper choice of candidates for these procedures has become prominent. Optimal practice in the assessment of patients not only ensures that patients are suitable for surgery but also optimizes their preoperative condition to achieve the best postoperative outcomes, as noted in arguments over standardization protocols among cardiovascular surgery units (Agnihotri et al., 2016). The incorporation of modern evaluative techniques is of prime importance in cardiothoracic surgery, particularly in advanced patient assessments. Advanced imaging modalities, including echocardiography and cardiac MRI, provide essential evaluations of cardiac structure and function, and the data derived from them enable surgeons to make informed decisions. Diagnostic imaging allows for proper evaluation of valvular disease, ischemic disease, and structural defects, and consequently optimizes the surgical team's ability to design individualized surgical plans. Furthermore, patient risk stratification models also aid in classifying individuals according to their operative risk, which influences preoperative counseling and perioperative management plans. Such intricate evaluations not only enhance surgical planning but also provide a deeper understanding of potential complications, ensuring that the surgical team is well-equipped to handle diverse situations within the operating room (Avidan et al., 2017). Successful intraoperative communication among the surgical team is crucial for patient assessment and evaluation, especially in the high-risk environment of cardiothoracic surgery. The use of formalized communication tools, such as TeamSTEPPS, has been shown to enhance teamwork and minimize risk from communication errors made intraoperatively. By establishing an open dialogue culture, workers are comfortable addressing issues about patient evaluations or complications without fear of retaliation. This psychological safety is critical to making patients safer and improving surgical outcomes, as it enables meticulous attention to detail during exams. Through the concerted effort of care teams facilitated by better communication, the general impact is a robust evaluative process that subsequently enhances the quality of care delivered in cardiothoracic surgery (Avidan et al., 2017).

12.3.2. Contraindications and Risk Factors

Risk factors and contraindications to cardiothoracic surgery are significant factors that can have a profound impact on the surgical approach as well as the patient's outcome. The existence of comorbid diseases such as diabetes mellitus, chronic obstructive pulmonary disease (COPD), and obesity may complicate interventions and make the surgeon more susceptible to postoperative complications. For instance, the healing of wounds in diabetic patients and increased risk of infection are compromised, for which consideration must be given to their preoperative overall general condition. Functional status and age are also strong determinants in risk assessment. Older patients generally have impaired physiological reserve, thereby predisposing them to poor outcomes, and therefore require a proper understanding of their personalized risk profiles in cardiothoracic procedures. Apart from inherent risk factors, there are specific contraindications that should be assessed cautiously before surgery. For instance, in the scenario of massive pulmonary embolism (PE), there is a particular challenge since it can lead to right ventricular (RV) failure and cardiogenic shock. In such a scenario, the risk of surgery may outweigh the benefits; therefore, alternative management strategies should be explored. Surgical teams must remain engaged in holistic risk stratification and construct multidisciplinary interventions to manage PE effectively. The decision to operate typically hinges on the timely assessment of these contraindications, which play a crucial role in determining patient mortality rates, bearing in mind that death in massive PE is up to 65% if inadequately managed (Bellis et al., 2018).

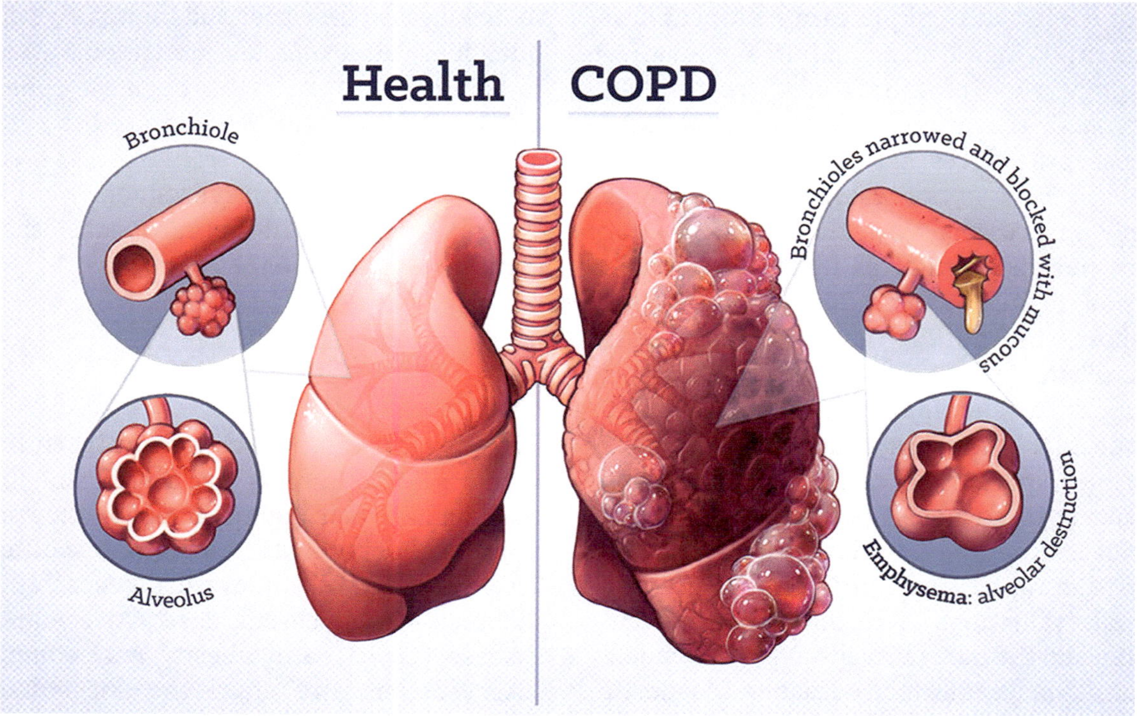

Figure 12.9. Chronic obstructive pulmonary disease (COPD).

Source: https://www.chandigarhayurvedcentre.com/wp-content/uploads/2022/12/HealthyvsCOPDlungs960px.jpg.

Risk minimization for cardiothoracic surgery is key in preoperative planning. Standardized processes for patient evaluation can accelerate contraindication and risk factor identification, thereby accelerating patient safety and surgical outcomes. For example, for minimally invasive mitral valve repair or replacement, meticulous preoperative assessment is essential to determine appropriate candidacy and optimize outcome. This involves careful consideration of available myocardial protection strategies and cannulation techniques to ensure optimal patient welfare during the procedure. The application of best practices based on evidence can significantly reduce the incidence of surgical complications, thereby providing an environment for enhanced patient care and facilitating more successful interventions in cardiothoracic surgery (Agnihotri et al., 2016) (Figure 12.9).

12.3.3. Preoperative Education and Preparation

Effective preoperative education and preparation are essential components of the care pathway for patients undergoing cardiothoracic surgery. The process serves multiple purposes, including the alleviation of anxiety in patients, promotion of understanding of the procedure, and compliance with postoperative protocols. Through effective preoperative education, patients can comprehend the anticipated risks and benefits of the procedure, ultimately enhancing their involvement in the process. This customized approach has the potential to be used in responding to some of the issues that may arise from surgery, such as estimated recovery periods, pain management procedures, and lifestyle changes that an individual may require after undergoing the surgery. By developing an open environment for communication, doctors can empower individuals, hence optimizing their overall surgical experience and outcome. The necessity of preoperative screening equipment cannot be taken lightly. Patients may arrive with undiagnosed pathology, that is, obstructive sleep apnea (OSA), which can compound perioperative risk. For example, studies indicate that nearly 90% of patients with moderate-to-severe OSA remain undiagnosed and are thus at greater risk of respiratory and cardiovascular morbidity in the operating room (Diamond et al., 2019). Utilization of a preoperative screening tool, for example, the STOP-BANG questionnaire, can be helpful in screening out these at-risk patients. The application of such equipment enables operating room personnel to provide more personalized anesthetic and perioperative care for the patient, thereby minimizing potential complications and enhancing safety. Preoperative teaching in the form of risk assessment and screening can hence significantly improve the surgical results of cardiothoracic operations. Preoperative preparation also extends to educational aspects as it typically involves optimization of the patient's physical status before surgery. These can include nutritional counseling, smoking cessation, and management of chronic diseases such as diabetes or blood pressure that can have significant impacts on recovery and surgical outcomes. Guidelines emphasize the need for individualized interventions to be created for each patient, ensuring physical and psychological preparation for surgery. Interprofessional working among healthcare professionals can facilitate this process, generating a shared practice that supports not only the surgical approach but also the overall well-being of the patient. Ultimately, thorough preoperative preparation is an essential part of optimizing the operating pathway for patients, confirming the role of anticipatory engagement in their cardiothoracic surgical experience (N/A).

Test Your Knowledge

1. Why is thorough cardiovascular and pulmonary assessment essential before cardiothoracic surgery?
2. How do risk factors such as comorbidities and medication use influence preoperative planning in cardiothoracic patients?

12.4. Surgical Techniques and Innovations

Learning Outcome

1. Define open-heart surgery vs. minimally invasive techniques
2. Discuss robot-assisted surgery advancements
3. Identify the use of imaging technology in surgery

Surgical techniques and advancements in cardiothoracic surgery have led to significant improvements, particularly in procedures targeting valvular heart disease. These include the development of minimally invasive procedures for mitral valve repair and replacement. These surgeries are performed using smaller incisions compared to open-heart surgery, resulting in quicker recovery periods for patients and a lower incidence of complications. More. Hospitals. Surgeons. In growing numbers, surgeons are embracing these new techniques, which strike a balance between effectiveness and patient care. Additionally, today's best practices dictate that meticulous patient evaluation and selection are key to the success of minimally invasive procedures, so that candidates will have the most ideal conditions for these new approaches to surgery. These developments not only elevate the levels of care provided to patients but also enhance overall efficiency in cardiothoracic surgery procedures, thus revolutionizing the field of cardiovascular surgery (Agnihotri et al., 2016).

Evidence for the deployment of minimally invasive methods in cardiothoracic surgery is also rooted in the growing consensus among practitioners on standard protocols. Optimizing outcomes in minimally invasive mitral valve surgery requires the implementation of optimal practices in patient evaluation and preoperative planning. Specifically, interventions involving more advanced cannulation methods and myocardial protection strategies have gained favor due to their ability to reduce the intraoperative risks associated with standard approaches. This harmony among the surgical community gives confidence to the surgeons and assists in creating a solid basis for training and implementation of these techniques in various clinical settings. Through the creation of a collective effort to incorporate these innovations, the specialty ensures that patients are offered evidence-based, higher-level surgical care aligned with contemporary medical standards, which ultimately leads to improved health outcomes and patient satisfaction (Agnihotri et al., 2016).

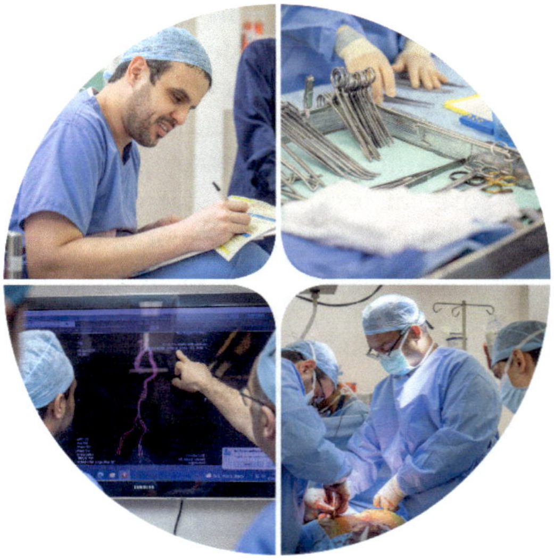

Figure 12.10. Surgical techniques of cardiothoracic.

Source: https://mmcts.org/images/MMCTS_cover-image.png.

Finally, innovation in surgical techniques within cardiothoracic surgery is also within the broader trend towards personalized medicine. As surgeons continue to refine their skills, emphasis on care plans tailored to specific patient characteristics is of utmost concern. Improvements such as robotic surgery and hybrid procedures, which combine traditional and innovative techniques, underscore the need to tailor surgical practice to meet diverse patient needs. Additionally, advancements in imaging technologies enhance preoperative diagnosis while providing real-time intraoperative guidance. The integration of these high-tech developments enhances surgical precision and promotes personalized interventions to improve patients' recovery patterns. By embracing these path-breaking surgical procedures, cardiothoracic surgery not only advances its medical practice but also sets a precedent for change in the medical sector as a whole, emphasizing the need for constant innovation in patient care delivery (Figure 12.10).

12.4.1. Open-Heart Surgery vs. Minimally Invasive Techniques

The choice between open-heart and minimally invasive approaches represents a critical milestone in the practice of cardiovascular medicine, with significant implications for both patient outcomes and postoperative recovery. Open-heart surgery, with its massive incisions and direct visualization, has been the gold standard for complex cardiac interventions, such as valve repair or coronary artery bypass grafting. This traditional approach provides surgeons with a wide range of exposure and sensitivity of touch, which can be crucial for okay repairs. However, the invasiveness of such procedures is likely to lead to more extended hospital stays, greater pain, and a more discomforting recovery process. Thus, even though open-heart surgery remains an essential component of cardiothoracic procedures, its shortcomings have prompted extensive research into less invasive alternative methods. On the other hand, less invasive surgeries cause minimal trauma to the body, generally made possible through improvements in surgical instruments and technology. These surgeries, such as robotic surgery and thoracoscopy, enable procedures to be performed through smaller incisions, resulting in reduced blood loss and fewer surgical complications. Recent best practices in patient evaluation are vital to the effective use of these techniques, particularly in complex cases such as mitral valve repair and replacement. Agreement on minimally invasive methods is gaining traction in the medical community due to evidence indicating faster recovery and improved outcomes. As noted by recent specialist opinions, promoting standardization of the process of patient selection and preoperative planning will enhance the adoption of minimally invasive techniques, and consequently, the quality of care being offered in cardiothoracic surgery (Agnihotri et al., 2016).

The development of minimally invasive techniques in cardiology is a testament to the rapid evolution within the field of cardiothoracic surgery. With ongoing innovations further enhancing surgery and postoperative treatment protocols, surgeons are increasingly able to utilize new technologies as a means to tailor interventions to meet particular patient requirements. The potential to reduce morbidity while maintaining efficacy places minimally invasive surgery at the hub of contemporary cardiothoracic practice. Furthermore, with the passage of time and the advancement of technology, it will have the capability to expand its scope from the repair and replacement of valves to a wider range of cardiac conditions. All these collectively point towards the revolutionary possibility that lies in the convergence of technology and surgical innovation at the intersection where the medical community focuses on maximizing patient outcomes by integrating both open-heart and minimally invasive procedures (Agnihotri et al., 2016).

12.4.2. Robot-Assisted Surgery Advancements

The integration of robotic surgical intervention in cardiothoracic surgery has revolutionized the field, offering a paradigm shift in addressing these complex procedures. Minimally invasive surgery (MIS), driven by the innovation of robotic technology, allows surgeons to perform precise cardiac interventions with enhanced accuracy and less trauma to adjacent tissues.

This advancement involves not only enhanced visualization with real-time imaging but also enhanced dexterity offered by robotic instruments, which are capable of moving more accurately than the human hand in small anatomical spaces. Consequently, patients experience less postoperative pain, a reduced hospital stay, and a shorter total hospitalization duration. Accordingly, not only have robotic-assisted interventions contributed to improved clinical outcomes, but the patient experience has also been enhanced, thereby making this approach an acceptable option for both surgeons and patients in cardiothoracic surgery, as indicated by scholarly trends in the field (Kshirsagar et al., 2023).

Furthermore, the new trajectory of robotic-assisted surgery points towards growing validity of these technologies in uses other than traditional ones. Early pioneers in cardiac surgery, robotic systems are safe and effective across a range of procedures, from urological to general surgical procedures. The growing interest in robotic surgery for cardiothoracic procedures, particularly coronary artery bypass grafting (CABG), is supported by evidence demonstrating its capability for successful revascularization with minimal complications.

While there is hope, currently, only a limited number of CABG surgeries are being performed using robotic assistance, and therefore, there is still scope for growth in this area. As the specialty becomes increasingly cognizant of the various advantages of robotic technology, its wider use is being called for in surgical procedures, thus enhancing the repertoire of modern cardiac surgery techniques (D'Auria et al., 2024). Forward, the improvements in robotic-assisted surgery look to redefine cardiothoracic interventions. Advances such as hybrid surgical strategies and augmented reality optimizations will continue to drive improved procedural outcomes. These cutting-edge methods mark a new chapter where robotics and artificial intelligence integrate, enabling even more precise and patient-centric care. With the ongoing training of new cardiac surgeons evolving to include such sophisticated techniques, it is of the highest importance that training programs accommodate a complete grasp of the technical and ethical principles of robotic surgery. With continued investment in technology and surgery, the next generation of cardiac surgeons will be well-positioned to develop even more sophisticated techniques, which are likely to improve patient outcomes and create new opportunities for surgery in the near future (D'Auria et al., 2024) (Figure 12.11).

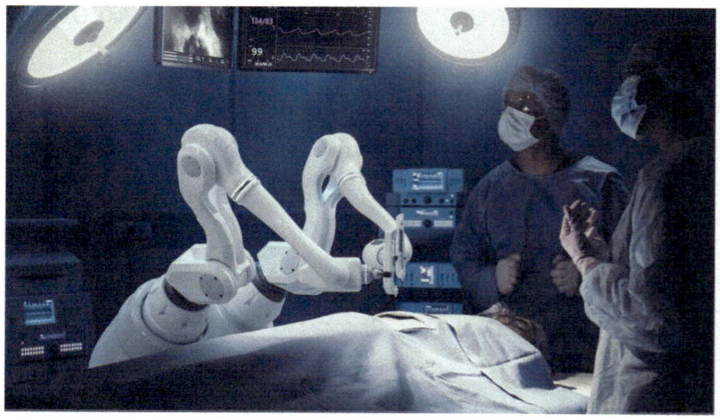

Figure 12.11. Integration of robotic-assisted surgery in cardiothoracic procedures.

Source: https://ca-times.brightspotcdn.com/dims4/default/370e8f6/2147483647/strip/true/crop/2430x1366+0+0/resize/1200x675!/quality/75/?url=https%3A%2F%2Fcalifornia-times-brightspot.s3.amazonaws.com%2Fd3%2F21%2F8adf3a6c4929baac3b00cdd7997d%2Frobotics-in-surgery.jpeg.

12.4.3. Use of Imaging Technology in Surgery

Imaging technology is a key component of cardiothoracic surgery, making surgery far more accurate and effective. New imaging modalities such as computed tomography (CT), magnetic resonance imaging (MRI), and three-dimensional (3D) reconstruction allow surgeons to visualize complex anatomical structures with unprecedented clarity. These technologies aid in preoperative planning by producing detailed images of the patient's heart and adjacent tissues, which are required to identify abnormalities and select the best approach for surgery. In addition, as the recent developments in 3D printing have demonstrated, surgeons can design precise anatomical models that represent unique patient pathologies. This method has been particularly groundbreaking for the treatment of congenital heart disease, enabling individualized surgical interventions tailored to a patient's anatomy and improving overall rates of surgical success (Anwar et al., 2018). Intraoperative imaging, particularly with the use of fluoroscopy and echocardiography, enhances real-time intraoperative decision-making in cardiothoracic surgery. These imaging techniques play a crucial role in visualizing complex structures, such as heart chambers and blood vessels, without posing a risk of complications. An example is intraoperative transesophageal echocardiography (TEE), which provides immediate feedback on the success of surgery, enabling surgeons to make in vivo corrections without the need for a second procedure. New technologies, such as Optical Coherence Tomography (OCT), have also found utility because they enable the precise assessment of stent location and the monitoring of the in-stent restenosis process during a procedure. The ability to monitor structural changes in real-time greatly enhances surgical outcomes and reduces the risk of complications following surgery (Deuse et al., 2009). The application of imaging technology in cardiothoracic surgery permeates not only the operating theater but also has implications in other areas such as training and interdisciplinarity. Advanced imaging is increasingly applied in medical training to teach surgical trainees about complex anatomical relationships and procedural planning. 3D-printed models from imaging data provide a sensory learning experience that significantly augments trainees' ability and confidence. Second, transparent imaging facilitates the transmission of advanced medical information to multidisciplinary teams, patients, and their families, ensuring a more enhanced understanding and cooperation among all stakeholders. Through these developments, imaging technology not only improves surgical planning but also enhances education and communication, ultimately yielding better patient outcomes in the cardiothoracic arena (Anwar et al., 2018).

Test Your Knowledge

1. How have minimally invasive and robotic-assisted techniques transformed cardiothoracic surgical procedures?
2. What recent innovations aim to reduce operative risk and improve recovery in cardiothoracic patients?

12.5. Postoperative Recovery and Care

Learning Outcome

1. Describe the monitoring and managing complications
2. Define the physical therapy and rehabilitation
3. Understand the long-term follow-up and patient outcomes

Postoperative care is key to ensuring optimal recovery after cardiothoracic surgery. This time is typically spent monitoring for complications associated with supportive treatments that promote healing. Patients are kept in an intensive care unit (ICU) facility during the initial days of surgery, where fluid management, vital signs, and pain are closely watched. Early mobilization is encouraged to reduce the risk of thromboembolism and to optimize lung function, a most critical concern due to the risk of future pulmonary complications after such invasive surgery. With the implementation of these preventive measures, patient outcomes can be significantly improved, resulting in reduced hospital stays and lower rates of reoperation. Multidisciplinary postoperative care management can lead to significant improvements in morbidity and mortality rates. Recent studies have shown that guidelines for quality improvement in institutions can reduce rates of operative mortality, highlighting the importance of goal-based management in patient recovery following cardiac surgery. Evidence has shown that effective interprofessional collaboration among surgeons, anesthesiologists, nurses, and rehabilitation specialists is essential to minimize the risk of complications in surgeries. The application of standardized protocols for monitoring and early intervention can lead to a more stable recovery pattern for patients, ultimately achieving the goal of better quality of care and patient safety in cardiothoracic surgery, as emphasized in ongoing research reports (Camp et al., 2008). Apart from routine postoperative therapy, management of some complications, such as upper-airway obstruction, is essential, particularly in children. Complication analysis following cardiac surgery has shown that derangements like extrathoracic upper-airway obstruction can significantly compromise the outcome of recovery. These are typical complications in patients who require intense sedation or are more likely to stay agitated during mechanical ventilation. Identifying such challenges enables the care agents to streamline postoperative practice optimally, such as instituting advanced sedation strategies and close monitoring. Addressing these factors during the recovery period can minimize the incidence of severe complications and equip healthcare providers with valuable data for optimizing postoperative care in high-risk categories, such as children undergoing cardiothoracic surgery (Delius et al., 2015) (Figure 12.12).

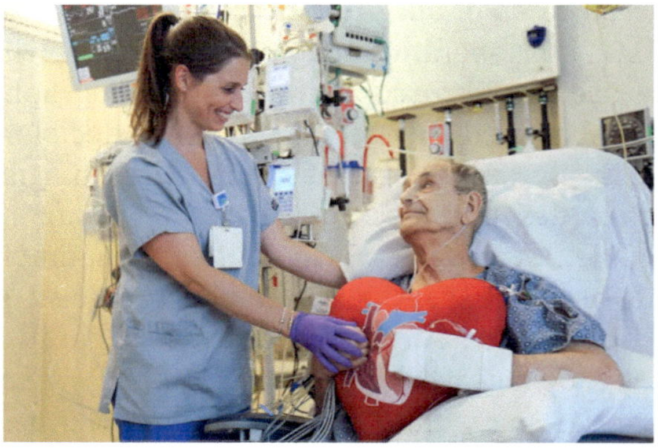

Figure 12.12. Tracks recovery for cardiac surgery patients.

Source: https://i0.wp.com/bwhheartandscience.org/wp-content/uploads/2019/08/ERAS.jpg?resize=860%2C574&ssl=1.

12.5.1. Monitoring and Managing Complications

Effective monitoring and management of cardiothoracic surgery complications are crucial for achieving improved patient outcomes and recovery. After surgeries such as coronary artery bypass grafting or valve replacement, patients can develop a variety of complications during the postoperative period. They can include arrhythmias, infections, and pulmonary complications, which need to be monitored vigilantly. Through the use of standardized protocols in patient assessment and postoperative monitoring, medical staff can detect and resolve potential complications at an early stage before they become uncontrollable, thereby enhancing patient care. This is consistent with industry best practices that advocate for thorough planning in postoperative care and assessment, as supported by the work of Agnihotri et al. (2016). Over the past few years, the concept of fast-track recovery pathways has garnered significant attention in the field of cardiothoracic surgery, significantly transforming the area of postoperative care. Fast-track recovery pathways aim to accelerate patient recovery and reduce hospital stays, which in turn helps reduce the risk of complications. However, as mentioned by Bingold et al. (2013), fast-track protocols must be sifted through to identify predictors of re-admission to the intensive care unit (ICU). Parameter knowledge, such as ASA classification and operation time, can provide surgical teams with information on who among the patients may be at greater risk of adverse outcomes, thereby allowing for personalized interventions and closer monitoring of high-risk patients. Not only does this data-driven approach maximize recovery pathway effectiveness, but it also maximizes healthcare practitioners ' effectiveness in terms of complications management in a high-risk case. The application of technology in postoperative monitoring systems has also transformed the management of surgical complications. With the assistance of advanced monitoring devices, such as telemetry for continuous cardiac monitoring and automatic systems for monitoring vital signs, real-time information can be accessed to alert medical teams regarding deteriorating cases. This enables quick clinical decision-making, which is crucial in mitigating the severity of complications. As cardiothoracic surgery evolves, the integration of standard monitoring practices with the latest technological advancements is poised to enhance patient outcomes and safety. By fostering an environment of continuous evaluation and practice improvement, surgical teams can enhance their ability to manage complications, ultimately leading to improved survival rates and quality of life for patients undergoing such complex procedures.

12.5.2. Physical Therapy and Rehabilitation

Rehabilitation and physical therapy constitute key elements of patient recovery in cardiothoracic surgery. Patients undergoing complex operations such as heart surgery or lung resections can suffer significant physical as well as psychological problems. Rehabilitation measures aim to restore the patient's functional ability, enhance quality of life, and minimize the risk of postoperative complications. These programs typically consist of exercise programs, respiratory techniques, and lifestyle modification education that allow patients to become actively involved in the process of recovery. Studies have shown that specially tailored physical therapy interventions can lead to enhanced pulmonary function and overall physical stamina, which are a necessity for patients who have undergone significant surgical stress. Through facilitation of prior mobilization and consistent re-escalation to physical exercise, rehabilitation is a cornerstone in the program of worldwide care in the cardiothoracic surgery category. Of particular interest in rehabilitation in the specialty is the emphasis on respiratory physiotherapy provided to individuals with diseases like CAP. Since intubation and mechanical ventilation are common in such patients, the role of physiotherapists becomes even more critical in maintaining respiratory status and preventing complications, such as atelectasis. As established in research, intensive care unit availability and delivery of respiratory physiotherapy, as well as after-hours care, significantly influence patient outcomes. With some proof provided that indicates a few hospitals provide after-hours physiotherapy services, there is a high degree of dependence on nursing staff for carrying out respiratory interventions. These dynamics underscore the critical necessity of integrating respiratory therapy into regular postoperative care to ensure that patients receive adequate support, regardless of day or night, and staffing (Hill et al., 2017).

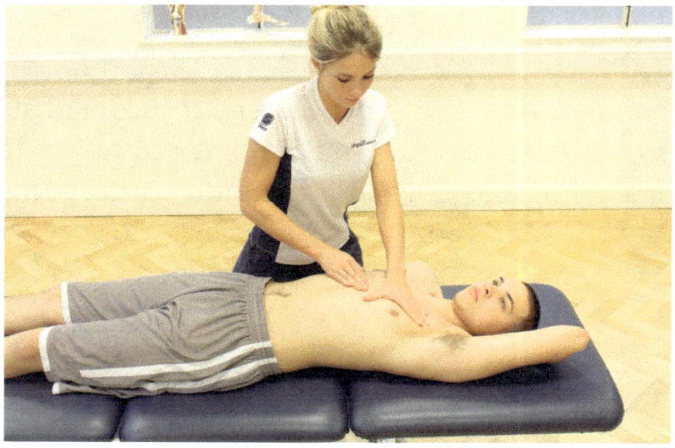

Figure 12.13. Rehabilitation and physical therapy for cardiac.

Source: https://www.physio.co.uk/images/cardiac-surgery/cardiac-surgery2.jpg.

Psychological support in rehabilitation programs should not be overlooked either. The majority of patients who have undergone cardiothoracic surgery are anxious, depressed, or show emotional distress, which makes it difficult to recover. Efficient rehabilitation should, therefore, incorporate not only physical therapy but also mental health care, facilitating an all-around recovery process. Interventions such as cognitive-behavioral therapy, mindfulness, and relaxation are valuable in overcoming mental resistance to rehabilitation. Reversing these elements enhances patients' motivation towards physical therapy, making their rehabilitation process more appealing. According to applicable health management literature, a comprehensive multidisciplinary care plan involving both physical and psychological support is required to optimize patient outcomes post-surgery, with an emphasis on the emerging knowledge related to the interdependence of body recovery and psychological well-being (Bonica et al., 2017) (Figure 12.13).

12.5.3. Long-Term Follow-Up and Patient Outcomes

Effective long-term follow-up in cardiothoracic surgery is crucial for understanding patient outcomes and the success of overall surgical interventions. Complete follow-up protocols enable clinicians to monitor the lingering effects of invasiveness on patients' health, particularly in diseases such as acute type A aortic dissection, which may demand repeated surgeries due to complications. The outcome of various strategies, including hybrid procedures for repairing the aortic arch, underscores the importance of meticulous postoperative care. The technique, which combines open and endovascular modalities, may lead to reduced cardiopulmonary bypass requirements and, presumably, improved early outcomes, as reported in studies where patients demonstrated excellent recovery despite the complexity of their situations (Brechtel et al., 2013). Therefore, robust follow-up mechanisms are crucial for controlling complications and enhancing patient survival and quality of life. The impact of chronic diseases on postoperative results cannot be exaggerated. For instance, patients with CKD have more complications after procedures such as TAVI. Findings reveal a high incidence of acute kidney injury (AKI) among CKD patients post-TAVI, with tremendous implications for postoperative mortality and morbidity. Specifically, the risk of 30-day mortality escalates disproportionately with AKI occurrence (Brecker et al., 2015). This justifies the integration of assessment of baseline health status in long-term follow-up programs. By carefully observing patients with pre-existing medical conditions, clinicians can tailor their therapeutic regimens and intervention timelines, which ultimately translates to improved outcomes and enhanced patient safety during the recovery process. Attempts at long-term follow-up also need to consider the quality of life, as survival does not encompass all aspects of outcomes in patients. The majority of patients undergoing cardiothoracic surgery have to deal with intricate emotional, psychological, and bodily concerns, necessitating an integrated approach to follow-up care. Repeat measurements through patient-reported outcome measures (PROMs) and clinician-rated assessments can provide relevant information regarding the perceived health status and quality of life of patients. Empowering patients to voice their needs and experiences fosters a healthcare giver-recipient interaction and has the potential to make follow-up care a more client-centered system. Thus, an overall approach towards follow-up not only enhances clinical outcomes but also goes a long way in improving life satisfaction in patients who have undergone cardiothoracic surgery.

Test Your Knowledge

1. What strategies are essential to prevent complications such as infection, bleeding, or respiratory issues after cardiothoracic surgery?
2. How does early mobilization and cardiac rehabilitation influence recovery and long-term outcomes in postoperative patients?

12.6. Ethical Concerns in Cardiothoracic Surgery

Learning Outcome

1. Understand the informed consent and patient autonomy
2. Define allocation of resources and access to care
3. Discuss end-of-life decisions and palliative care

The ethical problems in cardiothoracic surgery are multifaceted, affecting both the process of clinical decision-making and the broader healthcare system. Surgery must navigate a range of ethical obstacles, most fundamentally in the areas of patient consent and disclosure of risk associated with complex operative interventions. Informed consent thus becomes front and center, where patients need to be fully told about their conditions, the gravity of the operation, and potential outcomes before permission is given. The dilemma becomes even more acute when patients are potentially incapable of enjoying the fruits of their choices, such as cases of old age or intellectual impairment. This only serves to underscore the need for healthcare providers to adopt an empathetic approach, advising patients through their options while considering the extent of urgency of surgery versus the patient's right to make their own decisions. The second significant ethical issue involves fairness in the distribution of resources in cardiothoracic surgery. As procedures can be costly and consume a significant amount of healthcare resources, issues of effectiveness, affordability, and prioritization of maximizing patient outcomes arise. For instance, patients who require prolonged postoperative care are often subject to increased healthcare costs and resource utilization, as evidenced in studies examining determinants of postoperative length of stay (Almashrafi et al., 2016). The ethical responsibility of cardiothoracic surgeons also extends to ensuring that not only is care appropriate, but also equitable. This could involve hard talks on the triage of patients to be operated on in terms of recovery potential and quality of life following the procedure, and this raises questions regarding justice and society's values in healthcare allocation.

Another factor is that the ethical context of cardiothoracic surgery is complicated by the practical challenges inherent in surgical research and its translation into clinical practice. The lack of adequate numbers of high-quality randomized trials in the surgical literature is a cause for concern about the validity of evidence to inform surgical procedures and decision-making (Bhandari et al., 2008). Surgeons would struggle to justify their clinical choices without robust evidence, leaving them open to the threat of ethical conflict in selecting interventions that will not be maximally effective in all patients. The fundamental reliance on lower levels of evidence risks creating a disconnection between clinical practice and patient safety, underscoring the need for ongoing ethical debate regarding surgeons' responsibility to advocate for better research outcomes that prioritize patient care. Closing the gap between clinical practice and ethical research standards is therefore crucial to enhancing the level of care in cardiothoracic surgery (Figure 12.14).

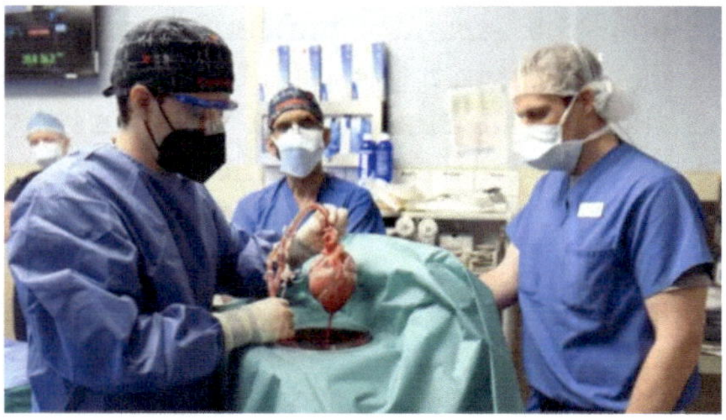

Figure 12.14. Ethical considerations in cardiothoracic surgery.

Source: https://ichef.bbci.co.uk/news/480/cpsprodpb/90AB/production/_122653073_073036943.jpg.webp.

12.6.1. Informed Consent and Patient Autonomy

Informed consent and patient autonomy are the guiding principles of cardiothoracic surgery, affirming the ethical obligation of care providers to inform their patients in a manner that empowers them with full knowledge of their healthcare choices as well as associated risks. Informed consent is not merely documentation but rather represents a display of respect for patients' autonomy in that it empowers people to make decisions regarding their health care on an informed platform. This is particularly crucial in cardiothoracic settings where complex surgical interventions like valve replacement or coronary artery bypass grafting are fraught with procedure-related risks. Surgeons need to engage patients in dialogue, not only explaining the benefits and risks but also other available treatments, which opens a field of shared decision-making that is critical to outcomes and patient satisfaction. At the core of the informed consent process is effective communication between the patient and the surgeon, an essential variable for minimizing the disparities of medical information comprehension. tailored approach to education and communication. Surgeons are responsible for ensuring that patients can describe their understanding of the recommended intervention, as well as the associated risks and benefits. In instances of specialized situations, this is even more critical, such as in the situation of discussing options with patients experiencing post-cardiotomy cardiogenic shock, where interventions like venovenous extra-corporeal membrane oxygenation (VV ECMO) can be presented as last options. Resolution of patient issues and confusion enables a more intense interaction that honors patient autonomy while also making them more informed about their care choices (Emin et al., 2017). Furthermore, the impacts of informed consent extend beyond individual autonomy to encompass broader ethical issues in the health system. For instance, as in the case of the newly emerging discipline of medical tourism, informed consent procedures become entangled, particularly when patients cross international borders to seek surgery that may be less expensive but may have different standards of treatment (Leggat, 2015). Surgeons must inform patients about the potential risks associated with accessing care from other regulatory environments and may also face greater challenges when patients seek follow-up care subsequent to surgery. This highlights the importance of a workable system that enables informed decision-making across various healthcare environments. Lastly, maintaining informed consent and patient autonomy in cardiothoracic surgery is not just compliance with guidelines in ethics, but also a commitment to patient-centered care that enables the patient to take a proactive role in managing their own healthcare decisions (Figure 12.15).

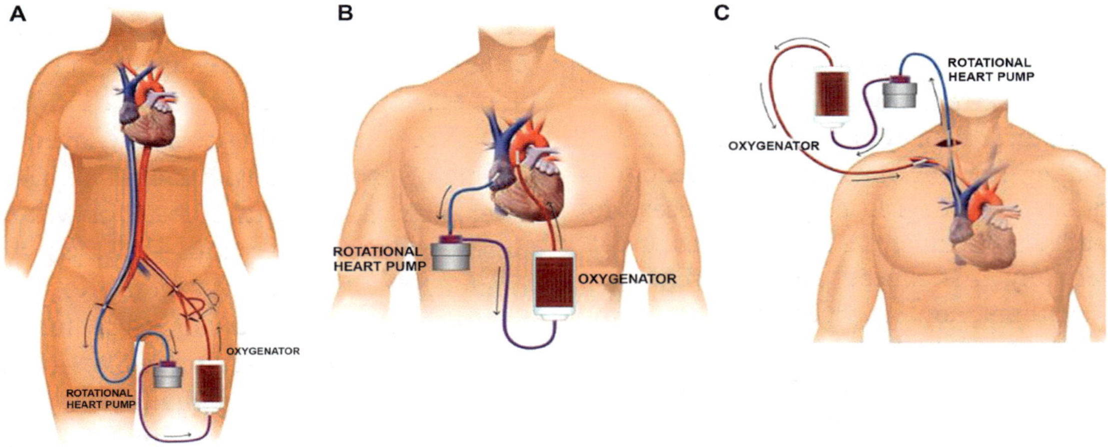

Figure 12.15. Venoarterial extracorporeal membrane oxygenation for cardiogenic shock and cardiac arrest.

Source: https://www.ahajournals.org/cms/10.1161/CIRCHEARTFAILURE.118.004905/asset/06ed997c-d899-4063-b747-ebf61723fcd6/assets/graphic/e004905fig01.jpg.

12.6.2. Allocation of Resources and Access To Care

Within cardiothoracic surgery, deployment of resources plays a pivotal role in patient access to intervention, with specific consideration for the availability of state-of-the-art medical technology. Ultrasound-guided central venous cannulation is an exemplary case in which technology is utilized to enhance procedural efficiency and safety. Clinical evidence has shown that the use of such a strategy reduces catheter placement failure rates, which is of utmost importance in emergency situations or in complex surgical cases. Specifically, research has shown that real-time two-dimensional ultrasound guidance is associated with a significantly lower failure rate compared to traditional landmark techniques, resulting in improved outcomes for patients requiring central venous access (Beverley et al., 2003). However, access to these high-technology devices can be unequal across different healthcare facilities, resulting in disparities in patient outcomes based on geographic and economic location. Further, the ethical aspects of resource distribution in cardiothoracic surgery should not be overstated. An equitable healthcare system demands that there should be open decision-making mechanisms and observance of the latest scientific facts. Complete data sets must be relied upon by cardiothoracic surgeons to guide their practices and optimize the use of resources. Audit and peer-reviewed standards of performance play a crucial role in ensuring a consistent level of care across institutions (Manche et al., 2003). Strict compliance with the utilization of hard data facilitates successful decision-making regarding resource allocation, ultimately enhancing patient access to the right surgical interventions. This fosters an accountability culture through information sharing, where patient management practices are enhanced to make quality care accessible to all, not a preserve of elite groups. In addition, cardiothoracic surgery resources cannot be separated from systemic variables, such as healthcare policy and the funding model. For example, funding limitations of hospitals can influence the degree of patient access to cutting-edge surgery. If the required resources are unequally distributed among privileged health systems, underserved patients may be disadvantaged by delayed treatment and access to diagnostic modalities. This disparity calls for policymakers to adopt comprehensive approaches that prioritize resource allocation according to patient needs over economic considerations. Addressing disparities is crucial to enhancing overall public health outcomes and ensuring equitable access to life-saving cardiothoracic surgery, enabling all patients to receive appropriate and timely care regardless of their background.

12.6.3. End-of-Life Decisions and Palliative Care

In cardiothoracic surgery, end-of-life care and palliative care become a vital issue for those suffering from severe cardiac illness. Palliative care is designed to enhance the quality of life in those with life-limiting illnesses through pain management, psychological distress, and other incapacitating symptoms from the initial diagnosis. This is particularly so for those with chronic cardiothoracic disease, such as congestive heart failure or pulmonary disease, where the extent of difficulty may radically affect daily activity. Indeed, a majority of patients are not given adequate help in controlling the disease until they are severely impaired. By incorporating palliative care early in the therapeutic process, medical professionals can align therapy with patient-specific goals, thereby optimizing symptom control and overall quality of life as evidence-based (Bakker et al., 2018).

The burden with which end-of-life decisions must be rendered so regularly in cardiothoracic surgery is illustrated graphically through the case of congenital heart defects, for example, hypoplastic left heart syndrome (HLHS). Parents who receive such a diagnosis are faced with an agonizing process of decision-making shortly after their child's birth, sometimes within days. Such burdens of decisions—such as avoiding immediate surgical treatment to choosing comfort care—can be too overwhelming for parents who feel ill-equipped to make such life-altering decisions. Healthcare providers play a crucial role here by providing clear and accurate information regarding diagnosis and treatment options. Effective communication and guidance enable parents to navigate these emotional waters, allowing them to weigh the potential benefits and drawbacks of each path and make decisions consistent with their family values and intentions (Coddington et al., 2012).

As patients enter the later stages of cardiothoracic disease, palliative care increasingly becomes indispensable. End-of-life care needs to be directed not just towards preventing pain, but also towards keeping patients and their families dignified and comfortable during the dying process. Access to specialist palliative care teams with the training and experience to cope with the complexity of physical, emotional, and spiritual distress can make a significant difference to the last days for patients and families alike. Furthermore, the fusion of palliative care with standard cardiac care encourages multidisciplinary practice, with medical, psychological, and family parameters coordinated together. This holistic practice enables more empathetic treatment, aligning with the inherent belief in prioritizing patient autonomy and making informed end-of-life decisions that are respectful and in harmony with the overall aim of sustaining quality of life (Bakker et al., 2018).

Test Your Knowledge

1. What ethical issues arise when deciding between high-risk cardiothoracic surgery and conservative management?
2. How does informed consent play a critical role in addressing patient autonomy and surgical decision-making?

SUMMARY

The progress in cardiothoracic surgery underscores the profound impact on patient care and the evolution of surgical practice. The implementation of new cardioplegic solutions, such as Custodiol-N, is a significant leap towards eliminating the harmful effects of ischemia-reperfusion injury. According to comparative studies, cardioplegic fluid design that enables personalized fluids enhances myocardial and endothelial function postoperatively, ultimately resulting in increased total coronary blood flow and myocardial ATP reserve. The significance of these findings rings true in the surgical community because they indicate a revolution in techniques applied in cardiopulmonary bypass surgery, and they emphasize the need for tailored solutions in a bid to yield the best results for patients who undergo complex cardiac procedures. Most importantly, studying such advancements is vital in addressing evolving challenges of cardiothoracic surgery. The shielding effect demonstrated by innovative cardioplegic solutions not only yields greater operative achievement but also provides insight into the broader impact of cardiopulmonary bypass on patient health. The reduction in oxidative stress markers observed in studies involving Custodiol-N further justifies the ongoing investigation aimed at optimizing the safety and efficacy of surgical interventions. By developing a deeper understanding of cardiac physiology and biochemical mechanisms, surgeons can refine surgical methods that minimize postoperative complications, thereby laying the groundwork for future breakthroughs in surgical technique. Ultimately, the focus on better cardioplegic solutions reflects a commitment to enhancing cardiothoracic surgery through empirical research and clinical practice. As technology continues to evolve, it is essential that surgeons stay abreast of new techniques and solutions that promote enhanced patient care. The established efficacy of solutions like Custodiol-N indicates that the industry is now trending towards personalized medicine, where therapy is tailored to the individualized biological responses of the patient. These innovations not only ensure enhanced safety in surgical procedures but also promote recovery, such that innovations in cardiothoracic surgery have direct applications in improving the quality of life for patients.

Cardiothoracic surgery encompasses a wide range of operations primarily aimed at the heart and thoracic space, with far-reaching effects on patient outcomes and healthcare systems. Among its significant advances are the use of new technologies, for example, autologous transfusion systems, which have transformed intraoperative blood loss management. Clearly, based on the analysis, these technologies entail considerable reductions in blood consumption, particularly in complex procedures such as vascular surgery and cardiothoracic procedures. The robust modeling outlined examines how processes such as preoperative preparation of surgery clinics, preoperative autologous donation, cell salvage during surgery, and cell salvage post-surgery can significantly redirect the determinants of surgical efficacy and expense, thereby enhancing healthcare resources in the National Health Service (Currie et al., 2005). Besides, the impact of cardiothoracic surgery extends beyond the operating theater. It has been shown that patients undergoing interventions like coronary artery bypass graft (CABG) experience detrimental breaks in their recovery, especially in sleep quality. Research determines a recurring rate of poor-quality sleep among patients both during and after intensive care admission, pointing to significant psychological impacts such as depression and anxiety. These findings underscore the necessity of more inclusive recovery pathways that account for the physical and psychological dimensions of postoperative recovery. The identified correlations between disturbed sleep and compromised health-related quality of life suggest an urgent necessity for interventions promoting better sleep as part of the recovery process (Caruana et al., 2016). In summary, the specialty of cardiothoracic surgery is characterized by the complexity of the procedures and the inherent need for a multidisciplinary approach to patient care. The convergence of emerging medical technologies with the psychosocial requirements of recovery provides an opportunity for enhanced treatment protocols. With the promise of streamlining surgical interventions and rehabilitating patients, continued effort must be made to refine such procedures while also addressing the complex challenge of postoperative recovery dynamics. For cardiothoracic surgery to remain at its prime, one must address innovation that encourages whole patient recovery, transforming the face of surgical care to be as nurturing as it is advanced in its technology.

KEY TERMS FROM THIS CHAPTER

- Aortic dissection
- Arrhythmia surgery
- Atrial septal defect (ASD) repair
- Cardiopulmonary bypass
- Coronary artery bypass grafting (CABG)
- Empyema drainage
- Esophageal surgery
- Heart transplantation
- Left ventricular assist device (LVAD)
- Lobectomy
- Median sternotomy
- Minimally invasive cardiac surgery
- Mitral valve repair
- Pericardiectomy
- Pleurectomy
- Pneumonectomy

CRITICAL THINKING QUESTIONS

1. **Which of the following is the most commonly used conduit for coronary artery bypass grafting (CABG)?**
   a. Saphenous vein
   b. Radial artery
   c. Internal mammary artery
   d. Cephalic vein
2. **Beck's triad (hypotension, muffled heart sounds, and elevated jugular venous pressure) is characteristic of:**
   a. Pulmonary embolism
   b. Cardiac tamponade
   c. Myocardial infarction
   d. Aortic dissection
3. **Which of the following is a minimally invasive procedure used to diagnose and treat thoracic conditions?**
   a. Thoracotomy
   b. Sternotomy
   c. Video-assisted thoracoscopic surgery (VATS)
   d. Open lung biopsy
4. **The most common indication for surgical valve replacement in adults is:**
   a. Infective endocarditis
   b. Rheumatic fever
   c. Aortic stenosis
   d. Mitral valve prolapse
5. **Which of the following is NOT a typical complication following open-heart surgery?**
   a. Post-pericardiotomy syndrome
   b. Arrhythmia (e.g., atrial fibrillation)
   c. Stroke
   d. Deep vein thrombosis of the lower limb only

Short Answer Questions

1. What are the common indications for coronary artery bypass grafting (CABG)?
2. Differentiate between open and minimally invasive mitral valve surgery.
3. What are the signs and symptoms of cardiac tamponade, and how is it managed surgically?
4. Name the commonly used conduits for CABG.
5. What is the role of cardiopulmonary bypass in open-heart surgery?
6. What are the surgical treatment options for a thoracic aortic aneurysm?
7. List the indications for lobectomy or pneumonectomy in lung cancer.
8. What is the difference between a thoracotomy and a sternotomy?
9. What is the role of video-assisted thoracoscopic surgery (VATS) in thoracic procedures?
10. What are the common postoperative complications following open-heart surgery?

Answers to Critical Thinking Questions

1. (c); 2. (b); 3. (c); 4. (c); 5. (d)

REFERENCES

1. Al-Attar, N., Coccia, R., Di Domenico, F., Nappi, et al. (2017). *Introductory editorial: Drug-eluting stents or drug-eluting grafts? Insights from proteomic analysis.* https://core.ac.uk/download/77601030.pdf (accessed on 12th July 2025).
2. Almashrafi, A., Alsabti, H., Aylin, P., Baskaran, et al. (2016). *Factors associated with prolonged length of stay following cardiac surgery in a major referral hospital in Oman: A retrospective observational study.* https://core.ac.uk/download/77011080.pdf (accessed on 12th July 2025).
3. Anwar, A., Barach, B., Bhatla, A., Biglino, et al. (2018). *3D printing is a transformative technology in congenital heart disease.* https://core.ac.uk/download/212858839.pdf (accessed on 12th July 2025).
4. Avidan, M. S., Ben Abdallah, A., Bollini, M. L., Dahl, et al. (2017). *Building a collaborative culture in cardiothoracic operating rooms: Pre and postintervention study protocol for evaluation of the implementation of teamSTEPPS training and the impact on perceived psychological safety.* https://core.ac.uk/download/129069724.pdf (accessed on 12th July 2025).
5. Badrkhani, S. (2019). *Comparing two surgical outcomes: Minithoracotomy or full sternotomy in coronary artery bypass grafting surgery.* https://core.ac.uk/download/215413077.pdf (accessed on 12th July 2025).
6. Bakker, S. E. (2018). *Implementing palliative care pre-cardiothoracic transplant.* https://core.ac.uk/download/220124441.pdf (accessed on 12th July 2025).
7. Bedford, M. A. (2024). *Developing an evidence-based practice framework for post operative cardiac surgery patients in the intensive care unit.* https://core.ac.uk/download/638454377.pdf (accessed on 12th July 2025).
8. Beverley, C., Calvert, N., Davidson, A., Hind, et al. (2003). *Ultrasonic locating devices for central venous cannulation: Meta-analysis.* https://core.ac.uk/download/59593.pdf (accessed on 12th July 2025).
9. Bhandari, M., Chaudhry, H., Einhorn, T. A., Mundi, et al. (2008). *How good is the orthopedic literature?* https://core.ac.uk/download/142041949.pdf (accessed on 12th July 2025).
10. Bingold, T. M., Huneke, P., Kiessling, A.-H., Moritz, et al. (2013). *Risk factor analysis for fast track protocol failure.* https://core.ac.uk/download/14529228.pdf (accessed on 12th July 2025).
11. Black, P. H. (1981). *Centerscope.* https://open.bu.edu/bitstream/2144/21093/1/Centerscope1981v12n1_web.pdf (accessed on 12th July 2025).
12. Bonica, M., Students of Health Management 721.01. (2017). *Healthcare management primer.* University of New Hampshire. https://core.ac.uk/download/215509297.pdf (accessed on 12th July 2025).
13. Brechtel, K., Kalender, G., Stock, U. A., Wildhirt, et al. (2013). *Hybrid debranching and TEVAR of the aortic arch off-pump, in re-do patients with complicated chronic type-A aortic dissections: A critical report.* https://core.ac.uk/download/17179841.pdf (accessed on 12th July 2025).
14. Brecker, S. J. D., Rahman, M. S., Sharma, R. (2015). *Transcatheter aortic valve implantation in patients with pre-existing chronic kidney disease.* https://core.ac.uk/download/77008396.pdf (accessed on 12th July 2025).

15. Bronicki, R., Checchia, P. A., Dodge-Khatami, A., Karamlou, et al. (2017). *Hematological and infectious complications associated with the treatment of patients with congenital cardiac disease: Consensus definitions from the Multi-Societal Database Committee for Pediatric and Congenital Heart Disease.* https://core.ac.uk/download/85216905.pdf (accessed on 12th July 2025).
16. Camp, S. L., Lobdell, K. W., Nussbaum, M., Reames, et al. (2008). *Quality improvement program decreases mortality after cardiac surgery.* https://core.ac.uk/download/pdf/82340064.pdf (accessed on 12th July 2025).
17. Caruana, N. (2016). *Sleep during and after cardiothoracic intensive care and psychological health during recovery.* https://opus.lib.uts.edu.au/bitstream/10453/43453/1/01front.pdf (accessed on 12th July 2025).
18. Coddington, J., Kirkpatrick, J., Toebbe, S., Yehle, et al. (2012). *Hypoplastic left heart syndrome: Parent support for early decision making.* https://core.ac.uk/download/77938974.pdf (accessed on 12th July 2025).
19. Currie, C. J., Dixon, S., Hind, D., James, et al. (2005). *Economic analysis of the implementation of autologous transfusion technologies throughout England.* https://core.ac.uk/download/56371.pdf (accessed on 12th July 2025).
20. D'Auria, F., & Santo, D. F. (2024). *Robot-assisted coronary surgery: A narrative review on the available data.* https://core.ac.uk/download/635776118.pdf (accessed on 12th July 2025).
21. David, G., Gunnarsson, C. L., Howington, J., Maddaus, et al. (2012). *Surgeons' volume-outcome relationship for lobectomies and wedge resections for cancer using video-assisted thoracoscopic techniques.* https://core.ac.uk/download/28942572.pdf (accessed on 12th July 2025).
22. De Bellis, A., D'Abramo, M., Frati, G., Greco, et al. (2018). *Surgical embolectomy for acute massive pulmonary embolism: State of the art.* https://core.ac.uk/download/188822613.pdf (accessed on 12th July 2025).
23. Delius, R. E., Green, J., Mastropietro, C. W., Sarnaik, et al. (2015). *Prevalence and risk factors for upper airway obstruction after pediatric cardiac surgery.* https://core.ac.uk/download/46960024.pdf (accessed on 12th July 2025).
24. Deuse, T., Ikeno, F., Robbins, R. C., Schrepfer, et al. (2009). *Imaging in-stent restenosis: An inexpensive, reliable, and rapid preclinical model.* https://core.ac.uk/download/323072828.pdf (accessed on 12th July 2025).
25. Diamond, B., Guerrier, G., Holliman, C., Marrero, et al. (2019). *A quality improvement project to determine the incidence and prevalence of obstructive sleep apnea, best practice anesthesia guidelines, and the incidence of perioperative cardiac and respiratory complications after the implementation of the STOP-BANG questionnaire.* https://core.ac.uk/download/301296636.pdf (accessed on 12th July 2025).
26. Emin, A., Kashani, A., Roussel, A., Fou, A. A., Hernandez, A. F., Rastan, A. J., Acheampong, B., et al. (2017). *Extra-corporeal membrane oxygenation for refractory cardiogenic shock after adult cardiac surgery: A systematic review and meta-analysis.* https://core.ac.uk/download/84341450.pdf (accessed on 12th July 2025).
27. Hill, A.-M., Berney, B., Brusco, N., Campbell, L., Chaboyer, W., Choi, et al. (2017). *After-hours respiratory physiotherapy for intubated and mechanically ventilated patients with community-*

acquired pneumonia: An Australian perspective. https://core.ac.uk/download/213606996.pdf (accessed on 12th July 2025).

28. Karck, M., Merkely, B., Radovits, T., Szabó, et al. (2015). *Custodiol-N, the novel cardioplegic solution reduces ischemia/reperfusion injury after cardiopulmonary bypass.* https://core.ac.uk/download/32585907.pdf (accessed on 12th July 2025).
29. Khakwani, A., Rich, A. L., Birkmeyer, Boudourakis, Campbell, Coleman, Baldwin, D. R., et al. (2014). *The impact of the 'hub and spoke' model of care for lung cancer and equitable access to surgery.* https://core.ac.uk/download/42493433.pdf (accessed on 12th July 2025).
30. Kshirsagar, A. Y., et al. (2023). *Advancements in minimally invasive surgery: Enhancing patient outcomes.* https://core.ac.uk/download/596247491.pdf (accessed on 12th July 2025).
31. Leggat, P. (2015). *Medical Tourism.* https://core.ac.uk/download/pdf/30672773.pdf (accessed on 12th July 2025).
32. Manche, A. (2003). *Why Audit?* https://core.ac.uk/download/46601838.pdf (accessed on 12th July 2025).
33. Reynolds, L. A., & Tansey, E. M. (2011). *History of British intensive care, c. 1950–c. 2000.* https://core.ac.uk/download/30696163.pdf (accessed on 12th July 2025).
34. Tilney, M. K. (2003). *Clinical audit: A synopsis.* https://core.ac.uk/download/46601845.pdf (accessed on 12th July 2025).

COLORECTAL SURGERY

13

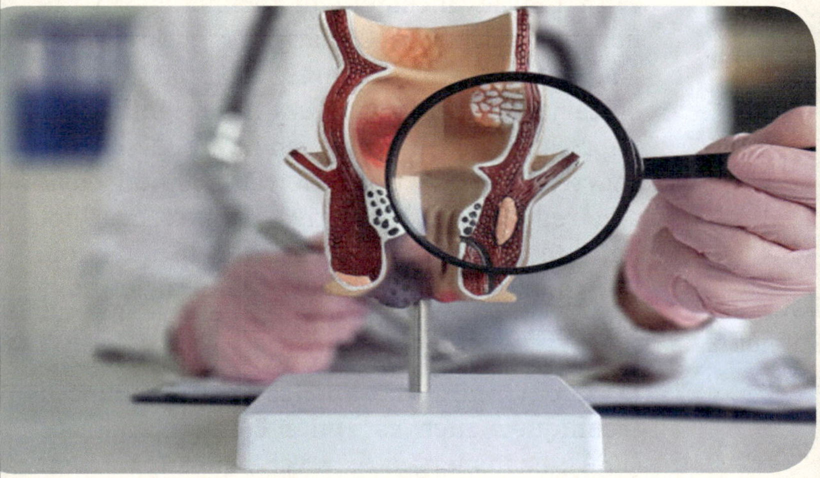

LEARNING OBJECTIVES

After studying this chapter, you will be able to:

1. Understand the anatomy of the colorectal system
2. Explain the indications for colorectal surgery
3. Discuss the types of colorectal surgical procedures
4. Focus on preoperative considerations for colorectal surgery
5. Learn about postoperative care and recovery for colorectal surgery
6. Evaluate the advances in colorectal surgery

Introduction

The overview of colorectal surgery is an essential guide for investigating the evolving face of therapy alternatives for patients with colonic and rectal disease. As a central branch of surgical oncology, colorectal surgery encompasses a range of procedures for managing diseases such as colorectal cancer, diverticulitis, and inflammatory bowel disease. Knowledge of such operations is imperative, especially in the context of the rising incidence of colorectal cancer, which highlights the importance of efficient and timely therapeutic protocols. An overview provides critical insight into the clinical rationale behind operations and highlights innovations such as minimally invasive surgery, which allows for faster patient recovery and improved surgical outcomes. One of the significant elements of the introduction is understanding the anatomical and physiological sophistication of the colorectal region. This sophistication not only influences surgical methods but also forms the basis of postoperative care strategies. Factors like the peritoneal cavity's special anatomy are of central significance in the delivery of site-specific treatment, particularly of peritoneal metastases. It has been suggested that intraperitoneal (IP) drug delivery can optimize treatment outcomes in malignancies of this area. The recognition of these pharmacokinetic advantages, as described in the literature, highlights their importance from a surgical perspective in colorectal malignancies. A balanced introduction allows for an increased understanding of how these mechanisms influence surgical therapy and patient outcomes (Braet et al., 2020). Secondly, the introduction must address the broader implications of colorectal surgery in the context of patient survivorship and ongoing care. The National Cancer Survivorship Initiative (NCSI) addresses the long-term effects of treatment on patients, with an emphasis on a surprisingly overlooked population within oncology (Brooks et al., 2014). This aspect of colorectal surgery emphasizes not only the acute surgical benefits but also the long-term patient quality of life. By examining the problems faced by patients who successfully recover from colorectal surgery, the introduction serves as a springboard to the presentation of necessary support mechanisms and rehabilitation programs. Thus, a good introduction provides readers with a comprehensive picture of the impact of colorectal surgery, both in terms of surgery itself and as part of a broader cancer therapy framework (Figure 13.1).

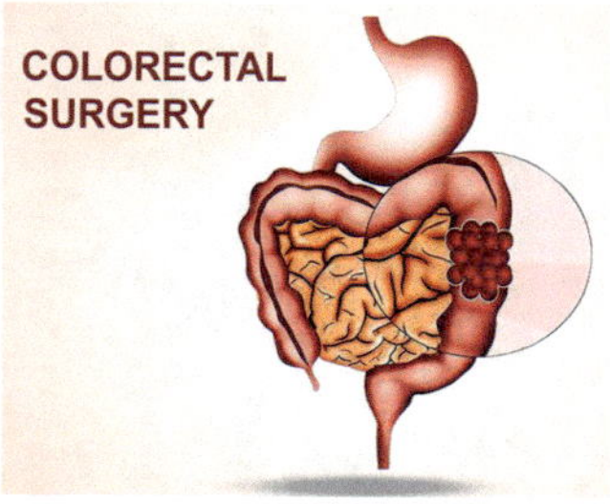

Figure 13.1. Colorectal surgery.

Source: https://res.cloudinary.com/drdawan/image/upload/colorectal-surgery-1554361577.jpg.

Definition of Colorectal Surgery

Colorectal surgery encompasses a variety of surgical interventions of the colon, rectum, and anus for various pathological conditions like cancer, inflammatory bowel disease, and obstructive disease. Both open and minimal invasive techniques are encompassed, and this allows surgeons to have the ease of selecting their technique based on the specific case needs of the patient as well as the type of disease. With the advancement of technology in the field of medicine, particularly in robotic surgery and endoscopic procedures, the precision and efficacy of colorectal surgery have significantly improved. Thus, patients can now benefit from shorter recovery times, fewer hospital days, and reduced postoperative pain. Hence, not only does it cure the condition in question, but colorectal surgery also seeks to improve the quality of life of patients by employing these methods for better outcomes of recovery. In recent years, the application of advanced techniques, such as Finite Element Analysis (FEA), has emerged as a valuable supplement to traditional surgical interventions. FEA can provide greater insights into the mechanical behavior of colorectal tissues during surgery, thereby enhancing preoperative planning and risk assessment. For example, simulations can present how surgical instruments interact with surrounding tissues, which in turn can ultimately refine surgical precision. Through various geometrical models of the colon and rectum, researchers aim to optimize surgical procedures, minimize trauma, and enhance the efficiency of these procedures. Such technological innovations represent a pivotal shift in the conduct of colorectal surgeries, where it is essential to integrate engineering principles into medicine for improved patient outcomes (Bici et al., 2017). Apart from this, technological improvements in surgical tools, such as the development of advanced endoscope positioning instruments, also indicate the advancement in colorectal surgery. These types of technologies are designed to minimize the pain associated with manual handling in minimally invasive operations. Research on evaluation has revealed that the addition of ergonomically engineered tools can significantly enhance the workflow of surgery. For instance, this has been demonstrated by a new one-handed controlled endoscope positioner, which facilitates manipulations during surgery, providing faster setup and reduced operating time without compromising safety or patient comfort. This reflects a broader trend in colorectal surgery, where the convergence of technology and surgical expertise creates a context in which improved surgical performance and patient satisfaction can be achieved (Bauwens et al., 2020).

Importance of Colorectal Health

The health of the rectum and colon is a crucial determinant of overall well-being, yet it is often not given due consideration in public health. The prevalence of colorectal cancer (CRC) is rising at a worldwide level, and hence, it is one of the prominent concerns of health agencies. The World Cancer Research Fund has identified some of the key dietary risk factors to be low fiber intake and high consumption of red and processed meat, highlighting the role of lifestyle components in the development of CRC.

To this extent, awareness and instillation of sound eating habits, along with regular physical activity, can work wonders towards avoiding this cancer. Interventions aimed at promoting dietary behaviors and increasing physical activity levels have also shown promise in reducing CRC mortality rates. Engaging patients in such lifestyle modifications is crucial to enhance their long-term health outcomes and quality of life, particularly among individuals who have undergone treatment for colorectal cancer, as highlighted in community health interventions (Cerin et al., 2013). Screening programs are crucial in ensuring colorectal health, enabling early diagnosis and improved outcomes for individuals with colorectal disease. Such programs can vary significantly in their effectiveness, depending on demographic circumstances, including ethnicity. A study on a population-based pilot fecal occult blood testing (FOBt) screening program has reported low levels of uptake, particularly among ethnic minority groups (Clay et al., 2025). This gap highlights a significant need for culturally sensitive health interventions that overcome barriers and facilitate increased access to screening. It is required that healthcare organizations are well aware of the diverse social contexts of their populations and make colorectal screening procedures sensitive to ethnic differences.

By creating strategic plans that account for these issues, healthcare providers can enhance access to screening, ultimately leading to improved colorectal health outcomes and fewer disparities in cancer care across diverse populations. Raising awareness of colorectal health may also allow individuals to take active steps towards prevention and early intervention. Educational interventions that describe the role of regular screening and lifestyle changes can potentially cause a revolution in public health. By drawing attention to the interrelationship between diet, exercise, and risk for colorectal cancer, the interventions can trigger a shift in attitude in society toward wellness and prevention. Healthcare workers must also actively encourage bowel health discussions to undermine stigmas surrounding colorectal health problems. This not only makes the occurrence of such a conversation an everyday event but also promotes early detection and treatment. Greater awareness leads to practices that can significantly improve the prognosis of patients undergoing colorectal surgery, enabling them to obtain maximum benefit from interventions tailored to their specific needs and circumstances (Cerin et al., 2013) (Figure 13.2).

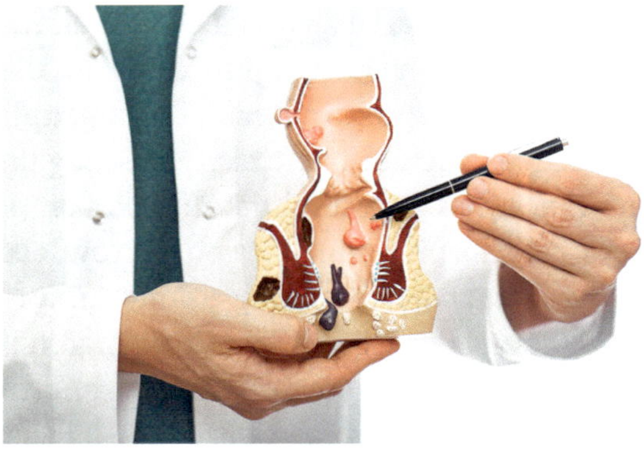

Figure 13.2. The Importance of colorectal cancer screenings and early diagnosis.

Source: https://www.inspirahealthnetwork.org/sites/default/files/2022-03/iStock-1296529394.jpg.

13.1. Anatomy of the Colorectal System

Learning Outcome

1. Describe structure of the colon and rectum
2. Define functions of the colorectal system
3. Discuss common diseases affecting the colorectal area

The anatomical structure of the colorectal system plays a central role in understanding its functioning and applicability to colorectal surgery. The system includes the large intestine, comprising the cecum, colon, rectum, and anus. All these structures play a vital role in the digestive process, facilitating the absorption of water and electrolytes, the formation of stool, and ultimately, the expulsion of waste. The colon, which has four sections in total—the ascending, transverse, descending, and sigmoid colon—performs peristaltic movements to move the fecal material towards the rectum. From an anatomical standpoint, the organization of blood vessels, nerves, and lymphatics in this region is complex, emphasizing the importance of precision in surgical operations. A thorough knowledge of this anatomical configuration is essential for surgeons, as it affects surgical planning and the management of potential complications in colorectal surgery cases. In colonic surgery, awareness of anatomical variations can significantly impact surgical outcomes. The mesenteric attachments and vascular supply to the colon, for example, can exhibit marked variability among different patients, which can become challenging in procedures such as resections and anastomoses. Moreover, the proximity of the colorectal system to surrounding organs, such as the bladder and uterus, requires precise dissection to avoid accidental damage during surgery. Knowing these anatomical subtleties not only reduces surgical risks but also maximizes the effectiveness of methods such as laparoscopic surgery, where accuracy is paramount. Therefore, surgery in this area must be undertaken with thorough planning that reflects the anatomical topography for the best patient outcomes. Additionally, the physiological behavior of the colorectal system should be considered when discussing its anatomy. The peritoneal cavity, for instance, creates a special environment that affects the administration of chemotherapeutic agents in the treatment of colorectal cancer. The intraperitoneal (IP) chemotherapy technique, which leverages the pharmacokinetic properties of this cavity, holds promise for treating peritoneal metastases, particularly in cancers such as ovarian and colorectal cancer. The complex interplay between the anatomy of the colorectal system and its physiological aspects makes it crucial to have a multidisciplinary process of planning treatment. Combining in-depth anatomical insights with advanced therapeutic modalities can lead to improved outcomes in colorectal surgery, particularly in managing metastatic disease (Braet et al., 2020). The knowledge of anatomy is thus crucial not just in surgery but also in oncological treatment modalities and patient care algorithms (Figure 13.3).

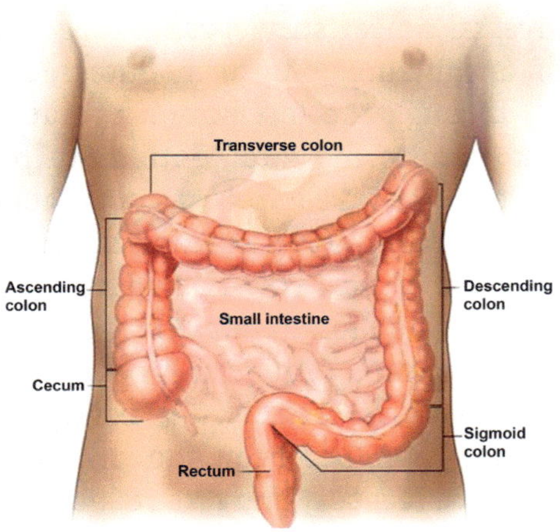

Figure 13.3. Anatomy of the colorectal system.

Source: https://www.surgeoncolorectal.co.uk/media/1041/colon-anatomy.jpg.

13.1.1. Structure of the Colon and Rectum

The colon and rectum are essential components of the human gastrointestinal system, primarily responsible for absorbing water and nutrients, as well as regulating and eliminating waste. The colon itself is most commonly divided into four sections: the ascending, transverse, descending, and sigmoid colon, which are specialized to perform different digestive and waste functions. The anatomical setup of these segments enables the adequate segregation of fecal content, which enters the rectum —a tubular organ that stores feces before excretion. This anatomy not only allows for adequate absorption of nutrients but also assists in body fluid and electrolyte balance control, and therefore the importance of having a knowledge of the colon's anatomy in relation to practice in colorectal surgery. The rectum is the terminal part of the large intestine, transitioning smoothly into the anal canal. Its design structure, lining, and muscular coat carry the most significance in the storage and expulsion of feces. The wall of the rectum has a dense muscular layer that assists in voluntary control during defecation, which reflects its role in both elimination and social behavior surrounding bowel movements. Innervation of the rectum, which is from the autonomic nervous system, influences rectal fullness sensation and urge to defecate. This structural-functional relationship is central to colorectal surgery, as understanding the anatomy of the rectum informs surgical interventions and repairs of defects such as rectal prolapse or cancer, thereby enhancing patient outcomes in this subspecialty. New developments in surgical training have highlighted the importance of learning the anatomy of the colon and rectum through new simulation techniques.

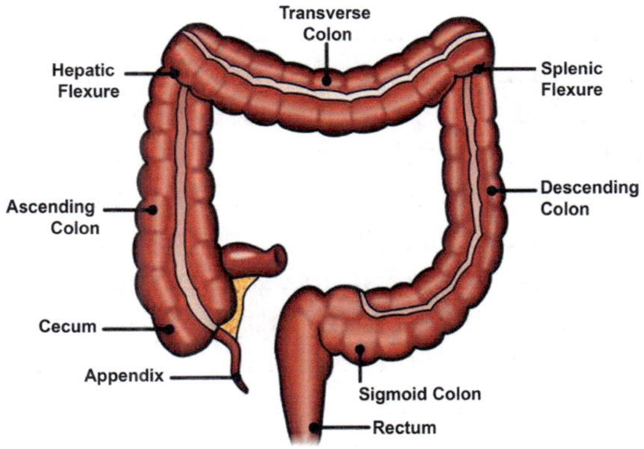

Figure 13.4. Structure of the colon and rectum.

Source: https://fascrs.org/ascrs/media/files/colon_0.jpg.

Virtual reality-based training systems offer an immersive platform for aspiring surgeons to acquire skills essential for laparoscopic rectal surgery. Such systems enable the simulation of realistic interactions between virtual computer-generated tissue and actual surgical equipment, providing both visual and tactile feedback to the trainee, thereby mimicking the intricacy of real procedures. Such technology integration not only enhances learning but also significantly lowers the learning curve for surgical residents. It speaks volumes about the efficiency of today's simulation tools in improving surgical education as well as proficiency in handling colorectal pathology, thus closing the gap between theoretical understanding of the colon and rectum structure and real surgical application in colorectal surgery (MA et al., 2013; Aggarwal et al., 2015) (Figure 13.4).

13.1.2. Functions of the Colorectal System

The colorectal system carries out essential functions within the human body, primarily the absorption and digestion of nutrients and the removal of waste. Located at the end of the digestive tract, the colon takes in water and electrolytes from indigestible food material and transforms it into a solid waste product known as feces. This process is crucial for maintaining homeostasis, as proper reabsorption of water prevents dehydration and enables the effective processing of nutrients. In addition, within the colorectal system, the bacteria play a critical role in fermenting indigested carbohydrates, producing short-chain fatty acids that are beneficial to colonic health and are utilized as an energy substrate by colonocytes. It is crucial to understand these fundamental functions, especially for surgical purposes, as damage or disease to these mechanisms can lead to severe health outcomes. In addition to its function in nutrient reabsorption, the colorectal system plays a significant role in modulating various aspects of physiology, including immune response and metabolism. The colonic mucosa serves as a defense against noxious organisms while allowing selective permeability to beneficial substances. This separation is crucial for maintaining gut immune homeostasis, particularly through interactions with the immune system by gut microbiota. Such a disturbance in these microbial communities has been shown in research to cause inflammatory disease, which can affect colorectal pathology, such as initiation of cancer. For instance, the enhanced immune competence of the colorectal system has led to the development of individualized treatment approaches, such as colorectal cancer survivorship care, with the aim of optimizing long-term outcomes after surgery through the integration of nutritional care and monitoring interventions to prevent the side effects of treatment, as documented in Haggstrom et al. (2019). Further, the colorectal system has a critical role in human health, as evidenced by its modulating effect on systemic immune function. Preoperative optimization of the colorectal setting, for example, with immunonutrition, has been shown to enhance postoperative recovery and also reduce infection rates, as seen in studies on patients with colorectal cancer.

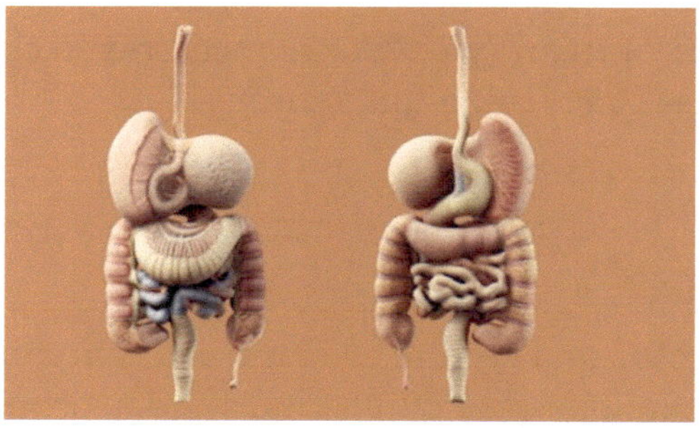

Figure 13.5. Functions of the colorectal system.

Source: https://images.unsplash.com/photo-1743767587835-7a80fe384236?crop=entropy&cs=tinysrgb&fit=max&fm=jpg&ixid=M3w3MDgyMDR8MHwxfHNlYXJjaHwxfHxsYXJnZSUyMGludGVzdGluZSUyMGFuYXRvbXklMkMlMjBjb2xvbiUyMGZ1bmN0aW9uJTJDJTIwZ3V0JTIwaGVhbHRofGVufDB8MHx8fDE3NDk4NTIxMDB8MA&ixlib=rb-4.1.0&q=80&w=500&?utm_source=numberanalytics&utm_medium=referral.

Preoperative oral immunonutrition is also included in the goal of maximizing the patient's immune capacity before undergoing extensive surgical procedures, such as colectomy. Such treatments highlight the potential for an active approach to colon surgery that addresses not only the resolution of the patient's acute surgical issues but also the support of general well-being and resistance to postoperative complications. These findings underscore the importance of a holistic understanding of colorectal functions in the development of successful surgical plans and survivorship care programs that prioritize long-term health outcomes for patients, emphasizing the interconnectedness of surgical approaches and integrative patient care, as noted by Agostini et al. (2017) (Figure 13.5).

13.1.3. Common Diseases Affecting the Colorectal Area

The colorectal area is susceptible to a variety of diseases, of which colorectal cancer is among the most potent health issues confronting the world. The tumor tends to develop from adenomatous polyps, which are the precursors that, if left unattended, can develop into cancer in the future. Risk factors for developing colorectal cancer include genetic predisposition, lifestyle factors such as diet and exercise, and the presence of inflammatory bowel diseases (IBD) like Crohn's disease and ulcerative colitis. The interaction among these factors is crucial in defining the etiology of colorectal cancer, with recent literature illustrating that modifiable health behaviors have a significant impact on disease prognosis and survival in patients undergoing treatment. The identification of these factors brings in its wake enhanced preventive interventions, affirming the efficacy of early detection and intervention of colorectal surgery. Beyond cancer, other disorders significantly affect the colorectal region, including diverticulitis and irritable bowel syndrome (IBS). Diverticulitis occurs when diverticula, small pouches that can form in the colon wall, become infected or inflamed. This condition is characterized by abdominal pain, fever, and changes in bowel habits. IBS, a functional gastrointestinal disorder, on the other hand, is diagnosed from abdominal pain, bloating, and changes in bowel habits without the resulting structural damage. Both diseases have overlapping symptoms, which makes it challenging to diagnose and create treatment avenues. Their management could include dietary modification, medication, and occasionally surgery for the reversal of complications such as abscess or bowel obstruction. The changing presentations and outcomes of these diseases highlight the importance of a multipronged approach in colorectal surgery. Moreover, the impact of colorectal disease extends beyond physical health, significantly influencing the patient's quality of life (QoL). Research has identified various factors, such as gender, co-morbidities, and psychosocial factors, to have significant effects on the quality of life of patients with colorectal cancer and other gastrointestinal disorders. Notably, modifiable factors like fatigue, social function, and emotional function significantly affect perceived QoL (Browne et al., 2011). Interventions such as psychological support and change management can make these changes, likely improving patient experience throughout and following treatment. Similarly, there is evidence that preoperative habits like exercise tolerance and body mass index (BMI) are significant predictors of survival following elective surgeries, indicating the intricate relationship between health behavior and disease outcome in colorectal surgery (Anderson et al., 2017). These kinds of relationships become crucial to define while developing patient-centered care models.

Test Your Knowledge

1. What are the major anatomical divisions of the colorectal system and their primary functions?
2. How does the structure of the colon facilitate absorption and movement of waste material?

13.2. Indications for Colorectal Surgery

Learning Outcome

1. Describe cancer treatment and prevention
2. Define management of inflammatory bowel disease
3. Explain the treatment of diverticular disease

The detection of indications for colorectal surgery is a crucial aspect of managing various colon and rectal conditions. Colorectal cancer is one of the most frequent indications for surgery at various stages. Endoscopic removal is regularly conducted in patients with early colon cancer (pT1), but guidelines emphasize the necessity for additional surgical procedures due to the danger of lymph node metastasis. A survey reported 72.3% of high-risk lesion patients were treated nonsurgically with endoscopic surveillance, with under-treatment concerns in some cases. This report indicates the complexity of clinical decision-making and necessitates careful evaluation of patients based on risk factors specific to individual cases, including age and comorbidities, and also exerts a significant influence on referral rates to surgery (Angeletti et al., 2018). In addition, patients with inflammatory bowel disease (IBD), including Crohn's disease and ulcerative colitis, represent another significant patient group requiring operation for colorectal surgery. The chronic inflammation of these diseases can lead to severe complications such as strictures, fistulas, and even dysplasia, which makes colorectal malignancy a possibility. In such instances, surgery can become imperative in an attempt to resect compromised segments of the bowel in an effort to treat symptoms as well as prevent further complications. The interaction between surgical management and medical treatment must be weighed judiciously, since premature surgery can result in unwarranted morbidity. In fact, total proctocolectomy and colectomy are typically reserved for individuals with diffuse disease or who are unresponsive to medical therapy, demonstrating the central role of individually tailored surgical planning and treatment (Breen et al., 2014). Furthermore, colorectal resection is also a treatment option for patients with complicated diverticular disease, particularly those who experience recurrent abscesses or diverticulitis. If conservative medical therapy cannot be successful, resection can already be performed to prevent further gastrointestinal upset as well as complications such as perforation. Decision-making in such situations is multidimensional; it must be taken based on the patient's overall health, the severity of the disease, and potential complications in the postoperative period. Further, determining the correct time for surgery has the additional effect of enhancing recovery to a great degree and reducing the chances of recurrence. Surgical standards stress the fact that early intervention enables more positive long-term prognoses, especially when using minimally invasive methods that reduce patient recovery periods and related risks (Breen et al., 2014) (Figure 13.6).

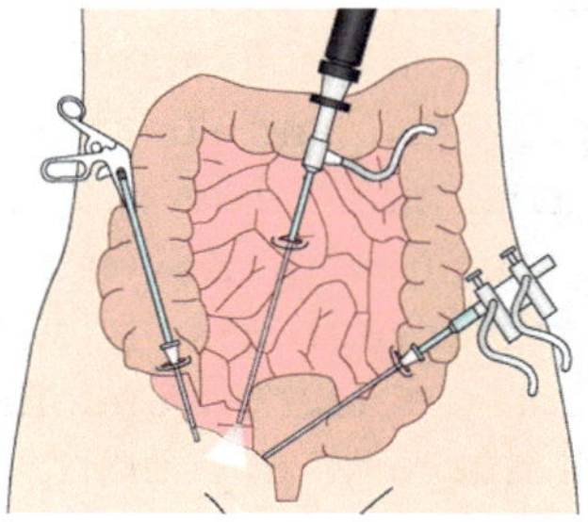

Figure 13.6. Laparoscopic colorectal resection.

Source: https://www.drsanatanbhandarkar.in/images/services/inner/18.jpg.

13.2.1. Cancer Treatment and Prevention

Effective treatment and prevention of cancer are crucial in improving patient outcomes, particularly in colorectal surgery. Early detection of colon and rectal cancers significantly enhances the chances of successful treatment. Diagnostic modalities, such as colonoscopy, fecal immunochemical testing, and CT colonography, are critical for early detection, as they enable the detection of premalignant lesions and asymptomatic cancers. Implementation of evidence-based screening guidelines will be paramount to ensure the maximum benefits of such interventions. In research, its follow-up shows that not only does following such guidelines decrease cancer death rates, but also presentations of advanced disease become reduced, ultimately meaning less intensive future surgical procedures, which will enhance patients' quality of life and survival rate. Aside from screening, it is also essential to understand the profound implications of nutritional status on surgical results, especially in patients who are getting colorectal surgery. Malnutrition is shown to impact postoperative recovery and complicate treatment regimens negatively. More importantly, patients with peritoneal metastases who undergo cytoreductive surgery and hyperthermic intraperitoneal chemotherapy (HIPEC) have significantly higher rates of postoperative complications, most importantly infections, when they are malnourished. An examination of 200 patients undergoing treatment in a clinical setting reveals that the incidence of infectious complications was disproportionate in patients who were deemed malnourished compared to those who were well-nourished. Hence, corrective nutritional interventions before surgery play an important role in cancer treatment and the possible prevention of postoperative complications, justifying the rationale for extensive preoperative screening and customized nutritional management (Carbonari et al., 2019). Furthermore, the incorporation of new surgical techniques and adjuvant therapies illustrates the evolution of colorectal cancer treatment paradigms, thereby maximizing overall effectiveness and safety in patients. Surgical techniques such as minimally invasive surgery and robotic surgery are increasingly popular, offering patients reduced recovery times and fewer complications. Further, incorporation of adjuvant therapy, including chemotherapy and targeted therapies, maximizes the effectiveness of treatments for recurrent cancer. Synchronization of operations with such therapies has given promising results in maximizing survival rates and reducing recurrence. These multidimensional therapies aim not only to eradicate established malignancies but also to minimize the chances of future malignancy, highlighting the importance of multidisciplinary planning of treatment within the cancer treatment pathway, particularly in colorectal surgery (Bracci et al., 2010).

13.2.2. Management of Inflammatory Bowel Disease

Management of inflammatory bowel disease (IBD), that is, Crohn's disease and ulcerative colitis, is multidisciplinary and is a two-pronged medical, nutritional, and surgical management. Early diagnosis and intervention are crucial in preventing strictures, fistulas, and even life-threatening bowel obstruction. Surgery is more indicated in later stages of the disease, particularly when medical treatment has failed or when complications have to be addressed urgently. Surgical treatments such as resection, strictureplasty, or colectomy can be an essential tool in symptom management and quality of life improvement in the patient with an extreme presentation of IBD. In the ever-evolving story of therapy modalities, that is, biologics, timing and choice of surgery are issues of ongoing research and clinical debate on the management of IBD. One of the most significant features of IBD management is the emphasis on multidisciplinary management, which involves collaboration among gastroenterologists, surgeons, dietitians, and psychologists. Nutritional therapy is also a significant feature of this disease because patients are malnourished due to a variety of factors, such as increased intestinal permeability and dysbiosis. Moreover, utilization of Enhanced

Recovery after Surgery (ERAS) protocols, which ensure quicker recovery and less postoperative complications, is an essential milestone in inflammatory bowel disease surgery of the colon. According to existing evidence, the utilization of ERAS guidelines has been shown to decrease systemic markers of postoperative inflammatory response and thereby enhance the surgical outcomes of patients undergoing IBD-related surgery, particularly those who develop complications in the postoperative recovery period (Horgan et al., 2015).

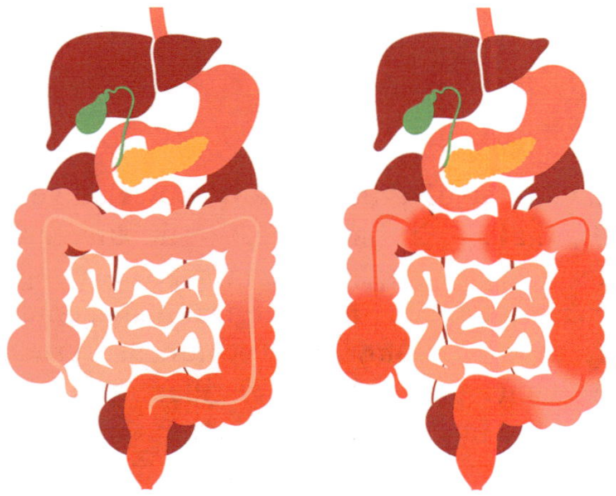

Figure 13.7. Inflammatory bowel disease (IBD).

Source: https://www.hopkinsmedicine.org/-/media/images/health/1_-conditions/stomach-and-gut/inflammatory-bowel-disease-graphic-large.png.

Finally, the care complexity for inflammatory bowel disease calls for highly reflective evaluation of patients' individualized parameters, including their condition overall, scope of intra-abdominal illness, and patient preferences. Decision-making must be a collaborative process with active patient involvement in his/her treatment regimen. Secondly, one has to be able to differentiate between IBD and imitator conditions, such as colorectal cancer, when developing care models, for instance, the increasing acknowledgment of diseases such as endometriosis affecting the bowel (Alexandrino et al., 2018). As the subspecialty of colorectal surgery continues to evolve, ongoing research into novel therapies and surgical techniques will undoubtedly lead to further improvements in the care of IBD, with the promise of enhanced outcomes and reduced complications (Figure 13.7).

13.2.3. Treatment of Diverticular Disease

Treatment of diverticular disease encompasses a spectrum of care tailored to the severity and nature of the disease. For uncomplicated diverticulosis, medical management, including increasing fiber intake, is typically recommended to promote regular bowel movements and ease straining during defecation. Conservative treatment aims at preventing progression to diverticulitis, which requires another treatment course. Surgical intervention is reserved only for patients with recurrent diverticulitis or those with complications, such as abscesses or perforations. The Italian Society of Colorectal Surgery emphasizes the value of evidence-based guidelines in the treatment of diverticular disease, noting that the guidelines should direct but not limit the standards of care provided to patients (Annibale et al., 2015). By adopting a patient-centered approach, healthcare practitioners can better align treatment modalities with patients' needs and preferences, thereby improving overall outcomes. In the management of acute complicated diverticulitis, accurate diagnosis is crucial to successful treatment planning. A good preoperative classification system is essential to determine the correct surgical strategy. Recent studies show the need for computed tomography (CT) scans to assess the severity of the disease. Outcomes in a sample of 152 patients show that high inter-observer agreement between radiologists is directly linked to clinical presentation and intraoperative findings, enabling proper surgical planning and approach (Brachini et al., 2019). The application of such classification systems not only assists in surgical planning but also enhances the predictability of postoperative outcomes. Thus, the introduction of advanced imaging techniques in diagnosis represents a milestone in surgical practice for diverticular disease, highlighting the importance of collaboration among radiologists, surgeons, and general practitioners to optimize treatment options. Besides conservative and surgical treatment, follow-up treatment remains an inseparable component of treatment for diverticular disease. Recurrence risk necessitates ongoing follow-up as well as possibly lifestyle interventions to reduce risk factors for flare of diverticular disease. Patients are often recommended to follow a diet high in fiber, maintain adequate fluid intake, and exercise regularly as preventive measures. Emerging guidelines suggest a growing consensus regarding education and lifestyle changes as preventive measures against the risks of diverticular disease flares. Continued research into long-term diverticular disease management can further individualize treatment regimens and optimize patient benefit. By adopting a holistic approach with a focus on proactive management, clinicians can reduce the burden of diverticular disease and enhance the quality of life for affected patients.

Test Your Knowledge

1. What clinical conditions commonly require colorectal surgery as a primary treatment option?
2. How do symptoms such as bowel obstruction or persistent bleeding help determine the need for colorectal surgical intervention?

13.3. Types of Colorectal Surgical Procedures

Learning Outcome

1. Describe colectomy and its variations
2. Define rectal surgery procedures
3. Understand the minimally invasive surgical options

Colorectal surgery constitutes various procedures to address ailments in the rectum, colon, and anus. The most common operations are resection, which is the removal of an ill part of the gastrointestinal system. It is primarily utilized to correct colorectal cancer, inflammatory bowel disease, and diverticulitis. Surgeons can either do open resection (OS), which involves a large incision in the abdomen, or laparoscopic surgery (LS), which involves small incisions and a scope for directed manipulation. Although OS has been the practice norm, the trend in the direction of LS is due to its benefits, such as reduced postoperative pain and shorter recovery time. However, economic analysis indicates that LS is generally more costly than OS (Group AHTA et al., 2008). This trend suggests the ongoing development of practice guidelines in colorectal surgery. Another critical type of colorectal surgical procedure is anastomosis, which is the joining of two ends of the bowel following a resection of a portion. This is a life-supporting procedure preserving gastrointestinal function and continuity after resections. Life-threatening complications like anastomotic leakage may occur, so careful preoperative planning and postoperative monitoring are necessary. The type of anastomosis—manual or mechanical—and location in the colon or rectum also influence clinical outcomes. Moreover, the improvements in technique, such as minimally invasive approaches, have decreased recovery time and complications. Such innovations have further emphasized the importance of technique and patient selection in optimizing outcomes in anastomotic surgery, underpinning the individualized surgical strategy for colorectal interventions. Endoscopic surgery is a rapidly growing field of colorectal surgery that has profoundly changed the treatment landscape. EMR and ESD have become increasingly common in the removal of large adenomatous polyps, with the potential to avert cancer development.

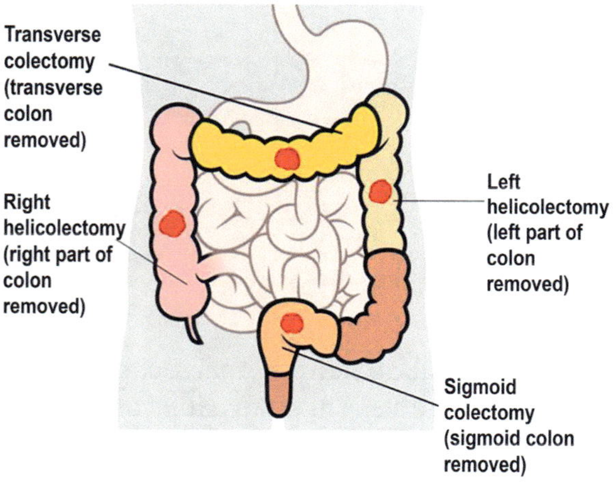

Figure 13.8. Types of surgery for colon and rectal cancer.

Source: https://www.cancer.ie/sites/default/files/2019-12/surgery%20types%20colon%20and%20rectal%20cancer.PNG.

These minimally invasive procedures eliminate the need for more significant surgical removal in the vast majority of cases, with patients experiencing decreased recovery times and less postoperative discomfort. Besides, refinements in endoscopic technology, such as chromoendoscopy and capsule endoscopy, enhance the diagnosis and treatment of neoplastic lesions. With further advances in these endoscopic methods, their application is expected to expand on a larger scale, potentially reducing reliance on conventional surgical avenues and reshaping the practice of colorectal disease management (Arebi et al., 2005). Thus, understanding of these advancements is essential to both the practice of surgery and patient management in colorectal surgery (Figure 13.8).

13.3.1. Colectomy and Its Variations

Colectomy, or the surgical excision of part or whole of the colon, is a significant procedure in the treatment of a broad spectrum of colorectal pathology, such as cancer, inflammatory bowel disorders, and bowel obstruction. Variants of the procedure, including partial colectomy and total colectomy, are tailored to the specific clinical presentation and extent of the individual patient's disease. The decision to undergo colectomy is generally dependent on several factors, including the nature of the underlying pathology, the patient's general condition, and the anticipated outcomes. Newer developments in surgical practice have enabled procedures like laparoscopic colectomy, which have the benefits of reduced scarring, less postoperative pain, and shorter hospitalization when compared to the traditional open procedure. Therefore, the choice between these surgical modalities is a trade-off between effectiveness and patient-oriented care and hence an essential priority in the specialty of colorectal surgery. Laparoscopic colectomy, in particular, has become a standout option due to its minimally invasive nature, which has a profound impact on recovery. Experiments have shown that this disparity can lead to reduced propofol and remifentanil consumption during anesthesia, as demonstrated in a study assessing the impact of transversus abdominis plane (TAP) block on analgesic requirements in patients undergoing laparoscopic colectomy (Jiang et al., 2018). The findings suggest that laparoscopic surgery not only minimizes the extent of the procedure but also optimizes perioperative management, ultimately resulting in improved patient outcomes. However, the effectiveness of laparoscopic versus open surgery remains a topic of ongoing investigation, particularly concerning cost-effectiveness and long-term results. While some research highlights shorter recovery times with laparoscopic approaches, the associated healthcare costs and intraoperative complexities can vary significantly, necessitating careful consideration when determining the best surgical approach for colorectal pathology. Comparative reviews of colectomy approaches on cost show the complexity of evaluating laparoscopic and open surgeries. Systematic reviews of published literature reveal that, although laparoscopic procedures are generally more costly to manage, they are associated with shorter hospital stays and comparable long-term outcomes compared to standard open resections (Group AHTA et al., 2008). Yet, these analyses reveal disparities, with some data indicating that open surgery is cheaper but more effective in certain patient populations. Such indecision underscores the importance of individualized patient evaluation and the need for evidence-based decision-making in colorectal surgery. As surgery technology becomes better and is increasingly refined, the potential of laparoscopic colectomy to be both economic and functional may alter the conventional modalities of colorectal therapy.

13.3.2. Rectal Surgery Procedures

Rectal surgery has evolved, embracing innovations that enhance the precision of surgical procedures and improve patient recovery. Minimally invasive procedures such as laparoscopic and robotic-assisted surgery have transformed the traditional approaches, making it possible for surgeons to perform complex surgeries with minimal trauma to adjacent tissues. All the innovations, including the incorporation of endoscopic devices, have been instrumental. For instance, a newly developed one-hand controlled endoscope positioning system has been designed to facilitate easier handling during procedure. This minimizes setup time, enhances ergonomics, and provides more control and efficiency for the surgeon during surgery. The average manipulation time for angular movements documented was impressively brief, illustrating the sufficiency of incorporating active zooming capacity in endoscopic surgery, thereby optimizing both the surgeon's and patient's operating experience (Bauwens et al., 2020).

Surgical techniques for the rectum are also being refined to address complex conditions such as rectal cancer, and precision in surgical margins can play a determinant role in survival rates. One of the newer procedures gaining ground is Total Mesorectal Excision (TME), designed to remove the entire mesorectum along with the cancer to minimize local recurrence. The conservative nature of TME requires a thorough understanding of the surrounding anatomy, with a special emphasis on preoperative imaging and meticulous surgical planning. The advancements have also highlighted the role of neoadjuvant therapies in conjunction with TME, where the tumor can be reduced prior to surgery, thereby ensuring that resection is safer and more effective. All these are imperative because they not only higher survival rates but also enhance the quality of life for patients post-surgery (Aalbers et al., 2022). Among the surgical procedures, the shift toward global treatment of complex rectal disease underscores the need for multidisciplinary care. The case of pelvic exenteration is the quintessential illustration of such complexity due to mass resections against a background of advanced cancer of the pelvis. Given the intricacies in identifying the organs and tissues involved, centralized treatment in specialized surgical units becomes warranted. The multidisciplinary integration of technological advancements in neoadjuvant therapy, diagnostics, and reconstructive surgery has improved recovery and patient outcomes. As rectal surgery continues to grow, future ongoing research and innovation in the specialty will be required, ultimately leading to further improvement in the management of challenging rectal diseases that demand not only surgical expertise but also greater interdisciplinarity across medical specialties (Aalbers et al., 2022) (Figure 13.9).

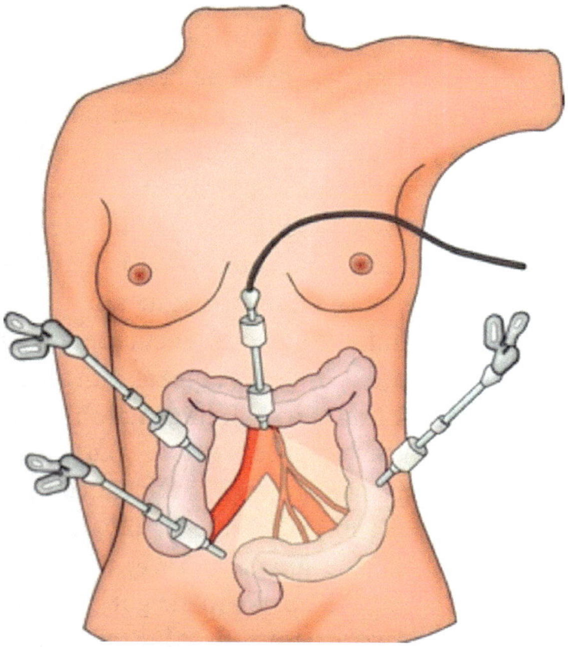

Figure 13.9. Minimally invasive rectal surgery.

Source: https://www.mdpi.com/jcm/jcm-14-01234/article_deploy/html/images/jcm-14-01234-g001.png.

13.3.3. Minimally Invasive Surgical Options

The development of minimally invasive surgical techniques is a significant milestone in the history of colorectal surgery. Traditionally, surgical interventions for disorders of the colon and rectum required enormous incisions, which were a hassle for patients and took months to recover from. Laparoscopic and robotic surgeries have made this trend obsolete by enabling surgeons to perform complex procedures through tiny incisions. These methods not only reduce tissue injury but also decrease postoperative scarring and pain, ultimately leading to a faster recovery and shorter hospitalization for patients.

This change in practice aligns with growing patient demand for less traumatic procedures and faster recovery, emphasizing the advantages of minimally invasive surgery in colorectal surgery. Additionally, evidence from the literature indicates that the adoption of these techniques is associated with improved postoperative outcomes, specifically reduced complication rates. Most colorectal surgeons have incorporated minimally invasive techniques, as indicated in the high number (87%) of respondents to a recent questionnaire that utilized these techniques on a regular basis (Dolan et al., 2017).

Furthermore, the integration of advanced imaging devices and surgical instruments has made complex procedures easier, such that they are performed with increased precision and visual information in real time during the procedure. Conversion to minimally invasive surgical techniques not only demonstrates surgeons' concern for improving patient care but also marks a transition toward evidence-based practices, with a focus on both safety and efficacy in colorectal treatment. Even though the benefits are evident, there are some hurdles to adopting minimally invasive surgery. Inconsistency in surgical training and exposure can hinder the overall adoption of such procedures across geographical areas, as indicated by global differences in surgical oncology training and practice (Are et al., 2016). These obstacles highlight the need for routine training and education to achieve competence in minimally invasive procedures among novice surgeons. In addition, the need for detailed postoperative care, including surveillance of systemic inflammatory responses, is highlighted prominently in colorectal specialty discourse (Dolan et al., 2017). By bridging training gaps and emphasizing the value of minimally invasive approaches, the field of colorectal surgery is well-positioned to further advance patient outcomes while bracing against the challenges of surgical oncology globally.

Test Your Knowledge

1. How do minimally invasive colorectal procedures differ from open colorectal surgeries in terms of technique and recovery?
2. What factors determine whether a patient requires a resection, anastomosis, or colostomy in colorectal surgery?

13.4. Preoperative Considerations

Learning Outcome

1. Define the patient assessment and evaluation
2. Describe preoperative preparation and education
3. Explain the risks and benefits of surgery

Optimal results in colorectal surgery demand efficient preoperative consideration. It is a diverse method of preparing patients physically and psychosocially for the operation. The central theme of such preparation is healthcare professional interaction, for example, surgeons, ostomy nurses, and mental health specialists. Recent research points towards the necessity of multidimensional collaboration in preoperative patient education for colorectal surgery, highlighting the importance of multiple viewpoints in shaping a comprehensive educational landscape (Cameron et al., 2011). The collaboration not only facilitates better patient comprehension but also helps mitigate potential issues that may arise, thereby creating a more supportive surgical environment with a significant impact on post-surgical recovery. A critical element of preoperative preparation is patient education regarding their unique procedures and potential outcomes. For colorectal surgery, the reality of ostomy creation itself, in some cases, presents a most unsettling experience for patients, while causing extreme worry and emotional duress. Studies reveal that early and focused ostomy care education is a prime determinant in allowing patients to adapt to changes in body image and, most importantly, in achieving better postoperative outcomes. Effective preoperative education can lower anxiety levels, enhancing preparedness on the part of patients to take charge of their own care post-surgery (Harris et al., 2019). Thus, providing individualized ostomy care information along with routine preoperative instruction is not only desirable, but increasingly it is deemed essential to the success of the patient following colorectal surgery. Moreover, psychological issues in the preoperative phase cannot be ignored. Anxiety has been shown to impair the ability of a patient to learn relevant information, which could lead to suboptimal attempts at postoperative management. Overcoming emotional and psychological barriers through targeted preoperative interventions is essential as a solution to educational efficiency and patient outcomes. Research highlights the complementarity of reduced anxiety levels and educational academic learning, suggesting that the implementation of formalized preoperative educational programs can contribute to creating a peaceful, more conducive learning environment for colon surgery patients (Harris et al., 2019). With active management of these emotional issues, healthcare practitioners can significantly improve the overall quality of care and help patients better deal with their recovery after surgery (Figure 13.10).

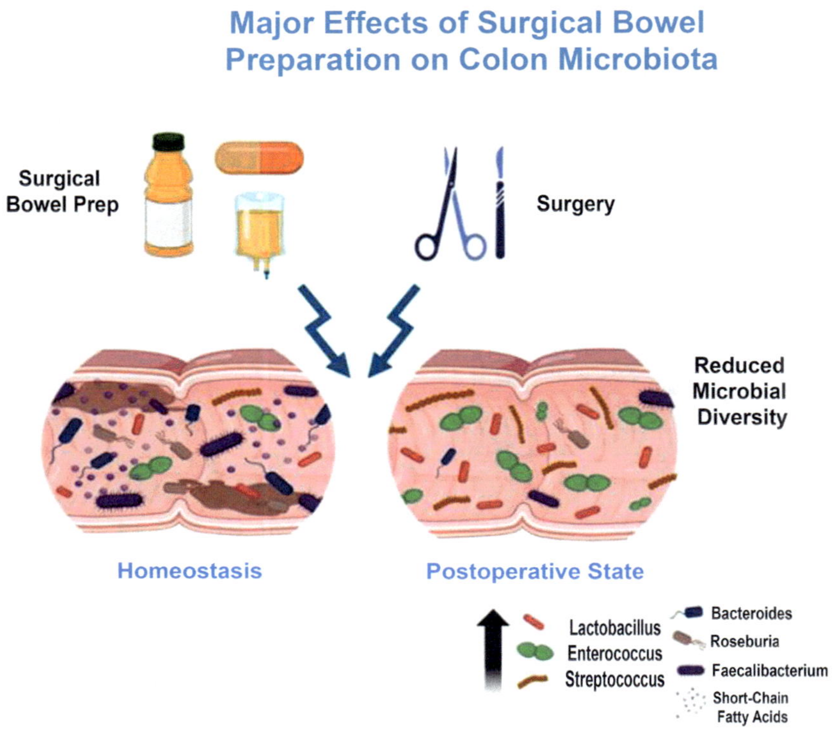

Figure 13.10. The impact of surgical bowel preparation on the microbiome in colon and rectal surgery.

Source: https://www.mdpi.com/antibiotics/antibiotics-13-00580/article_deploy/html/images/antibiotics-13-00580-g001.png.

13.4.1. Patient Assessment and Evaluation

Patient evaluation and assessment are essential processes in colorectal surgery, as they serve to guide each patient in receiving surgical treatment tailored to their specific needs. A good assessment will typically begin with a proper history, which will allow clinicians to gather significant information on the patients' symptoms, medical illness history, and family history for colorectal diseases. Physical examination typically precedes these steps of history taking, where clinicians evaluate for signs such as palpable masses or abdominal pain. The initial evaluation is significant because it helps determine the need for further diagnostic testing, such as imaging studies or colonoscopy, which are critical for diagnosing diseases like colorectal cancer or benign polyps. This master plan not only aids in accurate diagnosis but also serves as a benchmark for measuring the efficacy of treatment and long-term outcomes and thus serves as a firm ground for effective management methods. Once the preliminary evaluation is done, the measurement of patient-related factors becomes the determining factor in identifying the proper surgical technique. The patients' comorbidities, or health and age, all have essential roles in decision-making and anticipated operating outcomes. For instance, determining a patient's cardiopulmonary function is significant because compromised patients may have a higher level of surgical risk. Moreover, the choice between open resection and laparoscopic resection often appears to be based on individual assessments, as laparoscopic procedures are potentially more costly or technically complex, but may also be associated with shorter recovery times, according to a systematic review of economic evaluations (Group AHTA et al., 2008). Therefore, a comprehensive analysis enables health professionals to weigh the potential benefits and drawbacks of different interventions against one another, ultimately leading to informed clinical decisions that prioritize patient safety and quality of life. Last but not least, quality of life assessment following surgery is an essential component of the patient evaluation process in colorectal surgery. In addition to addressing physical recovery issues, the evaluations also encompass psychological and social aspects. Tools such as the EQ-5D are used to quantify the quality of life of patients in relation to their health, enabling the evaluation of health outcomes over time (Dowson et al., 2014). Through the union of quality of life measurement with cost-effectiveness analysis, clinicians are able to develop a better idea of how their surgical decisions impact the daily lives of patients. This holistic strategy not only makes intervention clinically effective but also promotes patients' overall well-being, which is crucial for achieving comprehensive postoperative outcomes. Thus, incorporating clinical and quality of life assessments into patient evaluation is a valuable contribution to the comprehensive treatment of patients undergoing colorectal surgery.

13.4.2. Preoperative Preparation and Education

Preoperative preparation and education are central in the surgical procedure of patients undergoing colorectal surgery. Such educational activities target the physical and psychological needs of patients, thereby reducing anxiety and improving recovery outcomes. Patients who begin colorectal surgery are bound to face various uncertainties regarding their medical procedures, potential physical changes, and recovery timelines. As seen, patients described that they needed to prepare themselves psychologically as well as physically for the surgery, seeking elaborate information about their condition and subsequent rehabilitation process (Bagnall et al., 2017). Being actively involved in this manner not only offers information to the patients but also allows them to be consciously engaged in their care process. Ultimately, an increased understanding of the surgical process can facilitate more robust coping mechanisms and facilitate recovery, supporting the hypothesis that well-informed patients are more likely to experience positive surgical outcomes. Utilization of multimodal preoperative practice education has been a major contributor to improving patient results. By embracing various modalities for delivering education—such as workshops, written documents, and interactive sessions—healthcare practitioners can effectively address the diverse needs of their patients. The qualitative analysis indicates that knowledge and participation are dominant themes underlying postoperative recovery; in relation to whether or not they feel informed, patients are likely to feel confident about their ability to take care of themselves (Bagnall et al., 2017). Additionally, the availability of personalized educational programs can help depersonalize the surgical process. These programs foster collaboration between patients and healthcare providers, enabling a team-based approach to recovery that aims to bridge the gap between patient expectations and the realities of surgery. Additionally, the emotional and social aspects of preoperative instruction should not be ignored. Patients frequently harbor significant concerns about quality of life post-surgery, particularly in contexts like stoma formation, which is a common outcome of colorectal procedures.

Research indicates that preoperative anxieties may stem from misunderstandings about stoma care, leading clinicians to avoid discussions that patients find salient. Addressing these concerns through early and open conversations about potential postoperative scenarios can significantly influence patient decision-making and long-term satisfaction. With the addition of guidance from peers who have successfully navigated similar experiences, patients can gain valuable information that encourages acceptance and adaptation to life after surgery. Last but not least, the delivery of equitable and compassionate preoperative education can be a significant dividend in enhancing the quality of life for patients contemplating colorectal surgery, highlighting the necessity for comprehensive preparatory programs in surgery (Figure 13.11).

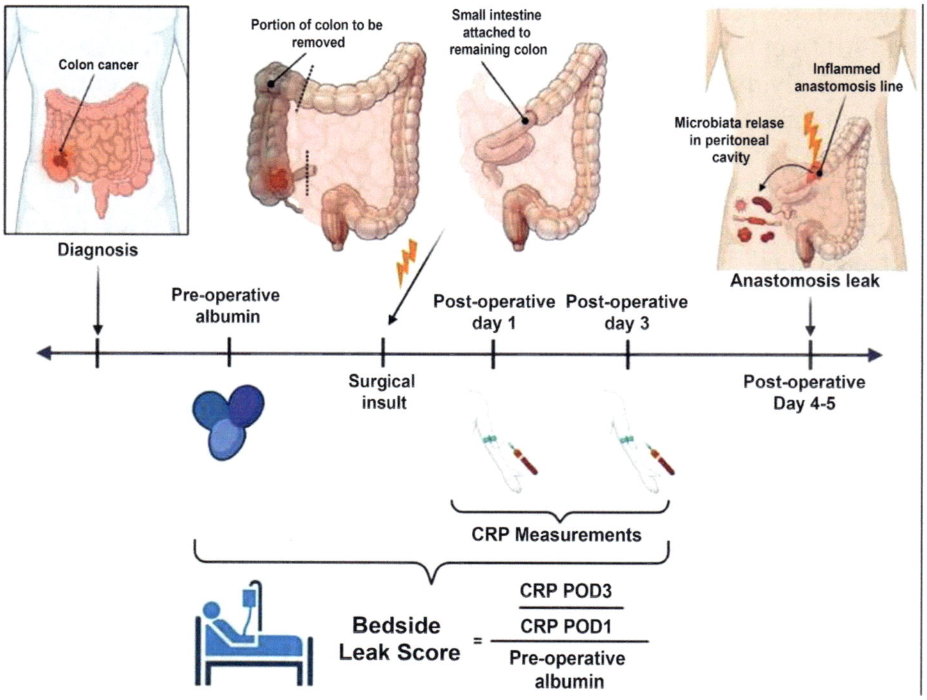

Figure 13.11. Colorectal surgery and proctology.

Source: https://www.frontiersin.org/_rtmag/_next/image?url=https%3A%2F%2Fwww.frontiersin.org%2Ffiles%2FArticles%2F1204785%2Ffsurg-10-1204785-HTML%2Fimage_m%2Ffsurg-10-1204785-g002.jpg&w=3840&q=75.

13.4.3. Risks and Benefits of Surgery

The decision to undergo colorectal surgery is typically a complex consideration of potential risk versus benefit, and thus it is critical to make patients aware of their individual circumstances. One of the most significant benefits of surgery may be eradicating cancerous tissue outright, a dramatic influence on survival rates for patients with rectal or colonic cancer. Surgical intervention can provide relief for symptoms secondary to malignancy, such as bowel obstruction or pain, thereby enhancing the quality of life of the patient. Not all patients may achieve the desired results, and surgical intervention, particularly in populations predisposed such as DMa, can be hazardous. Research indicates that patients with DMa have higher total postoperative morbidity and mortality when compared to the non-DMa counterparts, so patient selection is hence well-thought-out and preoperative workup comprehensive (Bateni et al., 2016). In addition to those risks associated with surgery in the context of colorectal surgery, the postoperative period presents its own array of issues with which recovery and general quality of life could be impacted. Patients have a risk of developing complications, such as infection, prolonged hospitalization, and readmission, each of which can detract from the perceived value of surgery. In the sample population that was under investigation, DMa patients had an alarming rate of complications, including significant morbidity and higher mortality than matched controls (Bateni et al., 2016). These findings support a crucial consideration: while surgery can be a life-saving intervention, it must be balanced against the threat of possible adverse consequences. Proper notification of patients about these risks, especially in relation to their general state of health and the purpose of treatment, is central to informed decision-making for surgery. Further, the higher age of colorectal patients also presents additional challenges in the determination of risks and benefits of surgery. With an aging population in society, it is essential to note the physical changes that occur, as well as the comorbidities associated with advanced age. Older patients may be considered more frail and with less chance of recovery than their younger peers; this ageist perspective brings significant undertreatment and mismanagement of their operative needs. Understanding the multi-faceted aspects of care in and for patients undergoing colorectal surgery, geriatric advances allow practitioners to create tailored treatment protocols that are better aligned with the abilities and health status of patients, ultimately leading to better outcomes and quality of life post-surgery. Surgery should therefore be approached from a patient-centered strategy with consideration that involves thorough risk-benefit analysis at an individual level.

Test Your Knowledge

1. Why are bowel preparation and nutritional optimization important before colorectal surgery?
2. What preoperative evaluations help identify risks such as infection, bleeding, or anesthetic complications in colorectal surgery patients?

13.5. Postoperative Recovery and Care

Learning Outcome

1. Describe the immediate postoperative monitoring
2. Discuss the long-term recovery and rehabilitation
3. Define the potential complications and management

The postoperative care and recovery process following colorectal surgery is critical to patient outcomes as well as the quality of healthcare delivery. This phase is characterized by the presence of a variety of biological markers, such as the systemic inflammatory response (SIR). Higher evidence supports the use of Enhanced Recovery After Surgery (ERAS) protocols, which augment perioperative care to minimize the physiological insult of surgical interventions. Evidence suggests that laparoscopic approaches, a component of ERAS, are most effective in reducing postoperative inflammatory markers, such as C-reactive protein (CRP) and interleukin-6 (IL-6) (Horgan et al., 2015). Targeting the underlying causes of the SIR through such protocols can ensure a faster recovery, fewer complications, and ultimately a better quality of life for patients after surgery. Ongoing monitoring of systemic inflammatory response syndrome has increasingly become an accepted aspect of postoperative care among surgeons. In a recent survey, a decisive majority of colorectal surgeons consistently report monitoring CRP in the postoperative period and actually using this marker proactively to inform clinical decision-making (Dolan et al., 2017).

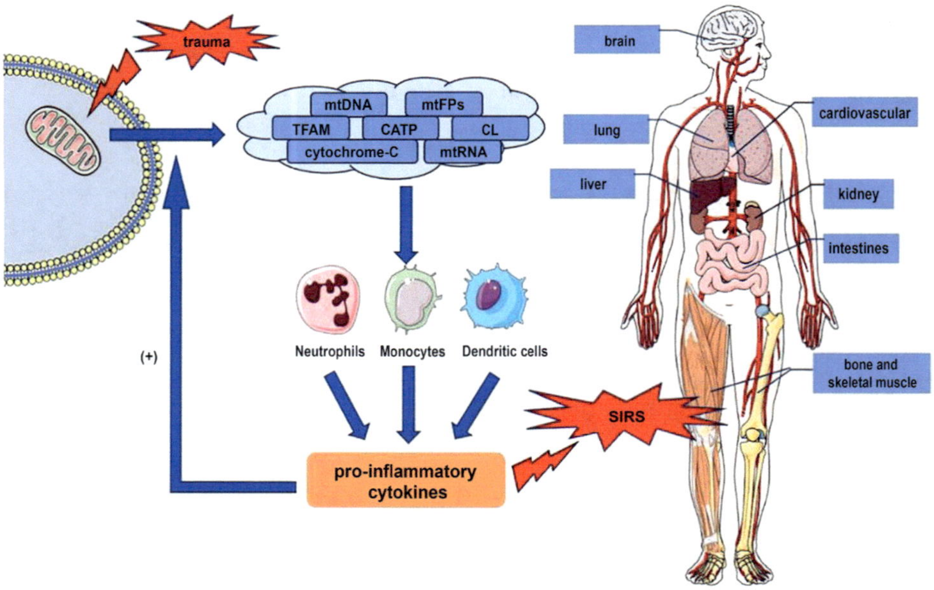

Figure 13.12. The role of mtDAMPs in the trauma-induced systemic inflammatory response syndrome.

Source: https://images-provider.frontiersin.org/api/ipx/w=1200&f=png/https://www.frontiersin.org/files/Articles/1164187/fimmu-14-1164187-HTML/image_m/fimmu-14-1164187-g001.jpg.

Against this background of high CRP and unfavorable postoperative outcomes, incorporating this practice into evidence-based care pathways is crucial for improving patient management.

Surgeons' recognition and responsive behavior are measures of a shifting paradigm, where the inclusion of biological markers in clinical pathways provides a more holistic approach to evaluating patient status and responsive adaptation of recovery methods. It ensures a smoother transition from surgical treatment to full recovery. Besides, proper postoperative care implementation encompasses not only the measurement of inflammatory markers but also an extensive array of supportive interventions aimed at enhancing recovery. Multimodal analgesia, early mobilization, and enteral nutrition support are all integral parts of ERAS protocols that have significant roles in patient recovery and satisfaction. The paradigm shift from the traditional to optimal recovery pathways based on hard clinical evidence all point to the necessity of holistic care in postoperative care following colorectal surgery. Combined, these elements provide a conducive environment for healing, thereby minimizing hospital stays and postoperative complications. Lastly, a focused and systematic approach to postoperative care after colorectal surgery is imperative for enhancing patient outcomes and upholding the importance of continuous improvement in surgical techniques (Horgan et al., 2015).

13.5.1. Immediate Postoperative Monitoring

The importance of postoperative observation after colorectal surgery cannot be overstated, as it is crucial in ensuring patient safety and improving surgical outcomes. Patients are typically admitted to a recovery room after surgery, where their basic vital signs, including heart rate, blood pressure, oxygen saturation, and respiratory rate, are closely monitored. These are preventive care measures that facilitate early detection of complications, including infection or hemorrhage, that can disrupt recovery. There have been findings from research indicating that patients who undergo extensive surgical procedures, such as CRS and HIPEC, have a very high rate of postoperative complications, thus validating the necessity of strict monitoring guidelines. By ensuring that healthcare providers are watchful for even subtle changes in key parameters, intraoperative monitoring is a valuable safety precaution against the onset of potential adverse events during the early recovery phase. Furthermore, the use of individualized postoperative care plans significantly enhances monitoring. Anesthesiologists and surgeons must communicate to develop tailored pain management strategies tailored to each patient's unique needs, particularly opioid use. Research has identified that a considerable number of patients develop chronic postsurgical pain, which often leads to long-term exposure to opioids, and thus recovery strategies are compounded. By employing multimodal analgesia methods that incorporate regional anesthesia techniques, doctors can reduce the use of opioids significantly. Not only does this avoid the risks of opioid dependency, but it also provides patients with a smoother and more enjoyable recovery experience. Enhanced recovery pathways with effective pain management can ultimately decrease complications, increase overall satisfaction, and facilitate early hospital discharge for patients undergoing colorectal surgery. Furthermore, nutritional status is another key factor in early postoperative care that directly influences recovery outcomes. Patients with conditions such as peritoneal metastases who are operated upon are typically at higher risk for postoperative infectious complications depending on their preoperative nutritional status. Evidence indicates that malnourished patients experience a far higher rate of complications, such as surgical site infection and bacteremia. Monitoring in the intraoperative period, therefore, needs to include assessment of nutritional needs so that immune-enhancing dietary support can be started early. This is an extremely valuable proactive approach, as it not only helps during the initial recovery period but also reduces the chances of a prolonged hospital stay and additional procedures. By carefully monitoring nutritional intake and utilizing targeted interventions, surgical teams can create a more robust recovery trajectory for patients undergoing colorectal surgery, thereby optimizing their overall health outcomes (Pozek et al., 2018; Carbonari et al., 2019).

13.5.2. Long-Term Recovery and Rehabilitation

Long-term recovery and rehabilitation following colorectal surgery is a multifaceted process that has a considerable bearing on the outcome for the patient. Recovery from surgery involves not only physical recovery but psychological and social readaptation. Patients may face a range of challenges, including pain management, dietary adjustment, and the possibility of complications such as infection or bowel dysfunction. Rehabilitation of this kind is thus indicated. This program must be patient-specific, and factors such as nutritional counseling, physical rehabilitation, and emotional counseling may be incorporated to enhance the recovery process. With these varied aspects of recovery in consideration, healthcare providers can significantly enhance the quality of life in postoperative patients. Pain relief remains a very much part of long-term recovery, and inadequate control may lead to chronic pain syndromes that complicate rehabilitation. It is remarkable to find that a considerable minority of patients experience chronic postsurgical pain, risk factors for which include preoperative opioid use, anxiety, and substance abuse. Reversal of these preoperatively would be vital in preventing the possibility of long-term opioid use, thereby working counterproductively to recovery processes. Application of multimodal analgesia protocols significantly reduces opioid dependency, thus the likelihood of persistent pain and addiction. Individually and collectively, surgeons and anesthesiologists can tailor intraoperative and postoperative pain control strategies not only to maximize recovery but also to facilitate the transition to long-term rehabilitation after colorectal surgery and enable patients to achieve optimal outcomes. Equally crucial to long-term rehabilitation is the integration of policies to promote patient self-management and enhance care coordination. Innovative policy frameworks can help facilitate prevention and the incorporation of palliative care, which can significantly impact the course of recovery in older patients undergoing colorectal surgery. Research has shown that effective patient self-management is linked to healthier outcomes, particularly when complemented by enabling interventions from care teams. Family caregivers play an essential role as well at this stage of rehabilitation, providing vital and emotional support. Future efforts must focus on expanding such care infrastructures and financing schemes to optimize recovery outcomes, establishing longer-term indicators of success that extend beyond the acute postoperative setting in addressing the multifaceted needs of recovering patients (Morton et al., 2015; Pozek et al., 2018).

13.5.3. Potential Complications and Management

Possible complications of colonic surgery can have far-reaching implications for patient recovery and overall outcomes. Of these, anastomotic leaks at the surgical site where two segments of the intestine are rejoined are particularly grave due to their potential to inflict severe morbidity and even mortality. Treatment of such complications typically includes prompt detection through accurate imaging and physical examination, as well as multidisciplinary management. The significance of strict compliance with clinical practice guidelines is emphasized by the fact that the Italian Society of Colorectal Surgery attaches great importance to evidence-based approaches for optimizing patient care while limiting complications. By following such guidelines, clinicians can maximize the likelihood of successful surgical outcomes while avoiding the dangers of serious postoperative complications that can occur, ultimately creating a guideline for optimal patient care management in colorectal surgery (Annibale et al., 2015). A further critical complication that arises in the course of colorectal surgery is postoperative infection, particularly surgical site infection (SSI), which can cause increased hospital stays and expense. Patients are at risk for inflammation and disruption of regular skin barrier defenses after surgical interventions, making them susceptible to infection. Effective treatment protocols must be applied efficiently to reduce the incidence of SSIs. This entails the use of prophylactic antibiotics administered before incision and meticulous surgical interventions that minimize tissue trauma and provide sterile conditions. Monitoring during the postoperative period also plays a central role in identifying early signs of infection, facilitating early intervention. As reiterated in the comprehensive guidelines on diverticular disease, evidence-based practice cannot be overstated, as rigid compliance with established recommendations can enhance the quality of care and reduce complication rates on the road to recovery (Annibale et al., 2015).

Aside from infection and anastomotic leak, metabolic complications such as electrolyte disturbances may also follow colorectal surgery. Reasons for these imbalances are the response to surgery stress, changes in fluid and dietary intake, and changes in bowel function that can prevent nutrient absorption. Electrolyte disturbances need close attention of the lab values, such as sodium and potassium, particularly in postoperative patients who are at higher risk. It is crucial that healthcare professionals initiate individualized treatment strategies, including proper fluid resuscitation and nutrition, to correct these imbalances in a timely manner. The subtlety of managing post-operative complications, such as metabolic imbalances, underscores the importance of adhering to proven surgical guidelines and protocols, as highlighted in the advanced surgery technology literature. By closely following guideline recommendations, patient care teams can reduce the risk of future complications and optimize outcomes for patients following colorectal interventions (Figure 13.13).

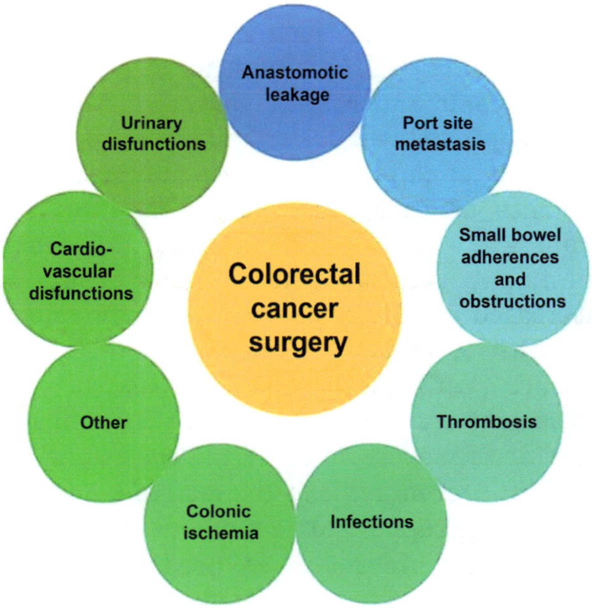

Figure 13.13. Potential complications associated with colorectal surgery.

Source: https://www.frontiersin.org/files/Articles/1452223/fsurg-11-1452223-HTML/image_m/fsurg-11-1452223-g001.jpg.

Test Your Knowledge

1. What measures are essential to prevent complications such as infection or anastomotic leakage after colorectal surgery?
2. How does early mobilization and dietary management influence recovery outcomes in postoperative colorectal patients?

13.6. Advances in Colorectal Surgery

Learning Outcome

1. Describe the technological innovations in surgical techniques
2. Define the role of robotic surgery
3. Discuss future trends in colorectal surgical practices

The landscape of colorectal surgery has been revolutionized with the advent of minimally invasive surgical approaches (MIS), which have transformed the way surgeons manage complex conditions such as enterocutaneous fistulas (ECFs). Current evidence suggests that laparoscopic and robotic surgery, as well as hybrid procedures, offer numerous benefits in terms of improved clinical outcomes. For instance, a systematic review of the literature from 2019 to 2023 confirmed that such minimally invasive interventions result in decreased morbidity and hospital stay among patients. Techniques such as vacuum-assisted closure (VAC) and extracellular matrix plug placement are also now acceptable options in specific scenarios. However, the consistency in surgical procedures and the lack of high-level evidence to support some methods ensure that standardized procedures are needed to further improve the safety and effectiveness of these interventions (Alava et al., 2025).

In addition to the improvement in the surgical technique, metastatic colorectal cancer (mCRC) management is also an aspect where improvement is needed. Given the five-year overall survival rate for mCRC of about 14%, however, there remains an urgent need for innovative treatment approaches that can improve patient survival. Recent progress in targeted therapy and emerging chemotherapeutic agents has promised to prolong survival and improve quality of life in patients with advanced disease. Not only do these advances highlight the complexities of mCRC, but they also underscore the importance of personalized therapeutic approaches tailored to individual patient profiles. Ongoing work in the same direction emphasizes the need for an interdisciplinary approach to colorectal cancer treatment, whereby surgery can be complemented by pharmacologic ingenuity to optimize patient care pathways (Coppola et al., 2024).

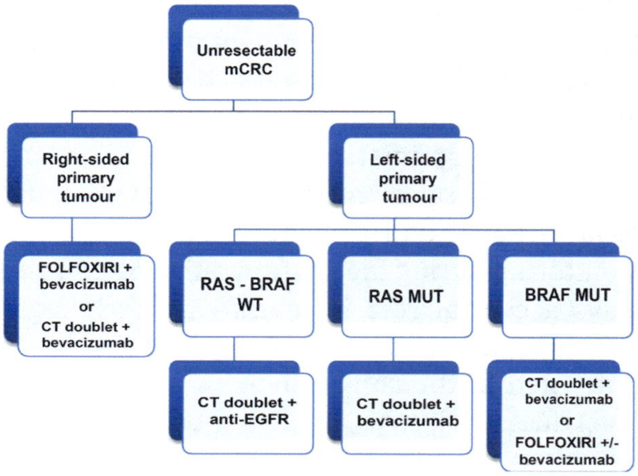

Figure 13.14. Advances in colorectal surgery.

Source: https://media.springernature.com/lw1200/springer-static/image/art%3A10.1007%2Fs12094-018-02002-w/MediaObjects/12094_2018_2002_Fig2_HTML.png.

Additionally, the application of precision medicine is rapidly emerging in colorectal surgery, enabling more tailored care strategies that target interventions based on a patient's unique genetic and molecular disease profile. This can significantly enhance the effectiveness of surgical and medical therapies, leading to highly individualized treatment plans with the goal of achieving improvement. Second, advancements in preoperative imaging modalities and biomarkers enable surgeons to make more informed decisions regarding surgical strategy and timing and thus enhance surgical planning. The intersection of new surgical techniques and precision medicine marks a new era in colorectal surgery, where patient-centered care takes precedence over all else. As technology continues to advance, the intersection of surgical innovation and novel therapies will most assuredly shape the future of colorectal surgery, increasing survival rates and improving the quality of life for patients (Alava et al., 2025; Coppola et al., 2024).

13.6.1. Technological Innovations in Surgical Techniques

The field of colorectal surgery has been transformed by a series of technological innovations that enhance surgical technique and outcomes. Minimally invasive surgery, such as laparoscopy, has become standard due to its ability to reduce postoperative pain and length of stay. Breakthroughs in endoscope development, with the introduction of devices that allow for more natural manipulation, have further reduced the effort required to perform surgery. A particular innovation is the one-handed controlled endoscope positioning device that enhances the ability of the surgeons to carry out procedures with accuracy and efficacy. This tool facilitates adjustments during surgery, making them extremely convenient, with a significant reduction in setup and manipulation times, leading to enhanced surgical workflows and patient outcomes (Bauwens et al., 2020). With the advancement of such technologies, there is an increased need for developing innovations that not only meet technical requirements but also place the greatest emphasis on the ergonomic involvement of the surgeon. Robotic surgery has brought a new sophistication to colorectal surgery. The systems enable surgeons to achieve greater precision, enhanced visualization, and the potential for performing intricate movements in small anatomical areas. By providing a three-dimensional view and increased maneuverability, robotic platforms facilitate procedures that would otherwise be cumbersome with traditional methods. Precision provided by robotics has been linked to lower complication rates and faster recovery times for patients, thereby improving overall patient satisfaction. The resulting high cost of these technologies, however, prompts critical evaluation of their value in clinical application. In this respect, the European Society of Medical Oncology's Magnitude of Clinical Benefit Scale is an important tool for measuring improvements in treatment options in a manner that focuses on patient-oriented outcomes (Aggarwal et al., 2019).

With more technological advancements taking place, emphasizing real-world evidence is even more essential when measuring their impact. Surgical innovations must be tested not only on traditional metrics, such as survival rates, but also on their overall value in terms of patient satisfaction and quality of life. Sustaining new models with a broader array of patient-based endpoints has the potential to reduce the risk of adopting low-value innovations while simultaneously uncovering high-value innovations. This can lead to a more sustainable adoption of new technologies in colorectal surgery. Furthermore, ongoing study and prudent review of new methods will provide a way to ensure that surgical innovation not only propels the specialty forward but also aligns very much with patients' needs and desires (Aggarwal et al., 2019).

13.6.2. The Role of Robotic Surgery

With the emergence of robotic surgery, colorectal surgery has undergone a complete transformation, characterized by increased surgical accuracy, reduced recovery times, and improved patient outcomes. Robotic surgery enables surgeons to perform complex, minimally invasive procedures with the aid of advanced technology that provides a three-dimensional view and enhanced dexterity. This enhanced capability enables the execution of advanced maneuvers within the confined area of the pelvis and abdomen, effectively revolutionizing the approach to treating disorders of the colon and rectum. By doing this, patients can benefit from lower complication rates and shorter hospital stays compared to open surgery. The advanced equipment provided by robotic systems enables better control during surgery, with the potential for improved preservation of surrounding tissues and organs, which is crucial in preventing postoperative complications and facilitating the earlier resumption of everyday routines. Robotic surgery has thus become a key feature of modern-day colorectal procedures. Robot-assisted surgical procedures have, in recent research, been found to be effective in the management of complex colorectal pathology, particularly the advanced pathology involving malignancies and enterocutaneous fistulas. Research has attributed the incorporation of robotic techniques to improved clinical outcomes, including reduced morbidity and shorter hospital stay, which enhances the overall postoperative patient experience (Alava et al., 2025). The precision of robotic instruments eradicates risks associated with conventional surgery, consequently minimizing complication rates such as infection and bleeding. Moreover, surgical resection using robotic systems has yielded promising five-year survival rates in well-selected cases, indicating the advantage of adapting these technologies in treating colorectal cancer. Not only is robotic surgery advantageous for patients in terms of improved survival, but it also enables surgeons to execute more complex procedures with greater ability and confidence. Additionally, implementing robotic surgery in colorectal surgeons' practices necessitates a paradigm shift in surgical training and interdisciplinarity. With the widespread use of robotic systems, surgeons will need to be specially trained to excel at the precise skills required by these procedures. Multidisciplinary teamwork among surgical subspecialties is also a necessity, where surgeons, anesthesiologists, and nursing staff work together to ensure optimum patient outcomes. Emphasizing education in robotic surgery is paramount, especially with its potential to change and establish new standards in the field of colorectal surgery. The combination of robotic support with comprehensive clinical strategies and individualized surgical plans yields enhanced survival and quality of life for patients with colorectal illness, particularly for those who present with complex cases such as synchronous colorectal liver metastases (Bolívar Sánchez et al., 2024). With increasing evidence for robotic surgery, its use in colorectal surgery will undoubtedly become more widespread, bringing future patients increasingly greater hope for curative treatments (Figure 13.15).

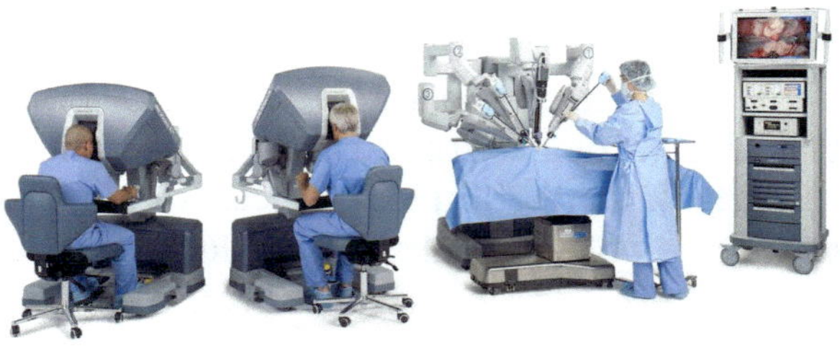

Figure 13.15. Robotic colorectal cancer surgery.

Source: https://cdnintech.com/media/chapter/46206/1512345123/media/image2.jpeg.

13.6.3. Future Trends in Colorectal Surgical Practices

With the evolving practice in colorectal surgery, the use of minimally invasive surgical techniques is the most significant trend revolutionizing the field. Laparoscopic surgery has become widely applicable because it lowers postoperative pain, hastens the recovery period, and reduces scarring compared to open surgery. This shift is supported by growing evidence that indicates improved patient outcomes, including reductions in hospital stay time and rates of complications. The increased ability of surgeons to use laparoscopic techniques and the development of more refined surgical instruments further facilitate this. Apart from that, with the advancing age of the population and the increasing prevalence of colorectal illnesses, there will be an increasing demand for such minimally invasive surgeries, hence further development and innovation of surgical procedures to improve patient experience as well as outcomes (Copeland et al., 2020).

Digital health technologies and telemedicine are bound to revolutionize the practice of colorectal surgery, maximizing preoperative assessment and postoperative rehabilitation. With the rise of telehealth platforms, surgeons can now conduct virtual consultations, facilitating early intervention and diagnosis, particularly for remote patients. Wearable health technology can also be used to remotely monitor patients who undergo surgery, facilitating the detection of early post-surgery complications. Such technologies not only transform the relationship between patients and healthcare providers to facilitate customized care but also optimize the utilization of resources within surgical units. Future developments in these areas will also increasingly involve data analytics and artificial intelligence, leading the way towards enhanced decision-making approaches and individualized treatment plans, ultimately leading to better surgical care (Cullum et al., 2004).

Precision and individualized medicine will significantly influence the future directions of colorectal surgery. With continuing advances in molecular biology and genomics, the potential for creating surgery with tailor-made strategies based on an individual patient's own genetic profile grows. Personalization can occur in preoperative planning, such as in the selection of the optimal surgery method or in the assessment of medical risk from postoperative complications based on genetic markers. Additionally, patient-specific anatomical knowledge, made possible through the use of 3D printing technology and advanced imaging modalities, can inform more effective surgical techniques. Ultimately, the convergence of personalized medicine and surgical advancements will likely improve patient outcomes, streamline care pathways, and contribute to the evolution of colorectal surgery techniques in response to the unique complexities of each patient's individualized needs (Copeland et al., 2020).

Test Your Knowledge

1. How have minimally invasive and robotic-assisted techniques improved outcomes in colorectal surgery?
2. What recent innovations are helping reduce postoperative complications and shorten hospital stays for colorectal patients?

SUMMARY

A critical appraisal of surgery for colorectal disease requires one to recognize that outcomes of surgery are multifactorial, particularly in populations of individuals with varied health backgrounds. The influence of metabolic syndrome on surgical outcome has been a focus of recent studies. Metabolic syndrome is proposed not to significantly influence the result of surgery for colorectal cancer, as indicated by a study wherein 73.1% of patients had zero complications whatsoever at 30 days following surgery. Additionally, the research found no statistical correlation between the components of the syndrome and the rates of surgical success, indicating that treatment of the patient may need to focus beyond metabolic factors to achieve optimal postoperative recovery and minimize complications (Ahmadi et al., 2017). This is one point that highlights the importance of an integrated evaluation of the patient based on an extensive range of comorbidities and predictors of surgical outcomes. Furthermore, the surgical context of colorectal cancer continues to evolve, most importantly in terms of the increasing number of elderly patients on whom such surgeries are conducted. With increased life expectancy, there is a consequent rise in surgical procedures among elderly patients who have additional cardiovascular and pulmonary comorbidities due to higher perioperative risks (Celentano et al., 2017). Yet, contemporary reviews suggest that laparoscopic procedures for this patient population are both effective and feasible, providing results as good, if not better, than those of traditional open surgery. This shift is a positive step in surgical technique, with greater emphasis being placed on minimally invasive approaches, potentially allowing longer recovery and reducing morbidity, a vital consideration where colorectal surgery is performed in the elderly patient. Finally, results from recent research emphasize the importance of continuously evaluating and refining surgical procedures in colorectal surgery, especially in light of demographic trends toward older populations. The observation that laparoscopic approaches deliver lesser morbidity while ensuring patient safety underscores the increased adoption of these approaches in elective surgery for colorectal cancer (Celentano et al., 2017). Meanwhile, the realization that metabolic syndrome cannot directly impact surgical results allows clinicians to hone their focus and allocate resources accordingly. Overall, this convergence of data provides a sound foundation for future studies and clinical practice improvement, ensuring that colorectal surgery remains robust and resilient to new healthcare challenges, ultimately optimizing patient care and rates of surgical success across a wide variety of patients.

In the field of colorectal surgery, there have been significant advancements in diagnosis, improving the accuracy of cancer detection. An improvement is also the employment of rapid evaporative ionization mass spectrometry (REIMS), which possesses high diagnostic accuracy to distinguish between adenomas, normal adjacent mucosa, and colorectal cancer. This technology has an area under the curve (AUC) of 0.96 between cancer and normal tissue, and 0.99 between adenomas and normal tissue, which emphasizes the accuracy of REIMS in the clinical setting. REIMS can also distinguish specific lipid profiles for every tumor feature and thus provide essential prognostic data on tumor differentiation and lymphovascular invasion. Such precise diagnostic capability can have a significant impact on treatment planning and operative outcomes, indicating a promising direction for enhancing patient care in colorectal surgery (Alexander et al., 2016).

Another vital aspect of colorectal surgery is watchfulness over treatment standardization and quality assurance, particularly in the case of rectal cancer treatment. The PROCARE project, launched by the Belgian Section for Colorectal Surgery, aims at addressing heterogeneity in diagnostic and therapeutic approaches to rectal cancer. In an effort to create universal guidelines and foster multidisciplinary coordination, the project aims to enhance patient outcomes by implementing uniform practices at healthcare centers. One of the central elements in PROCARE is the establishment of quality of care indicators (QCI), which cover a range of fields, including diagnosis, surgery, and follow-up. Through ongoing examination of these indicators through a prospective database, the initiative fosters an environment of accountability and practice development in colorectal surgery (Baert et al., 2011). In short, the dynamic nature of colorectal surgery underscores the importance of sophisticated diagnostic tools and standardized treatment protocols in patient care. The application of REIMS in operating rooms enables a high-tech approach to detecting and identifying colorectal cancers, paving the way for targeted treatment strategies. Concurrently, initiatives like PROCARE emphasize the importance of interdisciplinarity in standardization and the minimization of disparities in therapeutic outcomes. With these new techniques gaining ground, the future of colorectal surgery is brightened by increased patient satisfaction and improved results, as it attests to the synergy among technology, teamwork, and clinical excellence in modern healthcare (Baert et al., 2011; Alexander et al., 2016).

KEY TERMS FROM THIS CHAPTER

- Abdominoperineal resection (APR)
- Anal fistula
- Bowel obstruction
- Colorectal cancer
- Crohn's disease
- Hemorrhoidectomy
- Inflammatory bowel disease (IBD)
- Minimally invasive colorectal surgery
- Anal fissure
- Anastomosis
- Colectomy
- Colostomy
- Diverticulitis
- Ileostomy
- Low anterior resection (LAR)
- Pilonidal sinus

CRITICAL THINKING QUESTIONS

1. **Which of the following is the most common site of colorectal cancer?**
   a. Cecum
   b. Transverse colon
   c. Sigmoid colon
   d. Rectum
2. **Which surgical procedure involves removal of the rectum and anus with a permanent end colostomy?**
   a. Low anterior resection
   b. Right hemicolectomy
   c. Abdominoperineal resection (APR)
   d. Hartmann's procedure
3. **A patient with a history of diverticulosis presents with left lower quadrant pain and fever. The most likely diagnosis is:**
   a. Colorectal cancer
   b. Ulcerative colitis
   c. Diverticulitis
   d. Appendicitis
4. **Which of the following is a known complication of total proctocolectomy with ileal pouch-anal anastomosis (IPAA)?**
   a. Short bowel syndrome
   b. Pouchitis
   c. Bowel obstruction due to adhesions
   d. Fecal impaction
5. **Which investigation is most appropriate for screening average-risk individuals for colorectal cancer starting at age 45–50?**
   a. Capsule endoscopy
   b. CT abdomen
   c. Colonoscopy
   d. MRI pelvis

Short Answer Questions

1. What are the common indications for colectomy in colorectal disease?
2. Describe the difference between Crohn's disease and ulcerative colitis in terms of surgical management.
3. What is the TNM staging for colorectal cancer, and why is it important?
4. What are the risk factors for developing colorectal carcinoma?
5. How is a low anterior resection different from an abdominoperineal resection?
6. Describe the surgical options for managing diverticulitis.
7. What are the common causes of lower gastrointestinal bleeding in adults?
8. How is a rectal prolapse diagnosed and surgically treated?
9. What is the role of neoadjuvant therapy in rectal cancer?

Answers to Critical Thinking Questions

1. (d); 2. (c); 3. (c); 4. (b); 5. (c)

REFERENCES

1. Collaborative, P. C. P. (2022). Contemporary Management of Locally Advanced and Recurrent Rectal Cancer: Views from the PelvEx Collaborative. *Cancers, 14*(5), 1161. https://doi.org/10.3390/cancers14051161Abbas, M. A., Fung, A. K. Y., Aly, E. H., Goldberg, S. M., Card, G. V., Ross, N. P., Rojanasakul, A., et al. (2013). *Operative strategy for fistula-in-ano without division of the anal sphincter.* https://core.ac.uk/download/131024702.pdf (accessed on 12th July 2025).
2. Abdalla, A., Armuzzi, A., Verjee, A., Battersby, B., Beddy, D., Bentley, J., et al. (2018). *Patient decision-making about emergency and planned stoma surgery for IBD: A qualitative exploration of patient and clinician perspectives.* https://core.ac.uk/download/109947541.pdf (accessed on 12th July 2025).
3. Aberdeen Health Technology Assessment Group, De Verteuil, R., Fraser, C. M., Hernández, R. A., et al. (2008). *Systematic review of economic evaluations of laparoscopic surgery for colorectal cancer.* https://core.ac.uk/download/177130.pdf (accessed on 12th July 2025).
4. Aggarwal, A., Audisio, R., Banks, I., Collette, L., et al. (2019). *Towards an evidence-informed value scale for surgical and radiation oncology: A multi-stakeholder perspective.* https://core.ac.uk/download/200225252.pdf (accessed on 12th July 2025).
5. Agostini, M., Alfieri, R., Cagol, M., Castagliuolo, I., et al. (2017). *Immunonutrition before esophagectomy: Impact on immune surveillance mechanisms.* https://core.ac.uk/download/154325702.pdf (accessed on 12th July 2025).
6. Ahmadi, A., Alberti, A. V., Goulart, A., Mesquita-Rodrigues, A., Feliciano, C., et al. (2017). *The influence of metabolic syndrome in the outcomes of colorectal cancer patients.* https://core.ac.uk/download/154272615.pdf (accessed on 12th July 2025).
7. Alava, R. R. O., Hernández, K. S., Lopez, J. E. M., Miranda, L. A., et al. (2025). *Advances in minimally invasive surgical techniques for the management of enterocutaneous fistula: A systematic review of clinical and postoperative outcomes.* https://core.ac.uk/download/655504180.pdf (accessed on 12th July 2025).
8. Alexander, J., Balog, J., Darzi, A., Gildea, J., et al. (2016). *A novel methodology for in vivo endoscopic phenotyping of colorectal cancer based on real-time analysis of the mucosal lipidome: A prospective observational study of the iKnife.* https://core.ac.uk/download/77017517.pdf (accessed on 12th July 2025).
9. Alexandrino, G., Carvalho, R., Horta, D., Lourenço, M., et al. (2018). *Endometriosis: A rare cause of large bowel obstruction.* https://core.ac.uk/download/187249141.pdf (accessed on 12th July 2025).
10. Anderson, A., Boyle, T., Campbell, K., Courneya, K., Dignam, J., Haggar, F., et al. (2017). *A retrospective cohort study of the influence of lifestyle factors on survival of patients undergoing surgery for colorectal cancer.* https://core.ac.uk/download/74362645.pdf (accessed on 12th July 2025).
11. Angeletti, S., Antonelli, G., Berardi, G., Brescia, A., et al. (2018). *Clinical management of endoscopically resected pT1 colorectal cancer.* https://core.ac.uk/download/195777521.pdf (accessed on 12th July 2025).

12. Annibale, B., Bellini, D., Binda, G. A., Cuomo, R., et al. (2015). *Practice parameters for the treatment of colonic diverticular disease: Italian Society of Colon and Rectal Surgery (SICCR) guidelines*. https://core.ac.uk/download/54522076.pdf (accessed on 12th July 2025).
13. Are, C., Audisio, R. A., Berman, R. S., Cummings, B., et al. (2016). *Global curriculum in surgical oncology*. https://core.ac.uk/download/46580365.pdf (accessed on 12th July 2025).
14. Arebi, N., Saunders, B. P., Surgical Procedures, Endoscopic. (2005). *Endoscopy: An evolving specialty*. https://core.ac.uk/download/46602009.pdf (accessed on 12th July 2025).
15. Baert, K., Boterberg, T., Ceelen, W., De Ridder, F., et al. (2011). *Quality assurance of rectal cancer diagnosis and treatment – Phase 3: Statistical methods to benchmark centers on a set of quality indicators*. https://core.ac.uk/download/55726774.pdf (accessed on 12th July 2025).
16. Bagnall, A., Basse, L., Carney, K., Chelf, J., Cottle, L., de Aguilar-Nascimento, J. E., Dunn, D., et al. (2017). *Developing patient education to enhance recovery after colorectal surgery through action research: A qualitative study*. https://core.ac.uk/download/84144099.pdf (accessed on 12th July 2025).
17. Barone, C., Capussotti, L., Cognetti, F., Falcone, A., et al. (2014). *KRAS early testing. Consensus initiative and cost-effectiveness evaluation for metastatic colorectal patients in an Italian setting*. https://core.ac.uk/download/231747344.pdf (accessed on 12th July 2025).
18. Bateni, S. B., Bold, R. J., Canter, R. J., Meyers, F. J., et al. (2016). *Increased rates of prolonged length of stay, readmissions, and discharge to care facilities among postoperative patients with disseminated malignancy: Implications for clinical practice*. https://core.ac.uk/download/323069528.pdf (accessed on 12th July 2025).
19. Bauwens, K., Blanckaert, B., De Pauw, T., Dewaele, A., et al. (2020). *A novel hybrid 3D endoscope zooming and repositioning system: Design and feasibility study*. https://core.ac.uk/download/286549295.pdf (accessed on 12th July 2025).
20. Bici, M., Bini, F., Campana, F., Guachi, C., et al. (2017). *Finite element model set-up of colorectal tissue for analyzing surgical scenarios*. https://core.ac.uk/download/141694485.pdf (accessed on 12th July 2025).
21. Bolívar Sánchez, M. K., Castellanos, C. M., García Noriega, D. B., Massé Ponce, J. M., et al. (2024). *Combined clinical and surgical strategies for advanced colorectal cancer with hepatic metastases: Impact on survival and quality of life – A systematic review*. https://core.ac.uk/download/635338704.pdf (accessed on 12th July 2025).
22. Bracci, E., Pizzo, E., Vagnoni, E., van Ballegooijen, M., et al. (2010). *Cost-effectiveness analysis of a FOBT-based colorectal screening program*. https://core.ac.uk/download/1588874.pdf (accessed on 12th July 2025).
23. Brachini, G., Casciani, E., Cirillo, B., Costa, M., et al. (2019). *Differences between computed tomography and surgical findings in acute complicated diverticulitis*. https://core.ac.uk/download/227029115.pdf (accessed on 12th July 2025).
24. Braet, H., Ceelen, W., Remaut, K., Van Ramshorst, C., et al. (2020). *Intraperitoneal chemotherapy for peritoneal metastases: An expert opinion*.
25. Breen, D. J., Clegg, A. J., Colquitt, J., Cunningham, D., et al. (2014). *The clinical effectiveness and cost-effectiveness of ablative therapies in the management of liver metastases: Systematic review and economic evaluation*.

26. Brooks, J., Featherstone, V. A., King, N., Topping, A., et al. (2014). *Supporting people with active and advanced disease: A rapid review of the evidence.* https://core.ac.uk/download/19780349.pdf (accessed on 12th July 2025).

27. Browne, S., Campbell, N. C., Gray, N. M., Hall, S. J., et al. (2011). *Modifiable and fixed factors predicting quality of life in people with colorectal cancer.* https://core.ac.uk/download/151162659.pdf (accessed on 12th July 2025).

28. Cameron, M., Carr, W., Chelf, J. H., Elliott, J., Ely, M., Fearon, K. C. H., Poland, F., et al. (2011). *Multidimensional collaboration: Reflections on action research in a clinical context.* https://core.ac.uk/download/2780307.pdf (accessed on 12th July 2025).

29. Carbonari, L., Cardi, M., D'Agostino, C., Fonsi, G. B., et al. (2019). *Prognostic factors influencing infectious complications after cytoreductive surgery and HIPEC: Results from a tertiary referral center.* https://core.ac.uk/download/195777505.pdf (accessed on 12th July 2025).

30. Celentano, V., Chand, M., Cohen, R., Devoto, L., et al. (2017). *Colorectal cancer surgery in the very elderly patient: A systematic review of laparoscopic versus open colorectal resection.* https://core.ac.uk/download/154748144.pdf (accessed on 12th July 2025).

31. Cerin, E., Chan, W. Y. Y., Cheung, K. K., Fong, D. Y. T., et al. (2013). *Study protocol for "Moving bright, eating smart" – A phase 2 clinical trial on the acceptability and feasibility of a diet and physical activity intervention to prevent recurrence in colorectal cancer survivors.* https://core.ac.uk/download/360506755.pdf (accessed on 12th July 2025).

32. Clay, D., Gumber, A., Johnson, M. R. D., et al. (2025). *Ethnicity: UK colorectal cancer screening pilot – Final report.* https://core.ac.uk/download/49334.pdf (accessed on 12th July 2025).

33. Copeland, L. I. B. T., James, T., Duinkerken, M. S. I., Kelsey, G., et al. (2020). *Jefferson Digital Commons quarterly report: January–March 2020.* https://core.ac.uk/download/299811518.pdf (accessed on 12th July 2025).

34. Coppola, A., Dell'Aquila, E., Gallo, G., Giovinazzo, D., et al. (2024). Editorial: Future frontiers in the management of metastatic colorectal cancer. https://core.ac.uk/download/638805994.pdf (accessed on 12th July 2025).

35. Cullum, N., Dawson, D., Lankshear, A., Lowson, K., et al. (2004). What's the evidence that NICE guidance has been implemented? Results from a national evaluation using time series analysis, audit of patients' notes, and interviews. https://core.ac.uk/download/59840.pdf (accessed on 12th July 2025).

36. Dolan, R. D., Horgan, P. G., McMillan, D. C., McSorley, S. T., et al. (2017). Attitudes of surgeons to the use of postoperative markers of the systemic inflammatory response following elective surgery. https://core.ac.uk/download/84591739.pdf (accessed on 12th July 2025).

37. Dowson, H., Gage, H., Jackson, D., Jordan, J., et al. (2014). Laparoscopic versus open colorectal resection for cancer and polyps: A cost-effectiveness study. https://core.ac.uk/download/29139900.pdf (accessed on 12th July 2025).

38. Grazi, G. L. (2007). Liver resections: Complications and survival outcome. https://core.ac.uk/download/11162431.pdf (accessed on 12th July 2025).

39. Haggstrom, D. A., Robb, B. W., Tarver, W. L. (2019). Usefulness and usability of a personal health record and survivorship care plan for colorectal cancer survivors: Survey study. https://core.ac.uk/download/228066147.pdf (accessed on 12th July 2025).

40. Harris, M. S. (2019). Does preoperative ostomy education decrease anxiety in the new ostomy patient? https://core.ac.uk/download/215413071.pdf (accessed on 12th July 2025).
41. Horgan, P. G., McMillan, D. C., McSorley, S. T., Watt, D. G., et al. (2015). Enhanced recovery after surgery. https://core.ac.uk/download/42369931.pdf (accessed on 12th July 2025).
42. Jiang, M.-R., Li, T., Liu, G.-G., Liu, S., et al. (2018). Transversus abdominis plane block reduces remifentanil and propofol consumption, evaluated by closed-loop titration guided by bispectral index. https://core.ac.uk/download/323067899.pdf (accessed on 12th July 2025).
43. Morton, S., Dunn, W. (2015). Addressing the health needs of an aging America: New opportunities for evidence-based policy solutions. https://core.ac.uk/download/75783019.pdf (accessed on 12th July 2025).
44. Pozek, J.-P. J., Schwenk, E. S., Viscusi, E. R. (2018). Managing prolonged pain after surgery: Examining the role of opioids. https://core.ac.uk/download/213444274.pdf (accessed on 12th July 2025).
45. Swaminathan, D., Swaminathan, V. (2015). Geriatric oncology: Problems with under-treatment within this population. https://core.ac.uk/download/41992493.pdf (accessed on 12th July 2025).

PERIPHERAL VASCULAR DISEASE SURGERY

14

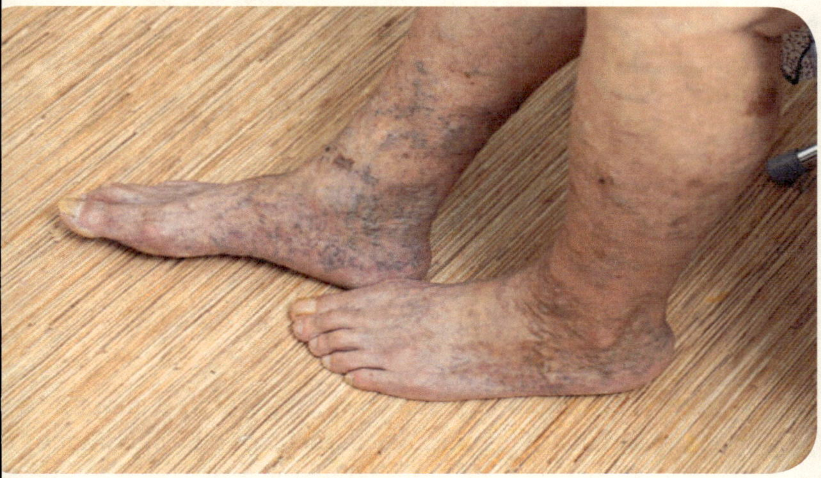

Introduction

Peripheral vascular disease (PVD) is a severe medical condition seen in millions of the global population. With obstructed or constricted vessels, PVD arrests blood flow, primarily to the lower limbs but also to other organs. PVD is more frequent with increasing age and is particularly common in individuals with risk factors such as diabetes, hypertension, and smoking. It is crucial for both the healthcare practitioner and the patient to be knowledgeable about PVD because the disease may readily lead to severe complications like limb ischemia and amputation. Surgical intervention is now a significant aspect of treating PVD as a strategy to restore blood flow and to provide alleviation for the symptoms that accompany this debilitating illness. In PVD surgery, there is a need to explore the cause mechanisms, intervening options, and patient outcome implications, and to integrate a broad perspective of the significance of such surgical procedures in today's medicine. Surgical treatment of PVD has evolved over the last few decades so that there are improved patient outcomes with less procedure morbidity.

LEARNING OBJECTIVES

After studying this chapter, you will be able to:

1. Understand the peripheral vascular disease
2. Explain the types of surgical procedures
3. Discuss the preoperative considerations for peripheral vascular disease
4. Focus on surgical techniques and innovations
5. Learn about postoperative care and recovery for peripheral vascular disease
6. Evaluate the outcomes and prognosis

Endovascular techniques, such as stenting and angioplasty, are increasingly popular because they are less invasive and have shorter recovery times compared to traditional open surgical procedures. These interventions target the precise location of the blockage, allowing for the successful restoration of blood flow with minimal destruction. Moreover, advances in imaging technology as well as instrumentation have allowed for more precise interventions through these means, which have been reflected in favorable outcomes. However, one must consider not only the technical aspects of the procedure but also the overall effects on patients. These are the risk of complications, the need for follow-up, and the long-term advantages implicit in successful surgical treatment of PVD, which all underscore the surgery's role in improving quality of life as well as functional mobility in the affected population. With every new development in peripheral vascular disease surgery, patient education and participation become central to successful treatment strategies. Involving patients in their care process encourages greater levels of treatment adherence and better overall health outcomes. Educating individuals about PVD, its risk factors, and how lifestyle modifications affect them can empower them to become proactive in maintaining their vascular health. Additionally, the intersection of multidisciplinary practice, such as vascular surgeons, interventional radiologists, and non-invasive specialists, ensures holistic patient care that accommodates specific needs. To this extent, then, this favorable trend underscores the importance of not only performing surgical procedures but also ensuring that patients are thoroughly educated and treated throughout their treatment process. Through its method of combining educational and surgical approaches to treating peripheral vascular disease, it is clear that quality care is a complex practice that relies on collaborative healthcare processes (Figure 14.1).

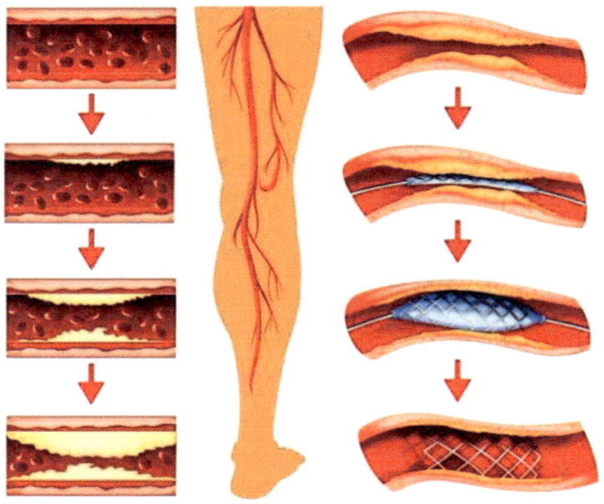

Figure 14.1. Peripheral vascular disease surgery.

Source: https://drtejasdharia.com/wp-content/uploads/2024/04/peripheral-angiography-and-angioplasty-2-1.jpg.

Definition of Peripheral Vascular Disease (PVD)

Peripheral Vascular Disease (PVD) is a common circulatory condition characterized by narrowing of arteries and veins, affecting areas beyond the heart and brain. PVD is primarily caused by atherosclerosis, a condition where fatty plaque accumulates within the walls of arteries, leading to reduced blood flow to the extremities. The clinical presentation of PVD may be variable, from asymptomatic to overt, such as leg pain with exercise, skin color change, or delayed healing. As PVD progresses, complicating factors like critical limb ischemia may develop, to which surgical intervention may eventually result, thus indicating the necessity for an awareness of PVD in relation to surgical treatment considerations. Knowledge of the pathologic basis of the disease is priceless to the management approach, particularly in surgical situations where restoration of blood flow is a top priority. Risk factors that predispose to PVD development are significant and include diabetes, hypertension, smoking, and family history of vascular disease. These risk factors lead to the vascular injury and reduced perfusion that characterize the disorder. In addition, PVD commonly comes with other diseases, such as chronic obstructive pulmonary disease and heart diseases, which will also complicate the case. Peripheral vascular disease, either as a complication of other systemic disease or as a separate pathology, should be clearly known to the clinicians. For instance, patients undergoing surgery with unrelated diseases may have unsuspected PVD, and this can heighten their risks, particularly those concerning postoperative outcomes like renal function impairment, as found in some studies that cited peripheral vascular disease as one of the primary risk factors (de Wolf et al., 2010).

The multidimensionality of PVD requires meticulous preoperative assessment to optimize surgical outcomes. Management of PVD ranges from non-invasive to invasive, with the choice depending on the severity of the disease. Lifestyle changes, medical therapy, and exercise therapy under supervision are typically initial interventions aimed at improving symptoms and function. Surgical treatment, though, remains an important option when patients have severe symptoms or life-threatening complications like critical limb ischemia. Procedures such as bypass grafting or angioplasty target the re-establishment of a normal blood supply to the affected tissues, profoundly enhancing symptoms and reducing the risks of severe complications. Notably, intervention trials such as pentoxifylline have resulted in symptom improvement in chronic critical limb ischemia, and the significance of effective therapeutic regimens for PVD management has even greater emphasis on it (N/A). By recognizing the multifaceted nature of the disease itself, alongside the potential routes of surgical treatment, healthcare practitioners can tailor more effective treatment programs for those suffering from peripheral vascular disease (Figure 14.2).

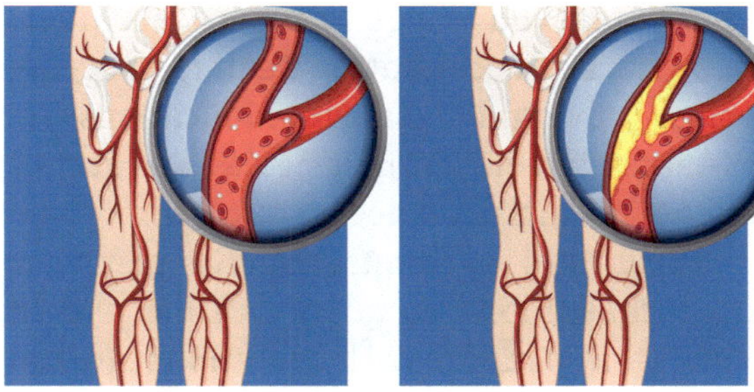

Figure 14.2. Lower extremity bypass for peripheral artery disease.

Source: https://vascularinstitute.com/userfiles/1625/images/3835_3nu4_180617.jpg?t=20201203021228.

Importance of Surgical Intervention

Surgery is a critical component of the treatment of peripheral vascular disease (PVD), as addressing the underlying anatomical and physiological issues that cause considerable morbidity and mortality in patients solves. With the reestablishment of blood flow to pertinent locations, procedures such as bypass grafting and angioplasty will alleviate symptoms of claudication, improve limb viability, and reduce the risk of life-threatening sequelae, including amputations. End-stage PVD patients may present with disabling pain during rest or non-healing ulcers and thus need prompt surgical intervention. Early application of these interventions not only enhances the quality of life in affected individuals but also provides an option to preserve limb function and prevent loss of mobility, which is critical to remaining active and independent. Moreover, the benefits of surgery extend beyond immediate symptom relief to encompass sustained health for PVD patients. Clinical evidence demonstrates that revascularization is very effective in reducing cardiovascular mortality, a common comorbidity among such patients. Given that PVD usually represents widespread atherosclerosis, successful surgery can immensely improve the overall cardiovascular risk profile. By correcting the profound blood flow deficiencies, patients achieve improved oxygenation of peripheral tissues, thereby accelerating healing processes as well as preventing further complications. This cross-talk between vascular health and surgery highlights the importance of integrating such procedures into a comprehensive treatment strategy that improves quality of life and life expectancy in patients with conditions affecting the peripheral vasculature (Acosta et al., 2020). Lastly, dynamic practice of vascular surgery emphasizes the value of tailored strategies in determining surgical treatment for PVD. Emerging imaging modalities and endovascular treatments offer personalized surgical options that minimize recovery times and optimize patient outcomes. Technological advancements have enhanced the surgical armamentarium, resulting in reduced morbidity during perioperative periods. The role of surgery is thus enhanced by the potential for personalized treatment programs that cater to the individual anatomical variations and clinical presentations of each patient. Such individualization represents a radical departure from traditional methods and demonstrates the ongoing development of surgery to improve patient therapy in peripheral vascular disease (et al., 2019).

14.1. Understanding Peripheral Vascular Disease

Learning Outcome

1. Understand the causes and risk factors of peripheral vascular disease
2. Describe the symptoms and diagnosis of peripheral vascular disease
3. Define impact on quality of life of peripheral vascular disease

Peripheral vascular disease (PVD) refers to a class of diseases characterized by reduced peripheral circulation, primarily due to atherosclerosis or the deposition of lipid cholesterol plaques within the arterial wall. Not only does the condition limit mobility, but it also often leads to pain, particularly on exercise, an illness known as claudication. The effects of PVD extend beyond physical suffering; patients face psychological and emotional upset stemming from lifestyle modifications and illness anxiety. The journey of patients with PVD is marked by delayed diagnoses and poor information regarding the disease, accompanied by poor management strategies. As documented by recent studies, the patients tend to downplay their symptoms or are passive regarding treatment decisions, which reduces their overall quality of life (Abaraogu et al., 2018).

Therefore, understanding further is crucial for effective patient care engagement and improving therapeutic outcomes. Moreover, the complexities inherent in the etiology of peripheral vascular disease underscore the need for specialized treatment interventions. Since the condition can range from mild intermittent claudication to severe critical limb ischemia, the patient's experience and needs are also very diverse. The majority of PVD patients are most likely to trivialize their symptoms at first, thus leading to delayed intervention and non-compliance with walking therapies (Abaraogu et al., 2018). Clearing such discrepancies in patient understanding allows for enhanced secondary prevention and active management of their condition. For candidates undergoing surgery, it is even more complicated, as misperceptions of surgical outcomes can influence patient satisfaction and adherence to postoperative measures. Therefore, enhancing disease understanding at each level of PVD is crucial to achieving congruence between patient expectations and clinical reality. The importance of what these patients are going through is also reflected in the field of peripheral vascular disease surgery, where decisions are made. Those patients who are more aware of their disease course are well-positioned to become involved in discussions about surgical intervention and the risks versus benefits. Inadequate understanding of PVD can lead to unrealistic expectations around surgery, placing additional stress on healthcare professionals. Also, as surgical techniques and outcomes continue to evolve, continuing education like PVD, along with in treatment modalities and lifestyle modification, is critical to promoting a more positive patient journey. This empowerment of knowledge not only improves the quality of life for PVD patients but also enables them to take an active role in their own care, making informed choices about their surgical procedures and overall health. The complexity of peripheral vascular disease must be given top priority in efforts to enhance surgical success and improve the overall health of patients with this condition.

14.1.1. Causes and Risk Factors

Peripheral Vascular Disease (PVD) primarily results from atherosclerosis, a condition characterized by plaque buildup in the arterial wall. This buildup of plaque causes narrowing of the arteries, resulting in a reduction of blood supply to the limbs and other extremities. Certain diseases, which also induce PVD, include inflammation of the blood vessels and blood clots, both of which result in poor circulation. Risk factors for the etiology of PVD include age, gender, and race. For instance, individuals over 50 years of age are incredibly susceptible to vascular complications, and men have higher incidence rates compared to women. Racially, African and Hispanic communities are more prone to PVD. Knowledge of such etiologic factors is crucial in planning appropriate surgical interventions and management strategies for affected individuals (et al., 2019).

In addition, lifestyle factors significantly contribute to the assessment of risk in Peripheral Vascular Disease. Among them, tobacco smoking is a significant modifiable risk factor and is also the cause of vascular damage and the pathogenesis of atherosclerosis. The harmful chemicals in cigarette smoke compromise endothelial function, thereby diminishing the blood supply within vessels. In addition, inactivity and poor eating habits increase the risk of PVD. Individuals who have a sedentary lifestyle are at higher risk of developing obesity, high blood pressure, and diabetes—conditions inherently linked with arterial well-being. Diabetes, especially, accelerates the development of vascular disease through the effects on blood sugar regulation and vascular structure. Awareness of these lifestyle etiologies is crucial for both prevention and management interventions by public health programs. Interventions tailored to promote healthier lifestyles could significantly reduce the incidence of PVD among groups (Acosta et al., 2020).

Finally, genetic factors are also involved in being at risk of Peripheral Vascular Disease because individuals with a history of vascular diseases among their family members are at greater risk. Genetic factors may influence lipid metabolism, inflammation, and vascular stiffness, all of which are essential for maintaining healthy blood flow. Paralleling genetic susceptibility, other comorbid disease conditions such as hyperlipidemia, hypertension, and metabolic syndrome exacerbate the impact of PVD. Furthermore, patients with a history of chronic kidney disease and cardiovascular disease are at higher risk, all emphasizing the necessity for strict screening protocols among risk groups. It is in comprehending the intricate interaction of those causes and risk factors that will guide the application of more effective treatment models and surgical techniques pivotal to the management of Peripheral Vascular Disease (et al., 2019) (Figure 14.3).

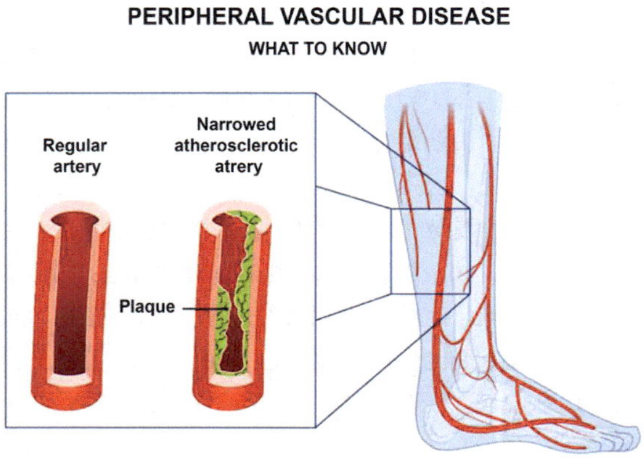

Figure 14.3. Causes and risk factors of peripheral vascular disease (PVD).

Source: https://media.post.rvohealth.io/wp-content/uploads/sites/3/2023/05/1711260-Peripheral-vascular-disease-1296x900-body-1024x711.png.

14.1.2. Symptoms and Diagnosis

The manifestations of peripheral vascular disease (PAD) are primarily due to impaired circulation to the lower limbs, presented as pain and discomfort that significantly impair patients' quality of life. Pain, best described as intermittent claudication, typically occurs in response to physical activity, such as walking, and is relieved by rest. Recurring pain may have a considerable psychological impact, as most patients feel frustrated and powerless due to their impaired mobility. Moreover, other individuals may underestimate or overlook such symptoms and delay visits for medical testing. Such delays can exacerbate the condition, which in turn leads to more severe complications, like critical limb ischemia, wherein the risk of losing the limb is profoundly heightened. Thus, symptoms of PAD must be found and described as a way of identifying them early enough, yet most patients lack an understanding of their disease, which is somewhat the cause of their ailment (Abaraogu et al., 2018). The diagnosis of PAD involves a combination of clinical evaluation and non-invasive testing. Physicians typically begin with a medical history and physical examination, then proceed to the Ankle-Brachial Index (ABI), a series of diagnostic tests that compare blood pressure at the ankle to blood pressure in the arm. An abnormal ABI value may indicate reduced blood flow typical of PAD. Additional imaging tests to be performed include Doppler ultrasound, computed tomography angiography, and magnetic resonance angiography, which provide more detailed information about the vascular anatomy. Regardless of all these powerful diagnostic tools, patient education of symptomatology and implications of PAD remains low. The inability to recognize symptoms leads to delays in seeking care, which ultimately impacts disease management and surgical outcomes.

This ignorance needs to be resolved to improve patient empowerment and treatment efficacy (Abaraogu et al., 2018). Besides that, the psychological and emotional dimensions of PAD living cannot be discounted in the diagnosis process. Powerlessness and anxiety regarding their future are further intensified by the patient's ignorance about their diagnosis and treatment options. It has been indicated by studies that insufficiently informed patients regarding the nature of their disease will most likely have unrealistic expectations of surgical procedures and outcomes. This makes them unwilling to engage in rehabilitation exercises that are very important in improving symptoms and quality of life. Encouraging a holistic understanding of the disease process can enable patients to be more engaged in the management of their treatment pathways and more capable of managing the complexity of the issues posed by PAD. Therefore, a patient-centered model of care enabled by education and psychosocial support is essential for reducing symptoms and improving the diagnosis and treatment of PAD (Abaraogu et al., 2018) (Figure 14.4).

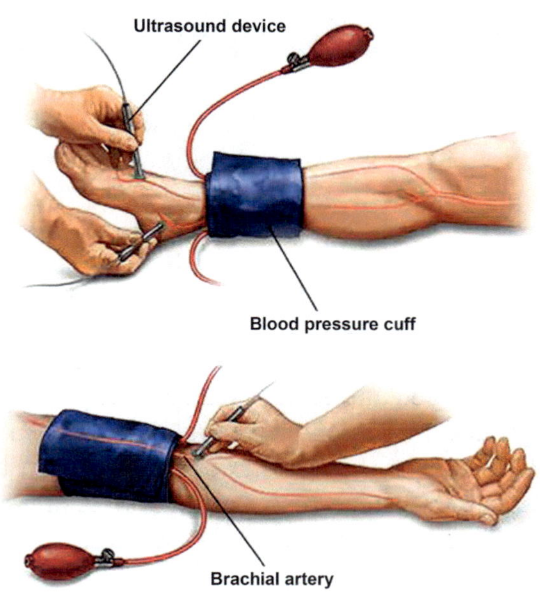

Figure 14.4. Ankle-brachial index.

Source: https://www.mayoclinic.org/-/media/kcms/gbs/patient-consumer/images/2013/08/26/10/58/my00074_im04412_mcdc7_anklebrachialthu_jpg.jpg.

14.1.3. Impact on Quality of Life

The impact of peripheral vascular disease (PVD) on an individual's quality of life is considerable, insofar as it considerably limits mobility and functionality on a day-to-day basis. The symptoms may involve intermittent claudication, the causation of pain associated with exercise, which can lead to severe restriction of walking and social activity. These restrictions not only affect the physical health of the individual but also have psychological impacts, leading to frustration, isolation, and concern for their health status. The National Institute for Health and Care Excellence highlights the value of supervised exercise programs as a first-line treatment for claudication, citing their efficacy in walking distance and function improvement, while simultaneously enhancing quality of life in patients (Cayton et al., 2015). Moreover, the subjective nature of living with peripheral arterial disease (PAD) reveals significant aspects of quality of life that lie beyond physical constraint. Patients frequently report helplessness in being unable to be active daily and frustration due to inopportune attacks of pain. Most patients are found to have insufficient knowledge regarding their disease, and this will lead to delayed diagnosis as well as poor compliance with treatment.

This ignorance generally causes unrealistic expectations regarding surgical interventions, with individuals becoming disillusioned when their experiences fall short of preconceived notions regarding surgery as a magic solution (Abaraogu et al., 2018). Thus, improving patient education and awareness of illness is paramount to promoting emotional resilience and general well-being. Additionally, managing PVD is closely linked to emotional and social well-being. Mobility-impaired patients also experience the deprivation of autonomy, which could become a turning point in their identity and interpersonal relationships within family life. Stigma towards PVD can also occur as a result of societal perception, causing patients to feel isolated and deprived of social contact opportunities. Physical capacity improvement interventions, through guided exercise, not only correct physical discomfort but also develop a sense of community and supportiveness among patients. By restoring individuals' mobility, such programs can significantly reorganize their social life and enhance overall quality of life. As individuals become increasingly capable of coping with the condition, they are more likely to report increased satisfaction with their lives, underlining the importance of integrated treatment strategies that focus on both physical and psychological dimensions of PVD living (Cayton et al., 2015).

Test Your Knowledge

1. What are the common risk factors that contribute to the development of peripheral vascular disease?
2. How does reduced blood flow in peripheral vascular disease lead to symptoms such as pain and tissue damage?

14.2. Types of Surgical Procedures

Learning Outcome

1. Define the angioplasty and stenting
2. Describe the bypass surgery
3. Explain the endarterectomy

Surgical procedures aimed at addressing peripheral vascular disease (PVD) are diverse, each designed to meet the specific needs of the individual patient and the disease. One common approach is endovascular surgery, which addresses narrowed or blocked arteries through minimally invasive procedures. Angioplasty and stenting, specifically, are gaining favor because they reduce recovery time and create fewer complications compared to open surgery. Angioplasty involves the introduction of a balloon catheter to widen the artery, while stenting consists of the insertion of a tiny mesh tube to keep the artery open. Secondly, advances in imaging technology have significantly enhanced the effectiveness of these procedures, enabling precise targeting of areas of difficulty and thereby improving patient outcomes. Open surgical methods remain vital in the treatment of severe PVD, particularly when endovascular techniques are not viable. Bypass surgery is also a standard method, wherein a portion of a healthy vein or prosthetic material is used to divert blood flow around the lesions. This procedure is also essential in patients with extensive arterial blockage threatening limb viability. However, open surgery has a more extended recovery period, and patients are susceptible to infections at the operative site. Existing evidence suggests that the choice between open and endovascular therapy should be guided by patients' general state of health, as well as by the location of blockages and the nature of vascular disease, thus stressing the value of tailored treatment regimens in vascular surgery (Carella et al., 2018).

Furthermore, the integration of new technologies and materials into surgical therapy can produce a significant impact on patient outcomes. For instance, antimicrobial-coated sutures have been among the strategies for reducing the incidence of surgical site infections, an essential concern in any operation. There is evidence to indicate that the application of triclosan-coated sutures reduces the incidence of such infections and is therefore beneficial in procedures of endovascular and open surgery (Carella et al., 2018). The importance of selective surgery extends beyond its direct implications; long-term survival and quality of life for the patient are also dependent on an effective surgical procedure. In the end, an acute understanding of varied surgeries, their risk, and rewards must be present to healthcare practitioners managing peripheral vascular disease patients, particularly when making decisions regarding options such as liver transplant for severe vascular impairment.

14.2.1. Angioplasty and Stenting

Angioplasty and stenting have emerged as the major interventions in the treatment of peripheral vascular disease, which primarily addresses the peripheral artery stenosis or occlusion due to atherosclerosis. The intervention is a catheter-based, minimally invasive one, wherein a catheter is inserted into the blocked artery, a balloon is inflated to compress the arterial plaque, and a stent is ultimately deployed to maintain the vessel patency. The development of drug-eluting stents and coated balloons has significantly enhanced the success of these treatments, enabling superior long-term results. These innovations have become necessary as they minimize the occurrence of restenosis, a frequent complication wherein the artery re-narrows after initial treatment. Their use in clinical situations represents a remarkable evolution in the management of symptomatic peripheral vascular disease, bringing with it prospects of a better prognosis and improved quality of life. The relevance of stenting and angioplasty is also underscored by new clinical trials, such as the RAPID trial, which evaluates the efficacy of pairing the Legflow paclitaxel-coated balloon with nitinol stenting in treating patients with superficial femoral artery (SFA) lesions. This study aims to determine whether the use of this novel balloon can effectively reduce the incidence of restenosis compared to uncoated balloons used conventionally in tandem with stenting. By targeting intermediate and long atherosclerotic leg lesions, the RAPID trial is poised to shed significant light on the efficacy and safety of the Legflow device as a potential alternative in contemporary vascular practice. The research emphasizes the continued evolution within the specialty of interventional techniques, with a focus on optimizing patient outcomes through the utilization of the most advanced technological integrations (et al., 2019). In peripheral vascular disease surgery, the resolution of postoperative complications such as restenosis is paramount. Drug-coated balloons, particularly the Legflow paclitaxel-coated balloon, have been proven to have a potential role in increasing patency rates and reducing the incidence of repeat procedures, thereby reducing overall healthcare costs and patient dissatisfaction. Both hemodynamic and clinical outcomes will be assessed in the RAPID trial, which will compare several endpoints, including the rates of target lesion revascularization and the intervention-related adverse events (de Boer et al., 2013). These comprehensive analyses ensure that continuous improvement and application of innovative techniques in stenting and angioplasty not only address short-term clinical needs but also fulfill the greater purpose of long-term vascular health for patients with peripheral vascular disease (Figure 14.5).

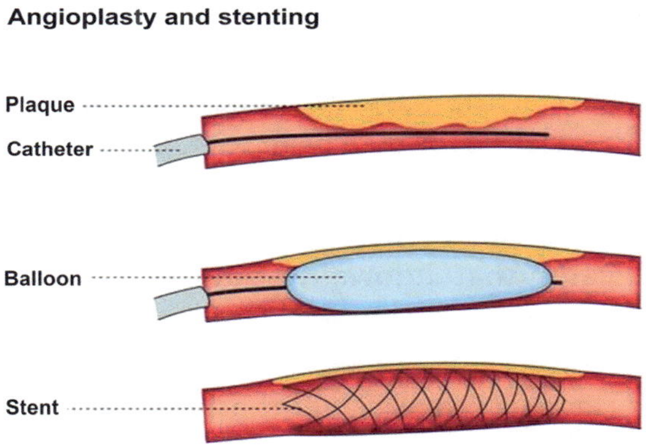

Figure 14.5. Angioplasty and stenting.

Source: https://www.cirse.org/wp-content/uploads/2018/08/Angioplasty600x440.jpg.

14.2.2. Bypass Surgery

Bypass grafting is a fundamental intervention for peripheral vascular disease (PVD) to ensure that an adequate blood supply is reestablished to affected limbs. It serves to provide an alternative path for blood to flow through and bypass blocked sites in the arteries. The blockages can result from atherosclerosis, leading to severe conditions like claudication and critical limb ischemia. With prudent pre-operative evaluation—including imaging studies and interviews with the patients—doctors schedule bypass operations tailored to the degree of the arterial devastation. Bypass surgery is highly effective in alleviating symptoms associated with PVD, thereby enhancing the quality of life and overall functioning in patients. Additionally, good results are associated with post-operative care, which is crucial for monitoring and controlling potential complications, ultimately reinforcing the importance of comprehensive surgical and follow-up procedures in managing peripheral vascular disease (Acosta et al., 2020).

While the benefits of bypass surgery are immense, it is essential to consider the risks and disadvantages that accompany this invasive operation. Complications arising from these include infection, graft failure, and deep vein thrombosis, which can compromise the efficacy of the surgery. Understanding these risks is crucial for both healthcare providers and patients when deciding between surgical options and medical management choices. Research indicates that informing patients regarding their specific prognosis and the likelihood of a successful outcome can allow for more informed decisions. Significantly, advancements in surgical techniques and technologies have also improved outcomes, but surgical candidates must be thoroughly screened for comorbidities that increase the risk of surgery. The relative balancing of potential benefits against inherent risks is a subtle consideration that must be addressed thoughtfully by both patients and surgeons (et al., 2019). In conclusion, bypass surgery remains a crucial component in the treatment of peripheral vascular disease patients. Not only does it try to reduce symptoms, but it also tries to enhance limb viability as a whole in patients with significant arterial obstruction. Successful treatment then by bypass would lead to improved mobility, reduced pain, and even limb salvage in severely ischemic situations. However, whether one should indeed undergo such a surgery or not must be decided with a complete understanding of the individual patient factors, clinical presentations, and what can be achieved postoperatively. This emphasizes the importance of multidisciplinary involvement by vascular surgeons, medical professionals, and the patients themselves with a view to optimizing treatment regimens. Overall, bypass surgery represents a significant advancement in the management of peripheral vascular disease, reflecting ongoing progress in surgical technique and patient care (Acosta et al., 2020) (Figure 14.6).

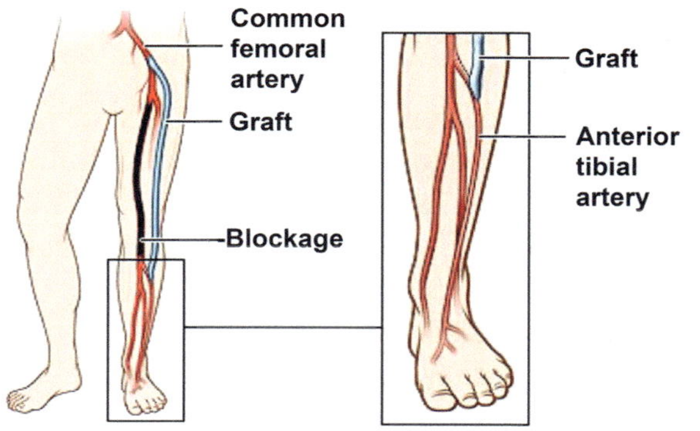

Figure 14.6. Peripheral artery bypass.

Source: https://cdn.bcm.edu/sites/default/files/styles/full_width_component_image_standard/public/media/images/h9991467-001b.jpg?h=637d6f66&itok=lN7UeFAT.

14.2.3. Endarterectomy

Endarterectomy is a severe surgical procedure primarily used for treating blockages due to atherosclerosis in the major arteries, particularly the femoral and carotid arteries. The procedure plays a crucial role in symptomatic peripheral vascular disease patients as it has the potential to prevent life-threatening conditions such as limb ischemia or stroke. The procedure involves the removal of deposits of plaque from the inner lining of the arteries and therefore achieves normal blood flow. The effectiveness of endarterectomy has been highlighted in various clinical studies, which affirm a dramatic improvement in patient outcomes, along with a reduced risk of future cardiovascular events. However, the decision to undergo surgery should be carefully weighed against potential risks, such as postoperative complications, and the overall condition of the patient, emphasizing the importance of a comprehensive preoperative evaluation. The selection of appropriate patients for endarterectomy constitutes the basis for optimizing surgical outcomes. Imaging plays a pivotal role in the selection process, and magnetic resonance angiography (MRA) is increasingly recognized as an effective modality for assessing arterial stenosis. A systematic review of the diagnostic accuracy of MRAs revealed high sensitivity and specificity for identifying patients with severe carotid artery stenosis suitable for surgery, particularly those with 70-99% stenosis, where maximum joint sensitivity and specificity of 99% were illustrated (Airey et al., 2002). Such accuracy is vital, as it helps surgeons determine whether endarterectomy is warranted, thereby impacting patient management strategies. Despite the variable literature on the use of MRAs in deciding on surgery, a call for further studies has been undertaken to optimize diagnostic accuracy and ensure that the results of surgical procedures are optimized. Despite the advantages of endarterectomy, the selection of patients is a multifactorial process depending on the presence of comorbid conditions as well as the overall functional status of patients. Potential for complications, despite the well-experienced operative teams, demands informed consent and considerable preoperative counseling. Technical innovations in the operations and postoperative care have also rendered endarterectomy a safer and more effective procedure. However, continued research into imaging modalities, including contrast-enhanced MRA development, may continue to refine candidate selection and enhance outcomes (Bath et al., 2000). Since peripheral vascular disease surgery is not static, an astute awareness of the risks and benefits of endarterectomy is essential for healthcare practitioners who aim to deliver high-quality, patient-focused care (Figure 14.7).

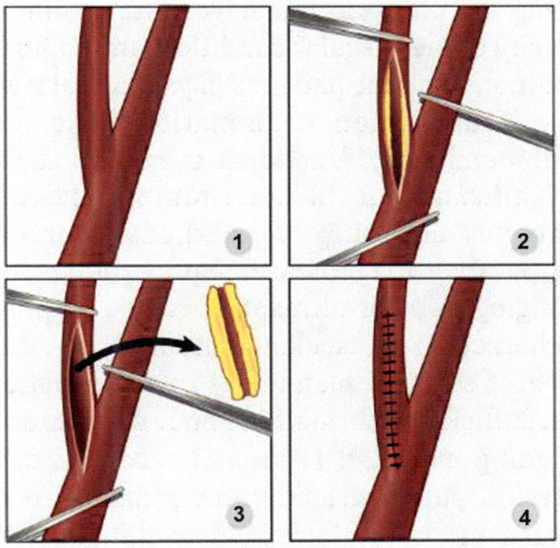

Figure 14.7. Endarterectomy.

Source: https://upload.wikimedia.org/wikipedia/commons/thumb/6/69/Carotid_Endarterectomy_svg_hariadhi.svg/1200px-Carotid_Endarterectomy_svg_hariadhi.svg.png.

Test Your Knowledge

1. How do minimally invasive surgical procedures differ from traditional open surgeries in terms of technique and recovery?
2. What factors determine whether a patient requires an elective, emergency, or reconstructive surgical procedure?

14.3. Preoperative Considerations

Learning Outcome

1. Explain the patient evaluation and selection
2. Describe the preoperative imaging techniques
3. Define the risk assessment and management

Preoperative care for peripheral vascular disease surgery is crucial in maximizing patient outcomes and minimizing complications. Adequate patient evaluation is extremely crucial during this phase, as it involves establishing the severity of the vascular condition, any comorbid conditions, and the patient's physiological status. Risk stratification examinations, including cardiopulmonary functional examination, play a significant role in determining anesthetic strategies and surgical methods. Moreover, preoperative diagnostic imaging studies such as angiography or ultrasound can be employed to characterize vascular anatomy and outline the best surgical planning. Providing patients with sufficient information about the operation, including expected risks and recovery times, fosters a patient-friendly environment, which in turn promotes improved compliance with preoperative instructions.

Concomitant with patient evaluation, optimization of medical management before surgery is a fundamental component of preoperative treatment for peripheral vascular disease surgery. Medication management related to conditions such as hypertension, diabetes, and dyslipidemia needs to be evaluated thoroughly and optimized correspondingly. The employment of antiplatelet therapy also warrants consideration; management of risks for thromboembolic complications, as well as prevention of excessive bleeding, is a delicate issue that should be followed closely. Prevention of complications of anesthesia is an interdisciplinary team effort, typically coordinated by surgeons, anesthesiologists, and cardiologists to coordinate planning of the patient's care. A comprehensive medical optimization plan is developed to minimize intraoperative and postoperative complications, thereby increasing the chances of successful outcomes. Furthermore, handling psychosocial problems is also part of preoperative management in patients who are to be operated on for peripheral vascular disease. Patients can be anxious and unsure about their surgical process, which can have a negative influence on their recovery and postoperative results. The use of psychosocial interventions like preoperative education and counseling can effectively reduce patients' anxiety and increase their knowledge about the surgical process. Moreover, it is crucial to assess the support systems accessible to patients post-surgery to prepare them for recovery. Effective communication of postoperative expectations and potential lifestyle changes is key to supporting patient resilience and compliance. Through such a strategy, holistic management of preoperative factors not only addresses medical factors but also encourages patients' overall well-being and preparedness for peripheral vascular disease surgery (Figure 14.8).

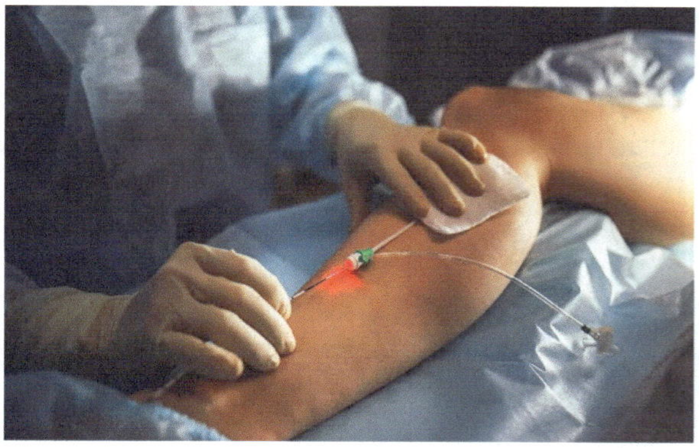

Figure 14.8. Vascular surgery.

Source: https://www.nhrcc.in/wp-content/uploads/2023/04/vss.jpg.

14.3.1. Patient Evaluation and Selection

The patient evaluation and selection process is crucial in the management of Peripheral Vascular Disease (PVD) and forms the basis for optimal surgical outcomes. The healthcare team must first perform a thorough evaluation consisting of the patient's medical history, symptoms that brought them into the clinic, and current comorbidities. Risk factors such as smoking, diabetes mellitus, and active cardiovascular disease are particularly pertinent, considering that they are key determinants of PVD severity and surgical decision-making. As some procedures have divergent results based on underlying pathologies, it is crucial to determine those patients who are most unlikely to benefit. As such, rigorous evaluation becomes the platform from which rational decisions are made regarding possible interventions and the treatment pathway as a whole. Diagnostic imaging and functional testing are among the selection criteria to check the extent of arterial obstruction, which is essential for recognizing the optimal surgical approach. Methods such as Duplex Ultrasound screening are applied in the examination of carotid and peripheral artery diseases, providing essential information on the grades of stenosis and occlusion. The quality of screening services plays a significant role in determining patient outcomes, as evidenced by studies comparing stroke disease evaluation standards. The diagnostic model created through the use of multiple modalities, such as angiography and Duplex scanning, enhances clinicians' perception of disease severity and aids in the formulation of individualized treatment plans. By optimizing these diagnostic protocols, clinicians can more accurately predict technical challenges and potential complications for surgery. Lastly, the decision to proceed with surgery involves a risk assessment that transcends teamwork among multidisciplinary teams comprising surgeons, radiologists, and general practitioners. Sufficient communication and coordinated care models ensure that all parties are aligned regarding the treatment goals. The collective efforts are further supported by the application of proven prognostic indicators that have been researched and tested through work conducted by institutions such as St. Luke's Hospital. Based on evidence-based standards, not only are the candidates chosen for surgery, but also realistic expectations about recovery and outcome are established. Patient assessment and selection, therefore, transcend simple consideration of clinical data to become an all-encompassing exercise prioritizing patient-centered care in the context of Peripheral Vascular Disease Surgery (Figure 14.9).

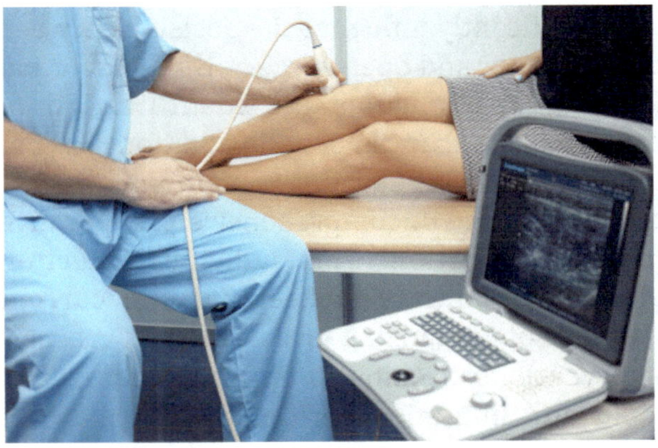

Figure 14.9. Duplex ultrasound screening.

Source: https://santancv.com/wp-content/uploads/2020/02/arterial-ultrasound.png.

14.3.2. Preoperative Imaging Techniques

Regarding preoperative planning in surgery for peripheral vascular disease, preoperative imaging modalities are necessary to diagnose and plan interventions accurately. Imaging modalities, including ultrasound, computed tomography (CT), and magnetic resonance angiography (MRA), provide detailed vascular anatomy and disease information. Ultrasound, particularly duplex ultrasonography, remains a first-line modality, with real-time visualization of blood flow and vessel morphology. CT angiography provides a detailed visualization, enabling three-dimensional reconstruction for the assessment of complex vascular lesions. The use of these new imaging techniques not only enhances the surgeon's knowledge about the area of interest but also informs surgical planning and patient management, ultimately aiming to reduce complications and maximize outcomes. Additionally, post-processing of the preoperative images enhances patient selection for surgery. The detailed evaluation of vascular anatomy enables the tailoring of methods based on individual anatomical variations and pathology identified through imaging studies. For example, the extent of stenosis or occlusion can significantly influence the decision between endovascular and open surgery. High-resolution imaging also enables the identification of comorbidities that can pose an additional risk to the patient during surgery, further emphasizing the importance of comprehensive preoperative patient evaluation. This judicious selection strategy is entirely in keeping with current methods of minimizing invasiveness in vascular interventions, seeking to optimize therapeutic yield and minimize perioperative risks. The development of imaging technology has further enhanced the accuracy of preoperative assessment in peripheral vascular surgery. Technologies like intraoperative ultrasound and fluoroscopy enhance real-time intraoperative decision-making, allowing intraoperative data to be responded to instantaneously. This ripple effect of improving accuracy also extends to postoperative patient care, such that continuous assessment using imaging modalities can lead to early intervention in the event of complications. With practitioners adopting these advanced methods, they significantly contribute to establishing a standard protocol for peripheral vascular disease treatment, ensuring that preoperative and postoperative pathways are well-documented and clinically established. The importance of standard practice in vascular surgery has underscored the crucial role that imaging plays in achieving successful surgical outcomes, as emphasized in current clinical research and best practice guidelines (Agnihotri et al., 2016; Poldermans et al., 2009).

14.3.3. Risk Assessment and Management

For peripheral vascular disease (PVD) surgery, and practical risk assessment and management are key components in optimizing patient outcomes. PVD is a multi-factorial condition that requires clinicians to thoroughly evaluate patient-specific factors such as diabetes, hypertension, and hyperlipidemia comorbidities before surgery. All of these factors can potentially complicate the surgery and post-surgical recovery process critically. A detailed evaluation also includes assessing the extent of arterial occlusion and the functional status of the patients, which further helps in tailoring the surgical strategy and predicting potential complications. The application of instruments to assess risk can facilitate the stratification of patients based on their likelihood of unfavorable outcomes, ultimately informing clinical decision-making and resource allocation in surgery. The application of systematic preoperative evaluation facilitates evidence-based practice, thereby ensuring patient safety and satisfaction. Further, PVD surgery risk management also extends beyond preoperative evaluation to intraoperative and postoperative factors. During preoperative planning of the surgery, an understanding of the likelihood of complications in the form of infection, bleeding, or thromboembolism is essential. Intraoperative monitoring and the use of newer vascular imaging technology can help minimize complications by allowing real-time assessment of blood flow and graft integrity. Postoperative management will require careful vigilance for the onset of complications, as well as an ideal rehabilitation regimen for problems like mobility and cardiovascular status. In addition, adjuvant pharmacotherapy will be carefully considered to address underlying pathologies and mitigate risks following surgery. As noted in more recent literature, the addition of specific vasoactive medications may have an adjunctive role in optimizing patient outcome, exceptionally when surgical revascularization cannot always be the ideal choice (Backer D et al., 2010). Ultimately, a thorough and systematic approach to risk management and evaluation in PVD surgery not only optimizes surgical success but also supports long-term health outcomes for patients. Multidisciplinary collaborative care models can enhance risk stratification and management processes by employing an interdisciplinary group of vascular surgeons, cardiologists, and rehabilitation physicians. Multidisciplinary collaboration enables clinicians to comprehensively address the multifaceted nature of PVD, thereby ensuring patient compliance and promoting lifestyle modifications essential for vascular health. Continuous monitoring of emerging evidence and technologies is vital in maximizing risk management protocols. Innovative testing and management programs ensure that all patients receive individualized, evidence-based care, effectively connecting surgery and patient recovery, and optimizing overall quality of life for patients living with peripheral vascular disease.

Test Your Knowledge

1. What preoperative assessments are essential for evaluating the severity of peripheral vascular disease before surgery?
2. Why is optimizing comorbid conditions such as diabetes and hypertension important before performing surgery for peripheral vascular disease?

14.4. Surgical Techniques and Innovations

Learning Outcome

1. Define the traditional surgical methods
2. Understand the minimally invasive approaches
3. Describe the advances in technology and materials

Innovations in surgical procedures considerably change the care of Peripheral Vascular Disease (PVD), improving patient outcomes and reducing complications. Technological advancements in minimally invasive procedures have led the way in transforming operations, offering high accuracy and reduced trauma. Methods like catheter-based interventions, as well as new endovascular techniques, obviate the large incisions characteristic of conventional procedures. This shift not only reduces recovery time but also reduces postoperative pain, hence promoting greater patient satisfaction and a quicker return to normal activities. With the improvement of operative methods, there is a general tendency towards tailored care, whereby treatments are designed according to the unique needs of individual patients without straying from standard clinical protocols. Advanced imaging tools have also made criticalsignificant contributions toward enhancing surgical techniques for PVD. High-resolution imaging technologies like intraoperative fluoroscopy and three-dimensional angiography provide clearer visualization of vascular anatomy to the surgeon, allowing for more accurate interventions. With these newer imaging tools, catheter and stent placements are performed much more accurately, minimizing misplacement and over-sizing complications. Additionally, the technologies enable real-time monitoring during operations, allowing for an instant assessment of the efficacy of the interventions conducted. From the literature, the integration of advanced imaging with surgical practice is critical in achieving better outcomes in minimally invasive surgery, thereby developing a culture where innovations can lead to improved outcomes for patients. Finally, the integration of robotic-assisted surgery into the domain of PVD represents a shift toward precision and efficiency in surgical treatment. Although primarily associated with cardiac surgery, robotic techniques are being increasingly adapted for vascular use and represent an attractive area for future enhancements in patient care. Surgical robots provide greater dexterity, enhanced visualization, and the ability to execute delicate maneuvers with a minimal invasive footprint. This technology has the potential to reduce recovery time and postoperative pain. Furthermore, continuous innovation in these technologies is crucial for establishing both endovascular and surgical techniques as effective means of treating complex vascular diseases. The future of PVD surgery lies in technology that combines innovation with progressive patient care, making surgery not only efficient but also humane (Figure 14.10).

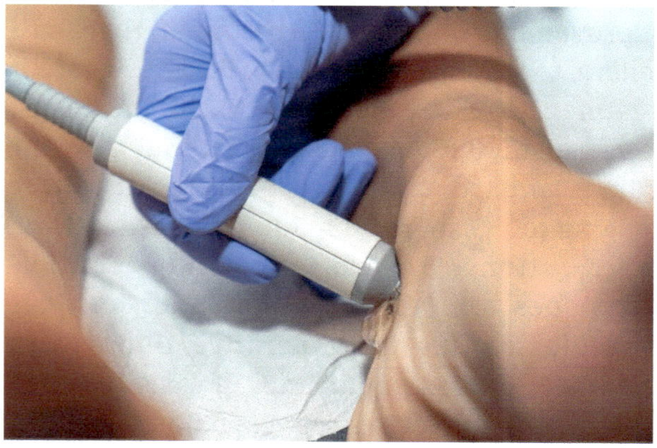

Figure 14.10. Surgical techniques for peripheral vascular disease (PVD).

Source: https://phoenixheart.com/wp-content/uploads/sites/628/2024/04/shutterstock_2419889963.webp.

14.4.1. Traditional Surgical Methods

Traditional surgical methods have long been the key to the management of peripheral vascular disease (PVD). These treatments encompass a wide range of interventions designed to restore a sufficient blood supply to the lower extremities, which can be severely compromised due to arterial blockage and stenosis. Bypass surgery is a common procedure that involves creating an alternative pathway for blood flow through a blocked artery. Surgeons typically employ grafts of the patient's native veins or artificial grafts to develop these bypasses, ensuring good perfusion to diseased limbs. Although this is an invasive treatment, it has been effective in increasing limb salvage rates and alleviating symptoms of PVD, thereby justifying the role of traditional surgical intervention in contemporary vascular practice (Becker et al., 2016). With accurate patient selection and surgery, these conventional methods are still the cornerstone in the battle against the devastating effects of PVD. Another seminal traditional surgical method is endarterectomy, a procedure designed to remove plaque deposits from the walls of arteries. The technique is especially beneficial to patients with severe stenosis, resulting in artery narrowing that may lead to critical ischemia. The procedure entails incision along the ailing artery and subsequent dissection and removal of atheromatous plaques with care. Through dilation of the arterial lumen, endarterectomy can significantly enhance blood flow and reduce cardiovascular morbidity. It is particularly suitable for patients with symptomatic PVD who are not yet good candidates for more complex surgical procedures. However, the success of endarterectomy is highly dependent on surgical expertise and patient condition. Therefore, conventional surgery continues to be an important instrument in the vascular disease armamentarium for both the short-term alleviation and long-term well-being of the vasculature (Ohiienko et al., 2015).

Even with the introduction of minimally invasive methods, conventional surgery continues to have its place in peripheral vascular disease treatment. As vascular surgeons refine these techniques, they have also begun adapting them to meet the evolving needs of patients. For example, advances in perioperative and anesthetic care have improved patient outcomes, making traditional surgeries safer and more feasible. In addition, while more modern techniques such as angioplasty and stenting are gaining popularity, traditional interventions remain important options in complex cases where less invasive methods are either ineffective or contraindicated. The use of time-proven methods in a multimodal treatment regimen reaffirms their continued value and applicability. As such, surgeons must possess training in both traditional and new approaches to deliver comprehensive care to patients with peripheral vascular disease (Becker et al., 2016).

14.4.2. Minimally Invasive Approaches

Minimally invasive techniques represent a significant improvement in the surgical management of peripheral vascular disease, encouraging shorter recovery times and improved outcomes for patients. Minimally invasive techniques typically employ smaller incisions than conventional surgery, and this decreases tissue trauma and is a trend in surgery today. With the application of high-tech imaging tools and sophisticated instruments, surgeons are now able to perform exact procedures with a lower risk of infection and complications from hospital stays. Additionally, the minimally invasive procedure facilitates a quicker recovery to normal activities, ultimately enhancing the quality of life for patients. With continued advancement in the practice, the evidence for its efficacy increases, especially in patients who may be at greater risk of complications from open surgical management.

One of the advancements in the minimally invasive vascular techniques has been catheter-based interventions, which have transformed the treatment of peripheral vascular disease. They are typically carried out under local anesthesia and can facilitate early mobilization after the procedure. Application of techniques such as balloon angioplasty and stenting has also gained prominence as a viable alternative to more invasive surgery. For instance, these techniques can effectively relieve peripheral artery stenosis, enhancing blood circulation and symptomatic relief for claudicant and critical limb ischemic patients. Further research on the creation of bioengineered materials and drug-eluting stents is also improving long-term outcomes by reducing restenosis. As cited in contemporary literature, agreement on the best patient selection and preoperative planning is crucial for achieving optimal results in minimally invasive vascular interventions (Agnihotri et al., 2016).

Beyond technological improvements, standard protocols of preoperative care after minimally invasive interventions are still necessary to optimize recovery. Effective management techniques have a significant impact on the success of surgery in general, involving close monitoring of patients to detect potential complications early on. Evidence suggests that meticulous postoperative care is associated with better outcomes, including fewer readmissions and improved long-term patency of the vessels (Agnihotri et al., 2016). Through the development of best practices that also encompass aftercare and surgical techniques, medical practitioners can optimize the therapeutic benefits of minimally invasive methods. Therefore, as the number of practitioners embracing this paradigm increases, the overall knowledge base regarding efficient treatment processes will continue to develop, ultimately enhancing patient care for peripheral vascular disease (Figure 14.11).

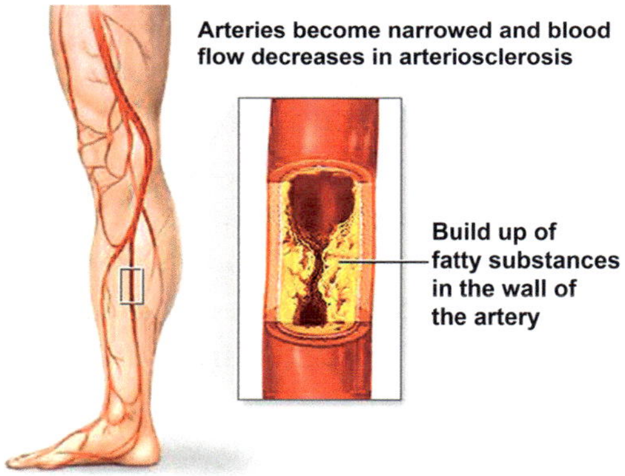

Figure 14.11. Stenosis in peripheral arteries.

Source: https://ssl.adam.com/graphics/images/en/18077.jpg.

14.4.3. Advances in Technology and Materials

Recent advancements in technology and materials have significantly transformed the landscape of peripheral vascular disease surgery, enhancing both procedural efficacy and patient outcomes. A noteworthy development is the emergence of minimally invasive surgical techniques, which have become increasingly viable due to the advancement of sophisticated imaging technologies and the refinement of catheter-based interventions. These approaches reduce patient recovery times and minimize surgical trauma, enabling a broader population to benefit from timely interventions. Furthermore, the advent of advanced biomaterials, such as biocompatible polymers and bioengineered scaffolds, has enabled the creation of more durable and effective vascular grafts, promoting higher success rates and longer longevity in peripheral interventions. The integration of these advancements not only addresses the immediate needs of patients but also supports long-term success in managing peripheral vascular disease, underscoring the necessity for continuous innovation in surgical practices. Moreover, technological advancements have facilitated the development of improved diagnostic modalities, including innovative imaging techniques and real-time intravascular ultrasound. These tools provide enhanced visualization of vascular structures, enabling surgeons to make informed decisions pre-operatively and during procedures. For instance, the use of three-dimensional imaging enables the precise mapping of vascular anatomy and pathology, which is crucial in planning complex surgeries. Additionally, the adoption of artificial intelligence in analyzing imaging data has streamlined the process of detecting vascular anomalies, thus facilitating early intervention. Such improvements are vital in managing diseases that often present asymptomatically until they reach severe stages. Enhanced diagnostic capabilities not only improve surgical planning but also contribute significantly to overall patient management strategies in peripheral vascular disease, thereby playing a crucial role in contemporary surgical practice. Finally, advances in technology have led to the refinement of surgical tools and instruments, enhancing their precision and effectiveness in peripheral vascular surgery. Innovations such as robotic-assisted surgical systems are revolutionizing how procedures are performed, offering unprecedented control and dexterity. These systems facilitate intricate maneuvers that are often challenging with traditional instruments, allowing surgeons to perform complex procedures with heightened accuracy. Furthermore, the development of specialized stents and drug-eluting technologies has provided surgeons with superior options for treating vascular lesions, contributing to reduced rates of restenosis. With the ongoing evolution of technological and material advancements, the field of peripheral vascular disease surgery continues to progress, resulting in improved clinical outcomes and a better quality of life for patients. The integration of these innovations signifies a promising future for the treatment of peripheral vascular conditions, reinforcing the commitment to enhancing patient care through surgical excellence.

Test Your Knowledge

1. How have advancements in imaging and robotic technology improved precision in modern surgical techniques?
2. What innovative surgical methods are emerging to reduce recovery time and postoperative complications?

14.5. Postoperative Care and Recovery

Learning Outcome

1. Describe the immediate postoperative monitoring
2. Explain the long-term recovery and rehabilitation
3. Understand the complications and management strategies

Postoperative care and convalescence are central components of the management of Peripheral Vascular Disease (PVD) following surgery. The postoperative course is marked by monitoring for potential complications such as infection, hemorrhage, and thrombosis. Proper care requires careful monitoring of vital signs and adherence to rules designed to minimize risks associated with surgery and anesthesia. With improved recovery, pain management measures become priority. Effective pain management not only enhances patient comfort but also enables earlier mobilization, which is crucial in preventing postoperative complications such as pulmonary infections and deep vein thrombosis. Effective protocols must be implemented for the avoidance of postoperative discomfort while minimizing the use of opioids, given their potential for causing side effects, especially among complicatedly ill patients. Thus, the initial management determines the direction of an optimal recovery process. Proper pain relief is combined with the risk of opioid addiction in a manner that becomes particularly complicated under PVD surgery. Postoperative pain has also been found to impact recovery negatively, and as such, it is of paramount importance for medical practitioners to have in place multimethod analgesic strategies. With multimodal pain treatment techniques that may include the use of non-opioid medications, one can alleviate pain without relying so much on opioids and thereby avoid the possibility of developing chronic pain and complications. Furthermore, in opioid-tolerant patients, one should be able to evaluate properly to avoid escalating doses that can lead to adverse effects. The perioperative surgical home model centers on the anesthesiologist as the organizer of this paradigm, with the intent of delivering an individualized analgesic plan to the patient, begun preoperatively and extended beyond discharge to maximize satisfaction and recovery outcomes of PVD surgery (Baratta et al., 2016).

Monitoring of patient mobility postoperatively is also encompassed, as ambulation following Peripheral Vascular Disease surgery is a crucial element of recovery. Early mobilization also stimulates the return of venous blood and reduces the risk of thromboembolic complications, a complication in vascular surgery. Physical therapy to gradually increase activity levels should be part of a successful postoperative rehabilitation program. The duration and the character of the rehabilitation are a function of the number of procedures performed and the patient's own state of health. Additionally, patient education is a key component of recovery, as it enables patients to be aware of potential complications in a timely manner, allowing for effective intervention. As healing progresses, careful evaluation of healing and restoration of function becomes paramount, with serial evaluation contributing to patients' long-term functional status. By integrating these into the care pathway, healthcare professionals can exert a significant influence on the quality of postoperative recovery for patients undergoing PVD surgery (Figure 14.12).

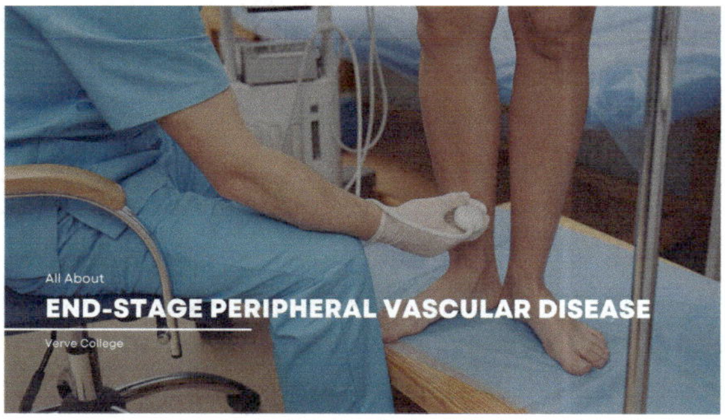

Figure 14.12. End-stage peripheral vascular disease.

Source: https://vervecollege.edu/wp-content/uploads/2025/01/End-Stage-Peripheral-Vascular-Disease-Symptoms-Causes-and-Risk-Factor.jpg.

14.5.1. Immediate Postoperative Monitoring

Postoperative observation shortly after surgery is highly critical in the recovery and treatment of patients operated on for peripheral vascular disease. It is the most crucial stage, as it allows medical officers to observe vital signs, examine the neurological status, and watch out for complications that may arise after surgery. Successful monitoring will aid in recognizing problems such as bleeding, thromboembolism, or graft failure—problems that can have a profound effect on patient outcomes. Furthermore, because fluid shifts and hemodynamics may be very significant with vascular surgery, close observation in a controlled environment will enable early intervention, which is essential for improving survival and decreasing recovery time. Adding new monitoring technologies can provide an additional level of protection, offering a more precise assessment of a patient's status in real-time during this critical timeframe. Control of postoperative pain is also a key element of immediate monitoring, particularly in patients who have undergone peripheral vascular disease surgery. Not only does control of pain enhance patient comfort, but it also provides for early mobilization, which is essential to recovery. Inadequate pain management may also lead to complications such as a delay in healing and a tendency to have more opportunities for chronic pain development. Opioid prescriptions, however, are traditionally bound by the risks of undesirable occurrences, especially in opioid-tolerant patients or those with prior medical conditions. In this context, anesthesiologists play an essential role in formulating an overall postoperative analgesic regimen that incorporates multimodal approaches designed to optimize pain relief and minimize risk of complication. Individualized care is a paradigmatic approach that prioritizes patient-specific care during the acute postoperative period (Baratta et al., 2016). For peripheral vascular disease surgeries, monitoring of cardiac and respiratory stability should also be done on an immediate basis postoperatively. Such patients are typically at greater risk of developing cardiovascular complications and therefore need careful monitoring of hemodynamic status in the postoperative situation. Having a rigid protocol for monitoring not only facilitates the detection of patients who require further cardiac intervention, but it also helps to judge overall surgical success. Additionally, respiratory function is crucial, particularly in those patients with underlying pulmonary comorbidities, where monitoring can aid in the early recognition of atelectasis or pneumonia (Poldermans et al., 2009). By implementing these multi-dimensional monitoring approaches, the healthcare providers can create optimal recovery environments, enhance patient satisfaction, and overall improve surgical outcomes in vascular intervention patients.

14.5.2. Long-Term Recovery and Rehabilitation

Long-term recovery and rehabilitation from peripheral vascular disease (PVD) surgery is a multifaceted process involving physical, emotional, and social recovery. Recovery outcomes in patients vary based on the extent of their pre-surgical health and their adherence to rehabilitation classes. Rehabilitation not only attempts to aid physical mobility but also to educate regarding the disease itself. The studies identify that restricted understanding of disease can generate unrealistic expectations of surgery and treatment, leading to distress and dissatisfaction on the part of patients regarding the healing process (Abaraogu et al., 2018). Therefore, a comprehensive rehabilitation plan should consider both physical exercises to improve circulation and mobility, as well as disease education for patients to establish realistic expectations regarding their healing process. Apart from that, emotional support plays a crucial role in the long-term rehabilitation process for post-surgery patients. The majority of patients experience powerlessness and anxiety over their health, primarily as they work with the uncertainties of having peripheral vascular disease. The emotional load triggered by such a response can hamper involvement in attempts at rehabilitation, causing rates of recovery to be low. Engaging patients in group support systems or one-on-one counseling can be vital in improving adherence to rehabilitation protocols and allowing them to proactively manage their condition (Abaraogu et al., 2018). In addressing physical as well as emotional demands, rehabilitation interventions can enable patients to control their lives and enhance their general quality of life following surgery. Finally, the importance of a multidisciplinary program for the rehabilitation of PVD patients cannot be overstated. Interdisciplinary programs that include a variety of healthcare providers, such as nurses, physical therapists, dietitians, and psychologists, contribute to an overall recovery process. The interdisciplinary approach to care emphasizes individualized treatment plans tailored to each patient's unique needs, considering the complexity of PVD and the resulting challenges. Studies indicate that patient-centered care raises rates of participation in rehabilitation, which results in increased mobility and overall health outcomes. In addition, following up on and reworking plans of care according to patient feedback provides ongoing improvement and demonstrates to patients that they are heard, which results in a more effective recovery process (Figure 14.13).

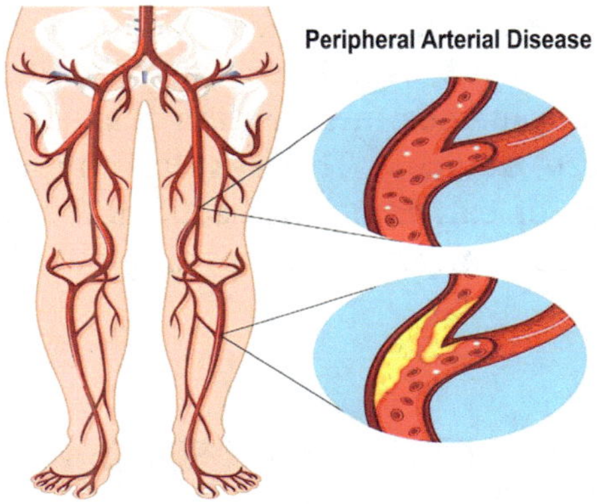

Figure 14.13. Peripheral arterial disease treatment.

Source: https://www.drsumitkapadia.com/wp-content/uploads/2025/02/pad.webp.

14.5.3. Complications and Management Strategies

Within the operative environment for peripheral vascular disease surgery, intraoperative and postoperative complications are likely, and they primarily have an impact on patient prognosis and recovery. Intraoperative complications typically include hematoma development and bleeding that may arise from the site of access, possibly leading to extended recovery or the need for additional surgical intervention. Postoperative complications are usually represented by infection and thrombosis that impair blood circulation and, in the most serious cases, produce limb ischemia. Effective treatment of these complications involves attention to a thorough surgical procedure, preoperative risk assessment, and postoperative monitoring to identify early signs of complications. The implementation of standardized procedures can reduce risks and enhance patient safety during surgical procedures. As a matter of emphasis on access site control of complications, many recent studies have determined the efficacy of closure devices (CD) in reducing the risk of hematoma and reintervention following femoral access for peripheral vascular interventions. Analysis indicates that patients provided with CDs were significantly less likely to develop any access site hematomas and complications requiring further intervention than non-users of these devices. The results support the concept of extending instructions for the use of CDs as a means of optimizing outcomes in select patient populations. With increasing evidence, it becomes increasingly clear that adopting new management strategies that involve the application of CD will help minimize complications and improve the patient's overall experience during recuperation (Conte et al., 2020). In addition to surgical interventions and device use, effective management practices also involve implementing comprehensive postoperative care practices, such as the enlightened use of anticoagulants and antiplatelet agents. These measures are crucial in preventing thromboembolic complications, particularly in high-risk patients with peripheral vascular disease. Persistent patient education about early warning signs of complications, coupled with clearly defined follow-up treatment, serves to empower the patient and enhance their involvement in the healing process. Additionally, the implementation of an interprofessional model with feedback from vascular surgeons, rehabilitation specialists, and nurses can lead to a more comprehensive plan of care, ultimately benefiting patients by offering better outcomes with fewer complications during the perioperative period (Acosta et al., 2020).

Test Your Knowledge

1. What key factors influence the speed and quality of a patient's recovery after surgery?
2. How does effective pain management contribute to improved postoperative healing and mobility?

14.6. Outcomes and Prognosis

Learning Outcome

1. Discuss on success rates of various procedures
2. Determinants of surgical outcomes
3. Describe the long-term management of PVD

The surgical treatment of peripheral vascular disease (PVD) yields valuable insights into patient outcomes and prognostic variables. Surgical interventions such as angioplasty and bypass grafting have been noted to improve peripheral circulation and alleviate the symptoms of patients with the disease. Prognosis following these interventions, however, is very heterogeneous based on an array of factors varying from comorbid illness to the extent of vascular injury. Follow-up management must be organized, with regular monitoring supplying medical practitioners with a means to assess quality of life as well as overall survival.

Furthermore, awareness of the typical outcomes that correlate with different approaches to surgery supplies patients and physicians with information for decision-making about treatment alternatives. The prognostic factors of outcome in PVD surgery cannot be overstressed. Patient-specific factors, including age, gender, and concurrent medical conditions like diabetes and hypertension, are relevant when making prognostications regarding success with surgery and survival. Systemic inflammatory processes that can possibly be quantified with specific scoring systems bring a helpful measure of risk stratification. Beyond assessing the present health status, these inflammatory markers may also provide anticipatory guidance on potential postoperative complications. Because these parameters play a significant role in determining late outcomes after PVD surgery, they need to be addressed during the preoperative assessment so that patient needs can be met more appropriately and prognostic expectations improved. In addition, comparing surgical outcomes between cohorts provides more information concerning the effectiveness of peripheral vascular surgery. Studies reveal that variations in procedural techniques and postoperative treatment can lead to disparate prognoses, underscoring the importance of evidence-based practice. For instance, patients undergoing revascularization procedures often exhibit variable success rates, which are often attributed to the degree of pre-existing ischemic damage. The addition of patient and tumor-related factors from broader surgical clinic oncology perspectives, as highlighted in research such as Benson et al. (2010), illustrates similarities in vascular bypass outcomes, and that markers for systemic disease have a significant role in predicting not only the immediate success of surgery but also long-term survival. Therefore, ongoing inquiry into PVD surgery prognostic variables remains crucial for refining treatment modalities and patient outcomes in this cohort (Figure 14.14).

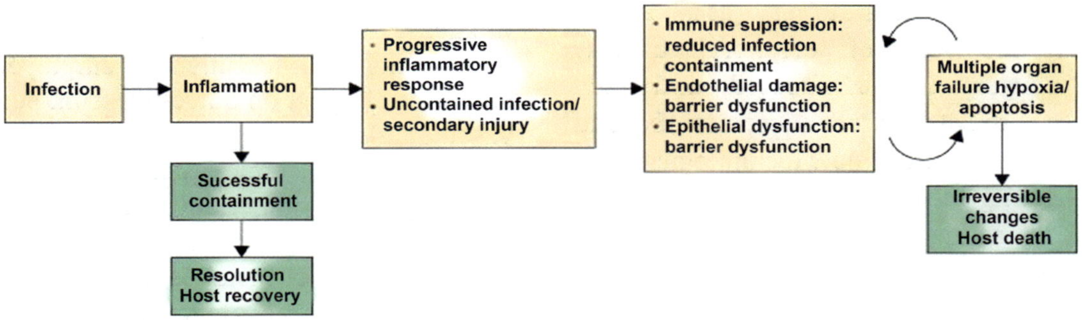

Figure 14.14. Systemic inflammatory response syndrome.

Source: https://ars.els-cdn.com/content/image/3-s2.0-B9780123742711000277-gr1.jpg.

14.6.1. Success Rates of Various Procedures

Evaluating success rates after surgery for peripheral vascular disease is crucial in determining the efficacy of interventional methods. Of these, Percutaneous Transluminal Angioplasty (PTA) has emerged as a front-runner treatment method. A review of 54 procedures performed at St. Luke's Hospital, Malta, indicates that PTA has good outcomes, particularly for femoro-popliteal stenoses, and can achieve a two-year patency rate of 93%. This high success rate testifies to the efficacy of PTAs in alleviating symptoms associated with peripheral vascular disease. Despite the encouraging result for stenoses, this is not the case for occlusions; the patency rate of iliac occlusions dipped alarmingly to 0%. This result calls for greater innovation in technique or adjunct treatments to improve outcomes for more complex occlusive lesions (Gatt et al., 1995). Similarly, under consideration are the rates of success for surgical revascularization. Bypass grafting remains a usual technique for those with severe peripheral vascular disease, particularly in situations where PTA is inadequate. The technique, which bypasses stenosed arteries by diverting blood flow, has been greeted with variable success depending on the variety of factors involved, such as patient populations, comorbidities, and the integrity of the prosthetic or vein graft utilized. Five-year patency rates for bypass grafts have been reported in the range of 50% to 85% in studies, and these rates are dependent on various factors.

Other variables, such as age, smoking, and diabetes mellitus, also play a significant role in the long-term success of grafts. Proper patient selection and comprehensive preoperative assessment are hence essential to maximize results and prevent complications with peripheral vascular surgery (et al., 2019). Ultimately, the world of peripheral vascular disease surgery is multifaceted, and each procedure is to some extent successful. Beyond PTA and bypass grafting, new technologies, such as drug-eluting stents and balloons, are being tested to determine if they can enhance patency and reduce the risk of restenosis. The application of novel technologies in the clinical environment holds promise, but the long-term stability and safety of these interventions should be thoroughly evaluated through multicenter trials and prospective long-term studies. Furthermore, determinants of success or failure of such interventions should be determined to optimize patient outcomes. While the specialty evolves, scientific research and clinical experience will continue to be essential in addressing the challenges presented by peripheral vascular disease and in the long run optimizing the success rates of various surgical procedures (Gatt et al., 1995).

14.6.2. Determinants of Surgical Outcomes

The multifaceted nature of surgical outcomes in patients with peripheral vascular disease eloquently underscores the importance of familiarity with numerous determinants. Influencing factors in patients, such as age, comorbidities, and lifestyle habits, rank highest among them. Older patients, for instance, have more advanced stages of peripheral vascular disease and thus a greater rate of complications. Moreover, surgical complications in patients with such comorbid conditions as diabetes mellitus and hypertension will adversely affect healing and recovery from surgery. Lifestyle factors such as obesity and smoking also contribute to surgical complications as they are well established to lead to vascular compromise and decreased wound healing. Therefore, it is crucial to optimize patient health before surgery by comprehensive assessment and maximum intervention to enhance operative outcomes in such a group. In addition to patient-related factors, the technical method employed has a significant impact on outcomes from peripheral vascular disease surgery. The choice between varying surgical techniques, that is, between bypass grafting and endovascular therapy, may determine long-term patency rates and the risk of complications. For instance, studies have shown that the utilization of newer graft materials, such as the Omniflow II biosynthetic vascular graft, can lead to improved graft patency and lower infection rates compared to conventional grafts. Such advancements reflect the need for the use of appropriate surgical modalities tailored to individual patients and the severity of their diseases. Furthermore, the surgeon's experience and skill with specific techniques will necessarily contribute to outcome predictability; thus, ongoing training and audit within surgical practice are essential. Postoperative recovery is a critical determinant of successful surgery, requiring multi-professional management to maximize recovery. Control of potential complications, for example, SSI, requires strict adherence to protocols intended to minimize infection risks. SSI may have a significant impact on the morbidity of patients and healthcare costs, and hence needs pro-active measures both pre- and post-operatively to reduce these risks. The synergistic relationship between environmental factors, such as operating room conditions and contact with prosthetic material, makes this aspect of surgical care challenging since biofilm formation and resistance among pathogens increase the challenge of treating the infection. Hence, prevention is key in the form of best patient optimization and the application of evidence from current research in surgical practice to deliver positive surgical outcomes in patients undergoing surgery for peripheral vascular disease (Chetter et al., 2015; Göncü et al., 2018).

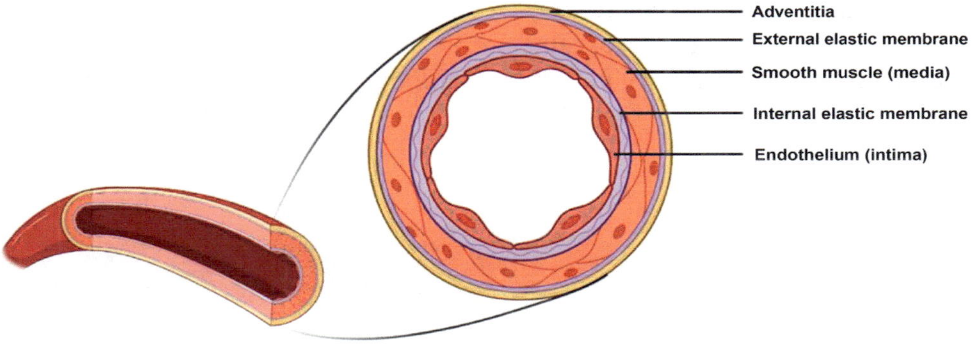

Figure 14.15. Small diameter cell-free tissue-engineered vascular grafts.

Source: https://www.mdpi.com/polymers/polymers-14-03440/article_deploy/html/images/polymers-14-03440-g001.png.

14.6.3. Long-Term Management of PVD

Management of Peripheral Vascular Disease (PVD) is multifaceted and encompasses both lifestyle changes and clinical management. The disease is associated with numerous symptoms, such as pain and walking limitations, which affect a patient's quality of life. Lifestyle change is the cornerstone of effective management, comprising smoking cessation, regular exercise, and a healthy diet. Such changes are not only crucial for alleviating symptoms but also for enhancing overall cardiovascular health. Education measures that serve to raise patients' awareness of their illness are of extreme importance here, and indeed many patients are found to lack understanding of the effects of PVD on their health, and therefore delays in appropriate treatment (Abaraogu et al., 2018). The incorporation of such measures leads to patient-directed care that supports the importance of active participation in disease control. Pharmacological management plays a crucial role in long-term PVD management, with symptom relief and prevention of disease progression as key elements. Antiplatelet therapy with aspirin or clopidogrel is the most widely used drug to avert cardiovascular events in PVD patients. In addition, statins are employed to manage dyslipidemia, lessening the risk of atherosclerotic complications once more. The efficacy of these medications underscores the importance of individualized therapeutic regimens, as drug reactions among patients can vary significantly. Finally, constant surveillance for disease activity and complications, including the potential need for surgery, is necessary in a bid to anticipate and counteract different patient needs (Acosta et al., 2020). Collaboration between healthcare providers and patients is crucial for ensuring adherence to pharmacological therapy and achieving optimal outcomes. Supervised exercise therapy is a central component of chronic PVD management, particularly among people with intermittent claudication. Supervised exercise therapy not only facilitates improved walking ability but also enhances patient empowerment by providing self-management strategies. Empirical evidence shows that evidence-based exercise can reduce symptoms and enhance the quality of life considerably. However, patient attendance in such programs is undermined by misperceptions regarding the nature of the condition and the treatment interventions. For example, misperceptions regarding aggressive surgical procedures may lead patients to underestimate the benefits of conservative management interventions, such as supervised exercise (Abaraogu et al., 2018). Effective education and communication, therefore, are essential in reconciling clinical reality with patient expectations. By addressing such challenges, health practitioners are able to provide adherence to exercise programs and achieve effective long-term management of PVD among their patients' populations.

Test Your Knowledge

1. What patient-specific factors most strongly influence the long-term prognosis after surgical treatment?
2. How do postoperative complications affect overall outcomes and survival rates?

SUMMARY

In a concise overview of the complexities that accompany peripheral vascular disease (PVD) surgery, it is evident that the introduction of new treatments and strategies influences patient outcomes. Surgical techniques, particularly bypasses, have evolved in terms of complexity, with the relevant consideration of selecting the appropriate graft material and method in relation to individual patient needs. Recent studies have shown the effectiveness of supervised exercise programs as a component of managing ailments such as intermittent claudication, thereby enhancing functional capacity and quality of life for patients. Such non-surgical interventions lend support to the utilization of exercise as a first-line treatment approach, emphasizing the need for an integrated management strategy for PVD that incorporates both surgical and rehabilitation practices (Cayton et al., 2015). The application of new materials, such as the Omniflow II biosynthetic vascular graft, yields promising results regarding graft patency rates and long-term success in femoro-popliteal bypass surgeries. Research indicates that this type of graft offers desirable patency rates, along with lower rates of aneurysm formation and infection, which are important for ensuring positive surgical outcomes. Notably, studies reveal cumulative primary graft patency rates that strongly favor the application of the above-knee bypass strategy, emphasizing the significance of tailored surgical planning (Göncü et al., 2018). Such studies enrich the existing controversy regarding the refinement of surgical techniques and materials in improving prognosis in post-surgery patients. Finally, the conclusion drawn from the overall evaluation of peripheral vascular disease surgery is in the direction of increasing recognition of individualized care strategies. Obviously, the realization of patient-specific profiles and optimizing surgical operations with corresponding clinical management is essential to maximizing recovery as well as long-term success rates. Increased research to further enhance present techniques and explore additional methods will enable practitioners to utilize the most advanced technology possible for the treatment of PVD. Blending evidence-based practice with new operative technology holds promise for a more optimistic future in vascular disease treatment, offering better outcomes for those suffering and improved quality of life in general (Cayton et al., 2015; Göncü et al., 2018).

In considering the field of Peripheral Vascular Disease (PVD) surgery, the key developments and strategies that characterize its evolution need to be emphasized. One of the key components of these developments is the application of endovascular techniques, which aim to restore blood supply by revascularizing through minimal intervention. These technologies, including minimally invasive angioplasty and stent placements, have brought significant improvements in terms of patient recovery times and outcomes. In addition, the success of interventions typically relies on a comprehensive understanding of patient pathology and the use of suitable devices tailored to the individual's vascular features. This customized treatment has maximized the success of interventions with minimal complications, underlining the importance of customized surgical techniques for PVD treatment. The use of drug-eluting stents, particularly those emitting everolimus, has revolutionized surgical therapy. These innovative stents are designed to minimize the risk of restenosis—a common challenge following vascular interventions. The study priorities around these stents recognize that their pharmacokinetics are critical to understanding therapeutic effectiveness. For instance, research has shown that levels of systemic everolimus after stent placement are significantly lower than with oral dosing, thereby enhancing its efficacy and safety in preventing vascular inflammation and promoting healing (Hausegger et al., 2012). This drug innovation in stent technology is a cornerstone of current PVD surgery, offering a solid solution to what would otherwise be a complex medical conditions. Additionally, the long-term benefits of these procedures cannot be overstated. Improved patient quality of life, along with the potential for decreased hospital readmissions and associated healthcare costs, underscores the necessity for ongoing research and clinical trials. Development of standard protocols and further inquiry into procedural efficacy across different patient populations remain vital areas of focus. As the prevalence of PVD continues to increase due to aging populations and chronic diseases, best practices based on the discoveries of contemporary studies, like the pharmacologic profiles of novel stents like everolimus-releasing stents, will eventually carry over to better patient outcomes (et al., 2019). Therefore, as the field of medicine continues to evolve, it is an absolute necessity that these points are the basis of decisions in future PVD surgeries.

KEY TERMS FROM THIS CHAPTER

- Amputation
- Ankle-brachial index (ABI)
- Atherosclerosis
- Carotid endarterectomy
- Critical limb ischemia
- Diabetic foot management
- Endovascular aneurysm repair (EVAR)
- Peripheral artery disease (PAD)
- Angioplasty
- Aortoiliac bypass
- Bypass grafting
- Claudication
- Deep vein thrombosis (DVT)
- Endarterectomy
- Femoral-popliteal bypass
- Saphenous vein stripping

CRITICAL THINKING QUESTIONS

1. **Which of the following is the most common symptom of peripheral arterial disease (PAD)?**
   a. Chest pain
   b. Claudication
   c. Headache
   d. Palpitations
2. **The ankle-brachial index (ABI) is used to assess:**
   a. Venous insufficiency
   b. Risk of stroke
   c. Arterial perfusion to the lower limb
   d. Pulmonary embolism
3. **Which of the following is a common indication for surgical revascularization in PVD?**
   a. Asymptomatic carotid stenosis
   b. Claudication that improves with rest
   c. Critical limb ischemia
   d. Varicose veins
4. **Which of the following is a contraindication to endovascular aneurysm repair (EVAR)?**
   a. Abdominal aortic aneurysm (AAA) >5.5 cm
   b. Short and angulated proximal neck
   c. No symptoms of rupture
   d. Patient older than 70 years
5. **Which of the following surgical procedures is most commonly performed for femoropopliteal occlusive disease?**
   a. Carotid endarterectomy
   b. Coronary artery bypass graft
   c. Femoral-femoral bypass
   d. Femoropopliteal bypass graft

Short Answer Questions

1. What are the risk factors for developing peripheral arterial disease (PAD)?
2. Define intermittent claudication and explain its clinical significance.
3. How is the Ankle-Brachial Index (ABI) measured and interpreted in PVD diagnosis?
4. Differentiate between critical limb ischemia and acute limb ischemia.
5. What are the indications for surgical revascularization in peripheral vascular disease?
6. Describe the surgical options for lower limb revascularization in PVD.
7. What are the common complications of femoropopliteal bypass surgery?
8. How is endovascular aneurysm repair (EVAR) different from open surgical repair of abdominal aortic aneurysms (AAA)?
9. What is the role of duplex ultrasonography in evaluating arterial insufficiency?
10. Describe the clinical presentation and management of atherosclerotic renal artery stenosis.

Answers to Critical Thinking Questions

1. (b); 2. (c); 3. (c); 4. (b); 5. (d)

REFERENCES

1. baraogu, U. O., Ezenwankwo, E. F., Dall, P. M., & Seenan, C. A. (2018). Living a burdensome and demanding life: A qualitative systematic review of the patients experiences of peripheral arterial disease. *PLoS ONE, 13*(11), e0207456. https://doi.org/10.1371/journal.pone.0207456
2. Acosta, S., Azuma, N., Bastos Gonçalves, F., Björck, M., et al. (2020). *Editor's choice: European Society for Vascular Surgery (ESVS) 2020 clinical practice guidelines on the management of acute limb ischemia.*
3. Agnihotri, A. K., Ailawadi, G., Barnhart, G. R., Farivar, R. S., et al. (2016). *Minimally invasive mitral valve surgery I: Patient selection, evaluation, and planning.* https://core.ac.uk/download/323076062.pdf (accessed on 12th July 2025).
4. Airey, C. M., Bamford, J. M., Berry, E., Cullingworth, J., et al. (2002). *Use of magnetic resonance angiography to select candidates with recently symptomatic carotid stenosis for surgery: Systematic review.* https://core.ac.uk/download/59922.pdf (accessed on 12th July 2025).
5. Andreetti, C., Borro, M., Cipolla, F., Defraia, S., et al. (2018). *Short-term one-lung ventilation does not influence local inflammatory cytokine response after lung resection.* https://core.ac.uk/download/158822841.pdf (accessed on 12th July 2025).
6. Baratta, J. L., Schwenk, E. S., Viscusi, E. R., Wenzel, J., et al. (2016). *Managing opioid-tolerant patients in the perioperative surgical home.* https://core.ac.uk/download/46975930.pdf (accessed on 12th July 2025).
7. Bath, P. M. W., Lees, K. R., Naylor, A. R. (2000). *ABC of arterial and venous disease: Secondary prevention of transient ischemic attack and stroke.* https://core.ac.uk/download/1633132.pdf (accessed on 12th July 2025).
8. Becker, L., Bellezo, J. M., Fair, J. F., Gaieski, D. F., et al. (2016). *Practice characteristics of Emergency Department extracorporeal cardiopulmonary resuscitation (eCPR) programs in the United States: The current state of the art of Emergency Department extracorporeal membrane oxygenation (ED ECMO).* https://core.ac.uk/download/299811653.pdf (accessed on 12th July 2025).
9. Belch, J., Boc, V., et al. (2019). *ESVM guideline on peripheral arterial disease.* https://core.ac.uk/download/286715349.pdf (accessed on 12th July 2025).
10. Benson, C., Brown, R., Compton, S., Cooper, T., Crozier, J., Dukes, H., Forrest, D., et al. (2010). Comparison of the prognostic value of tumor and patient-related factors in patients undergoing potentially curative surgery for colon cancer. https://core.ac.uk/download/91259.pdf (accessed on 12th July 2025).
11. Bhogal, R. H., Downing, R. (2011). The evolution of aortic aneurysm repair: Past lessons and future directions. https://core.ac.uk/download/pdf/1631327.pdf (accessed on 12th July 2025).
12. Buckley, B. S., Hannaford, P. C., McLernon, D. J., Murphy, J., et al. (2009). Five-year prognosis in patients with angina identified in primary care: Incident cohort study. https://core.ac.uk/download/4193237.pdf (accessed on 12th July 2025).
13. Carella, S., Onesti, M. G., Scuderi, N. (2018). Effectiveness of antimicrobial-coated sutures for the prevention of surgical site infection: A review of the literature. https://core.ac.uk/download/188823791.pdf (accessed on 12th July 2025).

14. Casavilla, F. A., Dvorchik, I., Fung, J. J., Iwatsuki, S., et al. (1997). Hepatic resection and transplantation for peripheral cholangiocarcinoma. https://core.ac.uk/download/12205423.pdf (accessed on 12th July 2025).

15. Cayton, T., Chetter, I., Harwood, A., Harwood, J., et al. (2015). A review of the potential local mechanisms by which exercise improves functional outcomes in intermittent claudication. https://core.ac.uk/download/151157091.pdf (accessed on 12th July 2025).

16. Chetter, I., Smith, G. (2015). Infection in prosthetic material. https://core.ac.uk/download/151157240.pdf (accessed on 12th July 2025).

17. Conte, M. S., Gasper, W. J., Hicks, C. W., Iannuzzi, J., et al. (2020). Antegrade common femoral artery closure device use is associated with decreased complications. https://core.ac.uk/download/288432601.pdf (accessed on 12th July 2025).

18. De Backer, G., De Backer, T., De Buyzere, M., Van Bortel, L., et al. (2010). Silence of the limbs: Pharmacological symptomatic treatment of intermittent claudication. https://core.ac.uk/download/55797842.pdf (accessed on 12th July 2025).

19. de Boer, S. W., Elgersma, O. E., Fioole, B., Heyligers, J., et al. (2013). Randomized trial of Legflow® paclitaxel eluting balloon and stenting versus standard percutaneous transluminal angioplasty and stenting for the treatment of intermediate and long lesions of the superficial femoral artery (RAPID trial): Study protocol for a randomized controlled trial. https://core.ac.uk/download/43288743.pdf (accessed on 12th July 2025).

20. de Wolf, A., Hamad, M., Martens, E., Schönberger, J., et al. (2010). Risk factors for deterioration of renal function after coronary artery bypass grafting. https://core.ac.uk/download/55796024.pdf (accessed on 12th July 2025).

21. Eichler, C. M., Nakakura, E. K., Tseng, W. W., Wang, L., et al. (2011). Complete and safe resection of challenging retroperitoneal tumors: Anticipation of multi-organ and major vascular resection and use of adjunct procedures. https://core.ac.uk/download/323073598.pdf (accessed on 12th July 2025).

22. Galea Debono, A., Gatt, A., Zammit, A. (1996). Carotid artery disease screening: Assessment of criteria. https://core.ac.uk/download/46601966.pdf (accessed on 12th July 2025).

23. Gatt, D., Mallia, D., Zammit, A. (1995). Five years of peripheral percutaneous transluminal angioplasty: The St Luke's Hospital experience. https://core.ac.uk/download/46601767.pdf (accessed on 12th July 2025).

24. Göncü, M. T., Toktaş, F., Yavuz, Ş., Çayır, A., et al. (2018). Long-term outcomes of Omniflow II biosynthetic vascular graft in lower extremity arterial revascularization. https://core.ac.uk/download/227060356.pdf (accessed on 12th July 2025).

25. Hausegger, K. A., Koppensteiner, R., Lammer, J., Mellon, S., et al. (2012). Pharmacokinetic analysis after implantation of everolimus-eluting self-expanding stents in the peripheral vasculature. https://core.ac.uk/download/55742996.pdf (accessed on 12th July 2025).

26. Kitsiou, A., Caforio, A. L. P., Porta-Sanchez, A., Vahanian, A., Iung, B., Carrera, C., Szymanski, C., et al. (2013). *ESC core curriculum for the general cardiologist (2013)*. https://core.ac.uk/download/55756305.pdf (accessed on 12th July 2025).

27. Ohiienko, M. M., Redko, S. I., Shyshchuk, V. D., Огиенко, М. М., et al. (2015). General questions of anesthesiology. https://core.ac.uk/download/141448194.pdf (accessed on 12th July 2025).

28. Pimienta, M., Edderkaoui, M., Wang, R., Pandol, S. (2017). The potential for circulating tumor cells in pancreatic cancer management. https://core.ac.uk/download/323077820.pdf (accessed on 12th July 2025).

29. Poldermans, D., Bax, J. J., Boersma, E., De Hert, S., Eeckhout, E., Fowkes, G., Gorenek, B., et al. (2009). Guidelines for pre-operative cardiac risk assessment and perioperative cardiac management in non-cardiac surgery: The Task Force for Preoperative Cardiac Risk Assessment and Perioperative Cardiac Management in Non-cardiac Surgery of the European Society of Cardiology (ESC) and endorsed by the European Society of Anesthesiology (ESA). https://core.ac.uk/download/55798032.pdf (accessed on 12th July 2025).

SURGERY IN TROPICAL DISEASES

15

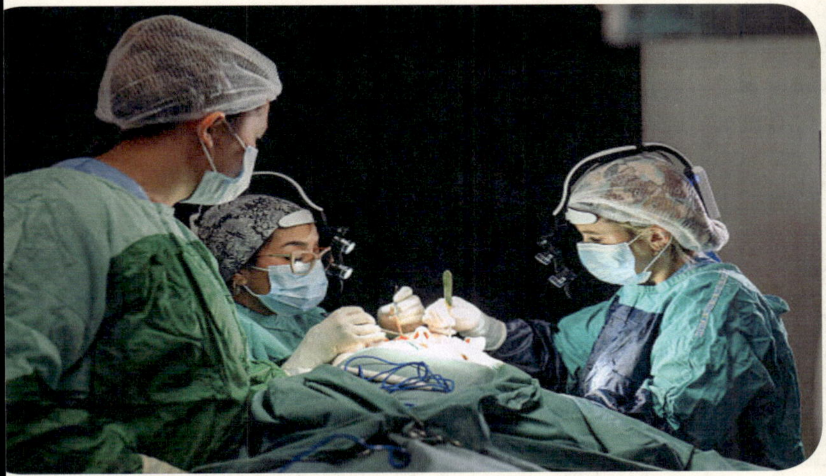

LEARNING OBJECTIVES

After studying this chapter, you will be able to:

1. Understand the common tropical diseases requiring surgery
2. Explain the surgical techniques in tropical medicine
3. Discuss the challenges in surgical care for tropical diseases
4. Focus on postoperative care in tropical surgery
5. Learn about case studies of successful surgical interventions
6. Evaluate the future directions in surgical approaches

Introduction

The geography of tropical diseases presents a unique challenge to health systems everywhere, particularly in regions where the interplay of risk is complicated by climate, socioeconomic status, and access to healthcare. Although the incidence of such disease grows, leading-edge surgical care becomes an essential element in intervention. Surgery's role in the treatment of tropical diseases cannot be overstated; such surgery is often necessary to minimize the complications of diseases such as lymphatic filariasis, schistosomiasis, and leprosy. The majority of these diseases, with a high prevalence in poor populations, need urgent surgery to prevent long-term morbidity and enhance the patient's quality of life. As recent health statistics indicate, the integration of surgical solutions into the public health system is crucial in the fight against both medical and social causes of disease in tropical regions, implying the need to address surgical resources among these impoverished populations (Matthew et al., 2021).

Inherent in the management of tropical diseases is knowledge about their multifactorial causes, typically implying that their surgical control becomes more complicated. Incubators in the form of resource-poor settings, a lack of skilled surgical personnel, and inadequate healthcare infrastructure present daunting barriers to effective treatment. Furthermore, most patients from the endemic regions may have advanced stages of disease due to late hospitalization, making surgical procedures even more challenging. Findings illustrate that the disease burden of diseases like lymphatic filariasis contributes to extreme morbidity, making surgery indispensable not only for physical repair but also for enhancing psychological well-being and social reintegration (Wu et al., 2020). This serves to illustrate that surgical intervention is never a single measure by itself; instead, it must be positioned in an overarching public health agenda that incorporates prevention, education, and adherence to care. It is thus imperative that multi-disciplinary interventions be emphasized in practice and healthcare policy in a bid to effectively address the challenges brought by tropical diseases through surgical intervention. The collaborative effort among surgeons, public health professionals, and affected populations plays a crucial role in introducing applicable and sustainable solutions pertinent to particular regional issues. Educational interventions targeting healthcare workers and the relevant populations have the potential to reinforce early intervention and improve surgical outcomes. Additionally, it is vital to invest in health infrastructure and the surgical workforce in order to enable a uniform supply of good quality surgical care. Ultimately, the establishment of surgical care for the management of tropical disease is an essential consideration for propelling global health equity and minimizing avoidable morbidity, and has a tremendous impact on the ultimate public health goals (Matthew et al., 2021) (Figure 15.1).

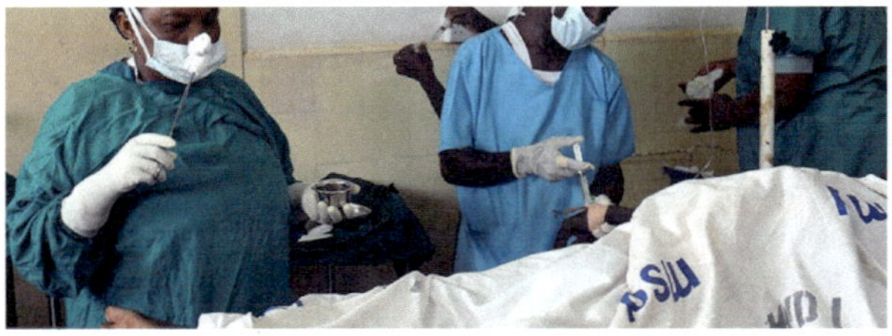

Figure 15.1. Surgery in tropical diseases.

Source: https://imaworldhealth.org/sites/default/files/styles/hero_image_country/public/program/image/https%253A/imaworldhealth.org/wp-content/uploads/2016/02/surgery_mw.jpg.jpeg?itok=6Bz_yWAD.

Definition of Tropical Diseases

The term "tropical diseases" describes infectious and parasitic diseases that are common in tropical and subtropical regions, primarily affecting economically disadvantaged populations. The diseases are typically specific to particular environmental factors, such as high temperatures, humidity, and specific ecological environments that favor the spread of the diseases. Examples of tropical diseases include malaria, dengue fever, and schistosomiasis, which heavily impact the public health infrastructure of the affected countries. Furthermore, their re-establishment in non-endemic areas, along with the emergence of drug-resistant forms, underscores the need for utmost vigilance and comprehensive understanding in both clinical and research contexts. Therefore, the term' tropical diseases' not only suggests their spatial distribution but also socio-economic factors that extend their scope, demanding a multidisciplinary approach to address such public health concerns appropriately. In addition to well-known infections like dengue and malaria, the tropical diseases group includes measles, which is less familiar, and taeniasis and cysticercosis, which illustrate the broad range of health problems associated with these illnesses. A significant finding from a Belgian study was 221 documented cases of taeniasis, primarily caused by the beef tapeworm *Taenia saginata*, with a remarkable percentage of mild or asymptomatic infections. Notably, the emphasis of this research was on the reality that tropical illnesses may manifest in non-endemic territories, particularly among international travelers or expatriates, as a global health concern irrespective of geographical location.

This provides a critical background in understanding the necessity for robust public health interventions, the allocation of research, and health infrastructure to control the risk of emerging outbreaks and minimize their transmission in various settings (Bottieau et al., 2019). Furthermore, co-infections tend to exacerbate tropical diseases, particularly with viruses like HIV, making management and treatment a complex affair. The drug-resistant TB case is a representation of the intricacy of these diseases, whereby incidences of multidrug-resistant (MDR-TB) and extensively drug-resistant (XDR-TB) tuberculosis escalate dramatically in the tropics. These drug-resistant strains present significant treatment modalities challenges and increase healthcare costs, primarily to communities already afflicted with few resources (Karim et al., 2010). The interconnectedness between tropical diseases and socio-economic determinants necessitates comprehensive surgical and medical interventions that address not only immediate healthcare needs but also support long-term improvements by enhancing local healthcare systems, investing in preventive services, and increasing community awareness about these diseases. On this front, understanding the definition of tropical diseases involves more than classification, necessitating an examination of their broader implications for global health.

Significance of Surgical Intervention

Surgery plays a pivotal role in the management of tropical diseases, particularly when other forms of management are ineffective or complications arise. The diversity of such diseases is likely to lead to acute presentations that require immediate and definitive surgical intervention.

A case in point is ascariasis, an *Ascaris lumbricoides* parasitic infection, for which surgery was required to manage an obstruction of the small bowel in an 8-year-old patient. Without laparotomy and enterotomy, the course of this complication would have resulted in catastrophic morbidity or death. The case highlights the crucial role of operations in the effective treatment of tropical diseases, which often present with acute complications that necessitate both medical treatment and surgical intervention to achieve recovery and prevent exacerbation (Liyew et al., 2025). Apart from treating the immediate cause of acute complications, surgery in the context of tropical diseases permits an improved quality of life for the afflicted individuals, particularly in resource-poor settings. The majority of tropical diseases, such as cystic echinococcosis, are likely to have severe long-term health consequences if left untreated. A Romanian study among children's patients highlighted that effective surgical treatment significantly minimized hospital stay time as well as associated complications. The complexity of such diseases necessitates a multidisciplinary approach that combines surgical techniques with medical therapy tailored to the patient's specific needs. The combination of surgical demonstrates an end-to-end approach that not only attempts to cure but also maximizes the overall well-being of patients fighting against the disabling aspects of tropical diseases (Mihai et al., 2025). Moreover, surgery is not just beneficial to an individual patient, as its significance extends to influencing public health policy for controlling and managing tropical diseases among multicultural populations. Infection transmission can be prevented by surgical intervention through reducing parasite burden among the population, and thus it is vital in endemic areas suffering from weak healthcare infrastructure.

The case of bowel obstruction with ascariasis and the management of cystic echinococcosis in children are two such examples that illustrate this dictum admirably. The operation serves as a vital link between moving patients from acute care to long-term health, and by doing so, contributes to the overall mission of public health interventions in tropical disease control. As noted in these cases, the use of surgical care as part of treatment practice serves not only to cure nearest health crises but also to instill an aggressive policy of community disease and health prevention in tropical environments (Liyew et al., 2025; Mihai et al., 2025) (Figure 15.2).

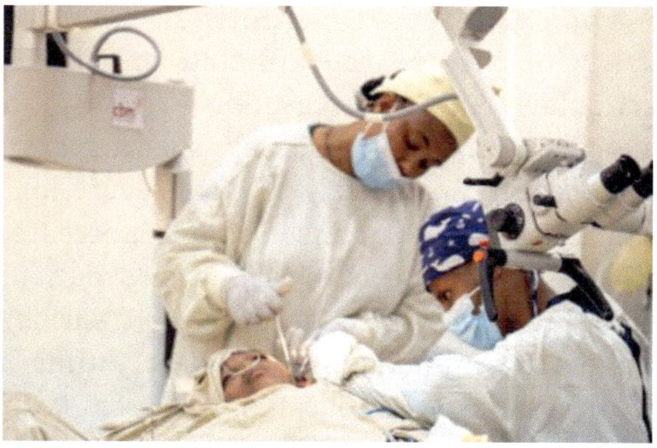

Figure 15.2. Neglected tropical diseases (NTDs).

Source: https://www.cbm.org/.imaging/mte/cbm-theme/articleTeaserTextContent-xl/dam/cbmORG/our-work/what-we-do/ear-and-hearing-care/ETH-24-Fekereab-Tezera-085-lpr.jpg/jcr:content/ETH-24-Fekereab%20Tezera-085-lpr.jpg.

15.1. Common Tropical Diseases Requiring Surgery

Learning Outcome

1. Define the schistosomiasis and its surgical implications
2. Discuss on lymphatic filariasis and surgical management
3. Lean about leprosy and reconstructive surgery

The incidence of tropical diseases in most regions of the globe often demands intervention by surgery, particularly with conditions such as tubo-ovarian abscess. This becoming increasingly common gynecological condition ranks second to pelvic inflammatory disease and has a pertinent bearing on women's health. Surgical interventions are necessary where conservative management is inadequate. A recent study found that patients with larger abscess masses—typically greater than 5.25 cm—have a higher propensity to require surgical intervention, guided by biochemical markers such as procalcitonin and white blood cell count (Gunkaya et al., 2025). Decision-making is an essential process, as prompt surgical intervention can avoid complications in the form of sepsis, which may arise from an infection left untreated. This underscores the urgency of recognizing symptoms early on. Pilonidal disease is also a common tropical illness in which an operation might be required. These abscesses could be due to the invasion of hair and skin debris in the buttock crease, which, in turn, becomes infected and inflamed. Incision and drainage would normally form the initial treatment, but where there are recurring infections or severe inflammation, one-stage excision under operation can be used very effectively. Single-stage excision is supported by evidence that not only accelerates recovery but also reduces the rate of disease recurrence, allowing for more efficient control of acute attacks (Gor et al., 2025). The success of the procedure is evident in the short hospital stays and high rates of recurrence-free healing of patients, with an encouraging future for therapy in the tropics. Identification of the surgical needs related to tropical diseases paints a broader picture in international health.

Tropical diseases, and especially parasitic infections, often lead to complications that need surgery. For instance, abscess formation due to prolonged infections, such as schistosomiasis, may require surgery in the form of drainage or removal to prevent health dangers. As these diseases are still significant health issues in areas of endemicity, improving surgical capacity and training for local healthcare workers is crucial. Such an initiative not only addresses the root issue of health but also renders healthcare systems in tropical environments more sustainable in the long term, bringing a future for improved patient outcomes and decreased morbidity from surgical needs related to tropical disease (Figure 15.3).

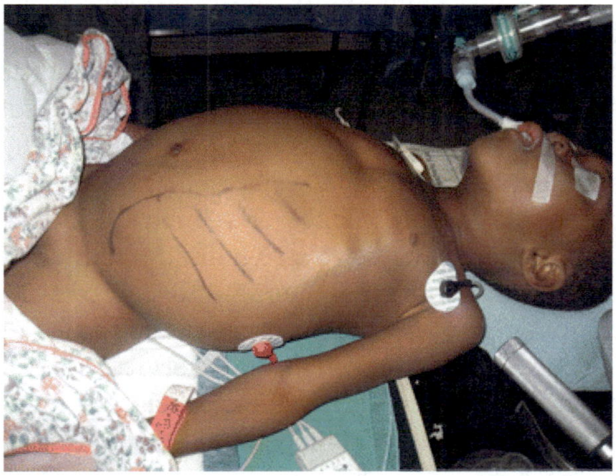

Figure 15.3. Tropical infectious disease medicine for surgeons.

Source: https://media.springernature.com/lw685/springer-static/image/chp%3A10.1007%2F978-3-319-49482-1_15/MediaObjects/331491_1_En_15_Fig3_HTML.gif.

15.1.1. Schistosomiasis and Its Surgical Implications

The health impact of schistosomiasis is most significant in regions such as Sub-Saharan Africa, where the disease is endemic and affects millions of people. Schistosomiasis is a neglected tropical disease (NTD) caused by parasitic flatworms of the genus *Schistosoma*, which inhabit freshwater environments. The parasite life cycle involves the use of freshwater snails as intermediate hosts, with human infection resulting from contact with infested water. The symptomatic presentation may range from gastrointestinal dysfunction to severe urinary tract complications that could necessitate surgery in the form of complications such as fibrosis, strictures, or ectopic pregnancy. In Ethiopia, for example, the endemicity of schistosomiasis highlights both the immediate health implications and long-term concerns related to sanitation and access to healthcare in managing such cases (Alemu et al., 2012). Schistosomiasis also has surgical implications, both elective and emergent. When patients experience complications from chronic schistosomiasis, surgical repair may be necessary to address specific anatomical and functional impairments. Schistosomiasis of the urinary tract can cause thickening of the bladder wall, for instance, which requires surgical repair to remove the obstruction and restore normal function. There are also cases wherein surgery is performed for the treatment or excision of fibrotic lesions that can predispose the patients to cancers like squamous cell carcinoma of the bladder. Not only do such surgeries improve the quality of the patient's life, but they also relieve the burden of disease symptoms, which can be particularly incapacitating in regions of limited access to healthcare resources and surgical expertise (Barnett et al., 2000). Against this backdrop of surgical considerations, the integration of community health programs into surgical management is crucial for efficiently managing schistosomiasis. Continuous sensitization and education programs with a focus on prevention, early diagnosis, and treatment are essential for reducing the need for surgery in the long run. Furthermore, improving healthcare infrastructure and reinforcing surgical capacity in endemic regions can assist in the implementation of timely interventions once complications arise. This dual approach not only enhances the effectiveness of surgery but also addresses the root causes of schistosomiasis transmission, thereby promoting public health resilience as a whole. Thus, as the science of tropical medicine continues to evolve, surgical interventions should be viewed in the context of the treatment strategy as a blend of preventive and curative methods for schistosomiasis (Alemu et al., 2012) (Figure 15.4).

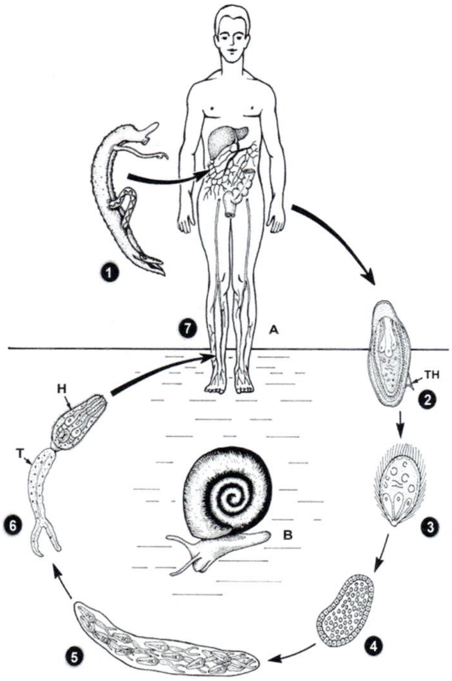

Figure 15.4. Schistosoma.

Source: https://media.springernature.com/lw685/springer-static/image/prt%3A978-3-540-48996-2%2F19/MediaObjects/978-3-540-48996-2_19_Part_Fig1-2822_HTML.jpg.

15.1.2. Lymphatic Filariasis and Surgical Management

The impact of lymphatic filariasis (LF) extends much beyond its immediate health implications, has a significant effect on the socioeconomic well-being of the regions involved. The mosquito-borne, neglected tropical disease leads to crippling symptoms in the form of lymphedema and hydrocele. As such, the patients are not just exposed to physical suffering but also suffer immensely from social stigmatization and ostracism. Surgical management of LF is crucial in alleviating these symptoms, particularly in individuals with hydrocele, which can be surgically cured by resection. In addition, surgical interventions are required for managing acute attacks and chronic sequelae of lymphedema, thereby providing patients with a better opportunity for readjustment in society. Successful surgery not only enhances the quality of life for individuals affected but also contributes to reducing the global LF burden in endemic communities, thereby addressing both the health and social dimensions of the disease. Robust public health strategies towards the elimination of lymphatic filariasis must accompany combined surgical management. Strategies such as mass drug administration (MDA) have been highly effective in reducing LF prevalence, as seen in Cambodia, where there was an overwhelming reduction in prevalence rates through targeted MDA campaigns and surgical interventions (Khieu et al., 2018). Inclusion of surgical services within primary healthcare systems is crucial for long-term success of LF management strategies. For instance, the establishment of reference hospitals, whereby specialized surgery for the treatment of hydrocele is offered, provides accessible care to those afflicted. Training local health workers in managing morbidity and performing surgical procedures ensures that healthcare systems become more responsive to LF complications, thereby making surgical management more efficient and sustainable in both urban and rural settings. For the final attainment of the benefits of surgical management in lymphatic filariasis, a multiagency response is required. Stakeholder agency involvement, like government health departments, local nongovernmental organizations, and international health organizations, is required to build upon resources and know-how in LF control programs. Public awareness campaigns for de-stigmatization of LF can also ensure community mobilization and acceptability of both medical and surgical treatments. The World Health Organization has also emphasized the importance of incorporating surgical interventions into broader public health strategies for controlling neglected tropical diseases (Engels et al., 2020). With the encouragement of a multidisciplinary approach combining surgery, public health policy, and community education, the effective management of lymphatic filariasis can be pursued more vigorously, paving the way for improved health care and quality of life for such groups (Figure 15.5).

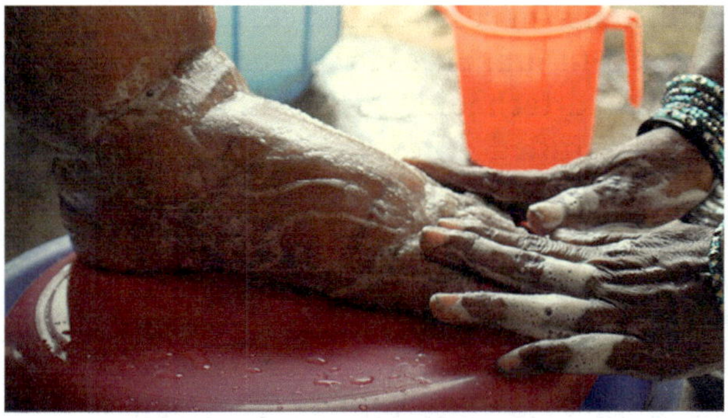

Figure 15.5. Clinical treatment of lymphatic filariasis.

Source: https://www.cdc.gov/filarial-worms/media/images/2024/05/LF-foot-leg-washing-demo.png.

15.1.3. Leprosy and Reconstructive Surgery

Treating leprosy in the realm of reconstructive surgery reveals a subtle interaction between a patient's physiological well-being and social status. *Mycobacterium leprae* causes leprosy, which is apt to cause radical physical deformities by destroying nerves to leave people with disabilities for fine motor organs and facial asymmetry. The conditions are compounded by the stigma attached to leprosy, whereby patients with the tropical disease are constantly exposed to social ostracism. Reconstructive surgery becomes the focal point of restoring not only physical function but also the psychosocial well-being of these patients, towards easing reintegration into society. Effective results in surgical operations play a pivotal role in the rehabilitation of the lives of leprosy patients, thereby offering a multidimensional intervention that not just tackles medical but also social facets of this neglected disease. Surgical interventions used in the correction of leprosy-related deformities have evolved significantly, keeping pace with advancements in reconstructive modalities. Current practices involve tendon transfer, skin grafting, and even flaps, which restore both mobility and aesthetics. Clinical evidence suggests that pre-operative and post-operative care with maximum attention can ensure acceptable functional results, thereby revolutionizing patients' quality of life. For example, studies indicate that reconstructive surgery significantly reduces secondary deformities and complications, enabling patients to resume productive everyday lives (Calongea et al., 2021). Moreover, surgery not only treats visible deformities but assists in psychological recovery as well, providing a sense of normalcy and self-assurance to individuals previously ostracized due to their condition. The reconstructive surgery setting for leprosy sufferers also needs to consider the overall implications of the availability of healthcare in tropical countries. Often, the surgery facilities that can treat such specialized reconstructive needs do not exist, particularly in low-resource settings. Moreover, the socio-economic challenges faced by leprosy patients might limit access to surgery, and an outreach and educational effort is needed to ensure that patients are treated in a timely fashion (Costa et al., 2006). Thus, enhancing leprosy patient surgery outcomes requires a multidisciplinary approach with trained healthcare professionals, adequate facilities, and supportive policies to reduce the disease burden. Not only does reconstructive surgery alleviate the physical effects of leprosy, but it also serves as a gateway to restoring dignity and acceptance in society, with significant implications for the overall management of tropical diseases through surgical care.

Test Your Knowledge

1. Describe the surgical indications and common operative procedures used in the management of intestinal obstruction caused by Ascaris lumbricoides.
2. Discuss the major tropical diseases that commonly require surgical intervention, such as amoebic liver abscess, filarial lymphoedema, tropical pancreatitis, and typhoid intestinal perforation. I

15.2. Surgical Techniques in Tropical Medicine

Learning Outcome

1. Define the traditional surgical methods
2. Discuss on minimally invasive techniques
3. Describe the innovations in surgical technology

The clinical context of surgical practice in tropical medicine presents a critical juncture between advanced surgical practice and the demands imposed by disease vectors associated with tropical diseases. Surgeons are often forced to operate across a spectrum of complex cases, frequently requiring innovative solutions, in populations where such diseases have been exacerbated by climate, socio-economic status, and limited access to care. Protein restriction diets, and so forth. Methods such as robotic surgery have emerged as possible substitutes, particularly for conditions such as pancreatic ductal adenocarcinoma. A systematic review has established that the results of robotic pancreatic surgery with vascular resection are equivalent to those of other surgical methods, but with longer operative times and variable complication rates, necessitating ongoing research (Ferrara et al., 2024). The incorporation of such advanced surgical technologies becomes imperative, especially as surgeons act on life-threatening ailments prevalent in tropical environments. In addition to advanced methods, accurate pre-surgical diagnosis cannot be overstated, especially in regions where there is limited health care. The incidental detection of renal masses, which is more prevalent in tropical conditions, necessitates rigorous evaluation to prevent unnecessary operations. Newer ultrasound technologies, including CEUS, have been identified as excellent agents for renal mass characterization. The modality has been shown to improve specificity in diagnosis, yielding sensitive characterizations that align with standard imaging modalities, such as MRI (Roussel et al., 2022). By enhancing the ability to differentiate between benign and malignant lesions non-invasively, these techniques considerably reduce the likelihood of patients undergoing unnecessary surgery and thereby optimize surgical outcomes and patient protection in tropical medicine. Furthermore, the ongoing development of surgical techniques in tropical medicine reflects the need for specialized training and resource allocation based on the region's specific requirements. Surgeons in the tropics must not only be highly skilled in advanced surgical procedures but also possess a sophisticated understanding of the prevalent diseases that confront them. With an increased emphasis on minimal invasive interventions, such as robotic surgeries, specialist training becomes a necessity. As noted in reviews of robotic surgeries, a considerable potential for benefits exists, provided that health systems invest in training and infrastructure for such refined techniques (Ferrara et al., 2024). Therefore, an all-inclusive approach that combines refined surgical techniques and advanced diagnostic modalities can make a significant difference in refining surgical practice in tropical medicine, with the ultimate goal of improving health outcomes for vulnerable populations (Figure 15.6).

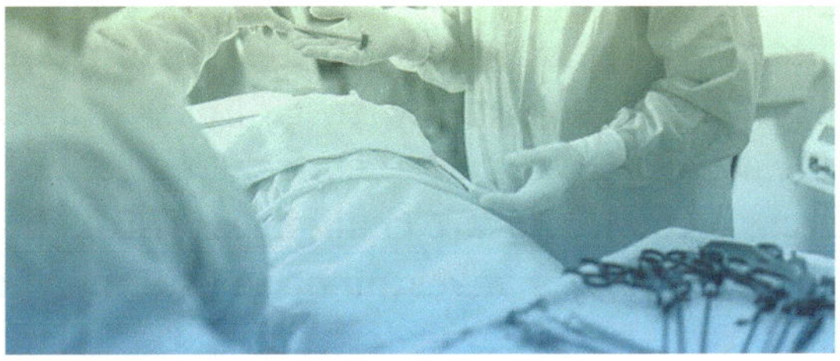

Figure 15.6. Surgical techniques development.

Source: https://pub.mdpi-res.com/title_story/title_story_17515245862202.jpg?1751444871.

15.2.1. Traditional Surgical Methods

Traditional surgery is a vital aspect of addressing most of the tropical diseases, particularly in third-world countries where advanced medical technologies are not readily available. Such conventional methods, traditionally borrowed from practice, have been adapted to address the development of diseases that are most prevalent in the tropics, such as schistosomiasis and lymphatic filariasis. Surgical interventions, including excisions, for instance, of lymphedema due to lymphatic filariasis and repair of schistosomal bladder damage, remain significant in the mitigation of morbidity. The technical simplicity and effectiveness of well-established surgical techniques render them suitable for application in rural health centers, where personnel with minimal training can employ basic equipment and local anesthesia in place of sophisticated surgical instruments. Despite technological advances in medicine, such procedures serve to underscore the areas of cultural context and regional expertise in the delivery of sustainable solutions to healthcare management of tropical diseases. The success of traditional surgical procedures in treating tropical diseases is attested to by their adaptability to local contexts and the emphasis on community-based care. Many classical approaches place significant importance on timely intervention to prevent further disease advancement, which is particularly important in highly endemic areas for vector-borne diseases and infectious diseases. For instance, implementing classical skin surgery for treating skin-borne tropical diseases, such as Buruli ulcer, not only results in clinical effectiveness but also enhances community involvement and trust in surgical operations. Further, traditional surgical interventions leverage herbal medicine and wound care knowledge to the fullest to improve positive patient outcomes while minimizing risks. Therefore, their implementation into contemporary medical practices can bridge gaps in healthcare access and offer much-needed services to at-risk populations of tropical diseases, as evidenced by sustained interventions throughout various low-income nations. Although conventional surgical techniques offer important advantages, their application also highlights the need for an overall strategy in the treatment of tropical diseases. Their integration with contemporary medical practice can improve the quality of care. For example, the combination of antique operations with new antibiotics can more effectively treat infections that occur in surgical wounds in diabetic patients, as recommended in contemporary diabetic foot care guidelines (Benjamin et al., 2020). But these antique measures also have their own complications, such as the possibility of ending up with complications arising from inadequate postoperative care and poor access to follow-up care. For the long-term development of traditional surgical practice to be sustainable, there must be collective action towards enhanced training of local health practitioners and increased financial investment to make everything feasible. This two-action approach would maximize the use of traditional surgical techniques, providing a window of opportunity for comprehensive and meaningful surgical coverage of tropical diseases.

15.2.2. Minimally Invasive Techniques

The introduction of minimally invasive surgery has revolutionized surgery, particularly in the management of tropical diseases, where patient populations and resource constraints present unique challenges. Traditional surgery induces a lot of trauma, lengthy recovery times, and hospital stays, all of which can be most disadvantageous in the low-resource setting. Through the use of techniques like laparoscopic surgery and high-end endoscopy, clinicians can now perform complex procedures with minimal incisions, resulting in less pain and a quicker recovery for patients. These benefits are paramount in tropical medicine, where rapid patient turnover and affordable treatment modalities are a priority in addressing diseases prevalent in a particular region. Minimally invasive surgery also enhances surgical efficacy and safety, two integral elements of tropical disease management. The precision offered by such techniques can minimize blood loss and decrease the risk of postoperative infection, both significant concerns in tropical areas where medical infrastructure may be limited. The ability to visualize internal anatomy through advanced imaging devices also allows surgeons to navigate challenging anatomical landscapes safely. This precision not only enables treatment but also reduces the likelihood of complications resulting from more invasive procedures, thereby improving overall patient outcomes and satisfaction in a field where these are paramount. The adoption of minimally invasive techniques in surgery for tropical illnesses serves as a model for addressing global health disparities.

As healthcare systems worldwide struggle to address both endemic diseases and resource limitations, the application of these techniques represents a mechanism for enhancing surgical care in regions that need it most. Development in surgical technology and training targeted to complement minimally invasive procedures can be pivotal for regions bearing a heavy burden of tropical diseases. These advances align with interventions aimed at reducing mortality and morbidity among vulnerable populations, demonstrating how modern surgical practices can be effectively reoriented to address local healthcare challenges. Throughout all this, increased investment in training and technology will be essential to guarantee further enhancement in surgical results across the tropics (N/A, 2015; Copeland et al., 2020) (Figure 15.7).

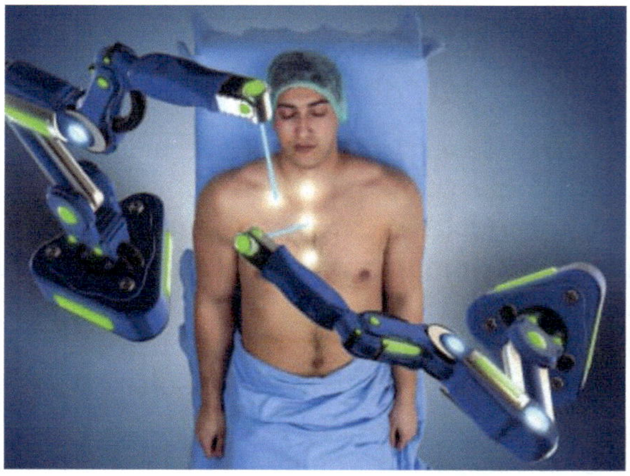

Figure 15.7. Advancement of minimally invasive device design.

Source: https://res.cloudinary.com/tbmg/c_scale,w_400,f_auto,q_auto/v1633321819/sites/mdb/articles/2021/features/MDB-1021-p12_fig1.jpg.

15.2.3. Innovations in Surgical Technology

The science of surgical technology has witnessed phenomenal advancements, particularly towards combating special issues resulting from tropical diseases. Technologies such as minimally invasive surgery have transformed the practice of surgery, with reduced recovery periods and fewer complications. This is particularly relevant in the tropics, where healthcare facilities can be remote and the disease burden, such as lymphatic filariasis or buruli ulcer, is considerable. These conditions are often characterized by vast morbidity, necessitating surgical intervention to prevent permanent disability. Recent developments, such as robotic surgery and telemedicine, have facilitated specialized surgical procedures in geographically distant areas, enabling patients to receive suitable treatment regardless of their location. These technologies would allow surgeons to perform complex procedures with precision and a better safety profile, emphasizing the key role they play in upgrading surgical outcomes in tropical disease management. Furthermore, with the integration of artificial intelligence (AI) and machine learning in surgical technology, the future also holds great promise for procedural development. AI can analyze vast amounts of data to enable diagnostic purposes and tailor surgical approaches to individual patient needs. In tropical diseases, where co-morbidities can complicate simple treatment, AI can recommend the most suitable surgical approach, thereby optimizing outcomes. Furthermore, advances in imaging technology, such as 3D visualization, enable enhanced preoperative planning and intraoperative navigation. These advances enhance the surgeon's visualization of complex anatomical structures, significantly improving accuracy during procedures. With continued development, these advances have the potential to reduce surgery complications for diseases that are more prevalent in tropical climates, ultimately contributing to better patient care and recovery rates. Furthermore, the role of collaborative partnerships in facilitating the dissemination of surgical innovations cannot be overstated. Surgical care organizations in low- and middle-income countries (LMICs) often try to increase access to advanced surgical techniques and training. When building local surgical capacity, such organizations spread knowledge and resources that incorporate innovative surgical technology. For instance, their impact on pediatric surgical programs has been substantial, as evidenced by cost-effectiveness in avoiding premature death and permanent disability in children with congenital anomalies (Uba et al., 2014). Programs established in partnership with global health foundations have led to efficient programs that integrate technological innovations in surgery into existing healthcare systems (Barnett et al., 2000). This joint approach not only fosters sustainable healthcare systems but also empowers local experts to effectively utilize innovations in surgical technology in combating the challenges of tropical diseases.

Test Your Knowledge

1. What is the role of incision and drainage (I&D) in managing tropical soft-tissue infections such as abscesses caused by Staphylococcus aureus or parasitic infestations?
2. How is the choice of surgical approach different in tropical gastrointestinal emergencies like typhoid perforation compared to non-tropical causes of bowel perforation?

15.3. Challenges in Surgical Care for Tropical Diseases

Learning Outcome

1. Describe the inadequate access to healthcare facilities
2. Discuss shortage of trained surgical professionals
3. Define financial constraints and resource allocation

The subtlety of surgical management of tropical diseases is also further jeopardized by the pervasive problem of antimicrobial resistance, which can largely endanger patient outcomes across such regions. In the endemic areas of tropical disease, promiscuous antibiotic overuse is caused both by excessive prescribing and by medical professionals' ignorance. Not only does this abuse lead to higher infection rates, which are often a source of surgical complications, but it also renders standard postoperative care measures less effective. To address these issues, a strategy centered on health education and professional development for healthcare workers is necessary. Besides, there is a need to place importance on evidence-based practice, especially when it comes to prescribing antibiotics. As highlighted in recent discussions, knowledge regarding the effectiveness of policies to address antimicrobial resistance is needed, as it directly affects the surgical management of tropical diseases and ultimately impacts the rate at which patients survive (Cornet et al., 2017). Another significant concern in surgical tropical disease care is the lack of access to resources and surgical expertise. In low and middle-income countries where tropical diseases are prevalent, there is often a lack of trained surgeons, substandard surgical facilities, and a scarcity of basic medical supplies. Not only are necessary surgeries unnecessarily delayed, but the possibility of complications is increased when surgeries are eventually carried out. Populations may be imperiled by the lack of timely and effective surgical care, which could address conditions such as lymphatic filariasis or neglected tropical diseases. Interventions that focus on building up surgical capacity within these areas must be directed at training the indigenous healthcare workforce and investing in infrastructure to achieve a long-term resolution. This is in addition to calls for universal summaries of existing policies addressing these gaps, highlighting equitable access to surgical care across all income settings (Aarestrup et al., 2015).

Secondly, patients in tropical disease-endemic regions should not be left behind by socio-economic determinants, which often affect the outcomes of surgical care. Many of the patients who are diagnosed with tropical diseases will also experience economic hardships that will deter them from seeking early medical attention or returning for postoperative follow-up. Cultural beliefs and practices will also interfere with the patients' decisions to pursue surgery, which leads to delay or denial of treatment. To resolve these issues, health workers must adopt a community-based approach with outreach and education that encourages early treatment-seeking behavior. A combination of human, animal, and environmental health through the application of the One Health concept can also ensure a wider appreciation of the issues in surgical care. Through tailoring interventions to socio-economic contexts and cultures, the effectiveness of surgical treatment for tropical diseases can be significantly improved (Aarestrup et al., 2015).

15.3.1. Inadequate Access to Healthcare Facilities

The availability of healthcare facilities is a major determinant in addressing the surgical needs of tropical diseases. In the majority of places where these diseases are prevalent, particularly in low- and middle-income countries, there is a lack of healthcare facilities. This limited access hinders timely intervention, with an increased morbidity and mortality associated with conditions requiring surgical intervention. Geographic barriers, such as remote locations and inadequate transportation facilities, also exacerbate this issue, often resulting in patients having to wait for treatment. In addition, the health facility inequity can reinforce situations in which surgical services become inaccessible or unaffordable, leading to reliance on limited access to basic services that can mitigate the catastrophic impact of tropical diseases on vulnerable groups. The effect of restricted access to healthcare is brutally exposed in maternal health outcomes. The obstetric emergency care by organizations such as Médecins Sans Frontières (MSF) opens the door to dramatic maternal mortality decline when access to high-quality care is improved. In Kabezi, Burundi, for example, MSF's programs have demonstrated an impressive 74% decrease in maternal mortality related to severe acute maternal morbidity because of emergency care provided (Baskett et al., 2012). However, the challenges that are context-specific, such as limited patient transfer systems and infrastructure disparities, remain and counteract efforts towards meeting maternal health targets as outlined by global goals. There is an urgent need to provide healthcare access in these regions to facilitate timely surgical interventions, ultimately protecting the health of mothers and infants in the event of potential threats from tropical diseases. In addressing these challenges, multi-faceted action must be taken, combining policy reform with community engagement to enhance healthcare infrastructure. It may include the development of mobile health units that enhance the scope of surgical capacity in remote areas, further strengthening a One Health approach as necessitated by the need for comprehensive policy review in various settings (Aarestrup et al., 2015). Investment in medical facilities, including training medical personnel and enhancing basic services, is crucial for current protocols that ensure the equitable provision of surgical care. These measures are essential in tropical disease control because the lack of equitable healthcare not only contributes to suffering at the personal level but also puts already compromised health systems in the developing world under undue strain, indicating a compelling necessity to improve health equity worldwide (Figure 15.8).

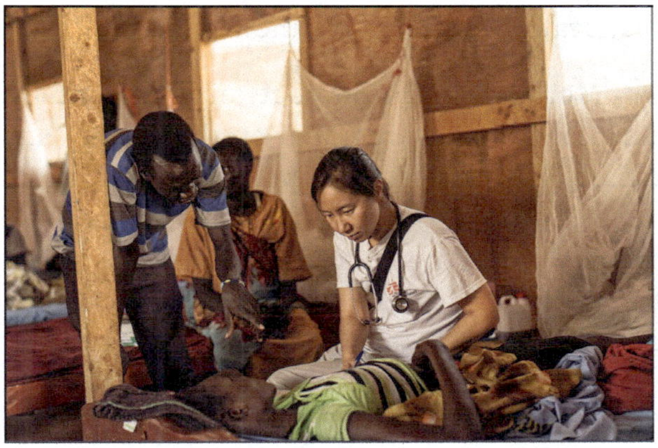

Figure 15.8. Médecins Sans Frontières (MSF).

Source: https://irishtimes-irishtimes-prod.web.arc-cdn.net/resizer/v2/LI7NC6EGPFATWZR3TS4IG7I6DY.jpg?auth=3c2add3ba4f955ac60e4e7a101307ddf9765476560c1129aa48b488f8feebcb8&width=1600&quality=70.

15.3.2. Shortage of Trained Surgical Professionals

The lack of qualified surgical specialists in the context of tropical disease substantially disables the potential for maximizing surgical requirements. The majority of low- and middle-income countries (LMICs) face a critical imbalance between the growing need for surgery and the inadequate provision of skilled surgeons. This deficiency is compounded by challenges such as limited access to surgical training and infrastructure weaknesses in the health sector, which discourage the development of a robust surgical manpower even further. Of concern here, residents of rural or underserved settings are disproportionately affected because these places most often lack either the facilities or trained personnel needed for safe surgery. As highlighted by recent studies, except for radical improvements in surgical training and healthcare policy, the global surgical burden is expected to continue increasing, underscoring the imperative for strategic interventions designed to enhance the workforce and reallocate resources (Matthew et al., 2021).

Moreover, the impact of substandard surgical training programs on the quality and efficacy of surgical care provided to patients suffering from tropical diseases can only be reduced by competency-based training. Most common surgical conditions of the tropics, such as cysticercosis and lymphatic filariasis, not only require urgent surgery but also a full understanding of the native practices of disease control. A lack of surgical training creates a void that leads to misdiagnosis, complications, and poor patient outcomes. Such excessive reliance on a small number of highly trained specialists puts pressure on them, fostering a culture of burnout and contributing to further attrition from the pool of health professionals. Such steps to increase educational pathways and mentorship prospects for future surgeons in underserved settings are vital in cultivating an educated surgical workforce with the capacity to deliver quality care to the most vulnerable populations (Semaan et al., 2020). Overcoming the shortage of trained surgical staff must be pursued through progressive measures aimed at capacity building in LMICs, particularly in the face of increased burdens from global health emergencies. The recent global pandemics, such as the one caused by COVID-19, have strained healthcare systems and worsened current inequities in access to surgery. While frontline health professionals reported greater stress and knowledge gaps in addressing the newer health challenges, it was realized that enhanced surgical education also needs to include ongoing professional education and psychological counseling for surgical teams. Integrated solutions should encompass partnerships with higher-regarded healthcare organizations, where they can offer the transfer of experiences and provide opportunities for experiential knowledge sharing. It should be prioritized to focus on the long-term sustainability of surgical training to create a strong surgical workforce that can address shifting healthcare demands while performing essential surgical interventions for tropical diseases safely and effectively (Matthew et al., 2021) (Figure 15.9).

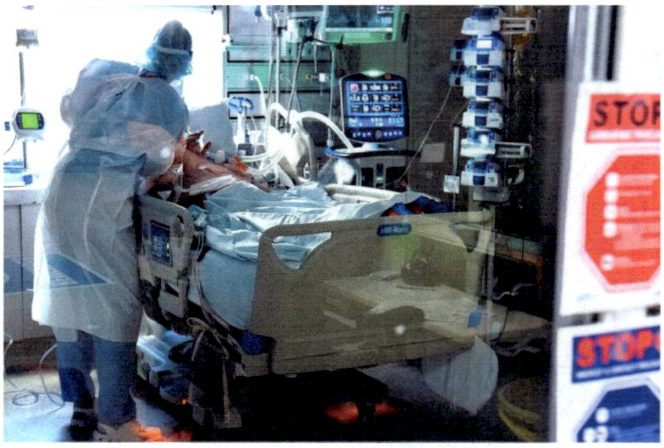

Figure 15.9. Shortage of trained surgical professionals in tropical disease.

Source: https://www.vmcdn.ca/f/files/shared/feeds/cp/2022/09/20220907110928-6318b8c744c955e5e4d89e39jpeg.jpg;w=1200;h=800;mode=crop.

15.3.3. Financial Constraints and Resource Allocation

Effective surgery for tropical diseases is generally limited by inadequate resources and poor funding allocation in healthcare systems in low- and middle-income countries. High priority for surgery, especially for tropical disease-affected regions, is primarily contingent on insufficient investment and funding in infrastructure, human capacity, and life-sustaining medical equipment. As pointed out in recent publications, insufficient financial assistance leads to stark disparities in the ability to access surgical care. It adds to the burden of otherwise treatable diseases through surgery. The mutual reinforcement of inadequate funding and wasteful resource utilization results in prolonged access to proper surgical care in a timely manner, further worsening health outcomes for these populations and hampering the process of universal health coverage in the tropics. In addition, integration of surgical services into national health plans should also emphasize financial sustainability to address the current deficit in care. The current accessibility of surgeries remains severely hampered by economic limitations that traditionally favor other health services over surgical needs. The COVID-19 pandemic has highlighted the importance of early diagnosis and equitable access to surgical care; however, economic disparities persist. For instance, less than 20% of the population in rural groups in low-income environments receive even primary surgical care since there are poor financing systems and management. Overcoming such budgetary constraints is crucial to improving resource utilization for surgical care, thereby enhancing outcomes for not only common conditions but also neglected tropical diseases within underserved populations. Importantly, the development of novel funding vehicles and partnerships is crucial for enhancing monetary support for surgical procedures and investing in resources in nations struggling with tropical diseases. Following the inspiration of international health agendas with universal health coverage and fair access, valuable interventions might include mobilizing public-private partnerships and tactical investment in facilities. These interventions can contribute towards a stronger workforce with surgical method training in tropical disease-specific procedures. Resource realignment and prioritization of financial allocation can significantly enhance access to surgical care, leading to improved health outcomes and a reduction in preventable morbidity due to tropical diseases. The requirement is to transform how surgical care financing is done, aligning the interests of local governments and international health organizations with the forging of lasting solutions to enhance surgical services in areas affected by tropical diseases.

Test Your Knowledge

1. What are the major barriers to timely surgical intervention for tropical diseases in low-resource settings?
2. How do coexisting infections and poor postoperative care increase complications in surgical management of tropical diseases?

15.4. Postoperative Care in Tropical Surgery

Learning Outcome

1. Describe the infection control and management
2. Understand the rehabilitation and recovery processes
3. Define psychological support to patients

Correct postoperative care is of very great significance in tropical surgery, whereby infectious complications are usual and can have direct relevance to patient outcomes. Because of the unique environmental conditions within the tropics, the site of surgery could be more susceptible to infection by other bacterial flora, particularly following surgery for tropical diseases such as Buruli ulcer. It is established that secondary-infected patients are prevalent in the postoperative period, with more than 60% of Buruli ulcers presenting with co-infection from bacteria such as *Staphylococcus aureus* and *Pseudomonas aeruginosa* before the start of treatment, leading to complicated healing processes (Pahlevan et al., 2013). Precautions taken to maintain careful monitoring and implement sound infection control procedures post-surgery are paramount in reducing these risks, allowing for maximal recovery while overcoming the insoluble problems posed by tropical pathogens. The risk of less-than-optimal postoperative care also lies higher in the context of tropical disease, in which patient reactions to surgery are less foreseeable. In the tropics, most patients are subjected to compromised immunity, often accompanied by malnutrition or co-infection, which is prevalent in the region. Such conditions make rigorous postoperative observation essential, complete with early detection and management of ensuing complications. For instance, strict adherence to asepsis and wound dressing after surgery can go a long way towards keeping the risk of infection to a minimum, leading to quick recovery. With improved effectiveness in their efforts, integrating proper postoperative care procedures into the systems under their influence, informed by the socioeconomic and environmental situation of tropical regions, is central to determining desired health outcomes (Fryer et al., 2011).

In addition to infection control, postoperative care in tropical surgery must also contend with the broader aspects of patient care, including psychosocial management and monitoring chronic conditions. Patients undergoing tropical disease surgeries may experience severe emotional distress as a result of their health condition, compounded by the socio-economic disadvantage suffered in these nations. Health workers should place more emphasis on crafting support care networks, promoting access to mental health, and addressing chronic illnesses that may indirectly affect recovery from the operation.

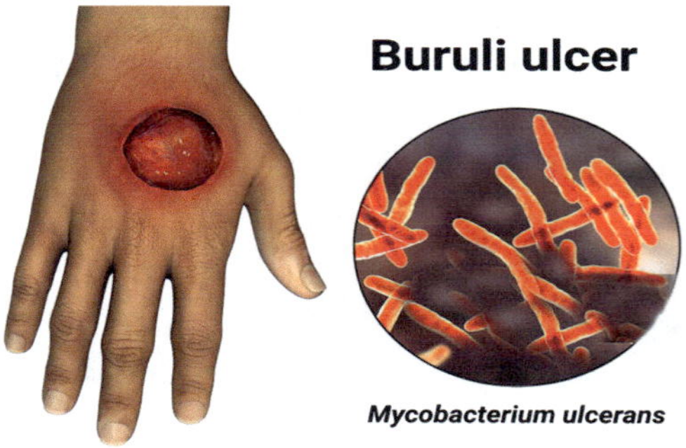

Figure 15.10. Buruli ulcer and *Mycobacterium ulcerans*.

Source: https://media.gettyimages.com/id/1481204520/vector/buruli-ulcer-and-mycobacterium-ulcerans-illustration.jpg?s=1024x1024&w=gi&k=20&c=Le2W_ycbEcDzTi3SsmRMss0_kKASzfUoHfQhLBMbXZU=.

Through embracing a whole-person approach to postoperative care, clinicians can improve recovery experiences, decrease re-admission rates, and ensure that patients are not only physically healed but also helped in terms of their psychology. This multidimensional approach is instrumental in strengthening health systems in the tropics, enabling the provision of improved surgical outcomes among vulnerable populations (Figure 15.10).

15.4.1. Infection Control and Management

Control and management of infection are central roles in the context of tropical disease surgery, particularly in light of the increased prevalence of infectious agents in endemic settings. The necessity in handling such infections lies in their potential to complicate surgical results and increase morbidity. Tropical diseases such as trachoma, for instance, which are primarily caused by *Chlamydia trachomatis*, can lead to preventable blindness and significant public health challenges in resource-constrained environments. Functional management processes must capture not just surgery but also an intersectoral strategy involving health education, community mobilization, and planning resources for initiating WHO SAFE strategies. The four strategy encompassing Surgery for trichiasis, Antibiotics for infection, Facial cleanliness, and Environmental improvement have been promoted to decrease trachoma's prevalence and as a result its companion surgical complications (Ismail et al., 2025). Hence, inclusion of infection control measures in the surgical procedure is essential for the achievement of optimal patient outcomes. Heterogeneity of infection care in tropical surgery is also augmented by unusual infections, such as Echinococcus granulosus, which results in hydatid cysts —a significant healthcare issue within regions where livestock is prevalent. Orbital hydatid cysts may present in patients and induce substantial visual impairment, and such cases require prompt surgical intervention. Treatment is usually surgical removal of the cyst, with or without the use of anthelmintic medication, such as albendazole, to treat the underlying condition. Interestingly, concomitant hydatidosis is a risk factor for recurrence and needs regular follow-up and good post-operative care (Pradhan et al., 2025). Thus, an interdisciplinary management approach that not only treats the surgical management of hydatid cysts but also emphasizes ongoing monitoring and preventive care is essential in preventing long-term complications and ensuring patient health. Proper infection control and treatment in the arena of tropical surgery ultimately demonstrates the significance of tailoring interventions to the appropriate epidemiological environment.

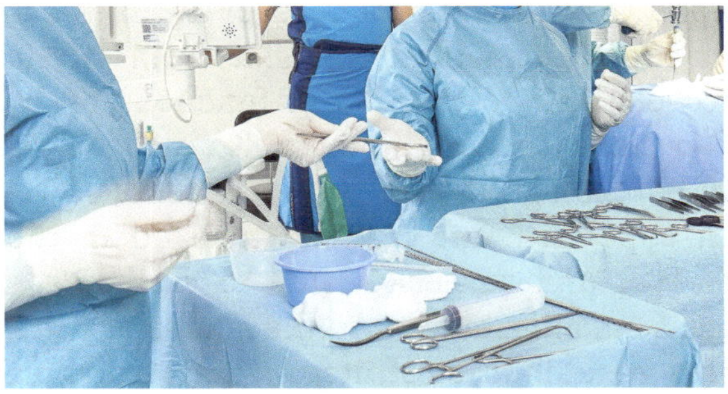

Figure 15.11. Infection control and management for tropical surgery diseases.

Source: https://www.getinge.com/siteassets/start/insights/articles/sterile-reprocessing/infection-control/hybrid-operating-room-infection-control-gloves-id-53572-cropped.jpg/cropbestbetmiddlecenter-1170x635--1740669445.jpg.

This involves exposing medical personnel to endemic local infections, information on the respective disease-causing pathogen life cycle, and transmission risk factors. Trachoma and hydatid disease, for instance, highlight the need for community education programs that educate individuals on environmental sanitation and preventive strategies to prevent the transmission of infection. Secondly, constructing the partnership among health departments,

NGOs, and local communities can significantly assist in the battle against infections. Thus, the operating environment in tropical areas can shift from reactive to preventive, resulting in substantial improvements in public health outcomes and the quality of surgical care (Ismail et al., 2025; Pradhan et al., 2025) (Figure 15.11).

15.4.2. Rehabilitation and Recovery Processes

The recovery and rehabilitation stages following surgical intervention for tropical diseases are integral to the overall success of treatment. In most cases, these operations have a significant physical and psychological impact on patients, and recovery is an all-out effort. Rehabilitation, aside from physical recovery and restoration of functions by way of special exercises and therapies, also includes the psychological recovery of patients so they can cope with the trauma involved in their diseases and surgeries. Due to variability in disease manifestation and the nature of patient cases, rehabilitation strategies must be tailored according to each case's specific requirements, with recovery mechanisms being maximally efficient and targeted. Moreover, the etiology of tropical diseases, which typically stems from determinants of health, makes rehabilitation the most challenging. In an effort to reverse long-term complications, public health initiatives aimed at combating diseases should include comprehensive rehabilitation and recovery interventions. For instance, as argued in the Global Burden of Diseases, Injuries, and Risk Factors Study (GBD), disease burden needs to be comprehended in a way that guides interventions that may lead to better rehabilitation outcomes (Alize et al., 2024). This integrated approach not only identifies the necessity of bodily healing but also emphasizes the importance of social support structures that can promote more effective recovery experiences and outcomes in various tropical environments. Lastly, the recent evidence of long COVID highlights the ongoing need to investigate rehabilitation processes in various patient groups affected by infectious illnesses. Following discharge from the hospital after tropical diseases like COVID-19, the majority of the patients experience prolonged recovery challenges that emphasize the importance of specialist rehabilitation (Rachael et al., 2022). Research into recovery patterns can inform best practices for individuals affected by tropical diseases, indicating that comprehensive rehabilitation must consider the paradigm shift in global health problems. Ultimately, successful rehabilitation and recovery protocols are essential not only for short-term patient outcomes but also for building resistance to future health adversity among patients with tropical diseases.

15.4.3. Psychological Support to Patients

The psychological impact of surgery on patients suffering from tropical diseases cannot be overstated. Operations, which are usually dictated by serious and chronic conditions characteristic of the tropics, can stimulate fear, anxiety, and apprehension in patients. These emotional responses are , which are further influenced by cultural perspectives on surgery, levels of healthcare literacy, and social stigmatization of specific diseases. Providing psychological counseling is crucial in mitigating these emotions as well as enhancing the entire operation process. Studies indicate that patients who receive proper emotional and psychological advice are less anxious and recover faster compared to other patients not undergoing counseling. By creating an environment of care that meets the psychological needs of surgical care, healthcare providers can optimize patient outcomes in the context of tropical diseases. In addition to individualized counseling, adequate psychological support also encompasses community outreach and education. In much of the tropical world, the stigma of disease and surgery can act as barriers to early medical care. Through raising awareness and knowledge through community interventions, health systems can de-mystify procedures, thereby reducing patient anxiety and creating a conducive environment. Additionally, engaging families in the psychological preparation of patients also helps build a solid support network that focuses on wellness outside the surgery. Public health initiatives that incorporate mental health education alongside physical health education have the potential to enhance patient resilience, enabling them to better cope with the challenges of their surgical experience. This combined strategy has the potential to bridge the void between medical care and psychosocial stability and provide a sense of solid ground for more enhanced surgical outcomes. Finally, the scope of psychological care is to the post-op period, where recovery from surgery may be impaired by underlying social and health histories prevalent in the tropics. Psychological distress, if untreated, can lead to complications such as prolonged rehabilitation times and high postoperative infection rates. The significance of multidisciplinary teams with mental health professionals in enhancing recovery protocols is then. Merging mental health screening into routine preoperative evaluation will detect patients at risk for emotional distress and allow individualized interventions meeting specific needs. Strengthening the psychiatric component of surgical care in tropical disease is not only about promoting better mental health, but is also essential to achieving optimal and long-term viable surgical results, a necessity given the special challenges in tropical environments detailed in Wu et al. (2020) and Matthew et al. (2021) (Figure 15.12).

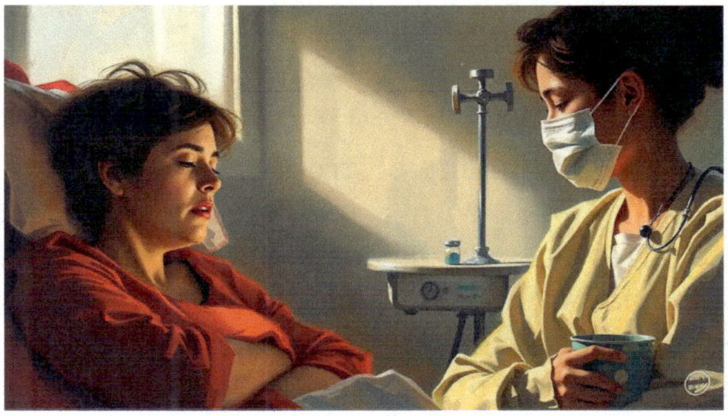

Figure 15.12. Anesthesia-and-mental-health-exploring-potential-cognitive-and-psychological-effects.

Source: https://neurolaunch.com/wp-content/uploads/2025/02/anesthesia-and-mental-health-exploring-potential-cognitive-and-psychological-effects.webp.

Test Your Knowledge

1. What factors make postoperative infection control more challenging in tropical surgical settings?
2. How does limited access to follow-up care affect recovery outcomes after tropical surgery?

15.5. Case Studies of Successful Surgical Interventions

Learning Outcome

1. Explain the case study on schistosomiasis surgery
2. Describe the case study on lymphatic filariasis treatment
3. Define the case study on leprosy reconstructive surgery

Surgical treatment of tropical diseases can be highlighted with a set of successful case scenarios that demonstrate good practice and outcome. A prime example is cataract surgery, which has considerably enhanced the quality of life for millions of people with visual disability, particularly in low and middle-income countries (LMICs). Because over 90% of those who are vision-impaired have treatable or preventable disorders, timely access to this highly cost-saving surgery is of crucial importance. There is evidence from literature to indicate that the implementation of community health programs that facilitate early detection and referral for cataract surgery can significantly reduce the incidence of blindness overall. Placing such a focus on eye health within these interventions has not only improved visual outcomes for these communities but, to a significant degree, also enhanced quality of life, underscoring the importance of continued investment in surgical interventions for tropical diseases (Matthew et al., 2021).

Yet another significant case study concerns the control of diseases such as lymphatic filariasis through surgery. Surgery, particularly hydrocelectomy, has been an effective procedure in the treatment of complications resulting from this disease. Hydrocele is a common outcome of lymphatic filariasis and can lead to stigmatization and discomfort. Research has proven that surgery not only alleviates physical complaints but also improves social reintegration and mental health status of patients. By conducting these surgeries within endemic countries, medical experts were able to address both the medical and psychological impacts of the disease. The inclusion of surgery within public health strategies effectively illustrates the multifaceted benefits of targeted surgical intervention in the prevention of tropical diseases (Gregory et al., 2020). Finally, the positive news about the surgical treatment of schistosomiasis implies that long-term improvement in the health of the public can be hoped for through precise surgical care. In particular, corrective surgeries for complications such as bladder or intestinal obstruction may significantly improve the health outcomes of patients.

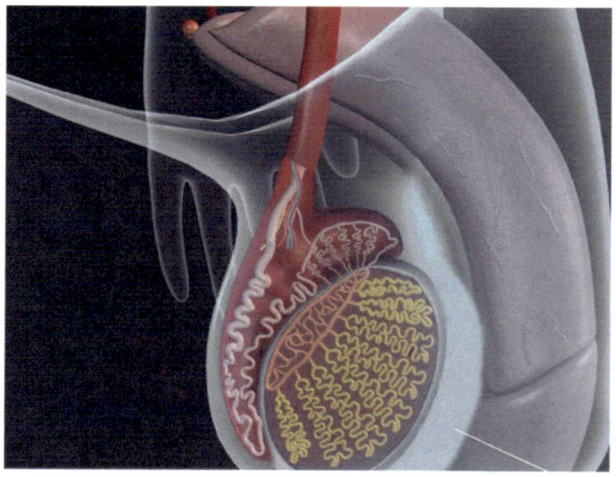

Figure 15.13. Hydrocele treatment.

Source: https://www.institutobernabeu.com/wp-content/uploads/2021/02/Hidrocele-LOW-1140x642.jpg.

The inclusion of such procedures within broader healthcare programs is proposed to reduce the frequency of secondary complications that arise from ongoing infections. In addition, by incorporating surgical treatment with preventive intervention and education on hygiene practices, communities will enhance overall health and alleviate the schistosomiasis burden in the population. It emphasizes the incorporation of surgical interventions with broader public health goals and highlights the role of surgery in addressing the challenges posed by tropical diseases (Matthew et al., 2021) (Figure 15.13).

15.5.1. Case Study on Schistosomiasis Surgery

Surgery for schistosomiasis is an attractive solution at the juncture of infectious disease treatment and surgery, particularly in cases of heavy morbidity due to the chronic presentation of the diseases. Schistosomiasis, caused primarily by trematodes of the genus Schistosoma, can result in severe complications, including hydronephrosis, splenic disease, and diffuse damage to intra-abdominal organs. In surgery, interventions can include procedures to clear obstructive pathology or lesions caused by parasitic infestations.

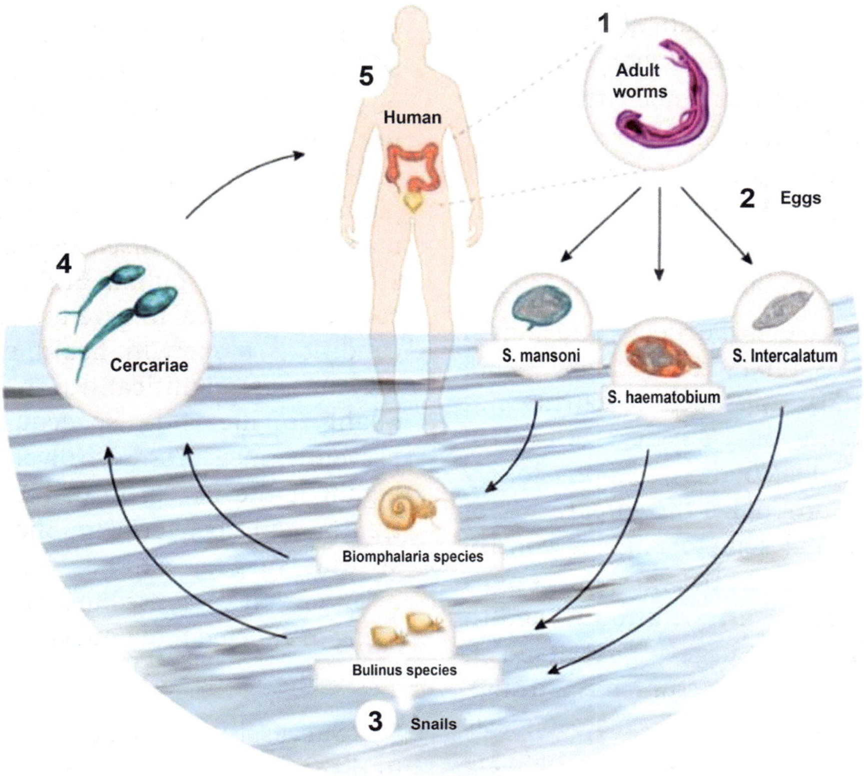

Figure 15.14. Schistosomiasis surgery.

Source: https://www.mdpi.com/tropicalmed/tropicalmed-06-00109/article_deploy/html/images/tropicalmed-06-00109-g001.png.

It is essential to interpret the broader epidemiological context, as surgical intervention must be in accordance with prevailing public health policy and available disease prevalence at the local level. Sophisticated geostatistical models, such as those applied in Tanzania, have been incorporated to enhance decision-making in medical and surgical outreach, highlighting the need for tailored practices across different geographic regions where schistosomiasis is endemic (Jake et al., 2024). Thus, integrating surgical practice into combined treatment approaches is vital in efficiently alleviating the disease burden. In addition to its contribution to resolving immediate surgical needs, the case study of schistosomiasis surgery also highlights the value of multidisciplinary treatment regimens that encompass medical, surgical, and prophylactic interventions. Traditional drug treatments are often hampered by drug resistance and chronic re-infection, making surgery an integral component for the treatment of advanced cases. Combining surgery with adjunctive therapies, such as phytochemical-loaded nanosystems, has tremendous potential for enhancing the efficacy and safety of treatments. Recent reviews also refer to the promise of such formulations to cure schistosomiasis, with potential therapeutic benefits of reducing parasite load and potentially improving patient outcomes (Soto et al., 2024).

Such overlap between surgery and novel medical treatments refers to the necessity of a multi-disciplinary approach to curing not only the immediate post-surgical effects of schistosomiasis but also the pathophysiology of the disease. Additionally, the integration of surgery into national schistosomiasis control programs highlights both the challenges and opportunities of international health interventions. Effective surgery goes hand in hand with adequate infrastructure, trained staff, and a thorough understanding of schistosomiasis epidemiology on the ground. Reports indicate that targeted mass drug administration (MDA) has the potential to reduce transmission. Still, surgical interventions must also be included as part of the treatment approach, particularly where morbidity is high. The implementation of World Health Organization guidelines, combined with the application of new geostatistical models, can inform more impactful programmatic decision-making. These interventions are crucial to ensuring that surgery, in addition to meeting acute medical needs, contributes to overall health control strategies against schistosomiasis with a view toward eventual reduction of the disease burden in affected communities (Jake et al., 2024) (Figure 15.14).

15.5.2. Case Study on Lymphatic Filariasis Treatment

The treatment of lymphatic filariasis (LF), a tropical disease primarily caused by parasitic worms, has proved the interlinking of surgical therapy and community-based health interventions. Surgery is apt to form the core of managing hydrocele and lymphoedema complications widespread among the infected population. For instance, hydrocele removal not only cures physical discomfort but also has a significant psychosocial benefit of preventing stigma due to externally perceivable manifestations of disease. Findings of recent studies carried out in Ethiopia indicate that corrective surgical intervention for secondary LF conditions, along with health education among the masses, significantly enhances patients' quality of life and also acquaints them with preventive measures. Such diversified approaches highlight the necessity of integrating surgical treatment into overall public health practice, so that surgery extends beyond procedural intervention to contribute to the overall well-being of affected individuals, particularly in low-resource settings (Alemu et al., 2012).

Successful lymphatic filariasis treatment in disease management situations requires an understanding of both the medical and social dimensions of treatment. While first-line therapies involve drug therapy, primarily with diethylcarbamazine (DEC) and ivermectin, the surgical intervention addresses the long-term consequences, critically impairing patients' quality of life. The stigma associated with filariasis highlights the need for effective treatment measures to promote community involvement. Initiatives implemented to raise awareness about the disease and the route of transmission have the ability to alter public perception and encourage individuals to seek treatment significantly. The integration of surgical intervention with strong public health communication holds potential in rural Ethiopia, where health resources are often in short supply. Stigma reduction alongside surgical intervention can help create a setting in which effective disease control and patient compliance with ongoing care may be achieved (Richens et al., 2004). Furthermore, the condition of lymphatic filariasis extends beyond short-term medical and surgical management; it requires ongoing surveillance and community support interventions. Ongoing surveillance of LF cases can inform targeted interventions and prevent recurrence through hygiene education, vector control, and health-seeking behavior. The effectiveness of surgical outcomes relies not only on the technical success of procedures but also on the rehabilitation and follow-up care that patients receive after surgery. The development of an integrated healthcare approach, leveraging the use of surgical skills as well as community health interventions, is thus needed to minimize the public health impact of LF. This model demonstrates the future effectiveness of surgery when integrated into a broader plan that involves prevention, treatment, education, and community engagement, ultimately enhancing the health environment of those affected by this neglected tropical disease (Alemu et al., 2012) (Figure 15.15).

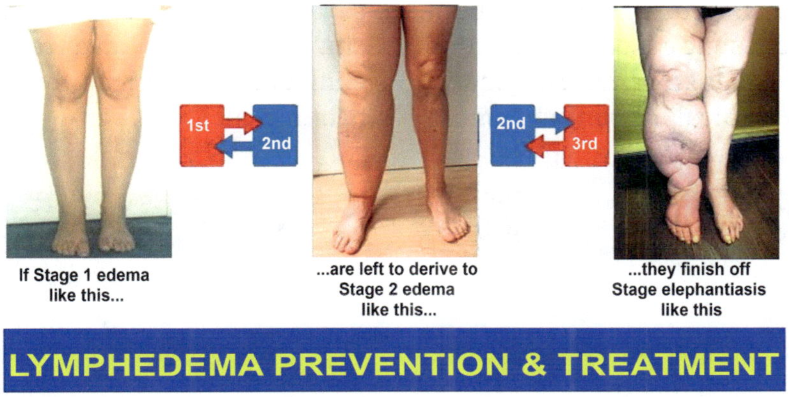

Figure 15.15. Lymphatic filariasis treatment.

Source: https://3.bp.blogspot.com/-hmJgLodmPi8/W7fnl2THFZI/AAAAAAAABc4/J5hxbmIVmFMsfGaBL3vRfqUJVHpT_iTjQCEwYBhgL/s1600/ENGLISH%2BLEG%2B1.1.jpg.

15.5.3. Case Study on Leprosy Reconstructive Surgery

Treatment of leprosy, or Hansen's disease, has evolved significantly over the past decades, more so with respect to reconstructive surgery to restore the disabling deformities induced by it. Antibiotic attempts at eradicating leprosy have not succeeded everywhere, and the majority of patients still carry with them long-standing physical disabilities secondary to nerve damage, most often of the ulnar nerve. Therefore, patients typically exhibit the characteristic ulnar claw hand, which significantly impacts their daily activities and overall quality of life. Offering these patients surgical interventions as part of their comprehensive treatment plan is crucial. Reconstructive surgery, in addition to restoring function, also helps in preventing social exclusion associated with visible deformity, hence enhancing patients' psychological well-being due to leprosy. Among many corrective surgical techniques available for deformity caused by leprosy, the *Zancolli lasso* technique is particularly effective and accessible. This technique addresses the challenging anatomic alterations that occur with ulnar nerve injury with the possibility of restoring finger flexion without jeopardizing overlying tissues. Since it enhances grip strength and arc of motion, the Zancolli technique allows patients to become more actively involved in their daily activities. Interestingly, the technique does not require sophisticated surgical skills and can be performed in smaller clinics, thereby making it accessible to underserved communities. The success of the Zancolli lasso technique underscores the importance of tailoring surgical techniques to meet the specific needs and circumstances of leprosy patients, ensuring that reconstructive surgery aligns with both medical and socioeconomic conditions affecting them. The role of reconstructive surgery in the treatment of tropical conditions, more specifically leprosy, extends far beyond the individual patient to encompass broader public health issues. Successful surgery can lead to a reduction in long-term disability, enabling the individual to be socially reintegrated, economically productive, and receive access to better healthcare facilities. The issue is getting such surgical services under total leprosy management programs. Cooperation among the healthcare workers, government, and nongovernmental organizations is key to ensuring access to care in the endemic regions. Furthermore, ongoing training and education of local healthcare personnel in performing such procedures is essential to the success of leprosy care. As illustrated by recent outbreaks in regions where leprosy has exerted a significant influence, investment in surgical care has the capacity not only to improve patient outcomes clinically but to advance global control and elimination programs for leprosy as a public health issue.

Test Your Knowledge

1. What key clinical decisions contributed to the success of specific surgical interventions in tropical disease cases?
2. How did multidisciplinary teamwork improve patient outcomes in documented tropical surgery case studies?

15.6. Future Directions in Surgical Approaches

Learning Outcome

1. Understand the research and development in surgical techniques
2. Focus on integration of technology in the practice of surgery
3. Define the global health initiatives and their impact

The evolution of surgical techniques in the treatment of tropical disease continues to change with much to report in the way of advances in patient care. With the percentage of minimally invasive procedures on the rise, surgeons today are better equipped to perform operations that minimize body trauma, decrease recovery times, and improve their patients' results. Technologies such as laparoscopic and robotic-assisted techniques are being employed increasingly in all sorts of settings, from the management of parasitic infestations and visceral diseases of organs encountered in the presentation of tropical diseases. As better and better techniques are developed, it also becomes increasingly challenging to apply them in conjunction with sophisticated imaging modalities, allowing interventions to become more targeted. This dual approach not only enhances the effectiveness of surgical treatment, but also addresses the complex character of diseases exacerbated by environmental factors that are incredibly trendy in tropical nations. Furthermore, the integration of pharmacological treatment and surgery is increasingly significant in the treatment of some tropical diseases. For instance, in spinal echinococcosis, where surgery has always been challenging, the development of adjunct pharmacotherapy would revolutionize the treatment procedures. Systematic analysis of recent literature has enlightened us to the reality that, despite the increasing sophistication of surgical procedures, they may not completely address the morbidity and mortality associated with such diseases. Consequently, the route forward lies in synergy between surgical interventions and medical treatments, which reduce infection rates or even promote healing, thereby generally improving the effectiveness of treatment regimens for illnesses such as cystic echinococcosis (Blum et al., 2013). Emphasis on an interdisciplinary approach has the potential to achieve dramatic benefits in terms of patient care and outcomes. Furthermore, early diagnosis and timely intervention are the key to the route forward in surgical practice against tropical diseases. The unethical character of such diseases as Buruli ulcer demands a shift in paradigm towards proactive care, where radical public health interventions are teamed with surgical expertise. Patients now present in the far-advanced stage, often very late, making surgery long and demanding. By investing in active case finding and community health education, as well as enhancing rapid diagnostic technology, the medical community can make early intervention a reality, thereby altering treatment streams. While surgery remains the primary treatment, acknowledging broader socio-economic and environmental determinants of diseases such as Buruli ulcer can facilitate more integrated responses that focus on early detection and management (Adjei et al., 2006). This broad perspective will be critical to maximizing surgical approaches in managing tropical disease (Figure 15.16).

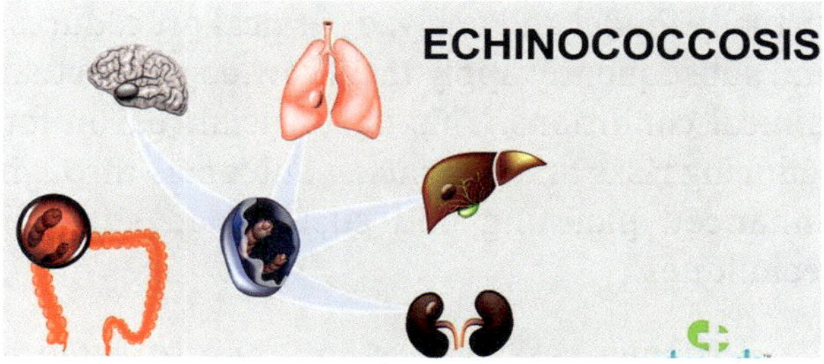

Figure 15.16. Echinococcosis causes symptoms and treatment.

Source: https://askthenurseexpert.com/wp-content/uploads/2023/09/understanding-echinococcosis-causes-symptoms-and-treatment-1.jpg.

15.6.1. Research and Development in Surgical Techniques

Refinement of surgical procedures is crucial to the success of surgical interventions, particularly in tropical diseases, where demand greatly exceeds the available means. The activity in this field is not only to develop new techniques in surgery but also to improve existing ones, aiming for better outcomes for patients. In low and middle-income countries, where the surgical disease burden is exceptionally high, surgical research inequities remain. For instance, despite Africa accounting for a vast majority of the world's surgical demand, it remains underresearched, producing fewer than 15% of the world's total surgical literature. This gap is a testament to the urgent need for focused programs that will accelerate surgical innovation through research and development to address the unique challenges of tropical disease surgery. Improving the quality and scope of surgical research will lay the groundwork for more effective treatments in these fields (Awuah et al., 2023). Utilization of modern technologies such as digital twinning, artificial intelligence, and big data analysis also brings new opportunities to enhance surgical procedures in developing regions. Digital twinning, for instance, is a cutting-edge method that enables surgeons to virtually model and analyze surgical procedures, and subsequently apply the knowledge in actual clinical conditions. This is a crucial reason for reducing risks and enhancing outcomes through enhanced planning and customized surgical techniques.

Although researchers continue to explore these technologies, the possibility of developing individualized surgical procedures that account for patients' specific needs in combating diseases in the tropics becomes increasingly feasible. Through the integration of traditional surgical practices with new technologies, the nature of surgery in low-income countries can be transformed, ultimately improving access to adequate and safe surgery (Rathore et al., 2021). Additionally, building research partnerships between international and local research communities is necessary to bridge the gap in research on surgical interventions for tropical conditions. The establishment of networks that facilitate knowledge sharing and resources can enhance local health worker training. It is essential for building capacity in surgery research and practice and promotes the development of localized solutions tailored to the challenges faced in the tropics. Inter Workspaces can also foster interdisciplinarity, combining inputs from fields such as data science, engineering, and public health to transform surgical practices. As we continue, governments, healthcare institutions, and medical schools must prioritize surgical research and its application to healthcare delivery systems to ensure gains made in surgical sciences that specifically address the growing burden of tropical diseases (Awuah et al., 2023).

15.6.2. Integration of Technology in the Practice of Surgery

Technology integration in surgical interventions has changed the landscape of surgery, particularly in treating tropical diseases, where resource limitations and limited environmental conditions are significant constraints. Robotic surgery, minimally invasive surgeries, and precision imaging are advancements that have enhanced the accuracy of surgery, increasing safety and patient outcomes. For instance, laparoscopic procedures enable surgeons to perform operations with , less invasive cuts, which shortens recovery time and reduces the possibility of infection—a substantial advantage in regions where medical centers may be overwhelmed. Also, technology supports sharing knowledge and best practices in disciplines like the Jefferson Digital Commons, an educational resource repository fundamental to sustained medical education in the tropics (Copeland et al., 2020). Accordingly, the use of technology not only supports the progression of surgical practice but also sustains the educative dialogue essential to addressing the unique challenges of the tropics. The benefits of new technology in surgery extend beyond mere operational efficiencies; they signify a new approach to interdisciplinary thinking. New technologies, such as telemedicine, provide remote consultations and post-surgical follow-ups, thereby making it possible to extend specialist surgical expertise to far-flung communities affected by tropical diseases. This capability is handy in settings where it is not likely to have trained surgical teams because it prepares local practitioners for guidance from distant specialists, who may be thousands of miles away. Technology can also conduct training sessions for local practitioners using virtual simulations and augmented reality environments. Accessibility of such computerized resources is key in enhancing skill sets and the quality of care in these populations, as observed from various activities reported in the literature

(Cornet et al., 2017). The incorporation of technology, hence, brings about better training and interprofessional practice that is crucial in fulfilling the surgical requirements of patients in the tropics. However, the successful implementation of technology within surgical practices also comes with a series of challenges that must be addressed carefully. Physical infrastructural constraints, particularly within low-resource settings prevalent in the majority of tropical disease hotspots, could hinder the applicability and functionality of advanced surgical technology. For instance, the reliance on stable electricity and internet connectivity to power technologies such as robotic surgeries or telehealth platforms is doubtful. In addition, there is an urgent necessity to continue investing in training medical professionals in the use of these technologies, or else this aspect might be neglected and yield disparities in patient treatment rather than advancements. Gaps in measures between technological advancements and practical applications remain key to maintaining the optimization of outcomes in surgical procedures for tropical diseases. As stakeholders move forward to find solutions, the lessons learned from current practices can influence future developments and create a stronger healthcare framework (Copeland et al., 2020).

15.6.3. Global Health Initiatives and Their Impact

Over the last few years, international health programs have gained traction, significantly influencing the healthcare scenario, particularly in the control of tropical diseases. Understanding disease burden prioritization helps nations create customized solutions for controlling endemic infections and enhancing the health status of populations. For instance, the Global Burden of Diseases, Injuries, and Risk Factors Study (GBD) systematically analyzes health statistics, promoting evidence-based strategies for addressing the complexities of disease patterns in populations at risk. Through analysis of various measures, such as years lived with disability (YLDs) and mortality, GBD informs public health strategies, one of which includes augmenting the potential of timely surgery intervention among tropical disease environments. This evidence-based approach promotes accountability among health policymakers and facilitates the coordination of international health targets, including the Sustainable Development Goals (Alize et al., 2024).

Surgical procedures are crucial in the treatment of conditions prevalent in tropical nations, where surgical coverage is often lacking. Global health interventions aim to provide a fairly equitable distribution of surgical services to low-income communities, ultimately enhancing access to interventions for tropical diseases such as schistosomiasis and lymphatic filariasis. Organizational-initiated interventions by organizations such as the World Health Organization are directed towards raising awareness about the contribution of surgical care to the control of diseases, as well as sensitizing local healthcare providers on best practices in surgical care. For example, there are management practices like preemptive surgery for diseases that are caused by neglected tropical diseases, which can reduce the suffering of the afflicted people and reduce long-term disability. These activities demonstrate how primary care and surgical services are interconnected, encouraging an integrated approach to preventing disease burdens (Manuela et al., 2023). Furthermore, global health initiatives play a crucial role in building local healthcare infrastructure through guaranteeing training programs and the delivery of resources. Spending on local surgeons and healthcare professionals' training programs builds a long-term talent pool that can address the particular challenges posed by tropical diseases. It not only enhances short-term health outcomes of communities but also renders health systems more resilient against future pandemics of disease. Moreover, the identification and handling of local factors that impact health, such as economic constraints and attitudes towards surgery among populations, become essential to the success of such campaigns. Through continuous cooperation between international organizations and local healthcare systems, global efforts in health can effectively undertake sustainable changes that lead to improved surgical results in tropical diseases, eventually reaching millions of patients afflicted with such diseases (Alize et al., 2024) (Figure 15.17).

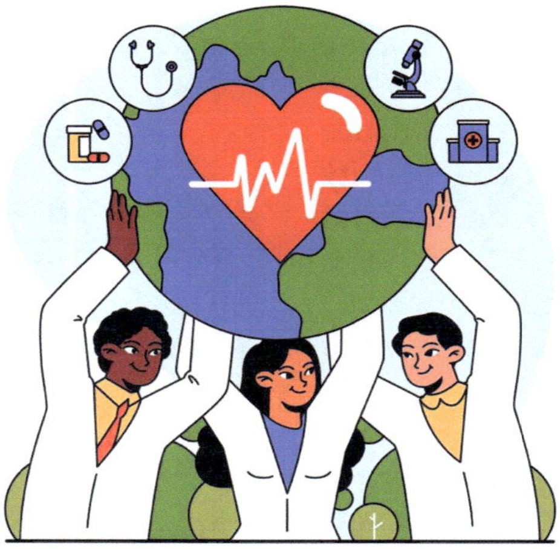

Figure 15.17. Global health initiatives.

Source: https://static.vecteezy.com/system/resources/previews/041/170/467/non_2x/global-health-initiatives-concept-flat-illustration-vector.jpg.

Test Your Knowledge

1. How can emerging technologies improve surgical outcomes for patients in tropical disease–endemic regions?
2. What innovations in training and capacity-building are needed to advance future surgical practices in low-resource tropical settings?

SUMMARY

Ultimately, the intersection of surgical intervention and tropical diseases is a fundamental area of medical practice that warrants greater attention from both public health and clinical perspectives. The management of NTDs often surpasses simple drug treatment; surgery plays a crucial role in the treatment of severe complications arising from these diseases. The financial cost imposed by NTDs, as documented in recent studies, confirms that a multifaceted strategy—not just medical expenditure, but encompassing financial stability—should be set at the forefront of healthcare strategies. The findings indicate that households that face catastrophic levels of health costs resulting from NTDs face severe financial hardship, which can amplify their exposure and drive poverty and disease cycles (Patikorn et al., 2024). Therefore, an overall strategy that includes surgical care can be a determinant in countering both the economic and healthcare impacts of these diseases. The global implications of climate change also pose a problem with the management of tropical diseases, particularly in terms of surgical needs. As the prevalence of diseases such as malaria and dengue continues to grow, the health systems must cope with heightened demands for surgical services. The changing environmental conditions not only increase the occurrence rates of diseases but also determine which populations are to be treated surgically, generally in areas where they are already resource-deprived (Pavia et al., 2024). It is crucial to combat NTDs effectively by establishing robust surgical procedures that are adaptable enough to withstand shifting climates and evolving disease patterns. This preparation would reduce morbidity associated with untreated illnesses and ultimately be part of the overall efforts in public health and disaster readiness. As a whole, the integration of surgical practices in tropical disease management is a vital aspect for improving patient outcomes and public health in such areas. With the development of refined surgical techniques and practices, the use by healthcare providers needs to be prioritized in diverse settings, especially in resource-poor settings that carry a heavy burden of NTDs. The evidence of the fiscal and health impacts of these conditions indicates the imperative necessity for targeted interventions and the need to include surgical capacities as a core element of a comprehensive approach. Addressing these issues through synergistic methods—financial assistance, surgical intervention, and climate resilience—is the promise of greatly enhancing the welfare of individuals afflicted with tropical diseases and thus laying the groundwork for sustainable health improvement globally.

In the evolving climate of tropical disease control, surgical interventions play a pivotal role in preventing the complications of certain endemic diseases. Outstanding features that emerge from the latest studies reveal surgery as an option for treatment but also as a preventive measure for the control of tropical diseases. For instance, the treatment of diseases such as lymphatic filariasis and cutaneous leishmaniasis typically requires surgical interventions to address disabling complications and promote the quality of life of affected patients. The adoption of effective surgical practices not only maximizes patient outcomes but also supports more generalized public health objectives by reducing disease transmission and facilitating recovery for communities (Matthew et al., 2021). However, health systems globally, especially in low- and middle-income countries (LMICs), face significant barriers, including limited access to surgical commodities and continuing professional development, that prevent the overall operation of surgical care in such regions. Another critical consideration in the argument over surgery within tropical disease is the necessity of robust, comprehensive healthcare systems with surgical services. Universal health coverage requires collective effort to equate surgical care with equity, accessibility, and integration into primary health services (Wu et al., 2020). This is particularly important since the majority of individuals affected by tropical diseases reside in underserved populations where healthcare systems are still inadequate. By placing an emphasis on integrating surgical services into overall health planning, countries are better able to enhance treatment and preventive options. Furthermore, increased public health investment in surgical care within the context of tropical diseases will not only improve individual health but also help decrease the healthcare burden of such diseases. Lastly, ongoing research and innovative approaches are necessary for maximizing surgical services for tropical diseases. The increasing prevalence of disease conditions such as diabetic retinopathy and other non-communicable diseases in the tropics signifies the need for novel surgical approaches. With the evolving patient population and dynamic patterns of tropical diseases, there is a need to develop an environment that fosters research and development tailored to the requirements of affected populations. Collaborative efforts among governments, non-governmental organizations, and academic institutions will help identify areas of necessity in terms of priority and resource allocation. By addressing these areas, the argument on surgery in tropical diseases can make a significant contribution to the course of health outcomes as well as attain sustainable development (Matthew et al., 2021).

KEY TERMS FROM THIS CHAPTER

- Actinomycosis
- Buruli ulcer
- Elephantiasis surgery
- Guinea worm disease
- Intestinal tuberculosis
- Leprosy deformities
- Parasitic obstruction
- Amoebic liver abscess
- Chronic osteomyelitis
- Filariasis
- Hydatid cyst
- Kala-azar complications
- Necrotizing fasciitis
- Schistosomiasis

CRITICAL THINKING QUESTIONS

1. **Which of the following tropical diseases most commonly causes intestinal obstruction requiring surgery?**
   a. Malaria
   b. Ascariasis
   c. Schistosomiasis
   d. Leishmaniasis
2. **Hydatid disease is caused by which organism and commonly affects which organ?**
   a. *Echinococcus granulosus* – Liver
   b. *Plasmodium falciparum* – Spleen
   c. *Entamoeba histolytica* – Colon
   d. *Wuchereria bancrofti* – Lymph nodes
3. **Which of the following is the preferred surgical treatment for a large liver hydatid cyst?**
   a. Simple aspiration
   b. PAIR (Puncture, Aspiration, Injection, Reaspiration)
   c. Pericystectomy or cystectomy
   d. Anthelmintics alone
4. **Which tropical infection is associated with chronic lymphatic obstruction and elephantiasis requiring debulking surgery?**
   a. Malaria
   b. Filariasis
   c. Amoebiasis
   d. Typhoid fever
5. **What is the most common complication requiring surgery in amoebic liver abscess?**
   a. Spontaneous rupture into the lung or peritoneum
   b. Massive ascites
   c. Splenic rupture
   d. Hepatocellular carcinoma

Short Answer Questions

1. What are the surgical indications in patients with liver hydatid disease?
2. How does filarial infection lead to elephantiasis, and what are the surgical options?
3. Describe the clinical presentation and complications of an amoebic liver abscess that may require surgical intervention.
4. What do *Ascaris lumbricoides* cause the role of surgery in intestinal obstruction?
5. When is surgical drainage indicated in patients with tropical pyomyositis?
6. What are the common surgical complications of typhoid fever in endemic regions?
7. How is a perforated duodenal ulcer due to tropical infection managed surgically?
8. What is the preferred surgical approach to a ruptured hydatid cyst?

Answers to Critical Thinking Questions

1. (b); 2. (a); 3. (c); 4. (b); 5. (a)

REFERENCES

1. Aamar, H., Siddiqui, J. A., Siddiqui, A., & Essar, M. Y. (2023). Neglected tropical diseases in Pakistan: challenges, efforts, and recommendations. *International Journal of Surgery, 109*(2), 143–144. https://doi.org/10.1097/js9.0000000000000186Aarestrup, F. M., Ahuja, R. B., Aidara-Kane, A., Zumla, A., Allegranzi, B., Allegranzi, B., et al. (2015). *Exploring the evidence base for national and regional policy interventions to combat resistance.* https://core.ac.uk/download/36779210.pdf (accessed on 12th July 2025).
2. Abdool Karim, S. S., Amor, Y. B., Balabanova, Y., Caminero, J. A., Centers for Disease Control and Prevention, Chan, M., Chiang, C. Y., et al. (2010). *Review of multidrug-resistant and extensively drug-resistant TB: Global perspectives with a focus on sub-Saharan Africa.* https://core.ac.uk/download/19085582.pdf (accessed on 12th July 2025).
3. Adjei, S., Amofah, G., Amofah, G., Andries, A., Aujoulat, I., Bentoucha, A., Darie, H., et al. (2006). *Mycobacterium ulcerans infection: Control, diagnosis, and treatment.* https://core.ac.uk/download/pdf/9416615.pdf (accessed on 12th July 2025).
4. Alemu, A., Aseffa, A., Deressa, A., Haileamlak, A., Yami, A., Aseffa, A., Bryceson, A. D., et al. (2012). *The burden of neglected tropical diseases in Ethiopia, and opportunities for integrated control and elimination.* https://core.ac.uk/download/16413153.pdf (accessed on 12th July 2025).
5. Awuah, W. A., Tenkorang, P. O., Adebusoye, F. T., Mehta, A., Ng, J. C., Asieduwaa, O. Y., Debrah, A. F., et al. (2023). The state of African surgical research capacity: Highlighting the current efforts, challenges, and recommendations – Editorial. *International Journal of Surgery, 109,* 91–93. https://doi.org/10.1097/js9.0000000000000216 (accessed on 12th July 2025).
6. Blum, J., Brunetti, E., Goblirsch, S., Neumayr, A., et al. (2013). Spinal cystic echinococcosis – a systematic analysis and review of the literature: Part 2. Treatment, follow-up and outcome. https://core.ac.uk/download/19496694.pdf (accessed on 12th July 2025).
7. Bottieau, E., Dermauw, V., Dorny, P., Luyckx, K., et al. (2019). Cysticercosis and taeniasis cases diagnosed at two referral medical institutions, Belgium, 1990 to 2015. https://core.ac.uk/download/287939837.pdf (accessed on 12th July 2025).
8. Burton, M. J., Ramke, J., Marques, A. P., Bourne, R., Congdon, N., Jones, I., Ah Tong, B. A. M., et al. (2021). The Lancet Global Health Commission on global eye health: Vision beyond 2020. *The Lancet Global Health, 9,* e489–e551. https://doi.org/10.1016/s2214-109x(20)30488-5 (accessed on 12th July 2025).
9. Calongea, W. M., Mereditha, P., Kouakou-Adonisa, K. A., Yaoa, C., K. M., N., & Assea, H. (2021). Reconstructive surgery for sequellae of *Mycobacterium ulcerans* infection (Buruli ulcer) of the upper limb. *Journal of Plastic Surgery and Hand Surgery, 55,* 339–344. https://www.semanticscholar.org/paper/ea791b7559f119ef8fac95ebf60f604b049c5d38 (accessed on 12th July 2025).
10. Cline, B. L., Asbury, C., & Gammino, V. M. (2000). The Edna McConnell Clark Foundation's Tropical Disease Research Program: A 25-year retrospective review 1976–1999. https://core.ac.uk/download/71350953.pdf (accessed on 12th July 2025).
11. Copeland, L. I. B. T., James, Duinkerken, M. S. I., Kelsey, G., et al. (2020). Jefferson Digital Commons quarterly report: January–March 2020. https://core.ac.uk/download/299811518.pdf (accessed on 12th July 2025).

12. Cornet, R., McCowan, C., Peek, N., Scott, P., et al. (2017). Addendum to Informatics for Health 2017: Advancing both science and practice. https://core.ac.uk/download/132585011.pdf (accessed on 12th July 2025).

13. Costa, D., Tortoli, E., Passidomo, D., Gaudiomonte, V., Grimaldi, A., Ostuni, G., Sisto, F., et al. (2006). *Ulcera del Buruli: la "nuova lebbra" Africana. Isolamento e identificazione di* M. ulcerans *in prelievi bioptici provenienti da pazienti del Benin* (Vol. 21). https://www.semanticscholar.org/paper/3ed82ff8e3c8d474625047ccc4bb3e70e12a1f6b (accessed on 12th July 2025).

14. Engels, D., & Zhou, X.-N. (2020). Neglected tropical diseases: An effective global response to local poverty-related disease priorities. *Infectious Diseases of Poverty, 9*. https://doi.org/10.1186/s40249-020-0630-9 (accessed on 12th July 2025).

15. Evans, R. A., Leavy, O. C., Richardson, M., Elneima, O., McAuley, H., Shikotra, A., Singapuri, A., et al. (2022). Clinical characteristics with inflammation profiling of long COVID and association with 1-year recovery following hospitalization in the UK: A prospective observational study. *The Lancet Respiratory Medicine, 10*, 761–775. https://doi.org/10.1016/s2213-2600(22)00127-8 (accessed on 12th July 2025).

16. Ferrara, V. Z., Martinino, A., Toti, F., Schilirò, D., Pinto, F., Giovinazzo, F., & On behalf of the Smageics Group. (2024). Robotic vascular resection in pancreatic ductal adenocarcinoma: A systematic review. *Journal of Clinical Medicine, 13*. https://www.semanticscholar.org/paper/1306c0b1ea0ef4e0ee9c94888d6eacd6214c9e18 (accessed on 12th July 2025).

17. Ferrari, A. J., Santomauro, D., Aali, A., Abate, Y. H., Abbafati, C., Abbastabar, H., Abd ElHafeez, S., et al. (2024). Global incidence, prevalence, years lived with disability (YLDs), disability-adjusted life-years (DALYs), and healthy life expectancy (HALE) for 371 diseases and injuries in 204 countries and territories and 811 subnational locations, 1990–2021: A systematic analysis for the Global Burden of Disease Study 2021. *The Lancet, 403*, 2133–2161. https://doi.org/10.1016/s0140-6736(24)00757-8 (accessed on 12th July 2025).

18. Ferreira, M. L., de Luca, K., Haile, T. G., Steinmetz, J. D., Culbreth, G. T., Cross, M., Kopec, J. A., et al. (2023). Global, regional, and national burden of low back pain, 1990–2020, its attributable risk factors, and projections to 2050: A systematic analysis of the Global Burden of Disease Study 2021. *The Lancet Rheumatology, 5*, e316–e329. https://doi.org/10.1016/s2665-9913(23)00098-x (accessed on 12th July 2025).

19. Fleming, K. A., Horton, S., Wilson, M. L., Atun, R., DeStigter, K., Flanigan, J., Sayed, S., et al. (2021). The Lancet Commission on diagnostics: Transforming access to diagnostics. *The Lancet, 398*, 1997–2050. https://doi.org/10.1016/s0140-6736(21)00673-5 (accessed on 12th July 2025).

20. Fryer, A.-K., Schoen, C., Radley, D. C., McCarthy, D., & How, S. K. H. (2011). Why not the best? Results from the National Scorecard on U.S. Health System Performance, 2011. https://core.ac.uk/download/71359185.pdf (accessed on 12th July 2025).

21. Gor, I. V., Popov, D., Skuridin, G. M., Yakhyaev, N. R., Zakharov, A. Y., & Pahomov, I. A. (2025). The position of primary radical surgery for pilonidal cysts in the acute inflammatory phase. *Ambulatornaya khirurgiya = Ambulatory Surgery (Russia)*. https://www.semanticscholar.org/paper/70e411b10ef4f7b995242909f7e4050fc68f03aa (accessed on 12th July 2025).

22. Gunkaya, O. S., & Bestel, A. (2025). The usefulness of serum procalcitonin levels in predicting surgical intervention in patients with tubo-ovarian abscess. *Revista*

da Associação Médica Brasileira, 71. https://www.semanticscholar.org/paper/f26abc678629d1ad0962dfbb3836a944cdaae785 (accessed on 12th July 2025).

23. Ismail, A. I., Saleh, A. H., & Abdulkadir, T. (2025). Spatio-temporal analysis of reported trachoma cases in Kano State, Nigeria (2013–2019). *Indonesian Journal of Health Research and Development.* https://www.semanticscholar.org/paper/19e40bf048d8b511cfbd1ee2ad56b5c3c254072a (accessed on 12th July 2025).
24. Kar Mahapatra, P. B., & Reddy, V. N. (2022). Reconstructive surgery of ulnar claw hand in leprosy patients by lasso procedure. *International Journal of Life Science and Pharma Research.* https://www.semanticscholar.org/paper/49f64fd4d8baf6fd45f054ed9bf2fcdc0bb2fa64 (accessed on 12th July 2025).
25. Khieu, V., Or, V., Tep, C., Odermatt, P., Tsuyuoka, R., Char, M. C., Brady, M., et al. (2018). How elimination of lymphatic filariasis as a public health problem in the Kingdom of Cambodia was achieved. *Infectious Diseases of Poverty, 7.* https://doi.org/10.1186/s40249-018-0394-7 (accessed on 12th July 2025).
26. Lipsky, B. A., Senneville, É., Abbas, Z. G., Aragón-Sánchez, J., Diggle, M., Embil, J. M., Kono, S., et al. (2020). Guidelines on the diagnosis and treatment of foot infection in persons with diabetes (IWGDF 2019 update). Diabetes/Metabolism Research and Reviews, 36. https://doi.org/10.1002/dmrr.3280 (accessed on 12th July 2025).
27. Liyew, E. F., Tollera, G., Mengistu, B., Chernet, M., Gidey, B., Maddren, R., Mayer, J., et al. (2025). Small bowel obstruction due to ascariasis in a child from southern Ethiopia: A case report. *Journal of Medical Case Reports, 19.* https://www.semanticscholar.org/paper/1fdf1e1d8552d7cf05d45134e07ab1ccd13d8d57 (accessed on 12th July 2025).
28. Mathewson, J. D., van der Spek, L., Matungwa, D. J., Samson, A., Coleman, H. L. S., & Rood, E. J. J. (2024). Challenges and motivating factors for integrating geostatistical models in targeted schistosomiasis control: A qualitative case study in Northwestern Tanzania. *PLOS Neglected Tropical Diseases, 18.* https://www.semanticscholar.org/paper/e09583ad41aa750b49d37e6823bc39aa8f15e189 (accessed on 12th July 2025).
29. Mihai, C. M., Lupu, A., Chisnoiu, T., Balasa, A., Baciu, G., Lupu, V., Popovici, V., et al. (2025). A comprehensive analysis of Echinococcus granulosus infections in children and adolescents: Results of a 7-year retrospective study and literature review. Pathogens, 14. https://www.semanticscholar.org/paper/0450c828a526dfd6a9433dae95b39155a0f63e75 (accessed on 12th July 2025).
30. Pahlevan, A. A., Wysocki, A. B., Paintsil, A., Shittu, A. O., Shittu, A. O., Bauer, A. W., Anku, B., et al. (2013). *Secondary bacterial infections of Buruli ulcer lesions before and after chemotherapy with streptomycin and rifampicin.* https://core.ac.uk/download/18261879.pdf (accessed on 12th July 2025).
31. Patikorn, C., Cho, J.-Y., Higashi, J., Huang, X. X., & Chaiyakunapruk, N. (2024). Financial hardship among patients suffering from neglected tropical diseases: A systematic review and meta-analysis of global literature. PLOS Neglected Tropical Diseases, 18. https://www.semanticscholar.org/paper/4b81ac5173ec5a8871433a4ec8d7c526294ddf42 (accessed on 12th July 2025).
32. Pavia, G., Branda, F., Ciccozzi, A., Romano, C., Locci, C., Azzena, I., Pascale, N., et al. (2024). The issue of climate change and the spread of tropical diseases in Europe and Italy: Vector

biology, disease transmission, genome-based monitoring and public health implications. *Infectious Diseases, 57*, 121–136. https://www.semanticscholar.org/paper/8db2bec1b4609afedf77a3db10f406c77958f40b (accessed on 12th July 2025).

33. Pradhan, E., Alrasheed, S., Melnyk, O. I., Azimi, H., Raeisi, S., Aghajani, A., Ashenef, B., et al. (2025). Hydatid cyst of the orbit: A systematic review with meta-data. *Barw Medical Journal*. https://www.semanticscholar.org/paper/93f611aa57c9e6d694af1922a1fd3a0890ab0be7 (accessed on 12th July 2025).

34. Rathore, M. M., Shah, S. A., Shukla, D., Bentafat, E., & Bakiras, S. (2021). The role of AI, machine learning, and big data in digital twinning: A systematic literature review, challenges, and opportunities. *IEEE Access, 9*, 32030–32052. https://doi.org/10.1109/access.2021.3060863 (accessed on 12th July 2025).

35. Richens, J. (2004). Genital manifestations of tropical diseases. https://core.ac.uk/download/1669842.pdf (accessed on 12th July 2025).

36. Roth, G. A., Mensah, G. A., Johnson, C. O., Addolorato, G., Ammirati, E., Baddour, L. M., Barengo, N. C., et al. (2020). Global burden of cardiovascular diseases and risk factors, 1990–2019. *Journal of the American College of Cardiology, 76*, 2982–3021. https://doi.org/10.1016/j.jacc.2020.11.010 (accessed on 12th July 2025).

37. Roussel, E., Campi, R., Amparore, D., Bertolo, R., Carbonara, U., Erdem, S., Ingels, A., et al. (2022). Expanding the role of ultrasound for the characterization of renal masses. *Journal of Clinical Medicine, 11*. https://www.semanticscholar.org/paper/2a35d877d3d5c531182ed55975da597df78b500d (accessed on 12th July 2025).

38. Semaan, A., Audet, C., Huysmans, E., Afolabi, B. B., Assarag, B., Banke-Thomas, A., Blencowe, H., et al. (2020). Voices from the frontline: Findings from a thematic analysis of a rapid online global survey of maternal and newborn health professionals facing the COVID-19 pandemic. *BMJ Global Health, 5*, e002967–e002967. https://doi.org/10.1136/bmjgh-2020-002967 (accessed on 12th July 2025).

39. Soto-Sánchez, J., & Garza-Treviño, G. (2024). Combination therapy and phytochemical-loaded nanosystems for the treatment of neglected tropical diseases. *Pharmaceutics, 16*. https://www.semanticscholar.org/paper/49ea3855d2b3e68d8041e979309030c296b56dd8 (accessed on 12th July 2025).

40. Uba, A. F., Christianson, A. L., Measham, A. R., Nandi, B., Warf, B. C., Murray, C. J. L., Adeyemi, D., et al. (2014). *Congenital anomalies in low- and middle-income countries: The unborn child of global surgery*. https://core.ac.uk/download/323070414.pdf (accessed on 12th July 2025).

41. Wu, A., March, L., Zheng, X.-Q., Huang, J., Wang, X., Zhao, J., Blyth, F., et al. (2020). Global low back pain prevalence and years lived with disability from 1990 to 2017: Estimates from the Global Burden of Disease Study 2017. *Annals of Translational Medicine, 8*, 299–299. https://doi.org/10.21037/atm.2020.02.175 (accessed on 12th July 2025).

INDEX

C

D

E

F

K

L

M

N

O

P

Q

T

U

V

W

Y